T0293018

Vice and Psychiatric Diagnosis

INTERNATIONAL PERSPECTIVES IN PHILOSOPHY AND PSYCHIATRY

Series editors:

Bill (K.W.M.) Fulford, Lisa Bortolotti, Matthew Broome, Katherine Morris, John Z. Sadler, and Giovanni Stanghellini

Volumes in the series

Vice and Psychiatric Diagnosis

JOHN Z. SADLER

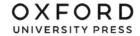

OXFORD
UNIVERSITY PRESS

Great Clarendon Street, Oxford, OX2 6DP,
United Kingdom

Oxford University Press is a department of the University of Oxford.
It furthers the University's objective of excellence in research, scholarship,
and education by publishing worldwide. Oxford is a registered trade mark of
Oxford University Press in the UK and in certain other countries

Published in the United States of America by Oxford University Press
198 Madison Avenue, New York, NY 10016, United States of America

British Library Cataloguing in Publication Data

Data available

Library of Congress Control Number: 2023945987

ISBN 978-0-19-887683-0

DOI: 10.1093/oso/9780198876830.001.0001

Printed and bound by
CPI Group (UK) Ltd, Croydon, CR0 4YY

Oxford University Press makes no representation, express or implied, that the
drug dosages in this book are correct. Readers must therefore always check
the product information and clinical procedures with the most up-to-date
published product information and data sheets provided by the manufacturers
and the most recent codes of conduct and safety regulations. The authors and
the publishers do not accept responsibility or legal liability for any errors in the
text or for the misuse or misapplication of material in this work. Except where
otherwise stated, drug dosages and recommendations are for the non-pregnant
adult who is not breast-feeding

Links to third party websites are provided by Oxford in good faith and
for information only. Oxford disclaims any responsibility for the materials
contained in any third party website referenced in this work.

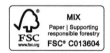

Contents

Preface and acknowledgments

An ambitious project like this one always requires many more people than a simple byline indicates. This project went on for so long I had to keep notes about who helped me, and indeed they came in handy as I wrapped up this book.

I should start with the people who gave me the green light—Oxford University Press—and specifically Martin Baum, Carol Maxwell, and Charlotte Green. I should give special mention to Charlotte, whose role for this book development spanned her marriage, delivery of children, and early retirement from OUP! Despite these distractions from my clearly less important work (!), Charlotte was a major figure in the fruition of this project. That my intermittent work on this book spanned some 15 years, as well as other people's major life transitions, is humbling. Ryan Morris and Karen Bunn picked up this project in its later stages, and I'm grateful for their stewardship toward a long-awaited conclusion. Martin Baum deserves special mention as an editor with extraordinary patience, on one hand, and confidence in me, on the other. I've known Martin for many years, and he's always been generous in encouragement as well as his forbearance in completing this and other projects. I hope the waits have been worth it!

I should mention a grant-funding organization, which remains anonymous, who enabled the majority of the research that went into the project. To these friends, I also hope the wait was worth it! Peer reviewers from the National Library of Medicine G13 grant mechanism were also helpful in their comments. People who wrote grant letters of support deserve thanks too, and for this a shout-out to Claudio E. M. Banzato, Michael First, and K. W. M. Fulford.

Several UT Southwestern administrative assistants provided substantive aid in chasing down library resources and compiling reference databases. My longtime assistant, Linda Muncy, provided essential and substantial assistance in the early years, aided by Aida Ramirez-Boyce, Hollee Nash, and Joey Santos at various stages. My current assistant, Ruth Vinciguerra, ushered this project over the finish line with great patience, and her meticulous attention to detail made it all the better.

The current Chair of the UT Southwestern Department of Psychiatry, Carol Tamminga, has been supportive of my work in multiple ways, and I am most grateful for her vision of a diverse psychiatry and her consistent resolve to fulfill it.

In the Volume 15, Number 1, 2009 issue of *Philosophy, Psychiatry, and Psychology*, I published an article, 'Vice and the diagnostic classification of mental disorders: A philosophical case conference', where a set of commentators explored my then-preliminary discussion of many of the themes in this book. This discussion was very helpful in developing the work, and I thank Gwen Adshead, Michael First, Jeffrey Geller, Chris Heginbotham, Stephen Morse, Nancy Potter, Lloyd Wells,

Christopher Williams, and Peter Zachar for their participation and diverse perspectives. With foresight, Chris Heginbotham recommended a 'third way' in dealing with vice and mental disorders, and while I wasn't completely sure what he meant at the time, I hope he will be pleased with the 'third way' I present in my conclusions for this book.

A large work of scholarship is bound to have spin-off projects in the form of articles or chapters written for other projects. In my case, I have published several papers through developing this *Vice and Psychiatric Diagnosis* project. All of them were contributory and readers of these papers will find plenty of original thought here, springing from these earlier publications. I thank Christian Perring and Lloyd Wells for the opportunity to write on the vice-ladenness of the DSM's Conduct Disorder concept; it was a great opportunity to clarify my thinking on this category and the insight into a misplaced emphasis on attention-getting manifestations of a disorder. I was surprised and delighted to be invited to contribute to the Patrick Singy and Steeves Demazeux book on the DSMs (*Diagnostic and Statistical Manual of Mental Disorders* publications); and my chapter on monomanias for that book crystallized my thinking about how single-symptom disorders can lead to feeble disorder categories. In the case of vice-laden single-symptom disorders, these insights helped me to consider naive, rather than informed, medicalization of vice. My colleagues of the time (2009), Fabrice Jotterand, Simon Craddock Lee, and Steve Inrig facilitated critical discussions contributing to a more nuanced view of the ethics of medicalization which clarified many analyses throughout the book. My current ethics colleague Elizabeth Heitman has served as a sounding board too. When Chaitanya Haldipur, James Knoll, and Eric v.d. Luft invited me to contribute to their book reappraising Thomas Szasz' work, I hadn't fully assimilated the cultural frames of the vice/mental disorder relationship, which were to inspire many of the conclusions in this book. I thank them for this opportunity.

A big, and perhaps the most fun chunk of this book was Chapters 4 and 5 on the intellectual history of relations between madness and morality. Building a historical account from secondary sources is challenging and intellectually tricky, and several history scholars helped me. Sander Gilman advised on references to madness in the Bible. Mael Lemoine was an enthusiastic sounding board for historiographic questions. Melvin Woody's wide grasp of the history of philosophy was a resource. Charles Curran advised me on the context and roots of Christian ethics. However, whatever foolishness exhibited here is all my fault, not theirs!

Another risky endeavor was delving into criminal law and its history, however essential for understanding the VMDR. I was lucky to have a sympathetic group of lawyers and legal scholars assist me at various turns. Foremost among this group was Dan Shuman (1949–2011), the M.D. Anderson Foundation Endowed Professor of Health Law at Southern Methodist University (SMU). Dan befriended me and guided me in the earliest stages of this book, through extended conversations about criminal law and psychiatric diagnosis. Dan combined the best of open-minded listening and rigorous criticism. William F. May introduced me to Roscoe Pound's work, so formative for Chapter 6. Bill Bridge helped me understand what criminal attorneys want from psychiatrists, a question many of my psychiatric colleagues have turned over. Steven Sverdlik assisted me with key elements in the philosophy of criminal law through presenting his own work in the context of the SMU Ethics Colloquium program. Gerben Meynen assisted me in thinking about free will in the context of forensic psychiatry. The SMU Forensic Group led by John Zervopoulos and colleagues in law, forensic psychology, and forensic psychiatry provided a generous sounding board for my ideas about the different modes of reasoning in criminal law and clinical psychiatry. My med-school friend Jaye Douglas Crowder lent a skeptical eye to my major theses, as well as generous amounts of cryptic humor. Later in my process my longtime lawyer-friend Tom Mayo and new lawyer-friend Duff Waring read substantive portions of this book to advise me in clarifying the basics of criminal law and process. I don't know if I got it just right, but they get credit for the improvements.

It turns out that talking about sex has always been a fraught topic. As will be apparent from discussions about the development of 'sexuality' and sexual disorders; throughout the Western history of morality, sexual relations have been contentious and regulated vigorously through various social forces and mores. Some of the paraphilic disorders posed paradigmatic examples of vice-laden mental disorders warranting understanding and analysis. In this regard, Ray Blanchard, Fred Berlin, Ken Zucker, Andrew Hinderliter, and the B4UAct community provided eye-opening insights. Thanks to them.

A collection of clinicians and scholars contributed readings of bits and pieces of the book, as well as tactful responses to critical ideas and grand theses. Molly Camp, Karen Maschke, and Bettina Fehr helped with reading the history material for its readability and coherence, and thanks to them. Theresa de Freitas and Saira Bhatti, in their growing passion for forensic and correctional psychiatry, critically compared criminal and psychiatric rehabilitation procedures for their paper for my philosophy of psychiatry resident elective. I give them credit for some of the crucial ideas in my own treatment of this comparison in Chapter 8. Jeffrey Geller's scholarship on impulse control disorders as well as our casual conversations on the subject were helpful in understanding these phenomena vis a vis the VMDR. Ken Schaffner provided encouragement and structure to my thinking about the idea of complex multi-causal folk-metaphysical assumptions. Alex Piquero provided insights into criminology science and practice at various stages, and his encouragement meant much. Fred Grinnell, Richard Wasserman, and Bob Fine helped me clarify my interpretation of the concept of sin in the Judaic tradition. Nancy Potter and Jennifer Radden always help me with the philosophy, and our friendship has nourished me for decades now. The North Texas Bioethics Network provided a hearing of my concept of the 'Enlightenment Split' and offered helpful comments, especially appreciated as my topic was far from most of their core interests. Last but not least, the

xviii   Preface and acknowledgments

fellowship of the Association for the Advancement of Philosophy and Psychiatry Executive Council provided helpful input, sometimes inadvertently, throughout the development of this book.

One's family is always important to a creative work. In this case, my sons Evan and Cole grew into smart, socially aware, empathic adults over the period of this project. Later, their significant others Jessica Wansart and Savannah Neiggemann chimed in over dinner table discussions about themes in this book. Along with my beloved wife Abbie, who knows how many dinner table conversations contributed to this project? They also put up with a lot of John's being stuck in a book or sitting in front of a computer. My sister Stephany and her husband Buzz provided much-appreciated interest and encouragement as well.

1
Introductions literal and metaphorical

1.1 The mystery story, the doorway, and the overture

Reading this academic book will be a long slog, so I'd best muster some intrigue from the beginning. To this end, I offer three metaphors: the mystery story, the doorway, and the overture.

While starting work on this book years ago, I began reading mysteries, thrillers, police procedurals, and more broadly, crime fiction—all with great interest. I don't think this was an accident. This book was inspired by a simple question—'Why does the diagnosis of some psychiatric disorders involve wrongful or criminal conduct?'—so crime fiction was a safe territory to explore this question, if perhaps elliptically. The crime fiction genre typically involves a mystery involving a primary protagonist—the police detective, private investigator, or occasionally the surviving victim, looking for the culprit. Commonly, the core characters pose a variety of psychopathologies, not just the villain, but also the hero(ine) and perhaps other key characters. Courageous but flawed characters are *de rigeur* for the genre. From this standpoint, such fiction would be of interest regarding my central question.

However, the crime fiction genre also poses structural elements that emerged in this book. Initially, the investigator is confronted by the crime, explores the crime scene, and most importantly collects and begins to interpret the evidence left behind—the ambiguous traces of what happened. This is followed by some preliminary conjectures about what happened, typically around motives for the crime, which require some chasing down and following up. Through this process, the investigator encounters a network of people who variously are suspicious, defensive, eager, collegial, prevaricating, angry, and seductive at different times and in degrees. The early conjectures fail to be supported, or fail to be conclusive, so the detective then embarks on a more extended investigative journey involving travel, a larger cast of characters, and often rummaging around in the dustbins of locale and history (e.g., 'cold' cases, other jurisdictions). Often the investigation discovers new crimes woven into the network of evidence, leading to hypotheses of links between crimes,

Vice and Psychiatric Diagnosis. John Z. Sadler, Oxford University Press. © Oxford University Press 2024.
DOI: 10.1093/oso/9780198876830.003.0001

or as likely, offering 'red herrings' (false leads) to the core crime. Looking for motives may give way to identifying opportunities for the perpetrator to act. New evidence, new leads, and new truths then provoke one or more twists—surprising turns of events—followed by the concluding solution(s) to the case.

This book presents a kind of mystery story that metaphorically follows many of these genre conventions. The opening chapters collect the bald evidence of the 'crime'—in this case the puzzle of wrongful or criminal conduct in psychiatric diagnostic categories. The essential evidence for the 'crime' is assembled, laid out, and examined. The middle chapters explore those dustbins of locale and history to find alternative ways of formulating the motives—the 'whys' of my research question, trying to find the motives that fit the evidence. Like in crime fiction, the evidence fits numerous hypotheses, and often the case turns on identifying the opportunity for the alleged offender to act. Likewise, the history of madness and morality in my early middle chapters identify multiple motives as well as opportunities to conflate madness and morality. The late-middle chapters recast the evidence in new lights, leading to insights into new 'crimes'—these being, in my case, new public policy and professional issues concerning vice and mental disorders. In the process of researching and writing this book, I had my initial guiding preconceptions. Ultimately, these preconceptions were turned upside down. This turnabout in my preconceptions lead me to conclusions which were far from what I had originally imagined—the 'twist' of the mystery story.

When I read nonfiction, especially philosophy and history, I hope for the 'wow' factor, the transforming insight(s) that change—often permanently—the way that I view some aspect of reality. This is the fun in reading and doing philosophy. Likewise, in my own writing, I try to provide a doorway into one or more alternative ways of seeing the world. This doorway metaphor figures into multiple literary genres, from fantasy fiction (such as C. S. Lewis's *The Chronicles of Narnia*) to pop philosophy (such as Daniel Dennett's *Consciousness Explained*). The success in the author's 'worldbuilding' makes for the wow factor. Our love of books is such that the doorway metaphor is apt for the transformative power of all reading. I can't speak for my readers, but I view mental illness and wrongful conduct in a dramatically different way today than I did 15 years ago when I started. I wish my readers to be similarly transformed by my goal of giving them most everything relevant to understanding the curious relationship between mental illness, criminality, and immorality. In my unveiling of facets of the world responsible for the current status of relations between these areas, the reader can think through her own investigation. My reader crosses a threshold into viewing the world of madness and morality in a different way and, perhaps, more than one different way.

For the musically inclined, the overture poses my third metaphor. In music, the overture, typically for an opera, provides a wordless, instrumental introduction to the main musical themes of the work, by necessity shifting the emotional tone of the work as motifs rise and fall. The overture, derived from the French '*ouverture*', or '*opening*', debuts the major themes in a synthetic, unified whole signifying both characters and action to come. In my view, the success of an overture is tied to the profundity of the music on conveying the emotional twists and turns of the drama to follow. The astute and experienced listener, merely by hearing the overture, may characterize the work as light or serious, comedic or tragic, and even anticipate much of the characters and action. The overture offers *clues* and suggests *context*, which returns us to the original mystery story metaphor. With these metaphors explained, I turn to my overture.

1.2 A historical moment as a doorway to the issues

> The criminal law represents the pathology of civilization.
>
> —Morris R. Cohen[1]

On April 16, 2007, a young South Korean immigrant, Seung-Hui Cho, aged 23 years, went on a rageful shooting spree at Virginia Tech University in the United States, killing 32 fellow students and faculty. In the months preceding the shootings, Cho's odd behavior had alienated and intimidated fellow students and faculty. Over the same period, Cho had accumulated, secretly, firearms and ammunition, engaging in target practice 40 miles off campus. In the preceding December of 2006, after two female students complained of being stalked by Cho, and his roommate noted his expression of suicidal thoughts, campus police escorted Cho to a psychiatric evaluation facility, the New River Valley Community Services Board.[2] There Cho was evaluated by a psychiatrist and found to be mentally ill and a danger to himself and others. However, he was ordered by the judge, Paul Barnett, to undergo outpatient psychiatric treatment rather than voluntary or involuntary psychiatric inpatient care. Cho never presented for the outpatient treatment.

A key record in the December 2006 visit, the 'Involuntary Commitment Process—Written Explanation' document obtained by the *Washington Post*,[3] is remarkable for the impoverished documentation of the 'Physician's Examination'. Other than a short checklist for behaviors like 'attempted suicide' or 'attempted homicide', the clinical note can be recounted in full:

> Oriented x 4. Affect is flat and mood is depressed. He denies suicidal ideation. He does not acknowledge symptoms of a thought disorder. His insight and judgment are normal.[4]

What is also remarkable is the complete absence of collateral information—from family, from faculty, from students, from campus police, from anyone, even though these people were, at least in theory, identifiable and available and, in hindsight, held important information.

Around the same time as these local events in Virginia, the British Parliament was in the midst, again, of negotiating reforms to their 1983 Mental Health Act, the law that governs mental health services for the British National Health Service. The planned reforms were both a response to public outcries for protection against the dangerous mentally ill, as well as an effort to strengthen patient safeguards, legitimate professional roles, and clarify treatment procedures.[5] The controversies around the Mental Health Act (MHA) preceded and followed its passing in 1983, and that same year the Mental Health Act Commission[6] was founded, in an effort to provide oversight for mentally ill patients who were involuntarily secluded and treated, to advise Parliament about the Act, and to propose revisions of the Act.

The most controversial aspects of the Act go back to February 15, 1999, when Jack Straw, the then Secretary of State for the British Home Office, recommended that Parliament modify the MHA of 1983 to enable 'indeterminate but reviewable detention of dangerous but personality disordered individuals'.[7] The basic idea was to use mental health assessments and facilities to detain potentially violent individuals before they could harm members of the public (preventive detention). The proposal was provoked by a series of high-profile crime cases and subsequent public outcry for more public protection. While there was a discussion of improving and expanding existing penal and forensic facilities to address the problem, the early phases of the debate seemed to favor the approach called 'psychiatric preventive detention'.[8] The debate focused on three aspects: (1) the ethics of preventive detention, (2) the 'dangerous and severe personality disorder' (DSPD) concept, and (3) the 'treatability' clause of the 1983 MHA.

The notion of preventive detention provoked protests from both the Royal College of Psychiatrists as well as service user (or mental health consumer advocacy) groups.[9] The gist of the concern was over the civil liberties of psychiatric patients, concerns about abuse or misuse of the detention, and for the psychiatrists' part, the insurmountable difficulty in the practical implementation of the practice, while at the same time holding psychiatrists accountable in case of the occurrence of a violent offense.[10] The concept of DSPD was also sharply criticized by the Royal College of Psychiatrists,[11] as it represented an invention of the courts and Parliament rather than a professionally recognized and scientifically validated diagnostic category. Such a vague construct was prone to misuse in the psychiatrists' view. Finally, the 1983 MHA had featured a 'treatability' clause, where involuntary confinement or treatment could be denied by psychiatrists if the condition had no effective treatment.[12] This feature had long been a focus of concern for some members of Parliament because it enabled known or potential offenders (e.g., 'psychopaths' or similar individuals with antisocial personality disorder or other criminal dispositions) to avoid hospitalization and seclusion. The DSPD moniker emerged as a legal-political shorthand to address dangerous individuals who were thought to have a mental disorder. This designation, however, had no official or scientific status within British psychiatry (or elsewhere), and British clinicians were upset, to say the least, at the idea of being held accountable for protecting the public from potential offenders, when the clinicians had little to no credible knowledge about the clinical features and treatment response of this population. Indeed, as the third aspect of the MHA revisions suggests, treatability has been one psychiatric method of determining who was eligible, or even justifiable, for involuntary detention and treatment. If psychiatry had nothing of treatment value to offer, then constraining the civil liberties, upon 'medical' criteria, of the potentially violent made no sense. The treatability clause, a 1983 requirement that detained individuals be able to benefit from treatment, kept many offenders, and would-be offenders, out of the psychiatric hospitals in the UK.

However, these two incidents on two continents, Cho's Virginia Tech University shootings and the debate around the MHA, in many ways represent a microcosm of the issues to be considered by this book. What should be the role of psychiatric diagnosis and treatment in the realm of crime? How do wrongful conduct and disordered or 'ill' conduct relate to each other? How should the relevant social institutions respond? What are the relevant social institutions? Are these institutions succeeding or failing?

1.3 Development of and context for the book

This book is an outgrowth of the research program that culminated in my 2005 monograph, *Values and Psychiatric Diagnosis* (VAPD).[13] In that thick text I aspired to present a broad survey of how values influenced psychiatric diagnosis and classification. I defined *values* broadly as beliefs or dispositions which were action-guiding and susceptible to praise or blame, following the lead of philosopher Hilary Putnam and others.[14] What became apparent very quickly in writing VAPD was that my queries into nosological values only peeked at the myriad value issues lurking within psychiatry and the mental health field. This book delves both more deeply and more narrowly into a particular value-laden domain in psychiatric diagnostic classification. For lack of a better description, I call this domain the vice/mental disorder relationship (VMDR). So what do I mean by the VMDR?

The term 'vice' I have remade into a philosophical technical term, having a particular meaning, though one close enough to the conventional meaning to be intuitive. 'Vice' as used in this book refers to human experiences and behaviors that fall into the domain of the wrongful AND the criminal. So while much will be made of criminality in this book, my domain of inquiry extends into wrongful conduct as well, and even wrongful thinking—'wrongfulness' in general. What qualifies as 'vice' in this book extends from the dramatic (e.g., gambling, theft, assaults, and molestations) to the realm of common human foibles (e.g., lying, losing one's temper, and cheating) and even into failures of virtue (e.g., failing to follow through with commitments, skipping school, and overeating).

What should be immediately acknowledged is that vice is a culturally relative concept, saturated with the vagaries, whims, and ephemera of historical era, culture, political will, fashion, and social convention. Indeed, if we consider 'criminality' as opposed to 'illness', we might recognize each as fundamentally different kinds of things.[15] 'Crime', for instance, presupposes an explicit sociopolitical context. If any concept counts as socially constructed, crime would be a thoroughly socially constructed one, perhaps even socially created, one. One could say that vice is social bound—its existence and meaning are fully dependent upon a social, cultural, and political context. Without a polity to define, frame, and regulate crime, there is none; only the 'state of nature' and anarchic human survival, to borrow Thomas Hobbes's withering appraisal.

Illness, on the other hand, while certainly subject to sociocultural influences, is a different, and a more conceptually complex phenomenon, at least in some ways. 'Illness' is also a sociocultural concept, as physicians and social scientists can provide many examples of physical and mental disorders which are socially framed and culturally relative.[16] However, illness can also be a primordially naturalistic, biological phenomenon. While the diseases of physical medicine may be subject to social and cultural variations of presentation, mental disorders are distinctive in their full immersion in sociocultural worlds.[17] To the degree that mental disorders are immersed in and shaped by societies and cultures; they also, Janus-faced, have biological, naturalistic aspects which psychiatric, psychological, and neuroscience research has increasingly explicated over the past 25 years. Mental disorders are, in sum, both naturalistic and social entities, with the relative weights of nature, nurture, and self-regulation of people with mental disorders generating ongoing, heated debate.[18] While vice no doubt has its own bionaturalistic aspects, its defining character seems primarily social, while disease and disorder appear to have a similar, dualistic character—both social and natural. However, even these generalizations require—and get—careful scrutiny, as they depend on our viewpoints about what people fundamentally are (what kinds of things people are) what philosophers call 'ontologies' or 'metaphysical assumptions', and everyone else calls 'human nature' or even more broadly, 'Nature'. The similarities and differences between illness and vice, however, rooted in ontological assumptions, are crucial topics to be explored in this book. For now I'll leave these issues as raised.

The American Psychiatric Association's *Diagnostic and Statistical Manual of Mental Disorders* (DSM), in a revised Fourth Edition[19] and now with a DSM-5[20] in use, has been the official diagnostic nomenclature for American psychiatric practice, research, education, and administration. I believe the DSM is a remarkable and powerful social document for a variety of reasons. As an official diagnostic manual, its categories enumerate and describe the full spectrum of psychiatric illness as it is understood by (at least) the American mental health professions, but indeed, the DSM reflects a broader Western biomedical understanding of mental illness.[21] Over the past 2 to 3 decades, the DSM has become progressively familiar to the American public as the standard bearer for what mental illness is, and means. The DSM has been subject to dozens, perhaps hundreds, of commentaries in the popular Western media over the past 30 years,[22] and its most common categories, disorders such as

Schizophrenia, Bipolar Disorder, Major Depressive Disorder, Posttraumatic Stress Disorder, (to name a few of them) have entered the common parlance as well as popular culture with magazines, newspapers, talk shows, blogs, social media, and the entertainment media as vehicles. Moreover, a DSM diagnosis is a fundamental unit for economic measures, health care funding, mental health care utilization statistics, even courtroom language.[23] The DSM has a 'gatekeeping' function—it legitimizes discussions of a person's mental condition, situates the condition in the context of scientific psychiatry, and provides explicit criteria for determining whether the person's condition qualifies as a legitimate disorder.[24] In my prior work I argued that the DSM was a de facto social or public policy statement, precisely because of its epistemological power in defining what counts as a mental illness for mental health professionals, the public, and policymakers.[25] At base, the DSM frames the discourse about mental illness. Looking to the future, we might expect similar social and epistemic power from future classifications of psychopathology, as well as international classifications of disease/disorders like those of the World Health Organization.

If we accept the DSM as a public policy instrument, the stakes surrounding any DSM diagnosis become substantially bigger. This is public policy that is not formulated in the public sphere, by voters, legislators, judges, or CEOs, but public policy developed largely behind closed doors among large panels of well-meaning clinical and research experts in the field of mental health.[26] Yet this document has profound social ramifications as noted above. A powerful public policy document developed and approved by a relatively small group of people—what better place to address broad, but pertinent social issues? What better place to do some good?

1.4 Chapter overviews

Hence, the focus of this book will be on how vice is involved in the DSM categories of mental disorders—What kinds of vice find their ways into diagnostic criteria? How has this happened? What is the significance of 'vice-laden' diagnostic criteria? The book will give some limited insight into why wrongful behavior and criminality find their way into a diagnostic manual dealing, presumably, with sicknesses.

Chapter 2 describes some of the particular instances of ambiguities and paradoxes in the DSM-IV-TR and DSM-5 regarding the VMDR. As this earlier material was written during the development of DSM-5, the emerging DSM-5 literature has been assimilated, as well as material drawn from online and other sources of emerging DSM thought, such as the DSM-5 Prelude Project.[27] As described earlier in this proposal, the social, professional, scientific, and moral significance of these paradoxes are raised. The chapter features numerous tables illustrating portions of the relevant DSM diagnostic criteria, contrasting them with prior editions, and provide a discussion of the context of the most recent changes. A description of the DSM developmental process sketches the scientific and practical considerations that constrain these efforts. The chapter concludes by exploring a variety of reasons for the DSM ambiguities regarding the VMDR from a scientific and nosological/nosographic perspective.

The general focus of Chapter 3 is the raising and elaboration of the philosophical-conceptual underpinnings of the VMDR in the DSM. The relationships between the guiding conceptual questions and the 'paradoxes' of the preceding chapters are sketched, building the background more explicitly for the analyses and arguments to follow in Chapters 8 and 9. This chapter is where the implicit and explicit assumptions of the various viewpoints concerning VMDR are discussed, along with the various kinds of value commitments involved. These understandings are organized into common themes, again leading to the more formative analyses to follow.

While in the middle of analyzing values and metaphysical assumptions about vice-laden mental disorders, I realized that in order to truly rethink the mad-or-bad problem, the muddling of vice and illness, a more formal consideration of history was required. As I was soon to find out, the particular 'history' I sought was not to be found. I wanted to see how the ideas about vice, sin, wrongfulness, and turpitude developed in Western history along with the concepts of sickness, injury, disease, and madness. A long Chapter 4 considers this parallel history of morality and madness, beginning in prehistory and carrying through to the mideighteenth century when the post-Enlightenment conceptions of mental illness and criminality gained cultural traction. Taken together, these two historical chapters build a profile of the development of sociocultural traditions regarding morality and madness, as well as the cultural responses in their blooming differentiations.

Picking up where Chapter 4 left off and 'psychiatry' was forming as a medical discipline, Chapter 5 sketches comparisons of the evolving American criminal justice, mental health, child welfare, and intellectual impairment systems beginning in the mid-eighteenth through the nineteenth and twentieth centuries, with a primary focus on the nascent VMDR. The evolution of this fourfold parsing of social deviance is discussed and situated in reference to other kinds of deviance-parsing, particularly relationships to poverty and racism. Considerations of the respective and fluctuating social roles for these institutions and systems are summarized. The bulk of the chapter describes the four key conceptual elements of historical context for the vice–mental disorder confounds (i.e., degeneracy theory, moral insanity, the 'criminalization' of intellectual impairment, and the description of deviant sexuality), and the development of the key DSM disorders of interest. The chapter concludes by drawing connections to the contemporary VMDR.

One could not imagine a discussion about vice without considering the perspective of the institutions involved directly in the social regulation of vice: law and jurisprudence, the perspectives from the criminal justice and penal systems, including the matter of juvenile criminality or 'delinquency'. Chapter 6 begins with a general summary of the structure and political aspects of law and jurisprudence in the United States. Notably, my analysis becomes narrower in limiting discussion to (mostly) the United States, the rationale being feasibility. The chapter then leads into discussions of mental health law as it overlaps with criminal law. A framework for the understanding of forensic psychiatry[28] practices is necessary as background to understanding the four key areas of the legal perspective discussed earlier: legislation implicating psychiatric practice, concepts of criminal culpability, the DSM forensic disclaimer, and courtroom-generated mental disorder categories. These latter issues are then connected explicitly to the development and status of the psychiatric nosologic categories discussed in Chapter 2. Consideration of penal and criminal justice perspectives highlight the ongoing political ambivalence about the proper role of penal institutions (e.g., protection of the public, punishment for wrongdoers, and reform of criminal offenders) drawing from Chapter 3. Review of empirical studies from the mental health research, law, and criminal justice literature concerning the VMDR clarify the issues raised.

From the very beginning of this introduction, the question of the public interest has been raised, and so an elaboration of the public viewpoint is another element of crucial background. Therefore, Chapter 7 summarizes findings pertinent to the VMDR in lay publications and media coverage. Of particular interest is an assessment of lay understandings of the VMDR, manifesting in social topics ranging from mass shootings, the dangerousness of mentally ill people, and forensic arenas like the insanity defense and sex offenders. These lay understandings are compared with the current knowledge from clinical and social science about the VMDR. Media studies of the public perception of crime, mental illness, and the mentally ill offender are reviewed, in addition to a review of popular media portrayals of mental illness and criminality. The mad-versus-bad confound in public perception will be explored from a review of sociological perspectives as well. A consideration of the controversial status of the insanity defense illustrates the mad-or-bad dichotomy from still another perspective. An assessment of what American psychiatric nosology faces in terms of public understanding of the VMDR is provided. This material contributes to the public policy considerations in the Chapter 9.

With all the ingredients in place, along with the demand of the conceptual questions, a formal analysis of the VMDR is undertaken in Chapter 8. Drawing upon the literature reviews, the chapter begins the philosophical analysis based upon the framing of the conceptual issues in Chapter 7, the scientific or nosological considerations posed in Chapter 2, and the practical and contextual considerations contributed by the other chapters. Four idealized accounts of the VMDR provide a focus and structure for exploring the conceptual issues: the 'coincidental' account, the 'medicalization' account, the 'criminalization (or moralization)' account, and 'mixed' account. These accounts are not intended to be 'straw men' to be set up and then criticized (as amalgams of ideas and positions, these accounts likely do not mirror a single author, theory, or perspective), but instead serve as heuristic devices for organizing the disparate and often inchoate thought about the VMDR revealed in the preceding chapters. The implications of policies, postures, and perspectives from preceding chapters are then considered in light of these four accounts. The coincidental account is the simplest—the idea that criminality and mental disorder are distinct entities that are not causally related but simply coincidental when they occur together. The medicalization account holds that traditional social deviance under the mental disorder rubric is not substantively different than criminal deviance, and both are subject to biomedical explanation and control. The criminalization-or-moralization account articulates the general view that other-infringing social deviance should be handled similarly: for example, criminality and mental illness behaviors that intrude on others is responsible conduct and should be handled by social structures that address crime and immorality, such as the educational, religious, and criminal justice systems. The mixed account mixes elements of the other three accounts in various, informal, ways. These accounts then pose a grid to examine the metaphysical and value assumptions involved in the actual debates about the VMDR, from the legal, psychiatric, criminal justice, historical, and lay perspectives. The laying out of the metaphysical and value assumptions for the various standpoints in the VMDR debate provide a transformative perspective on the VMDR, completing the chapter and leading to the summary conclusions in Chapter 9.

Chapter 9 pulls together the preceding material by considering two basic tasks, stated as '40 Theses': What are the implications of the preceding analysis for a future DSM, psychiatry, and the criminal justice system, and what are the implications of the analysis for VMDR-relevant public policy considerations? The former task will involve considering the congruence or conflict of values regarding the classification of psychopathology and criminal behavior. The latter will also require a consideration of differential political philosophies in understanding the criminality-mental disorder relationship. Why? Because the metaphysical and value assumptions clarified in Chapter 7 will only map onto particular political values and metaphysical assumptions in compatible ways.[29] For example, Thomas Szasz's Libertarian sympathies intercalate with his metaphysical beliefs about mental illness, which are that mental illness is a myth, a metaphor for 'real', physical illness.[30] Because deviance associated with a mythical mental illness is morally responsible, transgressive deviance called 'mental illness' should be handled by nonmedical institutions like the aforementioned educational, criminal justice, and religious systems. So for Szasz, political values and metaphysical assumptions align to form a sympathetic viewpoint with the criminalization-or-moralization account described above. The subsequent public policy considerations will then reflect the marriage of political considerations with medical-scientific ones in considering the role of psychiatry in VMDR public policy, and the role of public policy in VMDR-related psychiatric practice.

The book concludes with 40 'Theses', brief statements of conclusions, implications, and recommendations. A warning: Lovers of mystery stories, doorways to alternatives, and waiting until the fat lady sings, don't skip ahead. The puzzle has begun, and the best part is following the evidence and seeing how the mystery unfolds!

Notes

1. Cohen (1950).
2. Wikipedia, http://en.wikipedia.org/wiki/Cho_Seung_Hui.
3. *Washington Post* (2007).
4. Commonwealth of Virginia (2005, p. 4). (See citation inside the *Washington Post* (2007) story.)
5. Humphreys (2008); Hurley & Linsley (2005); Pilgrim (2012); Shaw & Middleton (2016).
6. Mental Health Act Commission (n.d.).
7. White (2002, p. 95).
8. ibid.
9. Tilley & Chambers (2005).
10. Moran (2002).
11. Royal College of Psychiatrists (2002).
12. See Grounds (2001); Moncrieff (2003).
13. Readers interested in the methodological aspects of my 'values' philosophical research can find detailed discussions in Sadler (1997; 2005). These methods are still relevant to this current work.
14. Putnam (1981, 1990a, 1990b); Sadler (1997, 2005).
15. In Chapter 8 I discuss in more detail the ontological assumptions (assumptions about 'human nature') of concepts like vice, criminality, and mental disorder.
16. Some examples of culturally relative illnesses include hypertension, anorexia nervosa, hypochondriasis, and *ataques de nervios*. See Mezzich (2002).
17. See for instance Crafa & Nagel (2020); Gagné-Julien (2021); Kirmayer (2018); Thornton (2017).
18. ibid; Sadler (2005, 2007, 2013).
19. American Psychiatric Association (2000).
20. American Psychiatric Association (2013).
21. Mezzich (1996); Mezzich, Parron, Kleinman, & Fabrega (1996); Sadler (2005, 2007).
22. Broad discussions of the DSM in pop media are in Bender et al. (2018); McGinty et al. (2016); and Rapley et al. (2011).
23. Frances (2010); Sadler (2005, 2013); Shuman (1989, 2002).
24. Sadler (2005).
25. Sadler (2002, 2005, 2013).
26. The process of building a DSM is discussed in Frances, First, & Pincus (1995) and Kendler (2013); DMS-5 (www.dsm5.org); Sadler (2005); Zachar et al. (2019).
27. www.dsm5.org, later assimilated by the American Psychiatric Association as http://www.psych.org/dsmv.asp.
28. Allan, Louw, & Verschoor (1995); Eigen (1991a, 1991b); Glueck (1916); Gold (2012); Mohr (1997); Pollack (1974); Prosono (2003); Quen (1983, 1994); Robitscher (1978); Tighe (1983); Watson (1992).
29. Political philosophies depend, in part, on metaphysical accounts of 'human nature' (Kymlicka 1990).
30. Haldipur et al. (2019); Schaler (2004); Szasz (1974).

2

Vice and the DSMs—the problems

> I cannot say I like the *commingling* of the *insane* and the *criminal* and to be
> *catalogued* with Sing Sing and Auburn . . . It tends to keep up a notion we
> strive to do away—that Asylums and Prisons are alike.
>   —Amariah Brigham to Pliny Earle, 1845 (in Grob, 2008b, p. 139)

2.1 Introduction—navigating values in diagnostic constructs

In this chapter, I will be introducing some philosophical tools to identify 'vice' concepts in *Diagnostic and Statistical Manual of Mental Disorders* (DSM) categories and criteria. This will require discipline on my part in systematically going through selected DSM categories, and discipline on the reader's part in working through a series of short analyses of DSM diagnostic criteria sets. The chapter poses tedious work for both writer and reader, but I know no better way to establish the vice-laden character of these selected DSM categories. These category discussions will provide the starting point for the material to follow, and that is why they are presented, in detail, this one time.[1] First, an illustrative example.

Vice and Psychiatric Diagnosis. John Z. Sadler, Oxford University Press. © Oxford University Press 2024.
DOI: 10.1093/oso/9780198876830.003.0002

On June 17, 2003, reportedly in response to a controversial symposium at the prior American Psychiatric Association (APA) annual meeting, the APA issued the following statement as a pronouncement for the public and press (text content reproduced here in full):

AMERICAN PSYCHIATRIC ASSOCIATION STATEMENT
DIAGNOSTIC CRITERIA FOR PEDOPHILIA
June 17, 2003
Arlington, Va.—Pedophilia, included in the American Psychiatric Association Diagnostic and Statistical Manual of Mental Disorders (DSM) since 1968, continues to be classified as a mental disorder. The DSM is the standard classification of mental disorders used by mental health professionals and provides clear, objective descriptions of mental illnesses, based upon scientific research. Pedophilia is categorized in the DSM-IV-TR as one of several paraphilic mental disorders. The essential features of a Paraphilia are recurrent, intense sexually arousing fantasies, sexual urges, or behaviors that generally involve nonhuman subjects, children, or other nonconsenting adults, or the suffering or humiliation of oneself or one's partner. An adult who engages in sexual activity with a child is performing a criminal and immoral act and this is never considered normal or socially acceptable behavior. Darrel A. Regier, M.D., M.P.H., Director, American Psychiatric Association's Division of Research states, 'there are no plans or processes set up that would lead to the removal of the Paraphilias from their consideration as legitimate mental disorders'.

The American Psychiatric Association Diagnostic and Statistical Manual of Mental Disorders, Fourth Edition Text Revision (DSM-IV-TR) criteria for Pedophilia (302.2) are:
  A. Over a period of at least 6 months, recurrent, intense sexually arousing fantasies, sexual urges, or behaviors involving sexual activity with a prepubescent child or children (generally age 13 years or younger);
  B. The person has acted on these sexual urges, or the sexual urges or fantasies cause marked distress or interpersonal difficulty;
  C. The person is at least age 16 years and at least 5 years older than the child or children in Criterion A.

Pedophilia generally is treated with cognitive-behavioral therapy. The therapy may be prescribed alone or in combination with medication. Some examples of medications which have been used include anti-androgens and selective serotonin reuptake inhibitors (SSRIs). Relapse prevention is also emphasized. However, the outlook for successful treatment and rehabilitation of individuals with Pedophilia is guarded.

The American Psychiatric Association is a national medical specialty society, founded in 1844, whose 35,000 physician members specialize in the diagnosis, treatment and prevention of mental illnesses including substance use disorders. For more information, visit the APA Web site at www.psych.org.[2]

This formal statement from APA sums up one of the issues to be considered in this book: some categories, as described in the DSMs, are both disorders and 'criminal and immoral act(s)', or the category phenomena substantively overlap as 'disorders' and 'criminality/immorality'. From one perspective, the occurrence that vice behavior (wrongful conduct) manifests along with mentally disordered behavior is no more surprising than the fact that criminal offenders get myocardial infarctions or asthmatic children tell lies. Sick people are complicated, just as healthy people are. What is important though about the case of the DSMs is that the very definitions of particular mental disorders include wrongful conduct (vice) as *core diagnostic features*. Vice is not just a simple coincidence of the complexity of people with mental disorders, but rather, partly *defining of* some mental disorders in the DSMs. If mental disorders are defined in terms of vice, this means, at minimum, we are shifting what we usually think of as 'illness' or 'disorder' into the realm of the moral and criminal.

The descriptive language of illness and disease has a limited general vocabulary for the varieties of suffering: terms like 'pain', 'incapacity', 'injury', 'failure', 'impairment', 'trauma', 'hurt', 'suffering', 'distress', and 'disability'. From the philosophical perspective, these words, and their associated concepts, share three things: (1) they are all negative value terms (words for undesired, unwanted human conditions); (2) they are accurately applied, in various combinations, to the full range of 'physical' diseases, injuries, and illnesses; and (3) they are all nonmoral in meaning. What does 'nonmoral in meaning' mean?

Years ago, the philosopher William Frankena[3] teased out an important distinction between moral and nonmoral value terms. For Frankena, moral values were values that had to do with rightness, wrongness, good, and evil. Nonmoral values occupied other sets of values—that in the medical setting involved terms like 'pain', 'suffering', 'disability', for example. In *Values and Psychiatric Diagnosis*, I defined 'values' as concepts which were action-guiding and involved praiseworthiness or blameworthiness.[4] Moral and nonmoral values are values. For example, evil people guide our action (we avoid them) and are blameworthy, whereas judicious people are action-guiding (e.g., we listen to them carefully) and praiseworthy (we think being judicious is something that should be praised and encourage ourselves and others to do).

Some people may be confused or annoyed when philosophers and bioethicists say that disease is 'value-laden'. This is a highfalutin way of saying that disease, illnesses, and injuries are 'disvalued'—they are things we don't want to have. To say something is a disease or injury is to imply a negative value—that a disease or injury is an undesirable state for the ailing person. This 'negative' evaluation of disease is common and taken for granted, especially in physical disease. Everyone agrees that the flu is a bad thing to have, so much so, the value judgement 'Flu is bad' is obvious, invisible, and never questioned. However, as Fulford[5] has pointed out, with mental disorders, no blanket consensus characterizes the negative versus positive aspects of clinical features of many, perhaps most, mental disorders. For instance, some people are fascinated by their hallucinations, enjoy getting high as often as feasible (or even when it is self-destructive) or seek to regain the energy of their manias. Mental illness engenders more disagreement—a dissensus—about the desirability or acceptability of the phenomena associated with mental disorders.

Furthermore, disease, illness, and injury are not just any undesirable situation: Getting arrested, failing to get a promotion, getting a divorce, and flunking a course are also undesirable situations, but they don't, in isolation, make for disease. Diseases, illnesses, and injuries involve particular kinds of disvalue. When we consider the diagnostic language (or descriptions of clinical features) of medical diagnoses like myocardial infarction, a fractured femur, scleroderma, or a third-degree burn of the arm, the clinical language we use is nonmoral, to use Frankena's distinction. To have a burned arm or a myocardial infarction has no implication of wrongdoing, at least as far as the clinical description goes. Any 'morality' that might be associated with the burn or MI patient is identified only through, perhaps, the circumstances that led to the injury or disease. For example, we might blame the burned individual because he smoked a cigarette while priming his car's carburetor, and we might blame the MI patient because of a lifetime of smoking, overeating, and being a 'couch potato'. The language of the features of illness, the language of pain, suffering, and disability, as well as other descriptive features of illness (ischemic changes reflected in the electrocardiogram, the formation of an eschar on the burn site) are *nonmoral* in meaning. To summarize, disease is generally defined in reference to nonmoral values. Outside the field of mental health or psychiatry, the value-ladenness of illness, injury, and disease is, overwhelmingly, *nonmoral*.

When we consider mental disorders in the DSM, however, we can recognize that some clinical features, diagnostic descriptors, and most concretely, diagnostic criteria involve moral values in describing the disorder. Examine the above-referenced criteria set for Pedophilia in DSM-IV-TR. Some individuals may meet the criteria by simply having sexual fantasies and preoccupation with sex with children. We could say some pedophilic individuals are 'conscientious' under the DSM-IV-TR criteria, if they don't engage in molestations. The DSM criteria require either distress by the fantasies and preoccupations, *and/or* acting upon their sexual fantasies about children. Other individuals may have adverse consequences (e.g., marital difficulties, getting fired because of viewing online child pornography) for their sexual preoccupations and problem behaviors and can qualify for the diagnosis of Pedophilia (and later, Pedophilic Disorder in DSM-5) on that basis as well.[6] However, Criterion B also notes that 'acting on' these fantasies, meaning actually molesting one or more children, fulfills this Criterion. When the individual engages in child molesting behavior, the situation moves into the realm of crime and criminality. At this point the 'wrongful conduct' moral aspect of the diagnostic criterion becomes explicit. One might wonder already, is the perpetrator's behavior in reference to a disease, illness, injury, or a crime/moral turpitude?

However, the moral-value content of the Pedophilia diagnostic criteria does not stop there. Let's say you were to tell your mother that you are having intrusive fantasies of molesting children. It's possible that she would wonder if you were ill. Perhaps more likely, she would be upset and perhaps outraged by your arousal and interest in such abhorrent images. She would react morally to your confession and might well consider the thoughts as wrongful or immoral. So for at least some people—and I would aver that this would be a LOT of people—thoughts and behavior of a pedophilic nature are wrongful and, thus, are cast in the language of wrongful conduct: 'evil', 'depraved', 'sinful', and 'exploitative', for example.

What may now be apparent for many readers is that wrongful thoughts and behavior are, like beauty and pornography, in the eye of the beholder. Stated 'academically', moral norms are culture-dependent. Some cultures permit, even encourage, sexual contact between children and adults,[7] but in these cases, such sexual contact is ritualized and socially constrained within particular, and approved, cultural purposes or worldviews. The realization that moral wrongfulness is culturally relative further complicates the issue of diagnostic criteria in a DSM. Not only do we have diagnostic criteria which imply moral wrongfulness for many people, we may not have any morally neutral territory—that is, relevant cultural universals, on which to ground normative healthy behavior[8] or even morally appropriate or acceptable behavior. DSM-IV Pedophilia, and DSM-5 Pedophilic Disorder, are defined as illnesses, but many people within Western culture view pedophilia as bad behavior—wrongful thought and conduct. When I refer to vice-laden diagnostic criteria now and later in this book this usage recognizes fully that the 'vice' aspect may not be shared by everyone—but I claim that *many* people would construe the criterion, descriptor, or clinical feature as involving wrongful thought or conduct. Vice-ladenness is a manifestation of social attitudes, beliefs, and traditions and, therefore, is subject to change. A key question, to be addressed later in this book, is *on what basis to establish* whether wrongful conduct is sick versus healthy wrongful conduct. I'll discuss more about this later.

When it comes to examining diagnostic criteria for moral-value terms and concepts, we should also recognize that using morality-laden diagnostic descriptors may be subject to varying interpretations by readers—whether mental health professionals or laypersons. What is an objectionable set of thoughts for one person may be the stuff of everyday mental life for another. Nabokov's *Lolita*[9] is a fiction classic partly because many readers can recognize, and perhaps even resonate with, Humbert Humbert's desire for the 12-year-old provocative Lolita, and other readers can recognize and perhaps even identify with these particular depictions of immature and mature sexuality. So does the eroticism sired by Nabokov as author and Humbert as fictional character render the both of them pedophiles or sexual predators?[10] Because of these ambiguities, using moral terms as diagnostic descriptors, then, poses an additional potential difficulty through introducing variability in diagnosis from one diagnostician to the next, as the criteria are applied by every clinician: from clinicians who are prudes, to ones who are sexually respectful, to ones who are sexual libertines. A clinician's own moral predilections, normative assumptions, and filters may partly determine whether a this or that patient meets moral-value laden diagnostic criteria.

In Chapter 1 I introduced my technical term 'vice' as a way of identifying morally wrongful thoughts and actions—incorporating both criminality and simple nonvirtuous thought and conduct. For now, and later in this book, I'll use 'vice-laden' to refer to diagnostic descriptions that harbor vice or 'vicious' meanings. At this point, it might be useful to take a closer look at DSM-5 diagnostic criteria to see how frequently 'vice-laden' criteria appear. In the following discussion, I have reproduced relevant portions of DSM-5 diagnostic criteria to examine specific details. For copyright reasons I cannot present every set of diagnostic criteria in the DSM, so I have selected examples carefully to illustrate both the absence of vice-laden criteria—categories that resemble conventional illnesses with nonmoral descriptors—and heavily vice-laden categories, as well as some in between—categories that are questionably vice-laden. Readers can examine the DSM-5 directly for the full criteria sets.

Before we proceed, a few words about methods are in order. How is it that one can identify vice-related values in diagnostic criteria? In *Values and Psychiatric Diagnosis* and an earlier article[11] I presented detailed methodological discussions about how to identify various kinds of values. I refer interested readers to these sources for more details. In short: values, as I mentioned earlier, are action-guiding attitudes or dispositions to act, which are susceptible to praise or blame. As one might imagine, language that describes vice would likely be susceptible to blame.[12] Values appear in texts, or 'discourses', in three basic ways.[13]

The first, the 'value term', addresses words whose concepts are indivisibly tied to values—one cannot define or use the word appropriately without expressing a value judgement. Value terms can be 'thin' or abstract and general (e.g., 'good', 'evil', 'right', and 'wrong'). Value terms can also be 'thick', meaning that these words or concepts mix evaluations and factual descriptions, and subsequently are rich, multidimensional words bursting with descriptive color and nuance, as well as value judgements. Examples of thick value terms are words like 'elegance', 'joyful', 'sullen', or 'decadent'. Mental health language is particularly rich with thick value terms, words like 'dysphoria', 'inappropriate', or 'manipulative' are good examples.[14] In contrast, typical 'factual' language is easily definable without a value judgement or evaluation—words like 'yellow' (a form of radiation with a wavelength of 580 nanometers perceptible to the human eye), 'automobile' (an enclosed motorized vehicle on wheels used by small numbers of people for land transportation), or 'hallucination' (a perception without a typical external stimulus).

Some value terms do double-duty: depending on how they are actually used in text or talk, some words can be evaluative or just factual. For instance, consider the word 'duty' in the following sentences: 'Dr. Garza showed up for duty in the emergency room.' 'It was his duty to care for the patients.' In the first sentence, 'duty' could easily be substituted by 'work' with no loss of meaning. In the second sentence, 'duty' means a moral-medical obligation, one that extends beyond mere work. 'Duty' in the second sentence is a value term—not so for duty in the first sentence. As revisited below, examining how words are used in practical communication is crucial to deciding if they depict a 'value' or not.

The second way values can appear in discourse (text or talk) is through a 'value semantic'. This notes that the meaning of a sentence implies a value judgement of some sort. My example from *Values and Psychiatric Diagnosis* was this sentence: 'John will do anything to get a grant.' As you can see, no value term appears in this sentence. However, in conventional usage, the speaker is suggesting that John is ruthless in grant-winning and perhaps even unethical in conduct. The example shows that even with no value term present, a sentence can indicate an evaluation. However, most value semantics appear transparently evaluative—as in this third sentence from DSM-IV-TR's Introduction: 'Our highest priority has been to provide a helpful guide to clinical practice.'[15] The sentence even includes two value terms: 'priority' and 'helpful'.

The third way values can appear in discourses is through implication: one can have a value *commitment* (the DSM-IV-TR Introduction sentence above is a good example), a value *entailment*, or a value *consequence*.[16] A value commitment explicitly endorses a particular disposition, action or range of actions. A value entailment occurs when the discourse implies that one or more values may be encumbered by, tied-up with, or necessarily associated with a particular viewpoint or perspective. In *Values and Psychiatric Diagnosis* I contrasted reductionism versus holism: to be a reductionist or to be a holist as a practitioner implies various ways one should make sense of the world—as a complex entity made up of component, discoverable parts (reductionist) or as a complex entity that must be considered as a unity (holist). The laboratory scientist is likely to be a reductionist, and her action may be guided accordingly, though only by implication, and the spiritual therapist may be a holist, whose actions, however different, are also implicitly guided by her larger perspective. Finally, the other implication: some values we encounter are value *consequences*: while not values per se, value consequences are the foreseen or unforeseen effects associated with a theory or practice. Stated a little differently, value consequences are the results of actions guided by our values. As noted in *Values and Psychiatric Diagnosis*, explicating value consequences was the reason for the ethical, legal, and social implications (ELSI) of the human genome initiative at NIH[17] and related programs, and it has become a model for considering ELSI for any big science program. ELSI programs attempt to foretell, and possibly forestall, the (adverse) value consequences of big science.

Of all these modes of values appearing in discourse, the value implications are the most difficult to identify—mostly because they refer to situations outside the meaning of the sentence, which value terms and semantics are limited to. Finally, consider 'vice' sorts of values. I earlier described 'vice' as referring to wrongful thought and conduct and criminality. For our interests here, we are not just identifying values—indeed, all of the symptoms of a disorder are negatively valued (e.g., things we don't want to have), but our question for this chapter and book is whether the values in the diagnostic descriptions are 'vice' (moral) values as opposed to the nonmoral values described above.

2.2 Vice-laden diagnostic concepts—some demonstrations

There are some other logical properties of values that we'll explain as we go—but for now, let consider some of the DSM diagnostic criteria in detail, to put some of this theory into practice. The remainder of this chapter will introduce our primary set of disorders of interest. Here, the case will be made for the vice-ladenness (or lack thereof) for each condition, but analyses of the why, how, and should-be questions will be left for later chapters. The primary focus in these remaining pages is to illustrate the utility of these theoretical tools in identifying vice-ladenness in diagnostic criteria.

The analyses that follow are limited in scope and in numbers of DSM categories under consideration. I have selected a subset of DSM-5 disorders, which, in my opinion, offer the most important cases of vice-laden categories, with important exceptions included (e.g., Schizophrenia, Sexual Masochism Disorder) as contrast-cases—examples which differ from vice-laden disorders (e.g., Schizophrenia) and for the case of Sexual Masochism Disorder, an example which poses curious evaluative properties. Of course, other DSM-5 disorders could be considered also, but as the reader will see, the list of vice-implicated disorders is long, even including my constraints. Perhaps readers will be inspired to consider additional disorders! I should also note that because of copyright constraints for DSM-5, I have only excerpted diagnostic criteria. In some cases, I have simply deleted less-than-relevant material from the DSM-5 text, setting this off in ellipsis (. . .), while in others I have summarized the significance of the criterion in terms of a key value term in the criterion, or the role of the criterion item in the criteria set (e.g., 'age requirements' or 'distinction from other disorders'). In these latter cases, the abstracted criterion is set off in brackets (e.g., [irresponsible conduct]).

2.2.1 Schizophrenia

For many, Schizophrenia is the exemplar mental disorder. While a disorder at the center of the psychiatric mainstream, Schizophrenia has had its own checkered history and controversies concerning its status as a disorder,[18] to its clinical features, to its etiology, which still is hotly debated.[19] A standard-bearing mental disorder, then, is a good first choice in considering vice in mental disorder diagnostic criteria and concepts. An excerpt, without subtyping, of the DSM-5 diagnostic criteria for Schizophrenia are listed in Table 2.1. Bracketed material is contracted, summarized criteria elements.

Table 2.1 Excerpt of DSM-5 Diagnostic Criteria for Schizophrenia 295.90 (APA 2013, pp. 99–100)

A. Two (or more) of the following, each present for a significant portion of time during a 1-month period (or less if successfully treated). At least one of these must be (1), (2), or (3):

    1. Delusions.

    2. Hallucinations.

    3. Disorganized speech (e.g., frequent derailment or incoherence).

    4. Grossly disorganized or catatonic behavior.

    5. Negative symptoms (i.e., diminished emotional expression or avolition).

  B. [impairment of functioning].

  C. [duration criteria].

  D. [differentiation from other disorders].

  E. [differentiation from other disorders].

  F. [differentiation from other disorders].

In considering criterion A, one should examine the definitions of the 'characteristic symptoms' as listed in Appendix C, the Glossary of Technical Terms in DSM-5.[20] Table 2.2 lists key excerpts of technical terms from DSM criteria for Schizophrenia which may disguise (or not) vice-laden meanings:

Criterion A lists the characteristic symptoms of Schizophrenia and requires two or more of the following five symptom areas. Delusion, one of these, is defined in Table 2.2, and describes a false belief which is culturally idiosyncratic and not amenable to contradicting evidence. While the full definition of 'delusion' is laden with value terms (e.g., 'false', 'incorrect', 'incontrovertible', or 'credibility') these terms do not describe wrongfulness, but rather, describe what might be called epistemic values, which are values that are concerned with securing credible knowledge.[21] In our culture, holding false or incorrect beliefs in and of themselves is not taken as morally wrongful, though culturally nonconforming belief may be perceived as wrongful by some (e.g., not believing in God). As they stand here, delusions as delusions hold little to no vice content.

Similarly, the full definition of 'hallucination' is also laden with epistemic value terms ('misperceived', 'misinterpreted', 'true', 'nonveridical', and 'false'), but these also fail to point convincingly to the meaning of 'vice', but instead refer to the truth-value of the hallucinated experience. If hallucinations represent a truth-failure, in our context of usage in clinical psychiatry this truth-failure is not deceptive (a lie), but rather represents a mistaken perception, an additional reason for hallucinations being out of the realm of vice.

'Incoherence' is also value-laden as a *disturbance*, but 'disturbance' is used as in a nonmoral medical impairment and not a moral one. Similarly, the full definitions of 'flat affect' and 'avolition', vice terms are absent, as are vice semantics. However,

Table 2.2 Excerpts from DSM-5 Glossary Definitions of Key Criterion Terms for Schizophrenia (APA 2013)

Delusion:

A false belief based on incorrect inference about external reality that is firmly held despite what almost everyone else believes and despite what constitutes incontrovertible and obvious proof or evidence to the contrary. The belief is not ordinarily accepted by other members of the person's culture or subculture (i.e., it is not an article of religious faith). When a false belief involves a value judgment, it is regarded as a delusion only when the judgment is so extreme as to defy credibility. . . . (p. 819)

Hallucination:

A perception-like experience with the clarity and impact of a true perception but without the external stimulation of the relevant sensory organ. Hallucinations should be distinguished from illusions, in which an actual external stimulus is misperceived or misinterpreted. . . . (p. 822)

Incoherence:

Speech or thinking that is essentially incomprehensible to others because word or phrases are joined together without a logical or meaningful connection. This disturbance occurs within clauses, in contrast to derailment, in which the disturbance is between clauses. . . . (p. 823)

Flat (affect):

A pattern of observable behaviors that is the expression of a subjectively experienced feeling state (emotion). . . . 'flat': absence or near absence of any sign of affective expression. (p. 817)

Avolition:

An inability to initiate and persist in goal-directed activities. When severe enough to be considered pathological, avolition is pervasive and prevents the person from completing many different types of activities. . . . (p. 818)

'avolition' might be construed as 'laziness' by some, except for the inclusion of 'inability' in the definition, which implies that individuals cannot help themselves and, therefore, cannot be 'lazy' in common usage.

Criterion B describes 'dysfunction' in terms of incapabilities in a number of spheres, none of which have vice or moral content. The remainder of the diagnostic criteria specify duration and distinctions from other conditions.

My conclusion is that the DSM-5 diagnostic criteria for Schizophrenia have little to no vice content. Schizophrenia is described in typically nonmoral value terms, specifying various impairments and incapacities.

2.2.2 Conduct Disorder

As a startling contrast, consider the diagnostic criteria for Conduct Disorder, one of the disorders of childhood and adolescence in DSM-5. Excerpts of these criteria appear in Table 2.3. Page numbers are provided for DSM-5 for readers interested in the full criteria sets. For copyright reasons, I have had to attenuate full quotation of criteria, and used brackets to summarize.

The diagnostic criteria for Conduct Disorder describe a litany of criminal behaviors and vice terms: 'bullies', 'threatens', 'intimidates', 'fights', 'harm', 'cruel', 'extortion',

Table 2.3 Excerpt of DSM-5 Diagnostic Criteria for Conduct Disorder (APA 2013, pp. 469–471)

A. A repetitive and persistent pattern of behavior in which the basic rights of others or major age-appropriate societal norms or rules are violated, as manifested by the presence of at least three of the following fifteen criteria. . . .

Aggression to People and Animals

1. Often bullies . . . .

2. [starts fights]

3. Has used a weapon. . . .

4. [cruelty to people]

5. [cruelty to animals]

6. [theft behaviors]

7. [engaged in sexual violence]

Destruction of Property

8. [set fires]

9. [damaged properties]

Deceitfulness or Theft

10. [forced domestic entry]

11. [frequent lying or conning]

12. [nonconfrontational theft—shoplifting, etc.]

Serious Violations of Rules

13. [keeps late hours without supervision]

14. Has run away from home overnight . . . .

15. Is often truant . . . .

B. [impairment of functioning]

C. [differentiation from other disorders]

'forced' (sexual contact), 'fire setting', 'destroyed', 'deceitfulness', 'theft', 'lying', 'cons', and 'truant', for example. Indeed, for Criterion A, every single subcriterion item involves wrongful or criminal conduct and, therefore, is incontrovertibly vice-laden. A set of specifiers describes some behavior patterns which have predictive value, and are vigorously vice-laden (*limited prosocial emotions, lack of remorse, lack of empathy, unconcerned about performance*, and *shallow or deficient affect*). The latter item, shallow/deficient affect, may be less transparent in its vice-ladenness, though it is defined in the context of 'insincerity' and 'manipulation'. The primary rationale for this specifier[22] is that these concerns enhance the prediction of adult antisocial behavior and psychopathy, and thus have prognostic and treatment-planning significance. One would not be surprised then, that the proposed modifier is also vice-laden to the core.

Criterion B, like that of Schizophrenia, specifies Conduct Disorder (CD) as causing impairment in psychosocial functioning—and through this criterion attempts to establish CD as a nonmoral, impairing disorder. CD may be the most extreme example of a disorder in DSM-5 where the vice-ladenness is complete.[23]

2.2.3 Oppositional Defiant Disorder

Like CD, Oppositional Defiant Disorder ((ODD), Table 2.4) is vice-laden as well, as a cursory examination of criteria A reveal: the patient reveals *argumentative/defiant behavior, or vindictiveness, often argues with adults, defies or refuses to comply, deliberately annoys others, and blames others.* While CD is defined in terms of primarily criminal behaviors, ODD is defined in terms of wrongful conduct and attitudes.

2.2.4 Personality Disorders

Antisocial Personality Disorder (ASPD) introduces the broader category of disorders called Personality Disorders (PDs), the latter briefly defined in DSM terms as 'an enduring pattern of inner experience and behavior that deviates markedly from the expectations of the individual's culture. . . [affecting] cognition, affectivity, interpersonal functioning, and impulse control . . . the enduring pattern is inflexible, pervasive, . . . and causes clinically significant distress or impairment . . .'[24] From this brief description, the vice-ladenness of PDs is not readily apparent.

The DSM-5 lists 10 different PDs, of which ASPD is one. The diagnostic criteria for ASPD are excerpted in Table 2.5. Often developmentally linked to CD, ASPD has a provocative history in Psychiatry, confounded by related concepts or categories like 'psychopathy'.[25] This history will be discussed more in Chapters 4 and 5.

The PDs section of DSM-5 has been among the most criticized portions of this and prior versions of the DSM.[26] The reasons for this are several, and not particularly pertinent to our considerations of vice in DSM-5 PD. Briefly, one issue was that multiple DSM-IV-era PD could be diagnosed in the same patient, a situation Skodol and Bender described as co-occurrence of PDs.[27] Moreover, DSM-IV-era PDs were found to be less stable, that is, patients would fluctuate in their qualification of a particular diagnosis, which is counter to the PD concept—a stable but dysfunctional adaptation over time. Finally, PDs tended to be phenomena that are graded in severity—PDs are 'worse' for some people compared to others, and the clinical

Table 2.4 Excerpt of Diagnostic Criteria for DSM-5 Oppositional Defiant Disorder (APA 2013, pp. 462–463)

A. A pattern of angry/irritable mood, argumentative/defiant behavior, or vindictiveness lasting at least 6 months as evidenced by at least four symptoms. . . .

Angry/Irritable Mood: losing temper, annoyed easily, often resentful

Argumentative/Defiant Behavior: argumentative, defiant, annoying, blaming others

Vindictiveness: spitefulness

8. Has been spiteful or vindictive at least twice within the past 6 months

B. [distress, impairment required]

C. [exclusion of other disorders]

Table 2.5 Excerpts of DSM-5 diagnostic criteria for Antisocial Personality Disorder (APA 2013, p. 659)

A. A pervasive pattern of disregard for and violation of the rights of others, . . . as indicated by three (or more) of the following:

1. [unlawful behaviors]

2. [deceitfulness]

3. [impulsivity]

4. [frequent fighting]

5. [recklessness]

6. [irresponsible conduct]

7. [guiltlessness]

B. [age criteria]

C. [relation to other disorders]

D. [relation to other disorders]

research on personality and PDs strongly supports the personality is better captured empirically through a dimensional (graded on a continuum) approach rather than as an either/or continuum, which was the DSM-III and IV approach.[28]

2.2.4.1 Antisocial Personality Disorder

What then, of the diagnostic criteria for ASPD in DSM-5? As with CD, we have an extensive list of wrongful conduct, or vices, to use my language: disregarding the rights of others, unlawful conduct, deceitfulness, aggressiveness (physical), irresponsibility, and lack of remorse after committing wrongful acts (Table 2.5). With the possible exception of impulsivity, or failure to plan ahead, all of these are vice-laden concepts.

Regarding impulsivity or planning failures, we can imagine examples where vice would be present (e.g., slugging your boss for saying no to your request for a raise or failing to pay much-needed child support to your ex-wife) or examples where no vice is involved (e.g., a batter prematurely swinging at the ball at a baseball game). Considering the DSM-5 criteria, ASPD is vice-laden to the core, identifying a population of people lacking virtue and exhibiting a cornucopia of persistent vices.

2.2.5 Impulse Control Disorders

In DSM-5, several disorders coming under the 'Disruptive, Impulse-Control, and Conduct Disorders' section are relevant to the issue of vice-ladenness. These disorders are differentiated in DSM-5 from other disorders associated with difficulties in inhibiting or controlling rash or poorly planned actions, such as substances abuse disorders, paraphilias, and others. Of the six categories under the Impulse Control Disorders NOS rubric, three are of primary interest regarding vice concerns: Intermittent Explosive Disorder, Kleptomania, and Pyromania. Conduct Disorder and ODD, also in this section of DSM-5, have already been discussed in Sections 2.2.2 and 2.2.3 above. Gambling Disorder (Pathological Gambling in DSM-IV-TR), also of vice-laden interest, will also be considered though this condition is now located in the DSM-5 Substance-Related and Addictive Disorders section.

2.2.5.1 Intermittent Explosive Disorder

Another of the DSM-5 impulse-control disorders, Intermittent Explosive Disorder ((IED) Table 2.6) poses intriguing difficulties in addressing the vice-ladenness of diagnostic criteria. IED's core features involve intermittent attacks of aggressiveness 'grossly' out of proportion to environmental provocations—referenced in the criteria as 'psychosocial stressors'. The episodes of aggression should not be attributable to another disorder.

So what's so intriguing? Well, episodes of interpersonal and property aggression, at first blush, would seem to qualify as morally wrongful acts. However, the DSM-5 authors make efforts to lead readers away from concluding that persons with IED are simply criminal offenders. How? In Criterion A, the putative IED patient must *fail to control* aggressive actions. The implication is that individuals with no intention of resisting, and simply proceed with deliberate aggressive acts, don't qualify for meeting this criterion, and the diagnosis doesn't apply. Reframed in the language of philosophy, IED patients represent failures of virtuous intention.[29] In order to ascertain whether the Criterion A has been met, however, the diagnosing clinician must make an appraisal of the patient's will or intent to resist the aggressive act. For Criterion B, the clinician must also make an assessment that the aggression is '*grossly out of proportion*' to the 'precipitating psychosocial stressors'. Multiple interpretations are possible here. One might be that to meet Criterion B, the perpetrator of the violence must be responding to less provocative stimuli than the average person. Another might be that the aggressive response is so disproportionate to the provocation that no justification for the acts is credible.[30] A third might be that the aggressive

Table 2.6 Excerpts of DSM-5 diagnostic criteria for 312.34 Intermittent Explosive Disorder (APA 2013, p. 466)

A. Recurrent behavioral outbursts … as manifested by either of the following:

1. [verbal aggression or physical aggression]

2. [a minimum number of episodes of destruction of property and/or physical assault]

B. [aggression disproportionate to provocation]

C. [outbursts are impulsive]

D. [distress/impairment]

E. [age requirements]

F. [relation to other disorders]

response is not understandable with regard to the provocation. That is, the response defies empathic understanding—the response falls beyond the cultural context of meaningful, motivationally credible responses.[31] Criterion C, new in comparison to DSM-IV and DSM-IV-TR, takes care to differentiate IED outbursts from deliberate or strategic use of aggression. This requires an inferential judgement on the part of the clinician, who must elicit from the patient one or more motives for the outburst or, much more difficult, establish the lack of a goal-directed motive. The clinician, in effect, must make a judgement of responsible guilt or innocence with the patient, and establish that the outburst was a response to a difficult-to-impossible-to-resist situation rather than a reasoned, deliberate, goal-directed action. The trouble here is the same trouble for judges and juries—the patient/defendant can simply lie or deny the deliberate intent. The demand for a clinician's implicit moral-responsibility judgement will be of interest in later discussions of free will and moral/criminal responsibility towards the end of this book. Criteria D and E invoke the clinical significance criterion for distress or impairment, adding 'financial or legal consequences' for those who may not have distress or impairment. The latter inclusion could be construed to undercut the requirement for a motiveless impulse in Criterion C, in that a patient can meet Criterion D by being indifferent to the impulsive actions, other than for the financial or legal consequences. Criterion E is likely a response to epidemiological evidence of impulsive aggression beginning in prepubertal children.[32] For Criterion F, the disorder must be distinguished from other mental disorders. More specifically, the aggression episodes must not be caused by ('due to') another disorder.

The intrigue of this criteria set resides in the interpretation and applicability of the criteria by a diagnostician. Often this may involve asking the patient if the victim(s) were deserving, but whether the patient pleads being overwhelmed by rage, or claims the victim asked for it, the potential for bias is powerful, depending upon which response the patient thinks the doctor is seeking.[33] Because illegality is implicated often in IED behaviors, this retrospective assessment of the patient's own intentions is subject to self-serving bias.[34] Moreover, the criterion requires a clinician to postulate an environmentally neutral context in which to assess this failure to resist. However, aggressive impulses are likely environmentally and meaning-driven. A soldier counter-assaulting the enemy who has killed a buddy may imply one measure of tolerance for impulsive aggression, whereas the same man assaulting his wife because of her low-cut dress' appeal to other men implies another measure of tolerance for aggression. Ascertaining whether Criterion B is met turns out to be a challenging and complex clinical task—perhaps an unfeasible one.[35]

Similarly, the assessment of responses out of proportion is complex and as much a *moral* judgement as any other kind of judgement; confounded by psychological versus moral justification. Justified violence varies not only because of contextual factors. The clinician's own viewpoint or value system regarding justified violence will in part determine whether Criterion B is met. The ethical question of justifying violent responses to provocation is addressed by the clinician as a final arbiter. Sherman, a bullied child on the playground may, having exceeded his limit of tolerance for cruelty, lash out aggressively at his tormentors, perhaps on multiple occasions. Is this the function of the failure of school staff to address school bullying, a function of the social power of group provocation, or is it a function of Sherman's aggressivity being 'grossly out of proportion' to the psychosocial stressors? This kind of complex causality confounds clinical determinations but also, as will become more important later, determinations of moral/criminal responsibility determinations.

In Sam Peckinpah's classic film *Straw Dogs*, the placid and loving husband played by Dustin Hoffman is driven by predatory locals to defend his wife and home through extraordinary and deliberate violence. The Afghan Taliban's impulsive violence against women is 'justified' by religious and cultural beliefs. Does that exclude diagnosis of IED? The nosological problem here is that the assessment of Criterion B, at base, is not medical, may be an *implicit exercise in practical ethics*, of determining whether violence is justified morally, and/or a *matching of inferred patient motivations against cultural conventions*. In the former application, the IED criteria are vice-laden, through the complicated value semantic described here. In the latter application, the IED criteria require a complex cultural and subcultural appraisal, as well as an interpretation of local circumstances and context—diminishing the reliability of the application of the criterion. Indeed, the difficulty in appraising the disorder has offered diagnostic difficulties.[36]

Criterion F for IED poses a special difficulty. While excluding other disorders in diagnosis is standard practice in the DSM, aggressiveness in intellectual disability (ID) populations is common,[37] leading thoughtful and experienced community psychiatrists such as Jeffrey Geller[38] to suspect disproportionately high rates of diagnosis of IED in the institutionalized intellectually impaired population (though my literature review could not identify data to this effect). Intermittent aggression in the ID population points to the serious difficulty in ascertaining whether Criterion C for IED is met—is the aggression part of the multietiological ID conditions, is it a separate disorder, and how does one establish a credible epidemiology?[39]

2.2.5.2 Kleptomania and Pyromania

Similar considerations about IED apply to 'Kleptomania', the DSM-5 term for people who compulsively steal, and 'Pyromania', compulsive fire-setters. Like IED, the criteria for Kleptomania imply that the patients cannot help themselves, and in that sense, the diagnostic criteria 'smuggle in' considerations of motivation in 'operationalized' criteria; see Table 2.7. Criterion D in Kleptomania explicitly excludes certain motivations (expressing anger or vengeance), and Criterion A emphasizes that the stealing is not motivated by need. The criteria create an image of theft without the usual 'vice' motivations, despite the transparent wrongfulness of theft. Unlike Gambling Disorder (formerly Pathological Gambling, discussed below) or IED, Kleptomania is described in terms of a particular behavior pattern in the B and C

Table 2.7 Excerpts of DSM-5 diagnostic criteria for 312.32 Kleptomania (APA 2013, p. 478)

A. [impulsive stealing of objects not out of need]

B. [anticipatory tension before the theft]

C. [release of tension following theft]

D. [exclusionary motivations]

E. [relation to other disorders]

criteria. This description implies that stealing is tension-reducing, satisfaction- or pleasure-inducing, or both.

Whether Kleptomania is interpreted to be vice-laden or illness-like may depend partly upon whether one interprets to the B and C criteria to mean stealing 'for the fun of it', which would imply vice, or interpreting the criteria, to mean that stealing is done in order to cope with, reduce, or otherwise soothe unpleasant feeling states. The latter interpretation suggests more a maladaptive, and ill, behavior pattern, similar to addictive processes (which will be considered shortly). The clinician is pointed to the tension-reduction interpretation in later criteria.

Similar considerations apply to Pyromania, where tension and/or anticipation of pleasure precede the fire-setting (Criterion B), and pleasure or relief follow the act (Criterion D); see Table 2.8. Criterion E provides vice-laden exclusionary criteria, as with Kleptomania, and again the reader of the criteria is led away from considerations of wrongful motivation in Criterion E (not because of 'sociopolitical ideology', to, e.g., conceal criminal activity or to express anger or vengeance).

The problem, from the DSM perspective, of invoking motivations (or lack of them) for diagnostic purposes is that contemporary psychology/psychiatry commonly recognizes motivation as a complex, multiply determined concept.[40] How is the clinician to 'rule out' the motivations for fire-setting from Criterion E's list?

The DSM-5 diagnostic criteria appear to have considered psychiatrist Jeffrey Geller's work on arson. 'Arson' as a property crime, historically reviewed by Geller, is

Table 2.8 Excerpts of DSM-5 diagnostic criteria for 312.33 Pyromania (APA 2013, p. 476)

A. Deliberate and purposeful fire setting. . . .

B. Tension . . . before the act

C. . . . attraction to fire and its situational contexts. . . .

D. [tension release, pleasure at fire-setting]

E. [exclusionary motivations]

F. [relation to other disorders]

found to be a complex phenomenon, occurring in a wide range of people with manifold reasons for setting fires.[41] In many ways 'pyromania' is defined by what it is NOT as much as by what it IS.[42] Fire-setting as a symptomatic behavior suffers from many of the problems that single-symptom disorders have historically exhibited: excessive comorbidities and imprecision.[43]

2.2.5.3 Gambling Disorder (formerly Pathological Gambling in DSM-IV-TR)

Sometimes called 'compulsive' gambling in lay settings, the person with Gambling Disorder indulges in gambling despite, and perhaps even in response to, adverse outcomes. The DSM-5 diagnostic criteria are excerpted in Table 2.9.

The full Criterion A(4) (see DSM-5 proper) is an excellent example of a sentence with a value semantics- no value terms, yet the meaning of the sentence, in ordinary usage and interpretation, is evaluative and, in these cases, a moral evaluation. In A(4) the practical meaning is close to 'preoccupied to the exclusion of other worthwhile activities' and implying a dose of condemnation for that.

Criteria A(7) involves a transparently morally wrong behavior (lying), with A(9) providing an example of a value semantic involving the exploitation of others in order to obtain funds. The use of 'get even' in A(6) may be misconstrued as vengeance seeking; I believe what is intended here is the gambler returns to recover lost funds.

The other criteria are more arguable as involving moral wrongs, and to my reading imply more nonmoral evaluations, such as A(2) restlessness and irritability, A(3) failure in efforts to control gambling, and A(5) gambling as a response to distress. Regardless, Gambling Disorder ends up being a vice-laden diagnostic construct.

Table 2.9 Excerpts of DSM-5 diagnostic criteria for 312.31 Gambling Disorder (APA 2013, p. 585, specifiers omitted)

A. Persistent and recurrent problematic gambling [distress/impairment requirement]:

1. [escalation of money risked]

2. [discomfort at efforts to reduce gambling]

3. [failed efforts to control gambling].

4. [preoccupied with gambling]

5. [gambling as relief from distress]

6. [returns to gambling to regain losses]

7. Lies to conceal . . . gambling

8. [functional impairment, losses]

9. [appeals to others to address gambling losses]

B. [relation to other disorders]

2.2.6 Paraphilias

> DSM-5's Paraphilias section describes a number of conditions which involve any intense and persistent sexual interest other than sexual interest in genital stimulation or preparatory fondling with phenotypically normal, physically mature, consenting human partners. (APA 2013, p. 585)

The paraphilias, historically called 'sexual neuroses,'[44] 'sexual deviations,'[45] and 'perversions,'[46] have a rich lineage in psychiatry, which will be briefly discussed in the historical chapters to follow. The paraphilic disorders are recognized as problematic within and outside psychiatric circles because of the often-fluid boundaries between the diversity of sexual tastes and arousal patterns that enrich humankind's sexual imaginations and activities, on the one hand, and the outer limits of sexual practices that may cause problems for oneself and other people, on the other.

I should note one of the most substantive changes in DSM-5 compared to prior DSMs. That change involves the formal distinction between paraphilias viewed, and named, as variations on human sexual diversity, and paraphilic disorders which are specifically stipulated as mental disorders involving impairment and/or distress.[47] In prior versions of the DSMs, simple engagement in paraphilic interests and arousal patterns qualified one for diagnosis as a disorder. In part owing to vigorous debate and criticism from sexually diverse communities and influential clinicians,[48] the distinction from paraphilias as normal variations in sexuality versus Paraphilic Disorders as pathological conditions was a new feature in DSM-5.

One of the paraphilias, Pedophilic Disorder, has already been discussed as an example of a vice-laden disorder. Several of the paraphilias involve victimization, or as the DSMs describes it, involve 'nonconsenting' others in their activities. For example, the voyeuristic person may invade others' privacy through his peeping; the patient with frotteurism may rub his crotch against others in the crowded subway; and the pedophilically disordered individual may molest children. For other paraphilias that do not directly involve nonconsenting others, like Fetishistic Disorder (erotic focus on inanimate objects like stiletto heels or underwear), Transvestic Disorder (erotic focus on dressing in the opposite gender), or Sexual Sadism Disorder (erotic focus on humiliation and/or suffering of others), the victims, if any, are those who suffer the emotional and social fallout from the patient's conduct—often, perhaps usually, the partners or spouses of the patient.[49] In this latter sense, that a disordered behavior may incur emotional and social fallout for others, paraphilias resemble many other mental disorders in the DSMs. Additionally, the focus on Paraphilic Disorders that involve victims directly permits a practical narrowing of focus for this book. For these reasons, and to closely serve the vice focus of this work, I will not discuss Fetishistic Disorder, Transvestic Disorder, and Sexual Masochism Disorder further.

2.2.6.1 The clinical significance criterion & victimizing behaviors

The paraphilic disorders—all of them—are among the most controversial of the mental disorders for a variety of reasons, which will be taken up in later chapters. Most of the disorders listed under the Paraphilia rubric involve wrongful conduct in the diagnostic criteria, through the value semantic of victimizing others, and, generally, the above disorders involve criminal sex offenses in many, perhaps most US jurisdictions.[50] What perhaps lies at the core of the paraphilia controversy is the role of the 'clinical significance criterion' (CSC)and the issue of false-positive (diagnosing a disorder when none is 'really' present) and false-negative (failing to diagnose a disorder when one is 'really' present).[51]

The clinical significance criterion (CSC) functions in past DSMs to establish that a condition is not a mental disorder unless it causes suffering, impairment, or problems in 'functioning': for example, problems with work and/or social relationships. The CSC is important for Paraphilias/Paraphilic Disorders because it helps to differentiate people who have diverse sexual desires who pursue diverse sexual practices with like-minded others (which we might call 'harmless sexual diversity'[52]), from people with diverse sexual desires and practices which harm others and themselves, which might be called 'harmful sexual diversity'. Complicating the harmful sexual diversity group, as a population, are two practical groups. One set of these make up the (for those who are caught with victimizing behaviors) the criminal sex offender population. The other set are those who engage in harmful sexual diversity but are not identified and prosecuted within the criminal justice system. Both groups, potentially, are individuals with a paraphilic disorder.

The CSC provides a requirement that actual distress or impairment before a diagnosis can be made. Over the DSM-III-R through DSM-5 period, the DSM diagnoses of Pedophilia and related disorders have varied in their handling of the CSC. In III-R, the patient must be 'markedly distressed',[53] in IV the standard 'distress or impairment' language is used,[54] in IV-TR, the 'markedly distressed' language reappears,[55] and in the DSM-5, the B criterion has been modified to include a CSC,[56] requiring the patient have actually molested a child, or have marked distress or interpersonal difficulty associated with the sexual urges for children.

The controversy concerns the role of molesting behavior alongside the CSC in diagnostic criteria sets from DSM edition to edition. If, on the one hand, one does NOT require a CSC for the diagnosis of Pedophilic Disorder, then the diagnosis of the disorder becomes tantamount to being identified as a childhood sex offender, or admitting to being one, thus making this criminality the same has having a mental disorder. This poses the ripe potential for individuals to be diagnosed as either false-negative (because his molestations have not been detected) or false-positive (because his molestations occurred for 'nonpedophilic' reasons, e.g., as a result of traumatic brain injury). On the other hand, if Pedophilic Disorder requires ONLY a distress or impairment (CSC) B Criterion, without identifying molesting behavior, then many false-negatives will occur because of the well-known tendency of pedophilic offenders to deny distress or impairment, even if it is present.[57] If BOTH a CSC and molesting behavior are required, then the bar is raised for diagnosis, and even more false-negatives may occur, because of denial of either or both conditions, with the putative benefit of diminishing false-positives, through raising the demands of the diagnosis. For DSM-5, Criterion B ended up enabling either acting on urges, OR encountering distress and interpersonal difficulty to qualify, keeping the diagnostic capture relatively broad.

Given these controversies about diagnosis with vice-laden criteria, and the high stakes at diagnosing the disorder, we should not be too surprised that eliciting frank and honest responses for criteria items, in diagnostic evaluations of patients, is an ongoing problem with Paraphilic Disorders.

2.2.6.2 Other paraphilias involving nonconsenting others

The following tables of DSM-5 diagnostic criteria excerpts for paraphilic disorders describe the particular behaviors. I have omitted the criteria for the above-described 'nonvictimizing' paraphilias. I will, however, briefly discuss the 'Unspecified Paraphilic Disorder' diagnosis, regarding its intent to capture other categories of disorder not specifically identified in DSM-5.

An initial review of these DSM-5 paraphilic disorders (Exhibitionistic Disorder, Frotteuristic Disorder, Pedophilic Disorder, Sexual Sadism Disorder, and Voyeuristic Disorder) indicates that an analogous approach to the issues around behavior and the clinical significance criterion has been applied to these disorders as well. That is, a behavior, distress or interpersonal difficulty which infringes upon others, is required for the diagnosis. Examining the particular behaviors, all involve sexually related transgressions of various sorts and would qualify as vice as I have defined it.

Tables 2.10–2.15 describe the criteria of these disorders for DSM-5.[58] Some global changes to paraphilia criteria as described in DSM-IV-TR should be noted. The big change was as the draft DSM-5 proposed that the A criteria define, for primarily research purposes, the paraphilic arousal pattern, while the B criterion establishes the condition as a disorder. This splitting of 'paraphilias' into human diversity conditions and secondarily into pathological conditions was formalized through this use of the A and B criteria. All paraphilic arousal patterns, then, for DSM-5, require a B criterion that specifies the reasons why the arousal pattern is a disorder.

Table 2.10 Excerpts of DSM-5 diagnostic criteria for 302.4 Exhibitionistic Disorder (APA 2013, p. 689)

A. [fantasies and behaviors about exposing one's genitals to others]

B. [acting out] with a nonconsenting person, or the sexual urges or fantasies cause [distress/impairment]

(Specifiers omitted, though they distinguish exposure to prepubertal children and/or mature individuals.)

Table 2.11 Excerpts of DSM-5 diagnostic criteria for 302.89 Frotteurism (APA 2013, pp. 691–692)

A. . . . recurrent and intense sexual arousal from touching or rubbing against a nonconsenting person

. . . .

B. [acting out] with a nonconsenting person or the sexual urges or fantasies cause [distress/impairment]

Table 2.12 Excerpts of DSM-5 diagnostic criteria for 302.2 Pedophilic Disorder (APA 2013, pp. 697–698)

A. . . . recurrent, intense sexually arousing fantasies, sexual urges, or behaviors involving sexual activity with a prepubescent child. . . .

B. [acting out] these sexual urges, or the sexual urges or fantasies cause [distress/impairment]

C. [age specifiers]

(Subtype specifiers omitted.)

Table 2.13 Excerpts of DSM-5 diagnostic criteria for 302.84 Sexual Sadism Disorder (APA 2013, pp. 695–96)

A. . . . recurrent and intense sexual arousal from the physical or psychological suffering of another person, . . .

B. [acting out] with a nonconsenting person, or the sexual urges or fantasies cause [distress/impairment]

(Subtype specifiers omitted.)

Table 2.14 Excerpts of DSM-5 diagnostic criteria for 302.82 Voyeuristic Disorder (APA 2013, pp. 686–687)

A. . . . recurrent and intense sexual arousal from observing an unsuspecting person who is [naked, undressing, having sex], as manifested by fantasies, urges, or behaviors

B. [acting out] with a nonconsenting person, or the sexual urges or fantasies cause [distress/impairment]

C. [age requirement]

(Subtype specifiers omitted.)

Table 2.15 Excerpts of DSM-5 diagnostic description of 302.89 Other Specified Paraphilic Disorder (APA 2013, p. 705)

This category applies to presentations in which symptoms characteristic of a paraphilic disorder that cause clinically significant distress or impairment in social, occupational, or other important areas of functioning predominate but do not meet the full criteria for any of the disorders in the paraphilic disorders diagnostic class. . . . [descriptions of atypical/uncommon paraphilic behaviors]

Table 2.16 DSM-5 draft diagnostic criteria for Exhibitionistic Disorder (APA)

A. Over a period of at least six months, recurrent and intense sexual fantasies, sexual urges, or sexual behaviors involving the exposure of one's genitals to an unsuspecting stranger.

B. The person is distressed or impaired by these attractions, or has sought sexual stimulation from exposing the genitals to three or more unsuspecting strangers on separate occasions. [2]

Specify type: [3]

Sexually Attracted to Exposing Genitals to Pubescent or Prepubescent Individuals (Generally Younger Than Age 15)

Sexually Attracted to Exposing Genitals to Physically Mature Individuals (Generally Age 15 or Older)

Equally Sexually Attracted to Exposing Genitals to Both Age Groups

Specify if:

In Remission (During the Past Six Months, No Signs or Symptoms of the Disorder Were Present)

In a Controlled Environment

Those reasons for establishing a disorder are: (1) that the arousal pattern causes distress or impairment OR (2) the patient has engaged in transgressive behavior with one or more victims. Regarding the latter, involving, as the DSM-5 people put it, 'nonconsenting persons' as a criterion constraint, considerations were given to having a minimum number of nonconsenting persons as a criterion point. The idea in developing this in DSM-5 was that although the minimum number varies from disorder to disorder, the derivation of a minimum number of victims intended to capture similar false-negative and false-positive rates across disorders, and, therefore, considers the variability of the perpetrator's sexual repertoire as well as opportunity to transgress in estimating the minimum number of victims. Table 2.16 provides an illustration from the DSM-5 draft criteria for Exhibitionism.[59] For example, the opportunities and frequency of behavior for Sexual Sadism Disorder patients is likely smaller than that for voyeuristic patients, hence the difference in minimum number of victims in order to qualify for the diagnosis. The specification of numbers of victims at all is intended to increase the precision of the diagnostic criteria, instead of relying on vague terms like 'recurrent' to describe criterion behaviors. However, these distinctions were ultimately abandoned for reasons unclear, and the DSM-5 criteria ended up as noted above.

The vice-laden quality of the DSM-5 draft criteria, like the DSM-IV-TR predecessors, is lent through the fact of the potential for, or actual participation in, victimizing nonconsenting others. From this standpoint there is little difference in these conditions from earlier editions. The clinical significance issue is handled as an either/or: patients can qualify if they have not offended but have distress or impairment or can qualify if they have offended.

Some comments on these categories are in order. The splitting of paraphilias into human diversity conditions and pathological conditions was at least in part in response to 'lobbying' of the DSM-5 committees from the lesbian/gay/bisexual/

transgender/queer and sadomasochism (S&M) communities. The contention was that human beings' sexual diversity is high, and without harm to others or self, classifying paraphilias as disorders was both inconsistent with other disorders as well as offensive to those involved in harmless personal activities.[60]

As virtually all of these conditions entail various sex-related offenses in one or more of the US states, they have to be considered as vice-laden, often having their own names as criminal activities: for example, peeping Toms, indecent exposure, and child molestation. Some may notice that Sexual Masochism Disorder was omitted. The condition is anomalous in that assigning victim status, or nonconsenting status, is more of a philosophical issue than a practical one. That is, the masochistic individual participates 'voluntarily' in that he seeks out the activities of choice, but what counts as voluntary in this setting is ambiguous. Is normative heterosexuality 'voluntary'? That is doubtful, along with other sexual orientations. These, however, do not involve punishment, humiliation, or pain as defining of the sexuality. So I will leave the victim/nonconsenting status of the masochistic individual as simply raised, and its ambiguous status as the reason for being omitted as a victimizing paraphilic disorder.

Similarly, Transvestic and Fetishistic Disorder are also omitted as victimizing/nonconsenting-related disorders. I acknowledge that individuals who have these disorders as a prevailing sexual interest likely inflict harm through eliciting emotional pain and interpersonal conflict in partners who don't share or appreciate their proclivities. However, other than from the clinical significance criterion, they (arguably) are of lesser harm to partners, and therefore of lesser interest to my analysis here. In terms of social approval by many people, they remain vices.

Finally, it should be noted that several of the sexual '-isms' listed in the Unspecified Paraphilic Disorder description would qualify as victimizing: telephone scatologia, zoophilia, and perhaps others, depending on who is being giving and who is receiving. For these and others, much of the vice-ladenness discussion will hold partially and perhaps equally.

2.2.6.3 New paraphilia-related proposals for the draft DSM-5

In the spring 2010 DSM-5 online draft criteria,[61] the Sexual Disorders Work Group proposed two new disorders for consideration. The first to discuss here is 'Hypersexual Disorder', with Table 2.17 reproducing the draft criteria set. Hypersexual Disorder is intended to address habitual/compulsive sexual behaviors that have been given a range of names: perhaps most prominently sexual addiction, but as the DSM-5 Work Group notes in its online explanation: 'The three primary putative pathophysiological models are sexual desire/arousal dysregulation, sexual addiction, and sexual compulsivity.'[62] As the accompanying literature elaborated,[63] these 'models' suggested mechanism relationships (e.g., linking the disorder to dysfunctions in desire or arousal, brain reward systems, or anxiety -related systems). While the proposal did not make the DSM-5 cut, it

Table 2.17 DSM-5 draft criteria for Hypersexual Disorder (APA)

A. Over a period of at least six months, recurrent and intense sexual fantasies, sexual urges, and sexual behavior in association with four or more of the following five criteria:

(1) Excessive time is consumed by sexual fantasies and urges, and by planning for and engaging in sexual behavior.

(2) Repetitively engaging in these sexual fantasies, urges, and behavior in response to dysphoric mood states (e.g., anxiety, depression, boredom, irritability).

(3) Repetitively engaging in sexual fantasies, urges, and behavior in response to stressful life events.

(4) Repetitive but unsuccessful efforts to control or significantly reduce these sexual fantasies, urges, and behavior.

(5) Repetitively engaging in sexual behavior while disregarding the risk for physical or emotional harm to self or others.

B. There is clinically significant personal distress or impairment in social, occupational or other important areas of functioning associated with the frequency and intensity of these sexual fantasies, urges, and behavior.

C. These sexual fantasies, urges, and behavior are not due to direct physiological effects of exogenous substances (e.g., drugs of abuse or medications) or to Manic Episodes.

D. The person is at least 18 years of age.

Specify if: [22]

Masturbation

Pornography

Sexual Behavior with Consenting Adults

Cybersex

Telephone Sex

Strip Clubs

Other:

Specify if:

In Remission (During the Past Six Months, No Signs or Symptoms of the Disorder Were Present)

In a Controlled Environment

remains viable as a research entity, generating 613 Google Scholar hits since 2013 on May 30, 2017.

The phenomenology of the proposed condition, and its cited clinical and research need, warrants raising the issue of vice-ladenness. The proposed disorder is intended to address individuals who encounter adverse consequences for engaging in relationship/marital infidelity, promiscuity, excessive masturbation, use of pornography, cyber- and telephone sex, and frequenting 'strip clubs'—nightclubs which feature various degrees of nudity and sexually related entertainment. Regarding the clinical need, the Work Group cited the growing demand from patients and clinicians to address the apparently growing problem of sexual 'addiction'.[64] The adverse consequences from this kind of sexual conduct range from relationship problems to increased risk of sexually transmitted infections, to at-work and at-home consequences for pornography users.

Table 2.18 DSM-5 draft diagnostic criteria for Paraphilic Coercive Disorder (APA)

A. Over a period of at least six months, recurrent, intense sexually arousing fantasies or sexual urges focused on sexual coercion. [23]

B. The person is distressed or impaired by these attractions, or has sought sexual stimulation from forcing sex on three or more nonconsenting persons on separate occasions. [24]

C. The diagnosis of Paraphilic Coercive Disorder is not made if the patient meets criteria for a diagnosis of Sexual Sadism Disorder. [25]

Specify if:

In Remission (During the Past Six Months, No Signs or Symptoms of the Disorder Were Present)

In a Controlled Environment

However, does the Hypersexual Disorder construct involve vice-laden semantics? It does point to a colorful (and prevailingly masculine) literary and lay vernacular ('womanizer', 'infidel', 'stud', 'philanderer', 'skirt chaser', 'ladykiller', 'wolf', 'rake', 'tomcat', 'Lothario', 'horndog', 'Casanova', 'seducer', 'Don Juan', 'lecher', 'playboy', and 'libertine', among many others). Referring to a man as any of these is not in praise of virtue. The behavior is frowned upon, at the least, by the orthodoxies of major religions and resented by women. Current (2022) US public views see this behavior as far more predatory, associated with sexual assault through the #MeToo movement. The question is, 'Does the involved behavior provoke negative moral appraisals from many people?' I believe the answer is certainly yes, though we should recognize that sexual behavior in general and promiscuity in particular has great cultural variability, and so one person's Lothario is another person's typical male.

The other DSM-5 proposed category of interest is 'Paraphilic Coercive Disorder'. Table 2.18 presents the draft criteria for this disorder from www.dsm5.org, as of May 2010. This condition, in essence, depicts a rapist who offends because of a deviant arousal pattern, as is the typical case with other paraphilias. Individuals with the putative Paraphilic Coercive Disorder have 'preferential arousal' to coercive sexual fantasies or coercive sexual acts. This disorder is directed towards serial rapists who reoffend presumably because of their preferential arousal pattern. Paraphilic Coercive Disorder also did not make the cut to DSM-5.[65]

The vice-ladenness of Paraphilic Coercive Disorder is not a subtle judgement. Rape, and serial rape are widely recognized and abhorred crimes, and so there is little question that these conditions qualify as vice-laden.

2.2.7 Other disorders involving vice

Having now presented a host of DSM-5 disorders that qualify unambiguously as vice-laden, let's consider some other DSM categories that pose more complex questions.

2.2.7.1 Substance-abuse disorders and behavioral addictions

In DSM-5, disorders related to drug abuse are grouped into three general categories: Substance Use Disorders, Substance-Related Disorders, and Substance-Induced Disorders. The last of the three refers to psychiatric complications of drug use, while the other two (i.e., 'Use' and '-Related') differentiate occasional users from habitual and drug-dependent individuals. The diagnosis of these conditions varies somewhat from disorder to disorder, based upon differential drug effects, use patterns, and impairment patterns. Table 2.19 excerpts the criteria for Alcohol Use Disorder, with its combination of compulsive use despite adverse consequences, along with particular features associated with the unique drug, make up the diagnostic profile and describe the addiction.

The older DSM-IV-TR distinction between Substance Abuse and Substance Dependence had been collapsed into a single category, 'Substance-Use Disorder', with the spring 2010 draft.[66] The rationale for the change was due to difficulties in differentiating the abuse from the dependence syndromes in practice and research, so a reasonable solution to this difficulty was to propose a single category with graded severity.[67]

For the purposes of a vice analysis, the problem is this: our culture is deeply ambivalent about the nature of drug abuse and addiction. Some people regard it as a moral failure, others as a self-control problem, while biomedicine and Alcoholics Anonymous and related 12-step recovery programs describe addiction as a 'disease'.[68] One could imagine people regarding these conditions as all the above as well. So from this perspective drug abuse disorders qualify as vice-laden under the moral-failure description. Yet examination of the particular diagnostic criteria betrays prominent

Table 2.19 Excerpts of DSM-5 diagnostic criteria for Alcohol Use Disorder (APA 2013, pp. 490–491)

A. A problematic pattern of alcohol use leading to clinically significant impairment or distress, as manifested by at least two of the following . . .

  1. [prolonged, large quantity of intake]

  2. [difficulty reducing use]

  3. [excessive seeking of alcohol]

  4. [craving]

  5. [functional impairment]

  6. [continued use despite adverse consequences]

  7. [reduction of activity in other areas of life]

  8. [alcohol use in dangerous situations]

  9. [persistent use despite adverse health consequences]

  10. [pharmacological tolerance]

  11. [pharmacological withdrawal]

biomedical features of Substance Use Disorder, in their references to tolerance and dependence phenomena, phenomena which have a powerful biological and extensive scientific evidence bases and indeed laboratory animal-based modeling.[69] That is, if you expose lab animals to repeated dosing for some drugs of abuse, they develop similar tolerance and physical dependence phenomena as do humans. These conditions illustrate, ultimately, the limitations of a strict vice/illness dichotomy, as the psychosocial factors and biological factors merge into a single morally, and nonmorally complicated syndrome. Because of this challenging feature of the drug abuse disorders to the issue of vice-ladenness in psychiatric categories, I'll return to this range of conditions later.

Before I leave this group of conditions, I do want to point out the nature of the diagnostic criteria sets in both DSM eras; the criteria sets largely refrain from moralistic and explicitly vice-laden terminology and go into some detail describing the kinds of behaviors that make up the syndromes. To use my language, while explicitly vice-laden behavior is infrequently described, the vice-laden conduct becomes vicious after being associated with the pleasure-seeking of drug use. For example, failure to fulfill role expectations is not, by itself, a vice; however, if one does so in the self-interested but shortsighted pursuit of pharmacological pleasure, then, many people would judge those failures as wrongful or vicious. Many of the substance-use disorder criteria, then, embody value 'entailments' to use my language—(see Section 2.1).

2.2.7.2 Attention-Deficit Hyperactivity Disorder

The attention-deficit-related conditions offer another kind of mix of moral-value laden diagnostic criteria/concepts. Table 2.20 describes excerpts from the DSM-5 diagnostic criteria for Attention-Deficit Hyperactivity Disorder (ADHD).

For the A.1. Inattention section, the DSM-5 includes a Note which states that the symptoms are not solely a manifestation of 'oppositional behavior, defiance, hostility, or failure to understand tasks or instructions'.[70] DSM-5 provides this Note again under A.2. 'Hyperactivity and Impulsivity' set of criteria options. The DSM-5 Work Group has taken some pains to remove connotations of moral wrongfulness from a criteria set which could be construed as naughty, moral-value laden criteria. A similar 'preamble' precedes the hyperactivity/impulsivity criteria options, to similar effect. It would be reasonable to surmise that this is an attempt by the Work Group to distinguish ADHD from Conduct Disorder, rendering ADHD less 'vice-laden' in effect, in contrast to the vice-saturated CD category. This stipulation requires the clinician to make a judgement about the motivational sources (or lack of them) of the inattentive/disruptive behavior. Indeed, moving the ADHD diagnostic criteria into the realm of the child not being able to help himself (or self-regulate) is required to move these behaviors out of the realm of the naughty, irresponsible, bad actor, and into the biomedical realm of disease/disorder.

Table 2.20 Excerpts of DSM-5 diagnostic criteria for Attention-Deficit/Hyperactivity Disorder (APA 2013, pp. 59–61)

A. A persistent pattern of inattention and/or hyperactivity-impulsivity that interferes with functioning or development . . .

1. Inattention: Six (or more) of the following [which adversely affect functioning]:

    a. [overlooks details, careless mistakes]

    b. [attentional focus not sustained]

    c. [not listening or attending]

    d. [fails to complete tasks]

    e. [mismanages tasks, disorganized]

    f. [avoids/dislikes complex tasks]

    g. [misplaces things]

    h. . . . easily distracted . . . .

    i. . . . often forgetful . . . .

2. Hyperactivity and impulsivity: Six (or more) of the following symptoms [which adversely affect functioning]

    a. Often fidgets . . . .

    b. Often leaves seat . . .

    c. [context-inappropriate running/climbing]

    d. [difficulty with quiet leisure activities]

    e. [frequent physical activity, driven]

    f. [talks too much]

    g. [impulsive responses to questions]

    h. . . . difficulty waiting his or her turn . . . .

    i. Often interrupts or intrudes on others . . . .

B. [age requirement]

C. [symptoms manifest in two or more settings]

D. [functional impairment]

E. [relationships with other disorders]

2.2.7.3 Pediatric Bipolar Disorder and severe emotional dysregulation

In the post-DSM-IV era, leading up to DSM-5 deliberations, two influential studies identified a dramatic increase in the diagnosis of bipolar disorder in children:[71] although as Ghaemi[72] has pointed out, this dramatic increase still represents a very small proportion of childhood mental disorder diagnoses. Considering the literature on this trend generated interest in the 'whys' of the increase, as well as the increased significance of the finding of persistent, nonepisodic irritability in some severely disturbed children, who otherwise might fit a 'pediatric bipolar disorder' diagnosis.[72]

The National Institute of Mental Health (NIMH) intramural research group led by Ellen Leibenluft at the time conducted a research program into a syndrome she

Table 2.21 Excerpts of DSM-5 diagnostic criteria for
Disruptive Mood Dysregulation Disorder (APA 2013,
p. 156)

A. [disproportionate and severe temper outbursts]

B. [outbursts are not developmentally appropriate]

C. [frequency requirement]

D. [chronically angry between outbursts]

E. [duration requirements]

F. [location requirements]

G. [age requirements]

H. [age of onset]

I. [relationships to other disorders]

J. [relationships to other disorders and relevant exclusions]

K. [other exclusions]

called 'severe mood dysregulation' (SMD),[73] which was later to be modified and included in DSM-5's Depressive Disorders section as Disruptive Mood Dysregulation Disorder (DMDD).[74] The original SMD syndrome involved 'severe, non-episodic irritability and anger outbursts, as well as symptoms of hyperarousal (specifically, those symptoms of attention-deficit hyperactivity disorder (ADHD) that overlap with the "B" criteria of mania)'.[75] To make a more complicated story short, this work in large part contributed to the DSM-5 coinage of 'Temper Dysregulation Disorder with Dysphoria' from the DSM-5 June 2010 draft criteria posted online.[76] The DSM-5 diagnostic criteria for Disruptive Mood Dysregulation Disorder (296.99) is excerpted in Table 2.21.

The DMDD diagnosis addressed several concerns. One was the potential for contributing to the explanation of the then-contemporary explosion of diagnosed cases of pediatric bipolar disorder, the latter an interesting question, but not relevant to my purposes here. Because the DSM-IV-TR and prior editions did not have a close-fitting category for these children, they were believed to be lumped in as Bipolar Disorder Not Otherwise Specified. Secondly, influential academic child psychiatrists such as Gabrielle Carlson[77] believed that DMDD was warranted as a separate diagnosis. Third, these children represent a significant challenge to clinical management without a diagnostic-specific evidence base and treatment literature.[78]

Setting aside the debate on pediatric bipolar disorder in order to pursue the vice focus here, the question for the DMDD category is whether it is vice-laden. Taking the perspective of a nonclinical layperson, the diagnostic description of DMDD raises the cultural trope of the spoiled-rotten child prone to temper tantrums to get his/her way. One can speculate that the public will view this condition as related to 'ordinary' temper tantrums which are viewed as ordinary misbehavior. Indeed,

Table 2.22 Excerpts from DSM-5 diagnostic criteria for Factitious Disorder Imposed on Self (APA 2013, p. 324)

A. Falsification of [illness, injury], or [self-induced] injury or disease

B. [the patient presents as] ill, impaired, or injured

C. [deception not driven by external incentives]

D. [relation to other disorders]

---

even the NIMH made this connection early, in a public health 'Science Update' headlining 'Daily or Severe Tantrums May Point to Mental Health Issues'.[79] A *Today's Parent* magazine article on DMDD announces 'Extreme Temper Tantrums May Signal Mood Disorder'.[80] While the DSM-5 clearly wants to emphasize DMDD as a condition of uncommon extremity, what counts as developmentally normative temper tantrums and what counts as extreme tantrums may not be transparent to the public.[81]

Criterion A1 formally answers this question; here verbal rages or physical aggression towards people or property certainly qualifies as wrongful conduct, and indeed, the entire disorder is built around this central symptom complex, similar to IED in adults (whose relationship, if any, to DMDD is yet to be determined).

2.2.7.4 Factitious Disorders

Among the most enigmatic of disorders in psychiatry are the factitious disorders, variously called over history as 'Munchausen's Syndrome', 'Polle Syndrome', and 'hospital hobos'.[82] The core of these conditions is the individual simulating, or self-inducing, illness in oneself or others (in the case of Factitious Disorder by Proxy) and then seeking medical care as a 'patient'. In examining the DSM-5 criteria in Tables 2.22 and 2.23, one can discern that the vice of deception is at the center of the diagnostic concept.

Less evident but ethically significant is the possibility that an individual with a factitious disorder may induce illness in others, including minors, with sequelae that may, and have included death for the victim of the illness-claiming deceit (see Table 2.23).[83] This condition, Factitious Disorder Imposed on Another (also known as Factitious Disorder by Proxy), in the setting of minors constitutes child abuse,

Table 2.23 DSM-5 diagnostic criteria for Factitious Disorder Imposed on Another (APA 2013, p. 325)

A. Falsification of [illness, injury], or [induced] injury or disease in another

B. The individual [presents the victim for health care]

C. [deception not driven by external incentives]

D. [relation to other disorders]

[diagnosis assigned to perpetrator]

---

and in the setting of spouses and elders, domestic violence, all crimes in many, per-haps most, states.[84] The definition of the disorder, with falsification and deceit as central, qualifies this set of disorders as vice-laden, and the potential for serious morbidity and mortality on the part of factitious behavior by proxy makes this vice-laden disorder an especially important, albeit uncommon, disorder for this book to consider.

2.3 Next steps

This chapter has laid out some core examples DSM vice-laden conditions to con-sider through the rest of the book. In the chapters to follow, these conditions are the ones to consider in what I call the 'Vice/Mental Disorder Relationship' (VMDR). The VMDR is the complex of relationships when a mental disorder is also vice-laden. Later chapters will be referring to these tables and criteria sets. I have, for better or for worse, kept my own comments about categories here to a minimum, and have limited my primary goal for this chapter to illustrate, through example, the vice-laden qualities of various categories and criteria. At this stage, we'll turn to some of the most interesting and challenging chapters, a consideration of the manifold con-ceptual issues that underlie these vice-laden categories.

Notes

1. These categories were selected for several reasons: (1) a preliminary analysis found them vice-laden; (2) many refer to important and relatively common phenomena; and (3) they situate the discus-sion of vice-laden diagnostic categories clearly, apart from more ambiguous examples of DSM-5 categories. I have omitted discussion of ICD categories because of the general agreement between the DSMs and the ICD Mental and Behavioural Disorders categories and the substantive length of this book focusing just on DSM categories and issues. Scholars interested in these can find much to think about in looking at the DSM-5- ICD connections. The current version of the ICD Mental and Behavioural Disorders classification is the 1993 ICD-10 (WHO 1992). The ICD-11 has been adopted as of 1 January 2022. (https://www.who.int/standards/classifications/classification-of-diseases). Pocai (2019).
2. APA (2003) online at: www.psychiatry.org.
3. Frankena (1973).
4. See Sadler (2005, Ch. 2), for a discussion of how to identify values in discourses. A video discussion by Sadler about identifying values in discourses can be viewed at https://vimeopro.com/user24832 613/psagacity/video/286424927. This work was built upon earlier methodological work in Sadler (1997). A more recent summary of this work, including a detailed example, is in Sadler (2013).
5. See Fulford (1989) for his early discussion of the logic of value terms. This work has been expanded and applied in subsequent publications (e.g., Fulford 1994, 2002, 2005, among others).
6. To avoid confusion, I am using the DSM-IV-TR diagnosis 'Pedophilia' here because it refers to the early APA Statement on Pedophilia. However, as will be seen, the current DSM-5 category for this pathological condition is 'Pedophilic Disorder' for reasons to follow later in the text (APA 2013).
7. See for instance Hage (1981).

8. See Davis (1996, 1998).

9. In recent years, sociocultural sentiment in the West has turned increasingly hostile to Nabokov, the Lolita story, and any sexual predation on minors, especially women, fueled by horrific revelations of hidden and/or condoned sexual abuse, generating social movements such as #MeToo in response. See Idov (2013).

10. See Sadler (2013) for a discussion of the controversy about pedohebephilic disorder, a proposed category for DSM-5 that attempted to add a disorder category for peripubertal children, which were older than the prepubertal children pertinent to classic Pedophilic Disorder in DSM-5.

11. Sadler (2005, Ch. 2; 1997).

12. In my current work on virtues in psychiatric diagnosis, I've realized that defining values as action-guiding and susceptible to praise or blame does not cover some of the negative kinds of evaluations values 'make'. Henceforth, I'm referring to values as action-guiding and susceptible to praise or criticism, the latter being a broader and more accurate characterization.

13. Sadler 2005.

14. See Potter (2009) for a detailed discussion of 'thick' value terms used in describing the psychopathology of Borderline PD.

15. APA (2000, pp. xxiii).

16. All of the discussion of identifying value terms to follow is drawn from Sadler (1997, 2005).

17. Watson (1990).

18. Szasz (1977).

19. Matheson, Shepherd, & Carr (2014).

20. APA (2013), beginning on p. 817.

21. Sadler (1997). The value-ladenness of the term, however, must be considered within the context of use, as noted earlier in the main text.

22. Frick & Moffitt (2010).

23. See Sadler (2014) for an extended discussion of the vice-ladenness of CD.

24. Adapted from DSM-5, 'General Diagnostic Criteria for a Personality Disorder' (APA 2013, pp. 646–647).

25. See Widiger (2006).

26. See for instance Bach, Markon, Simonsen et al. (2015); Brown (1992); Cloninger (1999); Millon & Davis (1995); Ford & Widiger (1989); Frances & Widiger (1987); Jablensky (2002); Livesley (1985a, 1985b); Skodol et al. (2015); Skodol, Morey, Bender et al. (2015); Tyrer (2005); Zachar et al. (2016); Zachar, Krueger, & Kendler (2016).

27. Skodol & Bender (2009).

28. Widiger, Frances, Pincus et al. (1991); Widiger & Frances (2002).

29. The kick on this is that assessing the veracity of virtuous intention is very hard to do.

30. An important distinction here is between moral justification versus psychological justification. A traumatized individual, say a soldier, may be psychologically 'justified' by the nature of his war trauma to be prone to violence. However, the moral justification for such violence may be independent of his psychological proneness. War crimes of various kinds might be explained by the incongruity between psychologically 'justified' actions and morally unjustified actions.

31. See Foucault (1999, p. 55) forward, on 'monsters'. The discussion of the Foucauldian monster will be taken up in Chapter 5, a concept marking the individual who commits the psychologically incomprehensible crime.

32. See Coccaro et al. (2004); Kessler et al. (2006).

33. A patient's expectations, perhaps obviously, in part shape her willingness to share information frankly. A patient needing the truth of her illness condition may well be more eager to share openly her motivations for behavior, as opposed to the felony defendant who risks imprisonment or worse in revealing motivations for behaviors.

34. See Simon & Shuman (2002), a book devoted to this issue.
35. See Sadler (2002).
36. Coccaro (2004).
37. See for instance Benson & Brooks (2008); Taylor (2002); Visootsak & Sherman (2007).
38. Geller (personal communication, 2008).
39. In clinical and institutional settings IED-like symptoms likely contribute to substantive expense in care of people with ID, from providing more intensive staff supervision to medicating patients with impulsive aggression.
40. Doley, Dickens, & Gannon (2015).
41. See Geller (1992a, 1992b 1992c); Geller & Bertsch (1985); Geller, Erlen, & Pinkus (1986).
42. See Geller (1992a, 1992b,1992c).
43. See Sadler (2015) for a conceptual critique of monomanias in psychiatric history up to the present.
44. Krafft-Ebing (1965).
45. APA (1968).
46. Stoller (1986).
47. APA (2013). See also Green (2002); Janssen (2013); O'Donohue, Regev, & Hagstrom (2000); Seto et al. (2006).
48. See Moser (2001, 2002, 2009); Moser & Kleinplatz (2005a, 2005b); First (2010); Wakefield (2011); Quinsey (2012).
49. American Psychiatric Association Task Force Report, 1999.
50. Douglas, Burgess, Burgess, & Ressler (2006).
51. For general discussions of the clinical significance criterion see Spitzer & Wakefield (1999); Wakefield, Schmitz, & Baer (2010). There was substantive debate about its value in the case of pedophilia/pedophilic disorder: see Blanchard (2010); First (2010); First & Pincus (2002).
52. Doing my preparations for this book, I learned much about the wide diversity of sexual practices described in the Humanities and Social Sciences. See for instance Nye (1999); Seidman, Fischer, & Meeks (2006).
53. APA (1987, p. 285).
54. APA (1994, p. 528).
55. APA (1994, p. 572).
56. APA (1994, p. 697).
57. Camilleri & Quinsey (2008); O'Donohue, Regev, & Hagstrom (2000).
58. APA (2013).
59. APA (2010).
60. See First (2010); Moser (2002); Moser & Kleinplatz (2005a, 2005b); Quinsey (2012); Wakefield (2011); Wollert & Cramer (2011), as well as Sadler (2013), for an overview and values-analysis.
61. See Blashfield, Keeley, & Flanagan (2014).
62. DSM-5 Sexual Disorders Work Group, DSM-5 online Rationale, last accessed 5/17/10.
63. Kafka (1997, 2003, 2010, 2014); Kafka and Hennen (1999, 2003); Kor et al. (2013); Moser (2011); Karila et al. (2014); Reid et al. (2012).
64. Karila et al. (2014).
65. See Agalaryan & Rouleau (2014); Balon (2012); Beech et al. (2016); Zinik & Padilla (2016) for reasons why.
66. APA (2010).
67. Hasin et al. (2013).
68. Heather (2013); Hill (1985); Jellinek (1960); Segal (2013).
69. See reviews by Willner (1997) and Koob (2014).
70. APA (2013, pp. 59–61).
71. Moreno et al. (2007); Blader & Carlson (2007).
72. Ghaemi (2010).

73. As will be seen shortly in the main text, the issue of episodicity in bipolar disorder has been considered crucial to this diagnosis, as opposed to continual waxing and waning of agitated, turbulent affects and behaviors.

74. See Leibenluft et al. (2003); Leibenluft et al. (2006); Rich et al. (2007, 2008); Stringaris et al. (2010).

75. APA (2013, p. 158); Towbin et al. (2013).

76. APA, DSM-5 Childhood and Adolescent Disorders Work Group (2010, p. 3).

77. Unfortunately, as of this writing, the APA has not maintained access to DSM-5 online deliberations. Carlson's view was also a personal communication from 2010.

78. See Balkissoon 2013, Margulies et al. (2012).

79. NIMH August 29, 2012, https://www.nimh.nih.gov/archive/news/2012/daily-or-severe-tantrums-may-point-to-mental-health-issues Last accessed 8/3/2022.

80. Today's Parent online, July 24, 2013, https://www.todaysparent.com/kids/extreme-tantrums/, last accessed 5/31/17.

81. See Clark (2002) for a discussion of how extremity of experience and behavior figures into attributions of psychopathology in the DSMs.

82. Nadelson (1979).

83. See Waller (1983).

84. Feldman and Eisendrath 1996.

3

Conceptual paradoxes in vice and mental disorder

Vice and Psychiatric Diagnosis. John Z. Sadler, Oxford University Press. © Oxford University Press 2024.
DOI: 10.1093/oso/9780198876830.003.0003

. . . medicine, professedly founded on observation, is as sensitive to outside influence, political, religious, philosophical, imaginative, as is the barometer to the changes of atmospheric density. Theoretically it ought to go on its own straightforward inductive path, without regard to changes of government or to fluctuations of public opinion. But . . . [actually there is] a closer relationship between the Medical Sciences and the conditions of Society and the general thought of the time, than would at first be suspected.

—Oliver Wendell Holmes, from Medical Essays 1842–1882,
quoted and edited in Grob (2008a, p. 3)

The practice of medicine is intimately tied to ethics; and the first thing that we must do, it seems to me, is to try to make this clear and explicit.

—Thomas Szasz (1960)

3.1 Introduction—the purposes of diagnosis and classification

I presented a detailed discussion of *Diagnostic and Statistical Manual of Mental Disorders* (DSM)-5 diagnostic categories in the prior chapter, to illustrate and support my claims of the vice-laden status of selected mental disorders. For this chapter, I will drill down more systematically to consider some of the philosophical or conceptual contributions or structures of vice-ladenness. This philosophical contribution has two general goals for the remainder of the book: (1) it frames conceptual issues to be considered in the brief historical context of Chapters 4 and 5, and (2) opens the opportunity for alternative conceptions and ways of classifying and diagnosing that will be considered in more detail for the concluding chapters of the book.

In *Values and Psychiatric Diagnosis* (VAPD),[1] I discussed at some length the distinctions between diagnosis and classification of mental disorders, as well as the purposes of each. Why reconsider these for a book about vice-laden mental disorder categories? One of the key reasons is the purposes of diagnosis and classification are important frames or contexts in which to consider the implications of vice-laden categories. Thinking about the DSMs in terms of purposes permits more systematic thinking through what vice-laden categories might mean and what significance they hold. Second, as discussed in *VAPD*, having multiple goals for diagnosis and classification might imply potential incompatibilities or conflicts between goals. Making these goals explicit contributes to systematic thinking too. Third, identifying goals and purposes help us discover how the DSMs *matter*, which might help us figure out how they matter *most*. Finally, in considering alternatives, keeping goals and purposes in mind enables us to consider the ethical and practical trade-offs involved in considering alternatives. Readers of *VAPD* will find much of this chapter's content familiar, making for a quick read.

3.1.1 Distinguishing diagnosis from classification

Before considering the DSMs' particular goals, let's consider the distinction between 'diagnosis' and 'classification' of mental disorders. Simply put, 'diagnosis' is both a noun denoting a condition, and a noun signifying a process of figuring out, as I put it in *VAPD*, 'what is going on' with a patient. That is, when a clinician encounters a patient seeking assistance, the practitioner must have a way, or process, for figuring out what the problem is, collaborating with the patient, and framing a potential solution for (or at least an approach to) that problem. Sometimes, the problem can be summarized in a name for a condition—typically a disease or disorder—but other times, the clinical problem may be more complex and may require a more complex description. As an example of the latter, I may know the diagnostic name (depression) and treatment, but if I ignore the barriers to my patient's access to that treatment, my holistic appraisal of the clinical situation will be incomplete, and my treatment efforts will fail.[2]

So we have one meaning of 'diagnosis', as a denotation for a disease or disorder, and another connotation of 'diagnosis', as the holistic understanding of the clinical situation. As implied, 'holistic appraisal' suggests the broader, more encompassing notion of diagnosis, and 'denotation' a narrower sense, including that of scientific taxonomy and practical taxonomies like the DSM and International Classification of Diseases (ICD) classifications. For brevity's sake, let's call the former sense of diagnosis-as-denotation (DAD), and the latter as holistic appraisal. Table 3.1 summarizes material from *VAPD* describing these various aspects or senses of 'diagnosis'.

These two senses of 'diagnosis', denotation and holistic appraisal, also imply syntactical differences. 'Diagnosis' as a term can be a kind of entity (in our case, the things are categories of disease or disorder) and name a process (finding out what's going on with the patient). Diagnosis can be an object of description and can be a

Table 3.1 Seven Senses of 'Diagnosis' as Holistic Appraisal

---

1. **Diagnosis as characterization**—viewing a particular set of clinical features as an example of a more general phenomenon.

2. **Diagnosis as disclosure**—the revealing of novel, unrecognized, or undiscovered features of the patient's ordeal or problem situation.

3. **Diagnosis as embedded observation**—the bilateral movement between figure (the patient) and ground (the context).

4. **Diagnosis as relevance**—the active selection of phenomenological features of the patient situation that are pertinent to the moral and practical goals of the clinic.

5. **Diagnosis as privilege**—the power of clinical expertise warrants the responsibilities of temperance and discretion.

6. **Diagnosis as rationality**—the deliberative and rational grounds for diagnostic actions.

7. **Diagnosis as ritual**—the normative or standard practices associated with diagnosis.

Adapted from Sadler (2005).

procedure or process (i.e., a verb): to 'diagnose' is to engage in a procedure of either denoting or holistically appraising. The distinction between 'diagnosis' as denotation and 'diagnosis' as holistic appraisal is important in understanding the many different purposes of diagnosis. Unfortunately, in everyday practice and discussion, the different meanings of 'diagnosis' are often interchanged, leading to confusion and unnecessary conflict. For example, thoughtful clinicians who are engaged in diagnosis (as holistic appraisal) may find themselves criticized by people concerned about the dehumanizing 'labeling' of patients—clearly a reference to diagnosis-as-denotation (DAD), divorced from the practical context of thoughtful, empathic practice.

Apart from such misunderstandings, the practical context of meaning of these two senses of diagnosis is important. DAD implies the trappings of scientific, or at least classificatory, inquiry, with its focus on shared features among groups of individuals, and intention to provide opportunities for scientific explanation and prediction. Diagnosis as holistic appraisal presupposes the particular practical, moral, and scientific activities associated with clinical practice—with caring for people, curing, and preventing diseases, disorders, impairments, and injuries. Importantly, one can be engaged with DAD, and never see a patient in need—think of the laboratory scientist investigating molecular mechanisms of a DSM disorder—but diagnosis as holistic appraisal requires the context of clinical care.[3]

3.1.2 Some purposes for diagnosis-as-denotation

The multiple purposes of DAD set the stage for a large share of the problems of vice-laden diagnosis. Having multiple purposes for a DSM, for example, facilitates the potential for conflict between purposes. What if the scientific interests regarding the technical language for a category interfere with public understanding of the category? What if a new scientific diagnostic category carries no prevalence or incidence rate for planning clinical services? What if the evidence for the validity of a new diagnostic category is thin, and a murder trial turns on the validity of said category? The latter example points toward detailed future discussions of vice-laden categories in the forensic or criminal justice setting.

3.1.2.1 The scientific classification of mental disorders

The history of the American Psychiatric Association's DSMs cannot be recounted here.[4] However, scholars agree that the founding of the United States' DSM was inspired significantly by the administrative need to track the course of patients through systems and levels of care.[5] By the latter half of the twentieth century, a number of factors suggested that American psychiatry needed more than a set of categories to facilitate clinical care and distribution of services: it needed a scientific classification of mental disorders to facilitate research, the development of and empirical testing of new treatments, and the discovery of potential causes for mental disorders.[6] For this and other reasons, concerns about the reliability (and at the time, and to a lesser extent, validity) of DSM diagnosis appeared, inspiring the development and release of DSM-III in 1980.[7]

The turn with DSM-III to criteria-driven, operationalized diagnosis is familiar now, through DSM-IV and on through DSM-5.[8] The DSM approach to diagnosis has dominated clinical research for over 40 years now. Michael Schwartz and Osborne Wiggins[9] wrote of the hegemony of the DSMs, and its ubiquity in clinical trials for new treatments. Only more recently, with the US National Institute of Mental Health's Research Domain Criteria (RDoC) classification for clinical neuroscience research has the DSM encountered a middling threat to its hegemony over US clinical research,[10] much less clinical practice. The RDoC classification was developed by neuroscientists and molecular biologists to address dimensions of behavior that map more closely onto anatomic pathways and molecular brain functions. As such it claims to be agnostic about traditional mental disorder or other psychological categories. However, the RDoC classification is still developing, and how, and if, its tools map onto categories relevant to clinical practice is uncertain, even years after its initial description.

In the meantime, clinical research and clinical practice demand a diagnostic rubric that, in principle, groups together similar sorts of disorders (and people) so that shared characteristics can be discerned, whether for treatment studies or etiological clues. For this purpose, the DSM and its international sibling, the ICD, reign supreme.[11]

3.1.2.2 A common language for clinicians

Related to the issue of categorizing mental disorders for the purpose of scientific investigation, but equally important, is a common language for practicing clinicians. Serving as a communication shorthand, one or more DSM diagnoses convey, in the ideal, much information about a particular patient in a very few words. Doctors assuming the care of a patient from a colleague depend on a diagnostic summary to prepare them briefly for what to expect from a new patient. Medical records require short summaries of the clinical encounter.

3.1.2.3 A common language for the public understanding of mental illness

Again, related to the above, the DSMs and ICDs provide a nomenclature that ultimately becomes appropriated by the lay public through media coverage and educational efforts. People who have heretofore not had a name for their particular distress or ordeal may characterize their experience as a 'mental illness' utilizing DSM terms.[12] However, the profundity in naming psychological conditions is the facilitation of the condition being assimilated into a patient's core notion of self or identity.[13] Not only do DSM categories constitute terms for lay discussion of 'mental illness', DSM concepts have become woven into the fabric of their identities, for better or for worse.

3.1.2.4 Diagnostic coding for billing, administration, and service planning

Each DSM or ICD diagnosis is accompanied by a diagnostic code number, along with modifiers to that number that encode variations on the condition. These numeric codes then may be entered into databases, used in billing mechanisms, feed statistical analyses to plot out service costs, issue billing statements, quantify service utilization, and establish baseline numeric data for planning mental health services. The diagnostic coding uses of the DSMs are not limited to administrative purposes but go into research endeavors, as well, such as epidemiological or 'big data' studies about rates of disorder in a population, or into scientific studies of health care systems, in evaluating service delivery in such systems and later, the development of mental health care policy.

3.1.2.5 Benchmarks for education

The DSM/ICD nomenclature and surrounding supportive material (i.e., text descriptions of clinical features of the disorder, associated features, and etiological information) also serve to teach beginning clinicians the fundamentals of their discipline. As an education benchmark, the DSMs structure medical perception—what clinicians notice and decide as pertinent, in addition to defining the irrelevant in clinical observation. In its educational function, like its use in the public sphere, the DSM classifications structure the perception of reality, and bring some phenomenological features of the clinical picture into sharp focus, while leaving other features of the clinical picture a blur, or even absent. This epistemological power[14] of the DSMs provides the cultural backbone for many of the conceptual paradoxes to be discussed below.

3.1.2.6 Benchmarks for courtroom use & expert witness status in forensic or criminal justice settings

This feature will be elaborated elsewhere in this book, but suffice to say at this stage, in the criminal justice setting, the use of DSM categories in identifying psychopathology in defendants and offenders, establishing credibility or even evidential admissibility of forensic testimony, and addressing issues of criminal and moral responsibility are all bound up with DSM categories, however much this has been lamented by DSM authors and critics.[15]

3.1.3 Some unintended consequences of diagnosis-as-denotation

When we characterize a phenomenon, we impose a particular point of view, assumptions, and constraints on the phenomenon. This feature of everyday life is illustrated by this joke:

> A man requests assistance from a feminist clerk in a bookshop: 'I found the "Women's Studies" section, but I couldn't find the "Men's Studies" section. Where is it?' The clerk replies: 'It's the rest of the bookstore.'

As with categories in bookstores, as it is in psychiatric diagnostic classification. This section addresses some of the unintended consequences associated with DSM categorization—consequences which will percolate through the discussion of vice-laden categories and their ramifications.

3.1.3.1 Reification

The philosopher Alfred North Whitehead discussed the 'fallacy of misplaced con-creteness'[16]—the idea that an abstract concept is falsely treated as if it were a concrete object or thing. 'Reification'—to make real—is the process whereby Whitehead's fallacy is committed. The DSM authors since DSM-III have been clear that the disorder categories are hypothetical, provisional entities—abstractions—yet an examination of how they are used suggests that they are 'reified': For example, a DSM mental disorder may be considered as real as the consolidation of bacteria and white blood cells in the lung are in constituting pneumonia. To reify DSM-5 Adjustment Disorder and call it a 'disease' seems inappropriate at the present time—Adjustment Disorder seems a maladaptive pattern of behavior and experience rather than a disease like pneumonia.[17]

Reification is a philosophical problem in psychiatry that I believe has received too little attention. In some ways it is a graded phenomenon—whether something is 'reified' depends in part on how well-established an abstract concept is in the culture or society. A good example of an abstract, theoretical concept that is so widely accepted that it seems a concrete fact is the 'electron'. No one sees, tastes, handles, or smells electrons, but most educated Westerners treat electrons as if they are real. In grade school, teachers demonstrate 'electrons' by running a brush through our hair, aligning them into a polarity that makes our hair stand on end.

Similarly, a common complication of reification of DSM categories is that discussions of reification can confuse the phenomenon as experienced by a person with the name or description given to the phenomenon. This is exemplified by a colleague, Phillip Slavney, saying in response to Thomas Szasz's *Myth of Mental Illness*: 'You'll have a lot of trouble convincing my patient that her depression is a myth.'[18] For Slavney, his patient has a primordial experience of profound sadness, discomfort, and disability that we label 'Major Depression'. However, that phenomenal experience is different from the DSM category of Major Depression. The phenomenal experience is concrete, while the category of Major Depression is an abstract, hypothetical entity. While the abstraction is dismissible, the phenomenal experience may not be.

The trouble arises when we commit Whitehead's fallacy and think the phenomenal experience is the same as the abstract hypothetical entity. One's misery is concrete—but the DSM name and description for that misery is abstract, hypothetical, and theory- and value-laden.[19] The ramifications of 'reifying' DSM categories are many. For one, to qualify for many mental health services you must 'have' a DSM diagnosis. For another, to qualify for National Institute of Mental Health (NIMH) funding, at least in past decades, you might well have to cast your research in the terms of a DSM category.[20] If you want to be reimbursed (by insurance) for mental health services you have received, you often must have a DSM or ICD diagnosis attached. In today's electronic medical records, even a prescribed medication must have an 'associated' diagnosis. If you want to join an online discussion group or public advocacy group that deals with your variety of psycho-emotional misery, then you probably will need to subscribe to a DSM category.[21] Whether or not you are responsible for your criminal conduct may depend upon, in large part, what reified abstract hypothetical category you are diagnosed with.

Of course, our institutions (e.g., legal, military, corporate, educational, public service, and online) need benchmarks upon which to depend, and because the DSM (ICD) is the recognized benchmark currently available, it goes to work in ways that are reifying and misleading.

3.1.3.2 Neglect of context

Many authors have lamented the 'reductionism' of denotative diagnosis in a DSM.[22] Reductionism used in this way is a negatively valued concept that describes the breaking down of a complex phenomenon into simpler components—whether these be simpler explanations, or simpler understandings, or shorter descriptions. DSM-IV authors talked about the 'loss of information' in using a DSM diagnosis (as denotation).[23] To say someone has 'Borderline Personality Disorder' conveys quite a bit of information but ignores much more—the entire historical-environmental-interpersonal surround is omitted. A denotated DSM diagnosis selects particular features of a person, describing them more-or-less accurately as of clinical relevance, but selects out, or marginalizes, one's personal circumstances, history, and other narrative, and even biological, circumstances in one's life. In *VAPD* I called this quality 'hyponarrativity', but one could just as easily describe denotative diagnosis as 'hypocontextuality'[24] to emphasize the limited context of circumstance associated with DSM diagnosis. The latter meaning here is more inclusive. Not only is the DSM 'hyponarrative' (impoverished regarding the patient's story) but impoverished in context—despite the attempts to restore some context through the DSM-III and IV multiaxial system.[25] However, even the latter has been discontinued in DSM-5.[26]

While we may fault hyponarrativity or hypocontextuality as reductionistic, such simplifying of complex phenomena poses crucial logical and practical advantages to scientific inquiry. The broad scientific endeavor depends not upon individualistic, unitary understandings of a single phenomenon, but rather groups phenomena together and searches for common features, rules of function, models of simulation, or laws, thus feeding scientific explanation and prediction.[27] Science proceeds from observing groups of phenomena and seeking commonalities. Through focusing on commonalities, one loses the rich complex uniqueness of phenomena—one cannot have science be both universalistic and particular at the same time.[28]

3.1.3.3 Focus on personal liabilities over assets

In psychology and increasingly in psychiatry, critics have emphasized that a 'positive psychology' is needed, one that addresses competencies, virtues, and resilience rather than only deficits and deficiencies, as in the classic 'psychopathology' concept in psychiatry. While DSM-III and DSM-IV provided some measure of competency or functional capacity through Axis V (adaptive functioning), the importance of positive mental health has appeared not just though experimental and clinical psychology,[29] but also through psychiatric genetics[30] and psychiatric epidemiology.[31] Community/social psychiatrists have recognized the issues of competencies and resilience through joining patients in promoting a recovery and self-management models for mental health.[32] The bottom line in these critiques is that mental health outcome is not simply a matter of symptom kind and severity.[33]

3.1.3.4 Promotion of convenience over rigor

Psychiatric training too often is driven by making DSM diagnoses before beginning clinicians have the requisite clinical skills to elicit credible clinical signs and symptoms. At least in the United States, residents enter training in psychiatry and immediately are placed in clinical care settings, where they are under substantial pressure to diagnose and treat patients—too often without engaged faculty support and instruction. DSM diagnosis becomes a checklist and a convenient shortcut. Residents often don't know what kinds of questions are appropriate to even elicit DSM criteria items adequately,[34] and progress through programs without detailed teaching and supervision in interviewing skills, eliciting subtle signs of psychopathology, much less detecting and capitalizing on personal assets and competencies.

3.1.3.5 Appropriation by the medical-industrial complex

Allen Frances among others[35] in his unofficial DSM-5 role as online process and content critic, has urgently pointed out the potential for new, unvalidated and untested diagnoses' potential for being appropriated and reified by (primarily) the pharmaceutical industry. The literature on pharma industry opportunism is substantive.[36]

3.1.3.6 Constrained funding for alternative approaches

Schwartz and Wiggins[37] have described the DSMs has exerting a 'hegemony' over psychiatric diagnosis. They mean, citing Tucker[38] and Kendell,[39] that the DSMs have 'come to dominate clinical research and practice in American psychiatry'.[40] A simple review of literature on any common diagnostic category in psychiatry of the past 40 years will reveal the depth and power of the DSM influence, and a similar review of US NIMH funding patterns will reveal the ubiquity of DSM diagnosis in psychiatric clinical research. The DSM's influence raises barriers for nosological innovation. Why? A reasonable possibility would be that study sections that approve clinical research grant funding are made up of several generations of researchers accustomed to DSM diagnosis, and innovators find it daunting to convince a

committee of scientists (with vested interests in the DSM approach) to fund alternative classifications of mental disorders.[41]

3.1.4 Some purposes for diagnosis as holistic appraisal

Figuring out a practical plan of action is a key challenge for any clinician facing a
patient in need of assistance. People, when ill, typically resort to self- or family care,
based on folk remedies or home-medical practices when the illness is mild. When
the malady is catastrophic or the patient's own resources are overwhelmed and the
patient doesn't know what to do to get well, the patient seeks assistance, often from
medical facilities. So healthcare-seekers come to clinicians for a novel appraisal of
the problem (i.e., to reinterpret the malady in the terms of their training, education,
and intellectual discipline) and hopefully receive a novel and effective intervention.
The patient's interpretation of the malady has failed, so the clinician reinterprets
the malady in light of other data and one or more alternative theories, models, or
formulations of the problem or case. One component of this reinterpretation may
be the diagnosis (as denotation), which then links the scientific evidence about that
diagnosis to this unique patient. However, this denotation is only part of the holistic appraisal a good clinician makes.[42] The denotation is a crucial ingredient, but
other factors may be as, or more, determinative of what healing actions take place.
If the patient has an allergy to a given medication, then alternative medications or
other treatments may be sought. If the patient has no funds to buy the treatment,
alternative means must be considered. If more than one set of credible treatments
are available, the patient and clinician enter a dialogue about what would suit the
patient best.[43] If ethical or moral constraints (like, e.g., confidentiality with an adolescent patient) pose challenges to the effective treatment, then other negotiations
occur. The diagnosis as holistic appraisal, as Juan Mezzich has put it, constitutes a
'psychiatry for the person'[44] rather than the psychiatry of a condition, which DAD
encapsulates. In summary, diagnosis as holistic appraisal captures the categorical
features of a malady (denotation) while assimilating the unique personal, historical, sociocultural, and moral circumstances, as well as the relationship-building,
with a unique individual.[45]

3.1.5 Some unintended consequences of diagnosis as holistic appraisal

The contemporary world of checklist-driven electronic medical records and care
pressures to be efficient make for a hostile environment for adherents of holistic appraisal. I find it difficult to identify the (negative) unintended consequences because

of my prejudice for holistic appraisal in clinical care. Nevertheless, the crucial unintended consequence of adherence to holistic appraisal in clinical care must be related to the costs of slowing down. Slowing down may well mean losing efficiency and increasing expense under holistic appraisal practices. The time involved in holistic appraisal is considerable, as the clinician spends time getting to know the patient as a person; grasps the hurly-burly of the patient's life and ordeals, considers the interpersonal context, including perhaps meeting significant others (e.g., family, friends, other clinical caregivers, attorneys, and case managers); reviews clinical records and comorbidities, selecting other studies (e.g., laboratory and imaging studies, psychological testing); and perhaps most difficult, interpreting all into a novel and effective understanding of the patient, a potential set of interventions, and negotiating the latter in a bilateral dialogue with the patient. That said, this frontend slowdown may pay off in greater efficiency later in the care arc.

Especially in the United States, where a relatively unregulated free market economy reigns supreme, and the cultural urge to judge most everything in terms of productivity and efficiency prevails,[46] the amount of clinical time and the steep financial cost of the holistic appraisal is perhaps the most important unintended consequence of this diagnostic philosophy. Not just a consequence, the cost of a thorough holistic appraisal is one that poses a major barrier to good diagnostic practice—clinicians simply don't have the time, or can't be paid for the time, required to perform a genuine holistic appraisal. Conscientious clinicians end up feeling that their care is compromised and subsequently experience moral distress—the sense that one is practicing below one's standards of integrity.[47]

A second unintended consequence is more metaphysical than practical. A friend and clinician colleague once told me, with his characteristic frankness: 'Your work is really interesting, but it makes me anxious to read it—it opens up problems I had never considered.' What makes everyone anxious about holistic appraisals is that each one tests us as clinicians and requires us to extend ourselves beyond our comfort zones and consider a clinical complexity that has few easy rules for interpreting and acting. The requirement to extend ourselves has several manifestations. One requires us to bridge the first-person and third-person knowledge gap, as John Searle puts it.[48]

First-person knowledge is what is delivered directly to me as an observer, which is the kind of knowledge captured in the clinical encounter by the clinician's own experience with the patient. Third-person knowledge, by contrast, is the kind of knowledge provided by science, where an individual (event, person, or circumstance) is studied as an example of a categorical phenomenon (e.g., a business failure as an event, a 'depressed' person, or exposure to battle as a circumstance) toward the end of generalizable knowledge of the categorical phenomenon. The clinical problem is deciding how my scientific knowledge (third-person) applies to this particular patient (first-person).[49] These judgments are often, perhaps usually, tacit, yet constitute the very essence of clinical practice skills, where the clinician is expected to extract an understanding of the patient that makes the difference for the patient's ordeal.

Related to the above is a perspective gap between clinician and patient.[50] Clinicians not only have to synthesize the clinical information and understand the patient's viewpoint for themselves, but also must communicate and ultimately have a dialogue with the patient in order to translate the clinical perspective into a sensible viewpoint suitable for the patient. Indeed, the reciprocity or give-and-take of understanding between clinician and patient contributes to the process of clinical as well as relational understanding. When the clinician explains something, and the patient feeds-back her understanding, then both augment their understandings.[51]

Diagnostic holism tends to place clinical experience on a pedestal, breeding skepticism about contrary scientific findings. This sets the stage for idiosyncratic or even dangerous practices, particularly if the clinician trivializes scientific insights or professional consensus. Clinical experience also generates 'clinical lore', alleged knowledge based upon clinical case experience, often legally recognized as a community practice standard, and when writ large across larger communities in textbooks and consensus statements, may either represent the fruits of hard-won wisdom or naive pseudo-knowledge based upon social contagion and charismatic leadership. Distinguishing these is often difficult to sort out.

Finally, just as the DAD may lead clinicians to premature closure in the clinical formulation, and a false confidence that they 'know the patient', so does holistic appraisal introduce its own potential for sloppy thinking. Simply because one has amassed a thorough amount of information and developed a substantive clinical intimacy and rapport with the patient, or a raft of patients, doesn't mean one has set the stage for inevitable treatment success. I'm reminded of an experience many years ago, where I was working in a community mental health clinic, where the clinical assessment roles were broken into stereotypic and rigid pigeonholes—the psychiatrist does medication assessment; the psychologist does testing; the social worker gathers a 'social history', for example. I remember the social worker giving me a substantive oral dissertation about the social history of the patient—but one that was a disengaged and rote set of facts without any reference to the patient's interests, values, current situation, or clinical problems. The social history had become a generic checklist item like the DSM diagnostic criteria can become checklist items. Synthesizing the information had become unfeasible. Don't forget the appraisal while doing the holism!

With this material as background, let's now consider some examples of conceptual issues relevant to the vice/mental disorder relationship (VMDR).

3.2 Vice-laden diagnosis and the cultural iconography of mental health

Religious men of the most irreproachable character, and women of unsul-lied purity of thought and habit, will use language, entertain ideas, and manifest conduct altogether opposed to their character in a sane state, and which become the source of the utmost pain and distress of mind when restored to reason.

—Anonymous (1887)[52]

In *VAPD* I catalogued a number of values wrapped up with the DSMs. Some had to do, like this book, with categories and diagnostic criteria, while others had to do with the values involved in building or creating the DSMs, as well as the cultural values in which the DSM project is embedded. As one might imagine, many of the values I identified as entangled with diagnostic categories and criteria were negative values—things we don't want to have or embody. Most broadly construed, these were the negative, and nonmoral, values described in the DSM's definitions of mental disorders—that mental disorders are associated with distress, disability, impairment, and the like. More subtly, the negative values exert themselves in other ways—one being extremes of a behavior or psychological trait—in being excesses or deficits of a trait. For example, being startled when being surprised by a loud noise is normal, but jumping out of one's skin and becoming assaultive, as in the 'exaggerated startle response' of Post-Traumatic Stress Disorder,[53] is an extreme manifestation of normative 'startle-ability'. As another example of the pathology of extremity, washing one's hands after going to the bathroom is an adaptive behavior. One who does it 300 times a day, as in Obsessive-Compulsive Disorder, is not engaging in adaptive behavior.

In *VAPD* I didn't catalogue the kinds of negatively valenced behaviors very well, and as I have learned in the ensuing years, this might have been a good discipline for later work.[54] A second thread about values in *VAPD* involved an idea that thinking about mental health and mental illness, one often, perhaps necessarily, has to make assumptions or presumptions of a normative nature.[55] This means that standards, and perhaps ideals, tend to get smuggled in—as contrasting values to mental disorders. For instance, if we consider DSM-5 Oppositional Defiant Disorder, even the name implies that, in some general and vague sense, psychiatrists think that children should not be trait-oppositional and, instead, should be, in some to-be-specified sense, *compliant* with adults—that children should, in some general sense, 'do as they're told'.[56]

I should acknowledge that the DSMs have never been created in response to a positive account of mental health—that is, what kinds of traits, beliefs, experiences, and behaviors a mentally healthy person should exemplify. However, the above examples imply cultural norms about behavioral health. So, it might be possible to describe an *implicit account* of positive mental health based upon the kinds of pathologies—deviation from normative ideals—that the DSM describes. That endeavor, while worthwhile, is not what I should attempt with this book, but simply to state, in a different way, my earlier *VAPD* point that the DSMs carry some sketchy, informal, implicit, and community-summated notion of what a good life is. The DSMs imply, but don't state, what it means to lead a good life: a life that flourishes, rather than languishes. Whether the DSMs should lay out an account of the good life is a matter for another time and perhaps another book!

3.2.1 The virtue/vice subtext of the DSMs & the example of the Seven Deadly Sins

In Chapter 4 I present a brief history of the VMDR, cast in the form of a comparative intellectual history of madness and morality. For this 'conceptual' chapter, however, some effort is needed to provide a cultural backdrop. The reader needs an introduction to other, non-DSM concepts that lurk in the cultural background as tacit knowledge about behavioral health. Such tacit background knowledge provides the commonsense context that give us the memes, the cultural tropes, the commonsense assumptions, the iconography for vice and virtue. In this regard, an entire book could be occupied by describing the cultural, religious, and literary moral worlds that frame our understanding of vice and mental illness and their relationships. That is too much for my purposes here, but some background about the cultural tropes that frame our experience of the sick and the bad can be an early step to understanding how some conditions came to be vice-laden disorders.

I have selected three topics of cultural context for this purpose here—many more would be possible—but these three are suitable examples in their own unique ways. The first, growing out of Roman Catholic tradition, is intriguing because of its medieval pedigree, and its persistent relevance to the present day. The second, (Section 3.2.2) the idea of 'common morality' is secular and contemporary in orientation and was selected because it provides a thesis of what are more-or-less agreed-upon tenets of morality in such a Western secular context. The third (Section 3.2.3), the critique from positive psychology, points to clinician blind spots in terms of virtue and vice, thus opening up some neglected domains of interest within the VMDR.

So on to the first consideration—the Roman Catholic concept of Cardinal Sins. What we know today as the 'Seven Deadly Sins' or Cardinal Sins have evolved in name and meaning since their medieval articulation. Inspired by passages from the Book of Proverbs,[57] the Sins are characterized as 'six things the Lord hateth, and the seventh His soul detesteth'. Around 375 AD, Evagrius Ponticus (Evagrius the Solitary), a Christian monk and scholar from the Roman province of Pontus, formulated what he considered the most significant eight thoughts or temptations in Christendom. Later translated into Latin for the Roman Catholic spiritual devotions (*pietas*), the original eight temptations were *Gula* (gluttony), *Fornicato* (lust), *Avaritia* (avarice or greed), *Tristitia* (sorrow or despair), *Ira* (wrath or anger), *Acedia* (listlessness or torpor), *Vanagloria* (vainglory), and *Superbia* (hubris or pride).[58]

In 590, Pope Gregory I revised Evagrius' list, condensing and revising it: *Luxuria* (extravagance), *Gula* (gluttony), *Avaritia* (avarice/greed), *Acedia* (listlessness/ torpor, and now sorrow or despair), *Ira* (anger), *Invidia* (envy), and *Superbia* (pride). These were adopted by Dante Alighieri for *The Divine Comedy*, which described the afterlife, stages of Hell, and allegorically, the way to God.[59] Since Dante, the Seven Deadly Sins have provided an ever-present religious, cultural, and literary bench- mark for how Westerners can be bad. Crucial to the link between the Seven Deadly Sins and historical madness, each sin was linked to a particular demon by German theologian Peter Binsfeld. For instance, Pride was linked to Lucifer, and Gluttony was linked to Beelzebub.[60] The Cardinal Sins are mirrored in the Roman Catholic Church today with the Cardinal Virtues, as listed in Table 3.2.

Table 3.2 provides a side-by side comparison of the Seven Deadly Sins, their op- posite Virtues, and the contemporary psychopathological symptoms and diagnostic categories related to the Sins. This comparison is not, of course, intended to imply a literal correspondence or even an adaptation of the Sins to DSM psychopathology, but only to illustrate the iconic power and cultural penetration of these tropes into our culture, including a scientific diagnostic manual of mental disorders. We'll see in later chapters that the penetration of powerful cultural tropes from history is a key to understanding the VMDR.

I leave the reader to examine the columns and correspondences for her own in- terest. I do wish to call attention to a few points that may only be 'read between the lines'. As mentioned earlier, commentators on the DSM have noted previously that many mental disorders have been characterized as disorders of excess, as well as de- ficiency.[61] As examples, euphoric mania can be understood as an excess of happi- ness, or pathological narcissism an excess of pride or hubris. What is remarkable is this: For each of the Seven Deadly Sins, a corresponding DSM psychopathology of excess—symptoms or disorders—may be recognized. However, what about excesses of *virtue*? Do these appear in the DSM?

These cultural correspondences, of virtue excesses leading to disorder, to my ex- amination, seem weaker compared to the correspondences of the Seven Deadly Sins to psychopathology. One could construe excessive Temperance with food as ano- rexia, and perhaps excessive Chastity as the inhibitions of Hypoactive Sexual Desire Disorder. Excessive Charity, as in giving away too much of one's wealth, could be a symptom of mania, but even in mania excessive charity is but one feature, and not a core feature, and not even one that is observed in all cases. I find it hard to conceive of excessive Patience, unless excessive patience means never taking action, but this is a stretch. One might be able to claim that excessive diligence character- izes Obsessive-Compulsive Personality Disorder (OCPD), but this does injustice to diligence—because to be diligent means to be productive-to-completion in one's work. The problem with OCPD is that the patient is not productive because of preoc- cupation with details. Similarly, there is no obvious disorder coupling with excessive Humility and excessive Kindness.

Table 3.2 Sins & Virtues in Roman Catholicism and in the DSMs

Sins in Pietas/Devotions	Seven Deadly Sins (Gregory I)	Cardinal Virtues	Associated psychiatric symptoms	DSM-IV/DSM-5 associated category	Notes
Gula (gluttony)	Gula (Gluttony)	Temperance	binge-eating anorexia impulsivity	Bulimia Nervosa (DSM-IV-TR) Anorexia Nervosa (DSM-IV-TR) Binge-Eating Disorder (DSM-5) Antisocial Personality Disorder (DSM-IV-TR) Antisocial/Psychopathic Type (DSM-5) Borderline Personality Disorder (DSM-IV-TR)	Bulimia and binge-eating suggest indulgence, while anorexia suggests "temperance" carried to an excessive degree. Impulsivity related to intemperate indulgences (sexual, emotional, etc.)
Fornicato (lust)	Luxuria (Lust, extravagance)	Chastity	paraphilic symptoms excessive sexual time/activity sexual violence	paraphilias (DSM-IV-TR/5) Hypersexual Disorder (DSM-5) Paraphilic Coercive Disorder (DSM-5)	paraphilic interests historically judged as "unnatural" desires Hypoactive Sexual Desire Disorder as an excess of Chastity?
Avaritia (avarice/greed)	Avaritia (Avarice/Greed)	Charity	"miserly spending style" (DSM-IV-TR)	Obsessive-Compulsive Personality Disorder (DSM-IV-TR)	miserliness omitted from DSM-5 dimensions
Tristitia (sorrow/despair)			symptoms of depression (especially cognitive ones)	mood disorders (bipolar/unipolar)	Overlap with Acedia in early use
Ira (wrath)	Ira (Wrath, Anger)	Patience	"failure to resist aggressive impulses" (DSM-IV-TR) aggressiveness aggression hostility inappropriate, intense anger or difficulty w/anger control	Intermittent Explosive Disorder (DSM-IV-TR/DSM-5) Antisocial Personality Disorder (DSM-IV-TR) Antisocial/Psychopathic Type (DSM-5) Conduct Disorder (DSM-IV-TR/DSM-5) Borderline Personality Disorder (DSM-IV-TR) Borderline Type (DSM-5)	Overlap with Gluttony as intemperateness

Acedia (acedia)	*Acedia* (Sloth)	Diligence	avolition various symptoms of inattention	Schizophrenia (DSM-IV-TR/DSM-5) Attention Deficit/Hyperactivity Disorder (DSM-IV-TR/DSM-5)	Obsessive-compulsive Personality Disorder as an excess of diligence?
Vanagloria (vainglory)			see Pride	see Pride
Superbia (hubris, pride)	*Superbia* (Pride)	Humility	narcissistic symptoms (grandiosity, entitlement, fantasies of unlimited success) self-centeredness	Narcissistic Personality Disorder (DSM-IV-TR) Histrionic Personality Disorder (DSM-IV-TR)
	Invidia (Envy)	Kindness	enviousness	Narcissistic Personality Disorder (DSM-IV-TR)

These Virtues carry with them a kind of implicit moderation—that is, to pursue Kindness, Temperance, Humility, and Patience is to pursue a moderate path of neither excess nor neglect. Indeed, Aristotle's doctrine of the mean explicitly theorized virtue as a midpoint between polarities of vicious excess or deficiency. The Sins, however, exemplify their own excesses, and some, like Anger, are rarely adaptive at all.[62] We'll consider the role of the virtues in psychopathology in more detail in Section 3.3.

3.2.2 Common morality as a cultural indicator & background DSM morality

One of the debated areas in contemporary moral philosophy is the idea of a 'common morality'. The basic idea is that all people possess a core set of moral dispositions that are the same. Where moral diversity kicks in is in applying the tenets of the common morality and how particular moral viewpoints are conceived, articulated, and defended. Robert Veatch sketches common morality as:

> The core idea of a common morality is that all humans—at least all morally serious humans—have a pretheoretical awareness of certain moral norms. The claim is that normal humans intuit or in some other way know that there is something wrong with things like lying or breaking promises or killing people.[63]

One of the most influential common-morality theorists is Bernard Gert. Gert notes:

> The existence of a common morality is supported by the widespread agreement on most moral matters by all moral agents. Insofar that they do not use any beliefs that are not shared by all moral agents, they all agree that killing, causing pain or disability, or depriving of freedom or pleasure from any other moral agent is immoral unless there is an adequate justification for doing such an action.[64]

Tom Beauchamp is another strong defender of common morality.[65] Beauchamp describes common morality as follows:

> I define the 'common morality' as the set of norms shared by all persons committed to the objectives of morality. The objectives of morality, I will argue, are those of promoting human flourishing by counteracting conditions that cause the quality of people's lives to worsen.

The notion of a common morality has been criticized,[67] and whether common morality stands as a universal is not the focus here. Rather, as with the Seven Deadly Sins, common-morality theorists provide a cultural template for prevailing Western moral themes. In other words, common-morality theorists describe a (particularly philosophical) moral iconography that helps frame the issues of the VMDR. Such an

Table 3.3 Bernard Gert's Ten Rules
of the Common Morality

1. Do not kill.

2. Do not cause pain.

3. Do not disable.

4. Do not deprive of freedom.

5. Do not deprive of pleasure.

6. Do not deceive.

7. Keep your promises.

8. Do not cheat.

9. Obey the law.

10. Do your duty.

Adapted from Gert (2004).

iconography provides another set of conceptual semantics against which to weigh the VMDR.

For brevity's and simplicity's sake, Gert proffers a common-morality list of the 'moral rules'.[68] These are listed in Table 3.3.

In contrast to the Seven Deadly Sins, Gert's rules do not transparently relate to DSM diagnostic categories. This is likely due to the focus on action in Gert's rules, rather than traits of character in the Seven Deadly Sins. Nevertheless, examination of Gert's ten rules indicates that the moral issues identified are quite familiar to clinicians working with patients, some more than others and some more derivatively than others.

For instance, while most clinicians don't worry commonly about whether their patients are going to kill someone, sometimes they do, and much effort it expended in addressing these concerns when they occur. More often, clinicians are listening to and addressing patients' angry fantasies about getting even with a provocateur. Such fantasies may include killing, but also, for example, causing pain, disabling, and depriving of pleasure. Many of these fantasies are not acted upon, but some are, and remorse over the harms one has caused others is a common consequence (e.g., hurting one's spouse, letting down one's children, exploiting one's boss, or failing to honor a promise). As a second example, clinicians often deal with patients' intentions, or regrets about, deceiving others. Patients often feel guilty about not honoring commitments (keeping promises), cheating, fulfilling their responsibilities, or even breaking the law. Indeed, most clinicians, I will venture to say, could recognize that Gert's ten moral rules spell out very common, perhaps even the most common, motivations for people to seek mental health care. This is to say that, in effect, many people seek mental health care when they, or others, find themselves failing to follow their internalized moral rules.

If the claims in the above paragraph have any kernel of empirical truth, then at the very minimum, mental health practitioners engage with the moral lives of their patients, explicitly or implicitly, on a daily, perhaps constant, basis. Further, the success of mental health interventions, for better or worse, might well be estimated, in the patient's eyes, against the success the clinician has in helping the patient achieve more adherence to Gert's moral rules. For example, I want to stop hurting my wife's feelings, or disappointing my children, or do a better job at work. Psychiatry and the DSM refer to these aims as improving 'functioning', but this masks the moral content that I have suggested here.

This shouldn't be too surprising. In *VAPD*, and earlier in this chapter, I argued that the morality of psychiatry is governed by implicit, undisclosed concepts of human flourishing and achievement of well-being.[69] However, such a realization that clinicians engage routinely with patients' moral conduct goes against the socialization of not imposing our 'values' on patients and that somehow our work should be value-free. We are instructed to not 'moralize' with our patients. These understandings that indeed, in some ways, we routinely address moral issues with our patients requires some special consideration about what kinds of moral engagement with patients are (morally) appropriate and professionally founded, and which kinds are not. This understanding also suggests that clinicians are already immersed in the arena of the management of moral choices, and consequently everyday work in psychiatry is virtue- and vice-laden.

The topic of virtue brings us to the critique of positive psychology, which is relevant to a philosophical understanding of vice in the DSMs.

3.2.3 The critique from positive psychology

> When psychiatrists and psychologists talk about mental health, wellness, or well-being, they mean little more than the absence of disease, distress, and disorder. It is as if falling short of diagnostic criteria should be the goal for which we all should strive.[70]

Influenced by the humanistic psychology movement of the 1960s and 1970s—but striking out on its own empirical path in the 1990's—the positive psychology movement intends to rebalance the prevailing deficit/dysfunction approach of conventional clinical psychology and psychiatry. In a 2004 manifesto for the field, Peterson and Seligman sketch out the theory and research behind positive psychology in terms of a 'Manual of the Sanities'[71] that 'focuses on what is right about people and specifically about the strengths of character that make the good life possible'(p. 4). The authors offer an explicit classification of character strengths as a corrective to the pathology-orientations to the DSM and ICD classifications of mental disorders. Their classification, in method, should be context-sensitive, meet careful methodological and descriptive criteria, and be empirically testable. Their 2004 Classification of Character Strengths is presented in brief in Table 3.4. Capturing Peterson and Seligman's (P&S's) 800-page tome is well beyond my constraints here, but their goals and findings to date are relevant to the vice-laden diagnosis question. Rather than the nonmoral values of illness experience, the positive psychology approach

Table 3.4 Peterson and Seligman's Classification of
24 Character Strengths

---

1. Wisdom and knowledge
   Creativity
   Curiosity
   Open-mindedness
   Love of learning
   Perspective

2. Courage
   Bravery
   Persistence
   Integrity
   Vitality

3. Humanity
   Love
   Kindness
   Social intelligence

4. Justice
   Citizenship
   Fairness
   Leadership

5. Temperance
   Forgiveness and mercy
   Humility/modesty
   Prudence
   Self-regulation

6. Transcendence
   Appreciation of beauty and excellence
   Gratitude
   Hope (optimism, future-mindedness, and future-orientation)
   Humor (playfulness)
   Spirituality (religiousness, faith, and purpose)

Adapted from Peterson & Seligman (2004).

suggests that cultivation of character traits associated with human flourishing completes, or rounds out, a clinical psychology otherwise preoccupied with incapacities and 'languishing'. Vice could be construed as a particular variety of languishing, and as such raises the question about the implicit conception of mental health in the DSMs. This is to say, what can be inferred about positive mental health by examining the failures and incapacities described by the various DSM disorders? Does a failure of one or more character strengths (or virtues) suggest psychopathology?

Interestingly, casual consideration of each of P&S's character strengths (in their inverse) evokes some DSM categories/criteria, while others, not. For instance, a failure of 'open-mindedness' might suggest the inflexibility of OCPD, or a failure of 'fairness' might suggest the interpersonal exploitativeness associated with Narcissistic or Antisocial Personality Disorders. On the other hand, the DSM doesn't have categories of psychopathology that deal with failures of creativity (like a 'banality disorder') or bravery ('cowardly personality disorder') or appreciation of beauty ('tastelessness disorder'). An amusing exercise would be to go on and contrive all kinds of disorders representing failures of P&S's character strengths—but I'm not recommending these disorders of virtue failure be added to the DSM lexicon! What character strength failures do raise, however, is the peculiar implicit vision of virtue that remains to be uncoded within DSM categories.

Closer examination, however, suggests that one superordinate category has perhaps the greatest significance for DSM/ICD psychopathology: Temperance, with its component strengths Forgiveness/Mercy, Humility/Modesty, Prudence, and Self-Regulation. Failures of these virtues imply the DSM-5 Cluster B Personality Disorders[72] (which have been debated in the literature as among the most moral-value-laden of the DSM mental disorders[73]). Virtue failures or associated vices of the Cluster B personality disorders would include, for example, 'callousness', 'arrogance', 'recklessness', and 'impulsiveness', which populate the Cluster B diagnostic criteria, and many of these fall into failures of temperance virtues.

3.2.3.1 Virtue failure, vice, and psychopathology
The interesting conceptual and historical question here is why failures of Temperance appear as personality disorders with such resonance, while other personality disorders occupy much more limited spaces of virtue failure. As regards Axis I disorders, one also sees virtue failures scattered among them—for instance, Hope failure would seem to line up with the 'hopelessness' of Major Depressive Disorder. Few, however, are defined as deeply by virtue failure as are the Cluster B Personality Disorders.

While it would be an interesting exercise to more carefully work through virtue failure and other vices in DSM-IV and/or DSM-5 categories, at this point in the book, I'll leave this conceptual issue as simply raised. The issue is this: What role should virtue failure or vice play in defining psychopathology?

A philosophical point and warning should be issued. Note that P&S's 'character strengths' as listed in Table 3.1 do not completely map on what I have as a *moral* value. Remember that values can roughly be divided into two kinds—moral, having to do with rightness and wrongness, good and evil—and nonmoral values, which are a diverse group, including epistemic values, like 'coherence', or pragmatic values, like 'utility' or aesthetic values, like 'elegance'.[74] When one examines the meaning of some of the character strengths, many of them are not, in typical use, moral values as such. For instance, we don't judge noncreative people as evil, or a banal creative work as dangerous (except perhaps in art-world hyperbole). Similarly, while we might well judge Citizenship as a moral good as typically used in discourse, Leadership may not qualify, because Teamwork is also crucial to human flourishing, and 'followers' are crucial members of teams. We need both captains and soldiers.

Recognizing this point, we might offer the conjecture that the Temperance group of character strengths then might be the most saturated with moral values, and indeed, forgiveness, mercy, modesty, humility, prudence, and self-regulation all likely qualify as moral values in ordinary use, and many in classical virtue theory in ethics. Are other groups of character strengths also rich in moral values?

The character strengths listed under 'Wisdom and Knowledge' would all qualify for what some philosophers call 'Intellectual' or 'Epistemic' virtues.[75] These are habits of mind that are associated with securing credible knowledge and/or wisdom. 'Wisdom' as a value in itself, along with others in this group, and may well do double-duty as both moral and epistemic virtues. Aristotle himself identified [practical] wisdom (as *phronesis*) as one of his key moral virtues.[76]

Similarly, we can cast 'bravery' from the Courage group as having moral and other meaning depending on the context of use. Rosa Parks exhibited moral bravery when she refused to move to the back of the bus,[77] but a neophyte skydiver probably has some other, nonmoral, brand of bravery in doing her first jump.

Examination of the 'Humanity' group of character strengths suggests traits that have substantive moral content in most contexts—love being good in the moral sense. Similarly, the Justice grouping also includes traditional ethical values that are familiar.

The Transcendence group poses a rich and diverse group of values. Appreciation of beauty or excellence most readily implies aesthetic, nonmoral values, but what about appreciation of moral excellence? Is that a moral value? As another consideration, it would seem inaccurate to universally characterize people without hope as morally deficient, and yet hope seems to accompany the morally excellent. Gratitude, while atypical in the classical moral virtues literature seems to be a term of moral praise (as 'I appreciate your moral goodness to me.'), and indeed, we often think of 'thankless' people as mean-spirited and callous—clearly morally deficient. Humor and spirituality also pose a mixed bag—they tend to march along with the morally excellent person, but humorless and spiritually adrift people are not typically branded as evil or immoral.

The insights of the analysis of P&S's character strengths as values suggests that some of these values (and their associated opposites/vices) are nonmoral, and indeed, their meanings have never been associated with mental or physical ailments proper. They are semantically separate. Others, however, particularly those in the Temperance group, have polar vices that fall into the domain of the DSM-5 Cluster B Personality Disorders, and indeed, the meanings fall into conventional Western notions of vice (e.g., irresponsibility, impulsiveness, and callousness).

So given the diversity of meaning of most of the remaining character strengths, it should not be surprising that their failures don't map onto DSM categories as dramatically as the Temperance virtue failures do. P&S note that the virtues follow a semantic structure that Wittgenstein[78] and Rosch and Mervis[79] have characterized as 'families' of concepts, and vices no doubt fit that description as well.

3.2.3.2 Flourishing, resilience, well-being, and mental health

These considerations prompt a reiteration of P&S's point about character strengths being distinctive traits, not simply antipathological but often uncorrelated or 'orthogonal' with psychopathological traits.[80] This observation suggests to me that the implicit positive values behind the DSM are normative in the standard sense—that is, psychopathology reflects the failure of typical capacities, competencies, states of comfort, and 'functioning'. As a branch of medicine, psychiatry has been occupied historically with restoring function and typical comfort—enabling flourishing—but not optimizing lives. Indeed, a great deal of bioethics debate today is focused on the role of biomedical enhancement as proper to the physician role. That is, should physicians be limited to restoring function and comfort, and leave 'enhancement'—exceeding ordinary human flourishing and excellence, to some other professional role?[81]

This question is suitable for another worthwhile albeit digressive discussion, but nevertheless leads to an additional consideration. P&S accuse the DSMs—legitimately, I think—as manuals of incapacities and function failures, overlooking positive mental health. They make the tongue-in-cheek assertion that the NIMH would be more accurately named the 'National Institute of Mental Illness' as the NIMH supports research (prevailingly) on disorders not health.[82] Their concern about the importance of positive mental health has been echoed in recent studies of human resilience and 'well-being', harkening back to Aristotle's *Eudaemonia*.[83] Recent research, led by sociologist Corey L. M. Keyes has indicated that mental health and mental illness, properly defined, are not poles of a dimension, but separate, psychometrically distinct but correlated dimensions with complex interactions.[84] Positive mental health and resilience can both be a protective or mitigating factor in mental illness-related disability, but also can be a preventive factor.[85] This recognition of the importance of mental health as a goal in its own right led the World Health Organization to rethink the meaning of mental health:[86]

> Mental health is defined as a state of well-being in which every individual realizes his or her own potential, can cope with the normal stresses of life, can work productively and fruitfully, and is able to make a contribution to her or his community.
>
> The positive dimension of mental health is stressed in WHO's definition of health as contained in its constitution: 'Health is a state of complete physical, mental and social well-being and not merely the absence of disease or infirmity.'

This work is important for the question of vice in diagnostic categories because it suggests that, in contrast to the traditions of psychiatry, (not to overlook medicine as a whole), cultivating resilience and positive [mental] health is crucial if clinicians are to be serious about therapies for diseases or disorders. That is, cultivating resilience and well-being in *patients* is important to disease or disorder outcome. Understanding these relationships tends to undermine the old distinction between therapy and enhancement—in a sense, therapy depends upon certain kinds of, or meanings for, enhancements (ones that foster resilience and well-being) and that clinical goals include not just the removal of impairments but the promotion of flourishing.

Perhaps not surprisingly, positive mental health appears to have a mitigating effect on criminal activity[87] and promotes prosocial behaviors.[88] Positive mental health, as exemplified by the character strengths, appears to be beneficial in a number of do-mains of human activity.[89] Indeed, P&S acknowledge that the field of positive psy-chology would not flourish if all it offered was ordinary wisdom of life experience, of the like 'every Sunday school teacher or grandparent already knew'.[90]

What is important for understanding the VMDR from the positive psychology cri-tique is the question the field raises about the social role of medicine. As mentioned earlier, the traditional notion of the medical healer is the individual who cares for the sick, not the well. Among the accomplishments of the positive psychology move-ment is the complicating of the strict therapy/enhancement distinction.[91] If interven-tions that promote human flourishing, like promoting a love of learning, or facilitate loving, competent interpersonal relationships; or improve humility, temperance, and self-regulation; indeed improve health, then it would seem that clinicians should ab-solutely be in the business of 'enhancements' and the promotion of such personal virtues. Conversely, this might also imply that clinician roles should include the re-duction or rehabilitation of vicious—vice-laden behaviors as well. Should they?

This question is one that will be addressed head-on in later chapters. Suffice to say at this stage, is that the critique of positive psychology and well-being theorists like Keyes suggests that the distinction between 'therapy' for moral and nonmoral bads is not quite as clear as we might have thought.

3.3 Omissions & commissions—paradoxes of clinical meaning

Up to this point the focus on the conceptual issues of vice-laden psychopathology has focused more on the fuzzy relationships between virtue, vice, character strengths, and the kinds of values we tend to view as disease- or disorder-related and the kinds of values we tend to see as governed by other generalizations (e.g., human foibles, character flaws, virtue failure, and the like). This section introduces a series of con-siderations that might be considered as nosological problems—that is, issues related to vice in diagnostic categories that are disease-classificatory in nature rather than semantic in nature.

The 'omissions & commissions' rubric in this section title refers to categories as vice-laden. Vice-laden categories that have found their way into the DSMs, ICDs, and other classification systems of psychopathology are 'commissions' of vice in the classification of psychopathology (i.e., some categories include, are committed to, vice concepts). On the other hand, other categories of human ex-perience and behavior that are also vice-laden, are, however, NOT classified as mental disorders. Vice-laden categories are, then, both committed and omitted. This section considers these and considers some of the reasons why here and in later discussions.

Chapter 2 listed an extensive dossier of DSM-5-proposed categories that are vice-laden—Conduct Disorder, Antisocial Personality Disorder, some of the

Paraphilias and Impulse Control Disorders, and so on. These categories are the 'commissions' of vice-laden psychopathologies, and the evidence for their vice-laden character was discussed in Chapter 2 as well. Chapters 4 and 5 will discuss some of the reasons why these and other vice-laden disorders have appeared, and persisted, to the present day. For economy's sake I leave commissions alone at this point.

For this section, the prevailing focus will be on the omissions of vice-laden psychopathology. The question is: Why are other vice-laden behavior patterns NOT classified as psychopathology? Some of these 'syndromes' have been proffered as disorders and rejected by the DSM committees, while others have been discussed in the literature, while still others again might be considered, but as yet, have not. Indeed, the central paradox of this section is that there are so many ways to be vicious, but so few have ended up as official mental disorders!

To make this discussion as straightforward as possible, a convention is needed for 'vice-laden behavioral syndromes that have not been classified as mental disorders' so that such a wordy phrase does not gratuitously lengthen any sentence by 11 words! My convention will be to use and abbreviation of 'vice-laden behavioral syndromes' (VLBS) of this kind, ones that have been forgotten, ignored, neglected, or excluded as potential categories of psychopathology, as well as potential categories in a psychiatric diagnostic classification system.

For this section, a logical first step is to consider the 'received view', the perhaps obvious reasons VLBS have not been classified as mental disorders, followed by a critical discussion of these allegedly obvious reasons. In keeping with the focus of the chapter, I'll limit my discussion to conceptual issues or problems, leaving the context, history, and understanding to later chapters. In the ensuing subsection, I'll consider putative mental disorders that qualify as VLBS that have in fact been proposed in the clinical literature, as well as categories that have appeared in the law literature (which is not limited by the DSM/medical psychiatry's constraints[92]). Some of the proposals from the law literature veer into comedic territory, at least from this psychiatrist's eyes, which leads naturally into a section of never-proposed VLBS conditions, and what I call some 'serious fun' in considering why these never-proposed conditions remain not proposed. Even this section will stop short of conclusions, as again the historical and pragmatic contexts of later chapters will be important in understanding the 'omissions'.

3.3.1 Obvious reasons for omissions of VLBS

Perhaps the most important reasons for not introducing this or that newly proposed disorder, VLBS or not, is nicely summarized in several papers by the DSM-IV Task Force group in the 1990s.[93] The details of their concerns needn't be detailed here, but the basic idea is new disorder categories should exhibit some minimum standards of scientific-empirical validity before the proposed category warrants classification as an official DSM mental disorder. That is, the proposed category should be validated through Robins and Guze's[94] classic five indices for validation of mental disorders: clinical description, laboratory studies, delimitation from other disorders, follow-up studies, and family studies. Alternatively, the proposed disorder category should meet some version of Cronbach and Meehl's[95] notion of construct validity. Briefly stated, a proposed diagnostic category should not be made official willy-nilly, but rather should be empirically established as a relatively distinct syndrome that intercorrelates with other clinically relevant descriptors and predictors.

That was in the DSM-IV era. For DSM-5, in Chapter 2, we mentioned some new vice-laden categories that are proposed for DSM-5, each with varying amounts of empirical validation (e.g., Hypersexual Disorder, Paraphilic Coercive Disorder). Many of these did not make it into the final manual for, among other reasons, lack of validation.

3.3.2 Review of some candidate categories of VLBS

With this introduction, we can consider some vice-laden syndromes that have been proffered as potential DSM disorders in the past DSM eras and indeed, more recently for DSM-5. DSM-5 has listed some proposal for new paraphilias (Paraphilic Coercive Disorder, Hypersexual Disorder) that were discussed as 'vice-laden' in Chapter 2 as well. I have selected some key proposals for discussion here (and omitted others) because they serve well as springboards to discussing some of the conceptual issues underlying vice-laden disorders.

3.3.2.1 Paraphilic Coercive Disorder

Originally considered for DSM-III-R in the mid-1980s,[96] and originally termed 'paraphilic rapism', the Paraphilic Coercive Disorder (PCD) syndrome intends to separate out a subgroup of rapists who are differentially aroused by violent sexual assault and a nonconsenting, resisting, victim. A 2010 series of articles in the *Archives of Sexual Behavior* focused on the DSM-5 Sexual Disorders Work Group progress reports, and three of those papers focused explicitly on reviews of this proposed disorder.[97] The disorder, even within the DSM-5 Work Group, appears to be controversial, not so much because it is, to use my terms, vice-laden, but rather because of scientific disagreements within the group about the interpretation and significance of plethysmography (penile strain-gauge) studies of rapists' arousal patterns, diagnostic overlap with Sexual Sadism (one of the DSM-IV-TR Paraphilias), and at least according to Knight,[98] concerns about the taxometric data supporting a dimension (a spectrum of the paraphilic arousal pattern) rather than a category (a bounded either/or taxon). Moreover, practical and ethical concerns about misuse or abuse within the courtroom or criminal justice system also persists with this round of proposals for PCD, as it did in the DSM-III-R era.[99]

My own critical response to the category is practical. It seems very strange to me to introduce a category for a subgroup of sex offenders defined by a particular response pattern to an artificial laboratory experience, while in the ugly world of rape 'practice', all (guilty) rapists are able to function sexually (develop and maintain an erection, with a potential for orgasm) while either violently abusing or restraining a perhaps equally violently resisting victim. So, the sexual-functional 'success' of the rape act seems to me to verify a deviant arousal pattern in the perpetrator—at least those who complete the rape act. The way PCD diagnostic criteria read to me, there should be a population of rapists out there who experience erectile or orgasmic dysfunction when their victims resist, because they don't have the disposition to paraphilic arousal. Sexual diversity being such as it is, people like this probably exist out there, but what status they hold as sex offenders is unknown. Rapists with erectile dysfunction seem so far from the gritty realities of rape crime, the entire distinction between paraphilic and nonparaphilic rapists doesn't make any practical or logical sense. How can the category not default to including *all* rapists that penetrate and ejaculate in their victims? One wonders if the plethysmography laboratory studies are ambiguous and mixed because they are heavily artificial, and perhaps, artifactual. To make a related point, no one would be surprised to find out that rapists have violent sexual fantasies, just as no one would be surprised to find out that loving husbands have tender fantasies of connubial lovemaking. The whole category and criteria set seem to redescribe the obvious in a rape offender. Regardless, PCD makes for a provocative example of a vice-laden disorder.

3.3.2.2 Pathological bias

Dunbar and others[100] have suggested various related categories of psychopathology that address irrational or delusional bias in individuals, described by Dunbar as 'Pathological Bias'. Dunbar describes a 'clinical triad' of pathological bias: preoccupation with the out-group, aversive arousal in relation to the out-group, and relationship-damaging behavior toward the out-group.[101] While Dunbar doesn't define 'out-group' in his 2003 and 2004 papers, the context of discussion implies that out-groups are social groups with cultural identities different from one's own. The symptomatic preoccupation with the out-group is described as 'fixed ideation or preoccupation with out-group persons', which are typically experienced as 'intrusive, provocative, and potentially disabling to the patient', establishing some impairment.[102] The symptom complex is associated also with avoidant and obsessive/compulsive thoughts and behaviors. Aversive arousal regarding the out-group is described as 'classic fight-or-flight' responsiveness involving 'contact-contingent anxiety or hostility'.[103] Relationship-damaging behavior for the out-group involves a sabotaging of opportunities to 'establish healthy intergroup contact',[104] which may involve various cultural sanctions with ingroup approval.

Carl Bell[105] addresses the issue of pathological bias within the framework of racism as a mental disorder, while Guindon, Green, and Hanna[106] propose a similar syndrome around the notion of 'intolerance', postulating an Intolerant Personality Disorder (IPD). The team describes a series of proto-diagnostic criteria for IPD as:

> A diagnosis of IPD should be considered when an individual does any combination of the following: (a) holds a rigid set of beliefs that assert the intrinsic superiority due to race, religion, culture, or gender of the person's own group (this could include self-perceptions that indicate a belief that his or her own group is somehow unique, special, more privileged, or more deserving than is another); (b) lacks empathy for one or more particular populations, such as, but not limited to, Latinos, African Americans, gays, lesbians, or women (conversely, the person may believe that only persons of his or her own group can truly understand him or her); (c) exhibits interpersonal behavior that ranges from covert or overt antagonism and hostility to exploitation toward one or more specific or targeted populations; (d) seeks to overtly or covertly block, deny, impede, or cancel the social, organizational, psychological, or financial advancement of someone of a group believed to be inferior; (e) uses power or other means to inhibit or prevent free expression of contrary or intolerable ideas; (f) has a sense of entitlement based on membership in a privileged group and believes that others should recognize his or her superiority without commensurate achievements or valid credentials; (g) manifests a pervasive pattern of disregard for the human rights of members of particular populations; and (h) shows lack of remorse as indicated by being callous or indifferent to having hurt, restricted, mistreated, or maligned members of selective populations.[107]

The IPD criteria describe the bigot, the racist, the homophobe, a substantial portion of perpetrators of hate crimes, and perhaps more than a few of us who tend toward righteous indignation as a trait rather than a state. In invoking my own Moral Wrongfulness Test,[108] individuals conforming to either Dunbar's construct, Bell's, or IPD would be viewed by many of us as involved in wrongful or morally bad attitudes and behaviors. So, indeed, these constructs would have to be judged as vice-laden.[109]

Tolerance, the virtue whose failure implies at least some of the IPD clinical features, is a complicated virtue and value. The practice of tolerance means the practice of permission and peaceful coexistence. As permissive, it doesn't require an 'acceptance' of others in the sense that one must agree or conform to others' viewpoints but does imply an acceptance of others' ability to hold their viewpoints and practice their [noninfringing] practices. Tolerance has strong American cultural roots because of the First Amendment to the US Constitution, and its place in the Bill of Rights:

> Congress shall make no law respecting an establishment of religion, or prohibiting the free exercise thereof; or abridging the freedom of speech, or of the press; or the right of the people peaceably to assemble, and to petition the government for a redress of grievances.[110]

Sometimes the value of tolerance is promulgated as a 'negative right', that is a right of noninterference, in the First Amendment's case, to assure that citizens can freely express their religious and other viewpoints and to assemble peacefully. To fail to respect the First Amendment is to give privilege to another viewpoint, religious or otherwise. The First Amendment is more a constitutional protection of tolerance than a proscription against intolerance. Intolerant people are free to assemble, voice their intolerant viewpoints publicly, and practice intolerant religions, provided they don't infringe upon others. This must have been a dicey Amendment to write because the value of tolerance seems to fit best as a virtue of the individual rather than a virtue for the collective. When we insist upon other's tolerance, then we begin to infringe on their own freedoms, and move toward intolerance ourselves. So, the Constitution doesn't say its citizens must be tolerant, it says that the government cannot pass intolerant laws.

The IPD and pathological bias categories pose related complexities. Does promulgating an IPD category promote, or depend upon, some of the self-same vices that are decried in the category description? By enacting an Intolerant Personality Disorder (IPT), are we as nosologists perpetrating a belief that our 'own [tolerant] group is somehow unique, special, more privileged, or more deserving than is another [intolerant group]' (IPT feature A above)? Moreover, by declaring IPD a mental disorder would we seek 'to overtly or covertly block, deny, impede, or cancel the social, organizational, psychological, or financial advancement of someone in a [intolerant] group believed to be inferior [e.g., pathological]' (IPT feature D above)? What about feature E above: '. . . uses power or other means to inhibit or prevent free expression of contrary or intolerable ideas'? Would not an IPT disorder serve this end?

The problem with categories of mental disorder centered on intolerance as a pathology is the categories themselves risk becoming tools of ingroup intolerance and vicious unto themselves, undermining tolerance while allegedly championing it.

3.3.2.3 Behavioral addictions

Early notices of the DSM5 online draft criteria included a discussion of the proposed transition of Pathological Gambling from the Impulse Control Disorders section to an expanded Substance Abuse Disorders section that would include 'behavioral addictions' or habit disorders.[111] The basic idea here is that some neuroimaging studies suggest that gambler's brains have similar arousal patterns to those addicted to cocaine when viewing videos related to their respective cravings. Pathological gambling has long segregated genetically with Substance Abuse Disorders[112] and treatment studies also support some similarities.[113] However, as Frances[114] notes, the expanded notion of behavioral addictions could include categories like sexual addiction, compulsive spending (a.k.a. credit card abuse), internet use,[115] and video gaming, Frances likens these behavior patterns to excesses of evolutionary adaptations, where pleasure-seeking is a 'ubiquitous part of human nature'. What makes the difference for Frances is whether, (invoking again the Clinical Significance Criterion), the compulsive pleasure-seeking is NOT rewarding and paradoxically unpleasant.

Whether or not one accepts Frances' account of human nature, the behavioral addictions manage to invoke associations to three of the aforementioned Seven Deadly Sins cultural tropes—gluttony, lust, and greed, as well as failures of temperance, chastity, and charity. These intemperances make the behavioral addictions somewhat unique vice-laden categories. Like the conventional addictions, the behavioral addictions are vice-laden through their intemperances and indulgences.

Holden's 2010[116] news item in *Science* makes much of the discussion about the neuroimaging similarities and putative neurobiological pathways between drug addictions and behavioral addictions. To use neuroimaging studies to study brain arousal pathways seems plausible as a nosological indicator. That is, in conditions that phenomenologically or phenotypically resemble each other (like compulsive pleasure-seeking behaviors), it is scientifically credible to use imaging and other biological studies to discriminate, for classification purposes, compulsive pleasure-seeking disorders from obsessive-compulsive anxiety disorders.

However, the behavioral addictions pose an excellent opportunity to discuss a common fallacy about assigning a pathological status to the condition with a biological pathway or explanatory nexus. The fallacy is this: We have a putative biological understanding, perhaps even the beginnings of a biological explanation for a condition, and therefore, this establishes the condition as a disorder. The likening of drug-addiction circuitry to excesses of behavioral-reward circuitry doesn't necessarily mean that the behavioral-reward excess constitutes a disorder. Why? Because all human behavior and experience, excessive or not, have neurobiological properties (how could it be otherwise?), and the mere presence of particular biological properties doesn't mean the condition is a disorder. Very smart people have neurobiological properties that may well be on the way to being identified, but we don't consider (yet) very smart people as being disordered. The obvious reason here is that smartness is socially valued, and even though it represents an excess of intelligence and therefore a statistical abnormality, we would not 'treat' smartness but rather would like to find out how to capture it and pass it on to others. What confers disorder or disease status on biological conditions are social value judgments, not biological pathways.[117] Further, social judgments about diseases or disorders are commonly propagated without much in the way of a biological explanation, not just in psychiatry (as with classical studies of schizophrenia) but in medicine at-large (as in the discovery of AIDS, where it was a disease long before we knew much about the biology of the condition). In summary, having biological correlates or even a robust biological explanation is neither necessary nor sufficient to award a condition disease or disorder status.[118]

Recognizing the fallacy of bioexplanation as determining disorder status, the question of whether behavioral addictions should be considered as mental disorders remains open, and subject to all the worries raised by Frances.[119] In a related thread, having a vice-laden condition isn't relieved simply by having bioexplanations. A criminal with an explained brain is still a criminal, until we change the social criteria for criminality. For help with determining whether vice-laden disorders should be disorders, we'll need to look at places other than biological ones.

The behavioral addiction proposal also raises the issue of the role of behavioral learning in the determination of disorder status. Let's say that people with behavioral addictions (pick your favorite pleasure) are found to rearrange their neurobiology because of repeated seeking and exposure to the pleasurable stimulus. That is, as McHugh and Slavney[120] suggest, addiction may be best understood as a learned behavior a la Skinnerian operant conditioning. Because, at least according to Skinner and colleagues, all of us have some potential for operant learning, and mammalian studies suggest the potential for compulsive ingestion and physical dependence on alcohol, cocaine, and opioids in all tested and unmanipulated (e.g., no gene knockouts) mammals, it stands to reason that most likely drug addictions arise in mostly intact brains and that neurobiological abnormalities are acquired through repeated use, rather than solely given through a biological endowment.[121] If Skinner is right, we acquire addiction behaviors through entrainment by habit with a (previously) normal brain. If true, the implications here for vice-laden addictive disorders is they are acquired by choice and volition, which could be construed as a failure of virtue.

3.3.2.4 Political Apathy Disorder

White[122] proposes a new diagnostic category for the DSM, 'Political Apathy Disorder'. The use of 'Political' here is specified to refer not to party politics but how 'resources of a society are managed'.[123] The core of the disorder is 'a pervasive pattern of failing to help reduce the suffering of others (particularly the underprivileged, oppressed, and poor) combined with overconsumption of society's limited resources'. White proposes a set of diagnostic criteria, including distress and impairment, along with a rating scale. White seems to explicitly endorse classification of failures of virtue as mental disorders when he writes:

> ... failure to achieve the characteristics necessary to live a constructive moral life that bene-fits society should be considered grounds for inclusion in the diagnostic nomenclature.[124]

As a failure of Charity, sufferers from 'Political Apathy Disorder' have vices, and indeed, it appears for White that such vices should be treated.

3.3.3 Omissions: having some serious fun with 'potential' categories of VLBS

Up until this point, 'commissions'—the inclusion or consideration of vice-laden categories has occupied this book's analysis. At this stage I walk a delicate line to indicate what might be called cautionary satire, hence 'serious fun'. While the putative categories may not be serious, much can be learned by considering them as possible DSM categories regardless.

Since DSM-III in 1980, the DSMs have lent themselves to satire by mock-disorder contrivances, casually and in print. One of the recent send-ups of the DSM turned out to generate sincere reader response about the seriousness of the problem. Ivan Goldberg, in an online mental health forum, contrived an 'Internet Gaming Disorder' as a mockery of the DSM, and his prank backfired when he got responses from sufferers.[125] (Indeed, in 2008, the issue of 'internet addiction' had already been raised for DSM-V.)[126] Public distress may be real, though it may not be due to a bona fide mental disorder. The story of Goldberg's 'Internet Gaming Disorder' is a cautionary tale: it demonstrates the embarrassing reality of the ease of medicalizing any undesirable mental/behavioral trait into an intuitively plausible candidate for a DSM mental disorder.[127] In this section I elaborate on this problem by considering some noncandidates for DSM inclusion—would-be cautionary tales about new diagnostic proposals.

My practice of the virtue of prudence fails me when I, with academic legitimacy and sincerity, consider what vice-laden categories might be, or could have been, in a DSM. So while the following are not serious proposals (at least at this point), their presentation points out some interesting omissions in the DSM approach to vice-laden disorders and point to some credible sociological hypotheses about what counts as a mental disorder.

3.3.3.1 White-collar antisociality

I'm grateful for Karen Maschke PhD of the Hastings Center for offering me 'stock market insider trading disorder' (which may be a subtype of 'white-collar psychopathy' or a 'Bernie Madoff syndrome'[128]) over a glass of wine at the 2009 American Society of Bioethics & Humanities annual meeting. One might speculate that the distress and disability associated with these conditions might have correlated with 2010 Congressional limits on corporate CEO bonuses.[129] More seriously, these would-be conditions are remarkable for their redistribution of DSM vice demographics. That is, moving DSM vice conditions away from the allegedly violent urban poor and into the curtain-wall skyscrapers of corporate malfeasance. Geoffrey White, of 'Political Apathy Disorder' fame, remarks about the latter trend in the abovementioned 2004 paper, while Hill and Maughan,[130] in a scholarly review of the psychosocial context of Conduct Disorder, characterizes disorders of conduct as having 'the strongest associations with psychosocial adversity'. The legitimate historical, nosological, and sociological question raised by 'Stock Market Insider Trading Disorder' is why wrongdoing by the urban wealthy tends to fall outside the current criteria for DSM vice-laden categories. One wonders about the possible pathologizing of the urban poor, leading to concerns about institutional racism as well. On the flip side, white male/white-collar offenders have to contend with the problem of having to be caught with your vice before it can be entered into a diagnostic formulation. Perhaps the slick psychopaths of the world evade detection and treatment through their 'successes'.

3.3.3.2 Sloth and Gluttony Disorders

Earlier I pointed to the relevance of the cultural tropes of the Seven Deadly Sins, recognizing that some of the seven were better represented in the DSM than others. One the most DSM-neglected Deadly Sins is 'Sloth', and given the widespread problem behavior described by sloth and its relatives (indolence and laziness to name two), one might postulate a Sloth Disorder and even link it to current youth-culture tropes (e.g., 'Slacker Disorder'). One might imagine Sloth Disorder intercorrelating with other health problems, notably obesity and deconditioning-related syndromes. If so, Sloth Disorder, through its connection to obesity, might well be one of the most important public health problems in a contemporary lexicon of mental disorders.

I wish I could claim to be the first to think of Sloth Disorder. In writing this I did a quick search on the Web, and to my dismay I found again that I'm just a Johnny-come-lately, and found an opinion piece on the Men of Order website [131] raising the issue, and an article by colleagues at my own institution in *Trends in Endocrinology and Metabolism* that raises the question of the link of Gluttony and Sloth to the metabolic syndrome and lipotoxicity.[132] This work raises the question whether Sloth and Gluttony should be lumped together as a Gluttony and Sloth Disorder, subtyped out, or perhaps split into a Sloth Disorder and a Gluttony Disorder. But these questions depend upon whether you are a 'lumper' or a 'splitter' in taxonomy!

This cautionary fable reminds us that vices have molecular-biological implications, as they always have, and that the fallacy of bioexplanation can be found just about anywhere vice and disease are discussed together.

It turns out that Sloth may have a historical precedent in DSM-III-R, where the Diagnostic Criteria for Passive-Aggressive Personality Disorder at least partially overlap with the Sloth concept. Table 3.5 excerpts the DSM-III-R criteria, while none discuss sloth, laziness, indolence, or the like, the individual described might well be

Table 3.5 DSM-IIIR Diagnostic Criteria for 301.84 Passive-Aggressive Personality Disorder

A pervasive pattern of passive resistance to demands for adequate social and occupational performance . . . as indicated by at least *five* of the following:

(1) procrastinates . . .

(2) becomes sulky, irritable, or argumentative [with unwanted tasks]

(3) seems to work deliberately slowly or to do a bad job [with unwanted tasks]

(4) [false claims of others' unreasonable work demands]

(5) avoids obligations . . .

(6) [false confidence in the quality of one's work]

(7) resents useful suggestions . . .

(8) . . . failing to do his, her, or their share of the work

(9) [critical] of authority

the kind of person Pope Gregory I had in mind when he adapted *acedia* or sloth into his list of Seven Deadly Sins.[133]

Passive-Aggressive Personality Disorder didn't make the cut to be a full-fledged disorder in DSM-IV, much less DSM-5. In DSM-IV; this condition was relegated to the appendix on 'Criteria Sets and Axes Provided for Further Study'.[134]

3.3.3.3 Pathological industry

From sloth one might consider a pathological excess of the virtue of diligence. I have called the idea of working to excess 'pathological industry' here, and we might recognize this condition as an 'overwork disorder' or possibly, a 'burnout disorder'. Here is one condition that is commonly recognized, yet so far has been neglected in the DSM-5 axis. 'Professional burnout' as listed in MEDLINE generates 5655 hits as of September 2010, and in PsychINFO under 'occupational stress' + 'burnout' as search terms I found 11,622 hits. These findings would seem to suggest a psychological syndrome involving distress, disability, and impairment[135] that we may know more about than many current DSM categories.

Maslach et al., authors of a commonly used assessment instrument, the Maslach Burnout Inventory, define 'burnout' as:

> . . . a psychological syndrome of emotional exhaustion, depersonalization, and reduced personal accomplishment that can occur among individuals who work with other people in some capacity. A key aspect of the burnout syndrome is increased feelings of emotional exhaustion; as emotional resources are depleted, workers feel they are no longer able to give of themselves at a psychological level. Another aspect of the burnout syndrome is the development of depersonalization (i.e., negative, cynical attitudes and feelings about one's clients). This callous or even dehumanized perception of others can lead staff members to view their clients as somehow deserving of their troubles. The prevalence of this negative attitude toward clients among human service workers has been well documented.[136]

An examination of the burnout literature reveals a substantial number of publications concerning academic medicine as the workplace of interest.[137] The syndrome appears to be endemic in academic medicine from administrator to faculty to student, as well as common among service industries in general, and is on the rise.[138]

One cannot help but wonder why this condition has not been considered in the DSMs. Perhaps this one hits a little too close to home for doctors and nosologists. Physician, heal thyself![139]

One might imagine other possibilities, indeed endless possibilities, for additional potential vice-laden DSM categories. For the sake of space and focus, we should move on to other conceptual considerations.

3.3.4 Omissions conclusions

The question of why some conditions come to gain consideration as DSM disorders and others is not a question for a historian, nor for a philosopher of psychiatry. Even for a historian in the seat of such a query, contemporary understanding is limited for the best of historians because of the lack of a historical (past) perspective. For contemporary analysis we need a cadre of sociologists; the whys and why-nots of vice-laden category inclusion would make for a real sociological mystery story.

What are the lessons of this discussion of vice-laden conditions that, as yet, have not made it into the DSM lexicon?

Perhaps the most important one is a recognition of an arbitrariness or perhaps even capriciousness about the appearance, or lack thereof, of DSM bona fide disorders. While conditions that meet the DSM definition of mental disorder AND meet some scientific standards of validity and reliability are important for consideration, categories like 'occupational stress' or 'burnout' teach us that scientific credibility is not crucial or perhaps, not even relevant. One would be tempted to claim monosymptomatic disorders like pathological bias or pathological industry would be disqualified because of comorbidity and overlap problems, but that doesn't seem to have resulted in the rejection of longstanding disorders like Kleptomania, Intermittent Explosive Disorder, or the various Paraphilias. As a white-collar psychopathy cluster of conditions prompts us, one wonders about the role of socioeconomic factors, power relations, and race and other kinds of discrimination as relevant to what sort of conditions get classified and which ones do not. Perhaps most of all it is not simple wrongdoing that qualifies some vice-laden conditions to appear in the DSM; indeed, not even qualifying as a mental disorder may be a requirement, as the putative Paraphilias/Paraphilic Disorders distinction in DSM-5 illustrates. The DSMs have no real policy approach to vice-laden conditions, and one can only conclude that one is needed if the variability of the medicalization of vice is to be managed.

3.4 Impoverished criteria, impoverished categories

One can consider the development of a descriptive diagnostic criteria set as an elaborate definition of a condition, and as such, the writing of diagnostic criteria serves as a philosophical-conceptual enterprise informed by the available empirical facts about the putative category. Like inclusion and exclusion criteria for prospective subjects in clinical research studies, diagnostic criteria delimit a population of people into those who exhibit the features (variables) of interest and exclude those who do not exhibit features (variables) that confound or otherwise don't belong to the putative category or concept.[140] Some thinkers in psychology, most notably Meehl,[141] emphasize that a role for theory in formulating testable psychological constructs is precisely in defining and delimiting concepts to be tested.

3.4.1 Richer and poorer criteria sets

A non-disorder example is illustrative, and indeed so classic its sources are obscure and is a standard in philosophy courses. Let's say the category we want to define and study is 'bachelors'. We want to capture the population of all 'bachelors' by developing 'diagnostic criteria' or a definitional construct, just like we want to write criteria for a diagnostic category that captures *all* examples of the disorder and eliminate (or at least minimize) false positives and false negatives.

A 'bachelor' is an unmarried man, right? Yes, and indeed if we had a single rule, a 'monocharacteristic', of the form 'Diagnose all unmarried men as bachelors', we would probably capture all bachelors. However, we would also capture a number of men that do not fit our conventional understanding of bachelors. Depending on when we think male children become men, we might capture some children by not specifying an age or maturity criterion. We would likely capture a bunch of widowers and divorced men because our definition doesn't exclude previously married men. We'd also capture some priests and men with other unmarried cultural roles that would test our boundary of bachelorhood. We'd also capture a lot of homosexual men, especially prior to the days of gay marriage. Including gay men as bachelors would seem to challenge the concept of bachelorhood as well. We need a richer criteria set.

The point of this example is we can get into trouble in defining a human condition too simply and with too few qualifiers and descriptors. The qualifiers identified for bachelors above could be adapted into diagnostic inclusion/exclusion criteria, and while likely not perfect, would eliminate, willy-nilly, a huge number of false-positive and false-negative diagnoses. That's the way diagnostic criteria sets should be written—with careful inclusion and exclusion criteria. Moreover, the diagnostic criteria should not simply restate or reformulate previous criteria, but identify distinctive clinical features that aggregate with other distinctive features.

Happily, the majority of the categories in the post-DSM-III era often exhibit these features, and this may be one of the primary reasons for the relative success of these manuals, especially in the setting of clinical research, where the DSM categories, if used rigorously, serve to reduce false positives and false negatives in research samples and thereby eliminate many confounding variables in research samples.

A second benefit comes with a rich, detailed, inclusion and exclusion- criteria set. This benefit is that detailed criteria diminish interdiagnostician disagreement, or increase 'interrater reliability'. The problem of diagnostic reliability was a primary motivator for the development of DSM-III as it did,[142] using 'operationalized' diagnostic criteria. How do multiple criteria in a set help reliability? Through reducing the involved diagnostic judgments of applicability. If we did not have a diagnostic rule for priests, some diagnosticians would diagnose the priest as a bachelor, while some others would not, compromising reliability.

As scientists have learned more about mental disorders, they have realized that phenotypes (observable characteristics) have limited utility in selecting patients for psychiatric research. This has led to a (largely) biological system theoretical structure of psychiatric research, the RDoC approach, which would require a substantial digression to discuss—and which I will simply acknowledge here.[143]

3.4.2 The impoverishment of vice-laden criteria sets

While the post-DSM-II manuals made strides in enriching diagnostic rules through reducing false positives and negatives and increasing interdiagnostician reliability, their wisdom was too often absent when vice-laden diagnostic categories were considered. Consider the comparison of the DSM-5 diagnostic criteria for Pedophilic Disorder[144] against the DSM-5 diagnostic criteria for Schizophrenia.[145] What is immediately evident is the greatly enriched and much more detailed criteria set for the Schizophrenia category. One might imagine that Pedophilic Disorder, with its core symptoms being (debatably) two, fantasies and acts, might prove to be an unreliable category with 'phenomenological heterogeneity' (i.e., would capture a wide range of individuals who may, or may not, represent what we mean when we consider the range of patients with disordered pedophilic behaviors). A variety of authors have noted substantive phenomenological heterogeneity for past/present DSM pedophilias and disorders.[146] While Schizophrenia certainly has its own phenomenological heterogeneity,[147] the narrowly circumscribed diagnostic criteria for this condition may well have permitted the growing recognition of the etiological heterogeneity of this (likely) group of disorders.[148]

I have described these kinds of criteria sets as impoverished, meaning that the criteria sets have only a few positive symptoms and few-to-no exclusionary criteria. DSM-5 disorder groupings that exhibit frequent impoverishment of diagnostic criteria for particular disorders include the Paraphilic Disorders,[149] the Impulse Control Disorders,[150] and Factitious Disorders[151] many of which qualify as vice-laden syndromes.

Why are some criteria sets impoverished, and others not? This has not been explicitly addressed in the literature, though a recent query to Allen Frances[152] supports some of the hypotheses offered here. First, the detail of criteria sets may represent the quirks or philosophical viewpoints of particular disorder Work Groups. That is, some Work Groups' consensus may have crystallized around shorter sets compared to others, taking into consideration other values like simplicity and brevity in formulating their criteria sets. Second, the impoverished criteria set may mirror a more impoverished research base or interest in research in classification for that particular group of disorders. The state of knowledge for some disorders may be small and insufficient information about clinical features, comorbidities, and etiology precludes more detailed criteria sets. Third, the impoverished criteria sets may genuinely reflect a paucity of co-occurring symptoms or signs. Fourth, the impoverished criteria may be a consequence of poorly describing a condition which is more suitable to a larger, more encompassing behavioral syndrome. The Paraphilic Disorders may simply not have many other symptoms other than fantasies and target behaviors.[153] However, this latter reflects on other issues to be discussed below, namely the problem of how to manage 'monosymptomatic' conditions and how such conditions fit into a diagnostic nosology: As primary disorders? As clinical features of a more encompassing disorder? As etiologically or phenomenologically heterogeneous categories awaiting further clarification and research?

The problem with phenomenologically impoverished categories and criteria sets is illustrated by the introductory fallacies associated with the 'bachelor' category. With general, encompassing criteria sets one risks capturing truly heterogeneous groups. Using the example of Pedophilic Disorder, casting a wide diagnostic net may include, and probably does include patients with substantial comorbidities,[154] patients with primary disorders of which pedophilic behaviors are secondary phenomena,[155] and substantive overlaps with other, in this case, criminal offenses.[156]

With this background, the Gender and Sexual Disorders Work Group for DSM-5 made some modest progress in this regard by adding criteria to the Paraphilic Disorder sets. For example, for Pedophilic Disorder, viewing of child pornography had been proposed as a diagnostic criterion.[157] However, this example raises is own difficulties. This addition may be more aimed at addressing detection or ascertainment issues in diagnostic criteria—the pedophilic offender may be motivated to obscure or lie about his mental life and behaviors in order to avoid punishment, constraints, recognition, or clinical care. If so, evidence of child-porn viewing—an operational criterion—may well diminish the ascertainment problem. However, with perfect ascertainment of symptoms, the correlation between pedophilic use of child pornography might overlap heavily with fantasies, and in this sense simply duplicates the fantasy as a phenomenological feature, adding nothing to diversifying clinical features of the syndrome. The false-positive and false-negative problems would still persist because distinctive features have not yet been identified, and no distinctive inclusion and exclusion criteria have been added. To make Pedophilic Disorder a true primary disorder, distinctive phenomenological features, etiological features, exclusionary criteria, and robust endophenotypic features would be most persuasive. In Chapter 4 we'll consider the legacy of 'monomanias' in classical psychiatric diagnosis,[158] and how this relates to our problem of impoverished criteria sets.

3.5 Hierarchy and comorbidity

In the recent DSMs, diagnostic categories have a hierarchical structure—some symptoms and disorders are higher-order and 'trump' other symptoms or disorders. For DSM-IV-TR and 5, three sorts of encompassing hierarchical commitments are made: the first rule could be stated as 'when faced with a psychiatric syndrome thought to be caused by substance use or abuse, diagnose the condition as secondary to substance abuse'. The second rule could be stated 'when faced with a psychiatric syndrome thought to be caused by a general medical condition, diagnose the psychiatric syndrome as secondary to the general medical condition'. The DSM-5 categories associated with these hierarchical rules are many, from Alcohol Withdrawal Delirium (292.0) to Major or Mild Neurocognitive Disorder Due to Another Medical Condition (331.83).[159] The third rule is less amenable to a simple statement, and therefore is not really a rule, but a trend. Some disorders have required, as an added qualifier in the criteria, the clinical features described in the other diagnostic criteria be 'not due to another disorder'. In many cases, this qualifier is intended to confirm the prior rules, as in DSM-5 Schizophrenia, where the E criterion reads:

> E. The disturbance is not attributable to the physiological effects of a substance (e.g., a drug of abuse, a medication) or another medical condition.[160]

In other places, the hierarchical rules imply that come conditions should be considered primary disorders, as in these D and E criteria for DSM-5 Major Depressive Disorder, Single Episode.[161]

The E criterion's rule promotes the diagnosis of Bipolar Disorder if a patient has both manic symptoms and depressive symptoms, and in this way assures that Bipolar Disorder is a 'primary' diagnosis, not just 'major depression with manic features'.

Outside of these sorts of hierarchical rules, the DSM-5 permits a large amount of comorbidities, that is, the diagnosis of multiple disorders in a single patient. For example, a patient could be diagnosed with Schizophrenia, Alcohol Use Disorder, and Antisocial Personality Disorder. The inconsistences in criteria and hierarchical rules in the DSMs have been cause for other discussions, though not particularly germane to my purposes here.[162]

3.5.1 Hierarchy and vice-laden conditions

The inclusion of hierarchy rules likely reflect the DSM architects' relative confidence that some disorders are primary etiologically (e.g., substance induced or medical disease induced). In the case of the parsing of the mood disorders, these judgments may be equally related to the desire to protect a category like Bipolar Disorder as a unique entity to stimulate more studies to adequately characterize it as a primary disorder. The DSM-IV-TR architects, however, were cautious rather than confident about applying hierarchical issues broadly, and laid out the significance of 'comorbidity' in these six relationships:[163]

1. Condition A may cause or predispose to condition B.
2. Condition B may cause or predispose to condition A.
3. An underlying condition C may cause or predispose to both condition A and condition B.

4. Conditions A and B may in fact be part of a more complex unified syndrome that has been artificially split in the diagnostic system.
5. The relationship between conditions A and B may be artifactually enhanced by definitional overlap.
6. The presence of conditions A and B may be a chance co-occurrence, which may be particularly likely for those conditions that have high base rates.

'High base rates' means here that conditions A and B are common, active conditions.

One can consider hierarchy rules as systematized exclusionary criteria. For instance, we exclude individuals with schizophrenia-like symptoms who have been abusing methamphetamine from the diagnosis of schizophrenia. What significance do hierarchical rules and comorbidities have for vice-laden conditions? We can consider, for the sake of simplicity, a couple of disorders, Pedophilic Disorder and Intermittent Explosive Disorder.

3.5.1.1 The example of Pedophilic Disorder

A substantive literature supports the idea that other conditions may cause or predispose to DSM-5 Pedophilic Disorder as in Frances, First, and Pincus's six relationships above. Because most of this research was done before DSM-5, under the older 'Pedophilia' diagnosis, I'll retain the older language in this discussion. A common finding is neuropsychological impairment has been found to be common in individuals with pre-DSM-5 Pedophilia.[164] Blanchard et al.[165] reported a disproportionate share of head injuries before age 13 years in pedophilic males over controls, as his group did in an earlier study.[166] Cohen et al.[167] found similarities in personality traits in pedophilic males and abstinent opioid-dependent patients, noting psychopathic traits and propensities for cognitive distortions. The research group concluded by asserting this evidence supported the idea of pedophilia as a behavioral addiction, sympathetic to work by Stein, Black, and Pienaar[168] as well as prior work from her group.[169] Some work has supported the potential for impulsivity as a core symptom in pedophilia.[170] Other neuropsychological abnormalities have been detected, including links with cortical-amygdaloid abnormalities.[171] Finally, a number of studies suggest that pedophilia, rather than being a distinct entity, is rather an option in a range of erotic preferences[172] as well as one pattern in a repertoire of sex-offender behaviors and demographics.[173] So is pedophilia a variation of a neuropsychological syndrome, a behavioral addiction, a variety of impulse-control disorder, or a subtype of a global disorder of sexual compulsion? Like the unspecified bachelor as an unmarried male, the pedophilia construct is broadly defined and therefore admits all kinds of people.

One should note that many of these studies are intended to identify biomarkers, phenotypes, and/or etiological features rather than validate or invalidate a diagnostic category. Finding a biological correlate, in itself, is not particularly helpful in validating a diagnostic construct if the putative validator does not discriminate the proposed construct from other constructs or other conditions. What these data do support is that pedophilia is both a phenomenologically and etiologically heterogeneous condition—not surprising given the impoverishment of the diagnostic criteria!

These data may also be consistent with an underlying condition, distinct from the pedophilia syndrome that may be driving 'pedophilia' as a variation—as described by Frances, First, and Pincus' Relationship 3, as well as a broader nosological construct, of which 'pedophilia' is a variation, as in their Relationship 4. More research is needed to find out what clinical features, if any, discriminate pedophilia from other conditions (or no clinical conditions) and, therefore, help develop discriminant validity, as well as what clinical features, if any, predict outcomes, responses to treatment, or other biological, psychological, or social features—predictive validity.[174]

The DSM-5 Sexual and Gender Identity Disorders Work Group has made a few proposed steps forward in setting the stage for more discriminant and predictive validity for Pedophilia through the breakdown of the Paraphilias into conditions and disorders (e.g., as in Pedophilia and Pedophilic Disorder), as well as adding an additional diagnostic indicator (use of child pornography), and the consideration of penile plethysmography as a laboratory diagnostic indicator[175] albeit the latter has been controversial as a DSM formal criterion.[176] As it stands, Paraphilias like Pedophilia are stuck with substantive comorbidities, raising the question of their place in the hierarchy of disorders, and whether they should be considered primary disorders, secondary disorders, or incidental features of other disorders.

The diagnostic splitting of Paraphilias/Paraphilic Disorders, however promising, does not address the issue of collecting a series of independent validators for clinical syndromes.[177] This means that good diagnostic indicators should not simply 'restate' a clinical feature, but rather identify qualitatively different clinical features.[178] In the case of Schizophrenia, flattening of affect, alogia, delusions, auditory hallucinations, and neglect of hygiene are qualitatively different, and relatively distinct, indicators. If they indeed quantitatively segregate 'schizophrenia' from other disorders, then they are empirically useful validators. In the case of Pedophilia, having fantasies about sex with children, having sex with children, viewing and masturbating to child pornography, and having penile erections in response to child sexual materials are all variations on the same phenomenological theme. A similar mistake, perpetuated upon Schizophrenia diagnostic criteria, might present three diagnostic indicators (1) 'experiencing auditory hallucinations', (2) 'being preoccupied with auditory hallucinations', and (3) 'expressing concerns about voices to others'. In both cases, criteria simply redescribe the same core phenomenon in different ways and do little to help one discriminate different kinds of conditions and predict future phenomena.

Are impoverished diagnostic criteria a problem only for vice-laden syndromes? No, but it just happens, as we noted, vice-laden syndromes just have too many categories with impoverished criteria, limiting their validity as constructs.

3.5.1.2 The example of Intermittent Explosive Disorder

Intermittent Explosive Disorder (IED) provides an interesting contrast case for the issue of diagnostic hierarchies. Like Pedophilia, IED has substantive comorbidities, and its role as a primary or secondary disorder is at question. However, unlike Pedophilia, its literature is more diverse, ranging from comorbidity studies, to nosological and epidemiological studies, to examination of a range of genetic, neurobehavioral, imaging, and psychological validators, to treatment studies. The psychiatric literature on IED of the past 25 years has been dominated by Emil F. Coccaro at the University of Chicago. Coccaro and colleagues have pursued what they call 'impulsive aggression' with missionary zeal,[179] performing an extraordinary range of studies on the phenomenon of impulsive aggression, utilizing a range of scientific research designs, theoretical constructs, and measures.[180]

Coccaro is critical of the manner in which IED has been classified since DSM-I on up through DSM-IV-TR. His research criteria for IED appear to have significantly influenced the DSM-5 criteria for the condition, however. He has presented a careful conceptual critique of DSM-III through DSM-IV-TR criteria for IED in several publications.[181] Key to the approach to IED is the distinction between 'impulsive aggression' and what he calls 'premeditated' aggression.[182] Impulsive aggression is unplanned, reactive, grossly out of proportion to any provocation, and not goal-oriented in the sense of having an objective for the violence. While not explicitly discussed, 'premeditated' aggression is likened to 'criminal' aggression[183] citing Barratt, Stanford, Felthous, and Kent,[184] Premeditated aggression is planned, deliberate, and goal-directed.[185]

Coccaro's critique of pre-DSM-5 concepts of IED has four themes. The themes are listed below, along with their putative rationales, as well as the potential effect on the pool of IED patients:

(1) The severity of the aggressive acts should be specified, as much as is feasible, in an operational manner. The specification serves to guide clinicians about what counts as explosive impulsive aggression, and thus both avoid false positives (including episodes of minor severity) and false negative (identifying threshold cases of explosive episodes). The impact on the pool of IED patients in respecting this guideline is unclear, as avoiding false positives reduces the epidemiological pool of patients, and avoiding false negatives increases the pool of patients. The net effect is an empirical question.

(2) A minimal frequency of explosive episodes should be specified, so as to set apart frequent episodes of impulsive aggression from occasional ones (to diminish false positives and thus reducing the pool of IED patients).

(3) The diagnosis of impulsive aggression should admit (not exclude) less severe instances of impulsive aggression apart from those 'explosive' episodes, as explosive behaviors are commonly accompanied by less severe impulsive aggression. Because explosive cases commonly have less severe instances of impulsive aggression, including them diminishes false negatives, and the effect of this change should be to increase the pool of diagnosed IED patients.

(4) Most relevant to the hierarchy issue, Personality Disorders such as Antisocial and Borderline Personality Disorders should NOT be exclusionary criteria because, in Coccaro's interpretation of the literature, there is no empirical basis to claim Personality Disorders 'trump' IED or other impulse control disorders. By removing this set of exclusions, the effect should be to reduce false-negative diagnoses and increase the pool of diagnosed IED patients.[186]

Barring dramatic empirical effects from Theme 1 in favor of reducing the pool of affected individuals, these principles, encoded in Coccaro's Research Criteria for IED (Table 3.6) should increase the pool of people with IED, and perhaps substantially, which turns out to be the case so far.[187]

Coccaro's rewritten IED criteria move in a desirable direction from the perspective of adding specifiers that help to homogenize the pool of diagnosed IED patients. The research criteria help to enrich the IED criteria and, while perhaps casting a wider net, the net effects would be a more reliable population of IED patients. The question of validity is also one that Coccaro has tackled, with variable, but on balance, positive results to my reading.

Coccaro's version of IED remains a vice-laden diagnosis, but the question remains whether IED should be a mental disorder, a complication of some mental disorder(s), or simply personal misconduct. His groups' and other mounting sets of studies showing increasing validity for his research IED construct and raise interesting policy questions for Chapter 9.

Table 3.6 Coccaro's Research Criteria for Intermittent Explosive Disorder

A. Recurrent incidents of aggression are manifest as verbal or physical aggression toward other people, animals, or property occurring twice weekly on average for 1 month.

B. The degree of aggressiveness expressed is grossly out of proportion to the provocation or any precipitating psychosocial stressors.

C. The aggressive behavior is generally not premeditated (e.g., is impulsive) and is not committed in order to achieve some tangible objective (e.g., money, power, and intimidation).

D. The aggressive behavior causes either marked distress in the individual or impairment in occupational or interpersonal functioning.

E. The aggressive behavior is not better accounted for by another mental disorder (e.g., Major Depressive/Manic/Psychotic Disorder; Attention-Deficit Hyperactivity Disorder), general medical condition (e.g., head trauma, Alzheimer's disease), or to the direct physiologic effects of a substance.

3.6 Metaphysical ambiguities

The Cambridge Dictionary of Philosophy, Second Edition,[189] defines 'metaphysics' as 'most generally, the philosophical investigation of the nature, constitution, and structure of reality ...'. For my purposes, 'metaphysical ambiguities' have to do with particular viewpoints about the nature of being human (ontology) and how we are to gain credible knowledge about reality (epistemology). Fundamental metaphysical questions include statements of the mind-body problem ('How is it that something immaterial, like the "mind" is connected to something material, the "body"?'), and questions about what is, and how to obtain knowledge. Metaphysical questions are prescientific in the sense that they address questions that science cannot answer, and indeed, provide the background assumptions for science to build upon. Science cannot answer a metaphysical question like What is evidence? because a fundamental tool of science—evidence—is presupposed in science's methods.

The key questions for this book are, at root, metaphysical: Are mental disorders moral? Do moral judgments belong in judgments of disease or disorders? If they do, how? Is wrongful conduct a disease? If not a disease, then what kind of thing is immoral or wrongful conduct?

3.6.1 Folk metaphysics and the DSMs

Perhaps the starting point for considering the metaphysical ambiguities is to recognize how metaphysical issues are situated in the DSMs. I've noted in *Values and Psychiatric Diagnosis*[190] that the DSM and ICD authors are not philosophers or metaphysical theorists, and, therefore, the kinds of metaphysical frameworks and assumptions made by them must represent a kind of 'folk metaphysics'.[191] A folk metaphysics is, at root, a bundle of culturally received set of assumptions about the nature of reality and human existence. As culturally assumed and taken for granted, folk-metaphysical assumptions may or may not, under scrutiny, be consistent and credible.

Folk metaphysics should be distinguished from philosophical metaphysics, the latter describing a systematic, deliberate effort to address the nature of reality and human existence. With this contrast, folk metaphysics is naive and taken for granted, a cultural 'received view', while philosophical metaphysics may be meticulously built up through years of systematic scholarly effort. So the DSMs' authors are folk metaphysical in that metaphysical assumptions are taken for granted, and not described, deliberated upon, and defended as would be the case in philosophical metaphysics. An example of philosophical metaphysical thinking by clinicians would be Kenneth Kendler's and Peter Zachar's work,[192] and philosophical metaphysics by philosophers would include Hegel, Kant, Hobbes, Heidegger, Hume, and Sartre. However, the focus here is *folk*, not *philosophical*, metaphysics.

The folk metaphysics (FM) of the DSMs play out in a number of ways. A simple example is illustrative for our purposes. The most explicitly relevant way FM plays out is regarding this metaphysical question: 'What kind of thing is a mental disorder?' A FM, conventional answer to this question is that mental disorders are natural kinds, that is, manifestations of deranged biological structure and function like diseases and injuries in physical medicine. Indeed, these FM assumptions are implied by formative DSM theoretical thinking, such as the Robins and Guze five steps to establishing diagnostic validity with mental disorder categories.[193] However, psychoanalysts and other psychotherapy theorists have argued that mental disorders are 'meaningful kinds' having to do with narratives, communications, ideas, schemata, introjects, and other manifestations of thinking, emoting, speaking, and relating to others.[194] From these two simple standpoints, mental disorders can be manifestations of Nature, and they can be manifestations of social-psychological communicative interactions. In a FM, this tension between two different kinds of things is ignored, or simply dismissed ('It's obvious they're both!') or naively reconciled ('Social relationships depend on the brain and therefore mental disorders are natural/biological.') In short, FM is presupposed, taken for granted, and largely unquestioned, as has been the case for the DSMs (excepting, of course, some philosophical studies of the DSMs performed by philosophers of psychiatry!).

This philosophical naivete in the folk-metaphysical DSMs, however, is mostly as it should be. Scientists, nosologists, and practitioners cannot formulate every scientific or clinical move based upon a rigorously thought-out metaphysical calculus. Nothing would ever get finished, as philosophers have been arguing metaphysics for (literally) millennia! However, as I hoped to demonstrate in *VAPD* and again here, recalcitrant problems in psychiatry and psychiatric diagnosis and classification suggest that more deliberate reflection is needed for the DSM's metaphysical assumptions and commitments.

When one takes seriously this dualism between mental-disorders-as-natural, and mental-disorders-as-social, one is getting into the realm of philosophical metaphysics. While the more crucial philosophizing about mental disorders will be left to later, nonbackground chapters, framing the metaphysical issues for the purposes of clarity may be useful at this stage of the book. The concept of FM will come up again in Chapter 8 and be elaborated in an effort to help understand both professional and lay attitudes and beliefs about mental illness and criminal conduct. This metaphysical ambiguity, what kind of things are mental illness, immorality, and criminality, will be examined in light of history in the next chapter, and in the realm of contemporary practice and policy, in the concluding chapters.

3.6.2 The DSM definition of a mental disorder—does it help with the VMDR?

A perhaps obvious place to start in consider the metaphysical ambiguities of the VMDR is with the DSM definition of 'mental disorder'. The focused question here is: Does the DSM-5) definition of 'mental disorder' help clarify the VMDR?

The DSM-5 definition of 'mental disorder' is reproduced here:[195]

A mental disorder is a syndrome characterized by clinically significant disturbance in an individual's cognition, emotion regulation, or behavior that reflects a dysfunction in the psychological, biological, or developmental processes underlying mental functioning. Mental disorders are usually associated with significant distress or disability in social, occupational, or other important activities. An expectable or culturally approved response to a common stressor or loss, such as the death of a loved one, is not a mental disorder. Socially deviant behavior (e.g., political, religious, or sexual) and conflicts that are primarily between the individual and society are not mental disorders unless the deviance or conflict results from a dysfunction in the individual, as described above.[196]

I provided a substantive discussion in *VAPD* about the DSM-IV definition of disorder and the problem of vice.[197] The gist of the problem is that 'dysfunction', still utilized in the DSM-5 definition, is employed to address which behaviors are 'in the individual'[198] and which are 'primarily a conflict between the individual and society'.[199] The problem is the concept of dysfunction has so far failed to make this distinction in any practical way. The problem is the manner of determining how dysfunction is 'in' the individual remains ambiguous. The approach of Jerome Wakefield, which appears to be the most favored one by DSM insiders, appeals to the findings of an evolutionary biology/psychology to ground dysfunction. Wakefield wants to ground dysfunction in the failure of evolved biopsychological mechanisms. The problem is in the application of Wakefield's approach. Which evolved biopsychological mechanisms are relevant to dysfunction have as yet not been identified, at least without controversy,[200] so the practical utility of Wakefield's account in making nosological decisions is severely limited. While others, including me,[201] have been critical of Wakefield's account for grounding dysfunction, whomever is right in theory ultimately doesn't matter, because the science is not there to support nosological judgments about the evolutionary basis of dysfunctions.

The second difficulty with the DSM definition vis-a-vis the VMDR is the severe difficulty in making practical clinical judgments about whether the patient's distress and impairment is a normative response to adverse social and environmental conditions or a problem 'in' the individual. Is the child with Conduct Disorder having a normative response to abuse, neglect, poverty, and social threat, or does the child with Conduct Disorder have a 'broken brain'?

The third difficulty is both definitions depend too much on causal judgments, and even worse, rely upon negative causal judgments. The clinician must rule out that the behaviors are NOT the result of an expectable (normative) response to a life event, NOT a culturally sanctioned response, and NOT the result of a conflict between an individual and society. These exclusions occur in a manual that is supposed to be 'atheoretical' with regard to etiology. Further, manifold difficulties exist just in ascertaining whether a response is culturally sanctioned. For instance, we don't know when a cultural sanction leaves off, and a legal sanction, as in a criminal offense, begins.

Finally, the demands upon a clinician in making a distinction between internal dysfunctions and culturally sanctioned behaviors is overwhelmingly complex. Consider the horrific stigma suffered by pedophilic offenders, illustrated vividly in the 2006 film Little Children.[202] How can a clinician separate the moral panic[203] associated with sexual predators and the response to sex predator laws?[204] The issue is especially relevant because sexual predators statistically contribute a trivial portion of child molestations.[205]

The metaphysical problem of the VMDR, is, as I've suggested, how the moral figures into concepts of mental disorder. The related ethical question is whether the moral SHOULD figure into concepts of mental disorder. Later in the book I'll be discussing four accounts which neatly frame the metaphysical issues in terms of the VMDR. Because this chapter is raising conceptual issues, I'll introduce these 'metaphysical accounts' of the VMDR here. They'll be important in the final chapters where the 'shoulds' of vice-laden mental disorders are addressed. These accounts are intended to organize and frame the literature, not to be 'straw men' to be set up and then criticized. Mostly these accounts map onto no single approach, author, and viewpoint. Rather, they more carefully describe and sketch how the VMDR has played out in the literature. These four accounts I call the (1) coincidental account, the (2) medicalization account, the (3) moralization account, and (4) mixed accounts.

3.6.3 The coincidental account

The question posed by the VMDR is 'What relationship does vice have to mental disorders?' One kind of relationship of vice to mental disorders is a coincidental relationship. That is, vicious thought and behavior manifests itself as an empirical accident of circumstance. Coincidental relationships occur all the time in ordinary life. I prepare to pull my car out of the garage, and an oncoming vehicle provokes me to delay my exit. The appearance of the other car is a coincidence.

In the domain of mental disorders and especially diagnostic criteria, some of the diagnostic criteria are crucial to the diagnosis, others contribute to the diagnosis but are not required in all cases, and other clinical features are associated with the diagnosis but carry no formal diagnostic weight, at least within the confines of the DSM system. Finally, some clinical occurrences may be purely accidental, and not related to the diagnosis at all. This discussion suggests there are four 'epistemic' kinds of diagnostic features in DSM diagnostic criteria:[206]

Essential diagnostic features: Clinical phenomena that are required for the diagnosis.

Contributory diagnostic features: Clinical phenomena that support a diagnosis, but are not required or invoked in every case.

Associated diagnostic features: Clinical phenomena that co-occur with the disorder, but carry no (formal) diagnostic weight in the diagnostic criteria.

Coincidental diagnostic features: Clinical phenomena that are not diagnostic features at all but accidental phenomena that happened to co-appear in the clinical context.

In DSM-5, the A criterion for a Manic Episode requires the patient to have a 'distinct period of abnormally and persistently elevated, expansive, or irritable mood ...' lasting 1 week or more.[207] This criterion would then be an example of an essential diagnostic feature.

For DSM-5 Manic Episode, the B criterion requires three or more of seven clinical features to meet this criterion, permitting the diagnosis to be made even if all of the seven features are not present.[208] These features include items like grandiosity, decreased need for sleep, and flight of ideas. Distractibility would be a good example of a contributory clinical feature.

In DSM-5, like earlier DSMs, each disorder is accompanied by a section on 'associated features supporting diagnosis'.[209] In the case of the Manic Episode, the DSM authors note that patients 'often do not perceive that they are ill ...' and later note that patients may be 'physically assaultive'. This lack of insight and physically assaultiveness are good examples of associated clinical features. Note that while physical assault could be judged a 'wrongful act', as an associated feature, assault does not contribute to a Manic Episode as a vice-laden mental disorder concept.

Finally, we can, with some amusement, note that wearing Mardi Gras headgear is not listed in the DSM-5 diagnostic criteria, and so as far as the DSM-5 is concerned, wearing of such headgear would be a good example of a coincidental feature. What is notable about this example is that, I would guess, most clinicians treating manic individuals in New Orleans would be able to claim that manic patients wearing Mardi Gras headgear are not only encountered, but perhaps even encountered commonly. Notably this criterion doesn't appear in the DSMs because of its local significance and social determinants, not because it indicates, in itself, a Manic Episode. Clinicians in South Dakota may never encounter a manic patient with Mardi Gras headgear. What this example illustrates, and 'wearing brown shoes' as another coincidental feature doesn't, is that psychiatric diagnosis depends upon multiple clinical features to make a diagnosis, and that clinical features can appear recurrently more as a manifestation of environmental context, even clinical features that are common. More succinctly, even coincidental features can be common, given the proper context. The danger with coincidental features is when diagnosticians become wedded to them because of their constrained world view and limitations of context. Indeed, we could conceive having Mardi Gras headgear as a diagnostic criterion if all the members of the DSM-5 Mood Disorders Work Group were from the New Orleans French Quarter. Allen Frances warns against the danger of provincial interests and experience finding its way into diagnostic criteria,[210] though in the form of research psychiatrists overly devoted to their esoteric worldviews!

This discussion sets the stage for the 'coincidental' account of the VMDR. The account is simple. A substantial number of people may be bank robbers, shoplifters, murderers, or child molesters not *because* they have a mental disorder, but simply happen to have a mental disorder at the time of their wrongdoing. The coincidental account means there is no phenomenological, substantively causal, or other determined relationship between the vice and the mental disorder. Just as men with ingrown toenails and psoriasis can be explosively violent, men with adjustment disorder with antisocial conduct can be explosively violent.

The coincidental account is important because the coincidental account can be mistaken. What appears to be an accident of fate can instead be a causal consequence of a chain of disorder-related events. This is the role of empirical research into associated features of the illness, and the validation of diagnostic criteria against other measures.

To simply use the coincidental account as a model, across the board, for the VMDR however, would be naive. We know that some mental disorders are causally connected with wrongful or immoral conduct, and so a more rigorous and nuanced account is needed.

3.6.4 The medicalization account

More familiar to clinicians will be the 'medicalization' account of the VMDR. While there are a number of definitions of 'medicalization', I prefer my co-authors' straightforward definition from our 2009 discussion: 'Medicalization describes a process by which human problems come to be defined and treated as medical problems.'[211] A detailed argument for our definition appears in that article. To medicalize vice would mean to define and treat wrongful thought and conduct as a medical problem. Immediately we recognize that the stuff of this book is, in large part, about the medicalization of vice. Indeed, a systematic and consistent 'medicalization account' of the VMDR might hold that some, or perhaps all, vice is a manifestation of a mental disorder, and ultimately vicious behavior would be subject to medical treatment and control, scientific advancements permitting.

The only spokesperson I have found in the literature that might endorse such a radical medicalization account as portrayed above might be Adrian Raine, a seasoned and productive investigator into the psychopathology of criminality, and a self-identified 'neurocriminologist'. The following 2001 statement comes very close to endorsing what I'm calling a pure medicalization account:[212]

> Criminal behaviour may be best construed as a neurodevelopmental disorder that arises early in life from a joint product of genetic, biological, and social forces, with conduct disorder as the age-appropriate manifestation of the adult outcome.

I should note that one needn't commit to a biological or other reductionistic account in order to have a medicalization account of the VMDR (e.g., claiming 'criminality

is little more than a disturbed biology'). Indeed, assuming Raine's quote is representative, his medicalization account is complex and multidetermined.[213] However,
characterizing criminal behavior as a neurodevelopmental disorder seems to be
metaphysically coming down on the disorder model of what I would call 'vice'.

What is troubling about a pure medicalization account is the potential for uncon-
trolled, proto-political power on the part of the medical-industrial establishment.
Social problems resulting in social deviance are pathologized, with affected individuals responsible for obtaining treatment. We already are worried about the price of
medicalization, as the growth of healthcare costs appears to be on a trajectory to
exceed our gross national product.[214] Normative conduct could be subject to market
forces even more than it is now, with the concern about rampant drug-company
manufacture of pseudo-disorders.[215]

What makes for the metaphysical ambiguities of the medicalization account is the
inconsistencies and seeming arbitrariness of its implementation in the DSMs. We
should recognize that for all of these accounts, no claims are made that the DSM Task
Force and Work Groups are subscribing to a particular account of the VMDR here.
The DSM Task Forces and Work Groups, as I have described above and elsewhere[216]
are simply acting in accord with their own collective folk-metaphysical assumptions.
Nevertheless, we have an interesting set of vice-laden disorders, with some conspic-
uously absent vice-disorder candidates as noted in earlier sections.

What might a more consistent 'medicalization' account look like? What vice-laden
conditions would qualify for inclusion of the DSMs would likely have to pass the
same sets of barriers and conditions as non-vice-laden conditions have to pass today.
That is, the disorder should, at minimum at an intuitive level, qualify as a mental
disorder as defined by the DSM corpus since DSM-III.[217] The proposed disorder
would need to have some substantive minimum of empirical studies that provide a
basis for the condition having a modicum of validity and reliability, and be clinically
relevant.[218] In this regard, a number of candidates considered earlier might qualify.

3.6.5 The moralization account

In contrast to the medicalization account, where any undesirable or morally objectionable behavior could potentially represent a disorder, the moralization account holds that undesirable or morally objectionable behaviors represent morally
accountable misbehaviors. The moralization account draws a bright line between
sick behavior—behavior that is a result of functional impairments of the brain/
body—and moral conduct that is responsible and autonomous. Under the moralization account, deviant behaviors, and especially deviant behaviors that impinge
on others, would qualify for condemnation as offenses, vices, character faults, or
personal failures—unless, of course, the person committed them under the most
clear-cut of medical circumstances—dementia, brain injury, or delirium. These
offending deviant behaviors may be simple vices, as we have previously discussed,

or they may be frank and deliberate crimes or they may fall into personal failures of virtue, like lying, chronic tardiness, or laziness. Wrongful, immoral, and criminal behaviors would qualify, but, depending on the societal norms, other thoughts and behaviors might qualify, depending on how the society handles particular instances of norm deviance. Homelessness, for instance, might be condemned as the failure to be responsible for job and home. Followers of minority religions may be condemned as soiled, heathen, or infidels. Depression may revert back to its ancient ancestor, 'acedia', meaning 'laxity of industry'.[219] Individuals with dissident political beliefs may be considered a threat to the public welfare. A pure moralization account marginalizes the contribution of disease (physical or mental) or disorder to any form of wrongful conduct. Under a pure moralization account, one can detect the potential for fascism in the suspect nature of nonconformity in any form, and the imposition of the state in behavior control.

The author in the literature that comes closest to presenting a pure moralization account of the VMDR is Thomas Szasz, well-known through his work on 'The Myth of Mental Illness' as article or book.[220] For reasons that I will discuss below, it would be unfair to claim, however, that Szasz would hold a 'pure' moralization account. While Szasz's position is closer to a pure moralization account than mainstream psychiatry's, Szasz does not describe the extreme values discussed above. Indeed, from the biographical perspective, his moralization account emerges in part from his *opposition* to Nazi fascism.[221]

For Szasz, mental illness is a metaphor for 'problems in living', and in this sense, his view of mental illness is not a 'pure' moralization theorist. He thinks people having 'problems of living' are worthy of assistance, whether through the education, criminal justice, or religious systems. He condones, even provides for counseling of people for problems in living, as has been his own practice. My reading of Szasz is not that he is unforgiving of human foibles, however construed, but rather he is unforgiving of ethical lapses being treated as disease:

> The idea that chronic hostility, vengefulness, or divorce are indicative of mental illness would be illustrations of the use of ethical norms (that is, the desirability of love, kindness, and a stable marriage relationship). Finally, the widespread psychiatric opinion that only a mentally ill person would commit homicide illustrates the use of a legal concept as a norm of mental health. The norm from which deviation is measured whenever one speaks of a mental illness is a *psychosocial and ethical one*. Yet, the remedy is sought in terms of *medical* measures which—it is hoped and assumed—are free from wide differences of ethical value. The definition of the disorder and the terms in which its remedy are sought are therefore at serious odds with one another. The practical significance of this covert conflict between the alleged nature of the defect and the remedy can hardly be exaggerated.[222]

He is especially unforgiving about the involuntary seclusion and treatment with 'metaphorical' disease[223]—that is, with psychiatric involuntary seclusion and treatment—and has dedicated his career to opposing such practices.

Both pure medicalization and pure moralization accounts have trouble accommodating the borderland cases of disease versus wrongful conduct. It turns out these borderland cases are where 'vice-laden' disorders dwell. The borderland cases also inhere in more 'mainstream' mental disorders like Schizophrenia and Bipolar Disorder where the affected individual can commit wrongful acts and be subject to an insanity defense. The extremity of pure medicalization and moralization accounts then leads naturally into a status quo which is the 'mixed account'.

3.6.6 The mixed account

The mixed account of the VMDR, as the name implies, involves elements of the prior three accounts. The mixed account is vividly exemplified by the American Psychiatric Association's official views on Pedophilia from a June 17, 2003 Position Statement:

> Pedophilia, included in the American Psychiatric Association's *Diagnostic and Statistical Manual of Mental Disorders* (DSM) since 1968, continues to be classified as a mental disorder. . . . An adult who engages in sexual activity with a child is performing a criminal and immoral act and this is never considered normal or socially acceptable behavior.[224]

Some disorders can be sick AND immoral, which in itself has a certain amount of intuitive appeal. The previously discussed disorders in this book have indicated the ubiquity of the mixed account, and the discussion to date has pointed out the difficulties with the mixed account. What kinds of things are mental disorders? What kinds of things are immoral or criminal acts? The next chapter discusses the answers to these questions in the past.

Notes

1. Sadler (2005).
2. See Sadler (2004) for an extended discussion of the functions of diagnosis.
3. ibid; Sadler (2005).
4. See Berrios (1996); Blashfield (2012); Blashfield et al. (2014); Decker (2013); Millon (2004); and Wallace (1994) for histories of diagnosis and classification in Psychiatry.
5. Blashfield (1984); Frances, First, & Pincus (1995); Wallace (1994); Sadler (2005). More on historical developments will be discussed in the next two chapters.
6. See especially Decker (2013).
7. Decker (2013); Frances, First, & Pincus (1995); Grob (1991); Kirk & Kutchins (1992); Sadler (2005); Wilson 1994. The problem of reliability—the constancy of diagnosis from clinician to clinician and moment to moment—was a major problem. The thinking was that if diagnosis in the DSMs was unreliable, then diagnosis could not be valid (e.g., measure or capture what it was intended to capture).
8. APA (2013).

9. Schwartz & Wiggins (2002).

10. Cuthbert & Insel (2013); Insel (2014); Insel et al. (2010).

11. See Sadler (2005, Ch. 3) for a review of the criticisms of the DSMs as scientific classifications of mental disorders. See also Cooper (2018); Kendler (2013); Nemeroff et al. (2013).

12. Charland (2004).

13. See Charland (2004); Radden (1994, 1996); Radden & Sadler (2010); Sadler (2007).

14. Sadler (2005).

15. APA (1987, 1994); Sadler (2005); Shuman (1989, 2002).

16. Whitehead (1925).

17. Peter Zachar has written a notable book on the issue of realism/antirealism in psychopathology (2014).

18. Philip Slavney (personal communication, 1992).

19. Sadler (2005).

20. Wiggins & Schwartz (2002).

21. Charland (2004).

22. Banzato (2004); Follette & Houts (1996); Harris & Schaffner (1992); Vailliant (1984).

23. Frances, First, & Pincus (1995).

24. Sadler (2005, Ch. 4).

25. Sadler & Hulgus (1994).

26. APA (2013).

27. Salmon & Kitcher (1989).

28. In Sadler (2005), I distinguished by 'universalism' (applying to all cases) and 'particularism' (specifying features of a single case).

29. Peterson & Seligman (2004).

30. Cloninger (2004).

31. Friedli (2009).

32. Davidson (2003); Davidson & Strauss (1992); Tondora, Miller, Slade, & Davidson (2014).

33. Sklar et al. (2013).

34. Zimmerman (1994).

35. Frances (2013).

36. See Blackwell (2017); Conrad (2007); Healy (2002 & 2004); Horwitz & Wakefield (2007); Lane (2008); Mehlman (2009); Rodwin (1993, 2011); Rothman & Rothman (2003); Sadler (2013).

37. Schwartz & Wiggins (2002).

38. Tucker (1998).

39. Kendell (1988).

40. ibid, p. 1301.

41. Blackwell (2017).

42. Sadler (2004, 2005).

43. Sadler & Hulgus (1992).

44. Mezzich (2007).

45. Sadler (2004, 2005).

46. In my 2005 chapter on Technology from *VAPD*, I developed an argument from Heidegger and Albert Borgmann about how our technological world drives our thinking in terms of the values of efficiency, productivity, and progress prevailing over most any other kind of value, be it artistic, emotional ties to family and friends, or spiritual ones.

47. Campbell et al. (2016); Peter (2013).

48. Searle (1992).

49. In *VAPD* (2005) and in a chapter for an anthology (Sadler 2004) I made some effort at describing the values which characterize diagnosis as not just practically effective, but also aesthetically beautiful, as in 'beautiful work'—an aesthetics of diagnosis.

50. Sadler (2007).
51. Nancy Potter (2009) has written insightfully about this process of 'uptake'.
52. Anonymous (1887, pp. 1283–1284).
53. Butler et al. (1990).
54. Pickard (2011).
55. In a positive sense, we compare values of mental disorders against typically assumed beliefs about the life well-lived, or eudaimonia (Sadler 2005).
56. Potter (2016).
57. Proverbs 6:16–19, Coogan, New Oxford Annotated Bible, 2001. See also Newhauser (2007).
58. Thomson 1993.
59. ibid.
60. Arp (2014).
61. Clark (2002); Sadler (2005).
62. See Aristotle (2014); Thurman (2006).
63. Veatch (2003 p. 189).
64. Gert (2004 p. 8–9).
65. Beauchamp (2003). See also Beauchamp (2014); Trotter (2020).
66. Beauchamp (2003), p. 260.
67. DeGrazia (2003); Rhodes (2019); Turner (2003).
68. Gert (2004).
69. Sadler (2005).
70. Peterson & Seligman (2004), p. 4.
71. ibid, pp. 3–4. For more recent and critical discussions of positive psychology, see Banicki (2014); Niemiec (2019); Niemiec, Shogren, & Wehmeyer (2017); Park & Peterson (2006).
72. DSM-5 Cluster B Personality Disorders consist of the Antisocial, Borderline, Histrionic, and Narcissistic Personality Disorders.
73. See for instance Charland (2006, 2010); Potter (2013); Reimer (2013); Zachar & Potter (2010).
74. Sadler (1997, 2005).
75. Baehr (2006); Fairweather & Zagzebski (2001); Greco (1993).
76. Aristotle (1984).
77. Brinkley (2000). Mrs. Parks was an African-American woman from Alabama who came to symbolize the US Civil Rights movement when in 1955, she refused to relinquish her seat on the bus to a white passenger, despite instruction from the bus driver to move to the 'colored section'.
78. Wittgenstein (1953).
79. Rosch & Mervis (1975).
80. Peterson & Seligman (2004, p. 4).
81. Jotterand (2014). Regarding this point, I don't want to imply an equivalency between the concept of 'enhancement' and ordinary human flourishing. Jotterand makes the point that enhancement takes capability beyond that of species typicality. Flourishing, on the other hand, can simply mean living a good life, which medicine would, uncontroversially, like to facilitate.
82. Peterson & Seligman (2004, p. 4).
83. See Friedli (2009); Keyes (2014).
84. Grzywacz & Keyes (2004); Keyes (2002, 2005, 2007, 2014); Keyes & Grzywacz (2005); Westerhof & Keyes (2010).
85. Friedli (2009).
86. WHO (2014).
87. Friedli (2009); WHO (2014).
88. Keyes (2014).
89. Peterson & Seligman (2004).
90. ibid, p. 9.

91. The blurring of the distinction between therapy and enhancement is not new in physical health either; for example, public health interventions like fluorinated water for caries-resistant teeth or waste management or vitamin use, are all interventions which tip over into making people better than 'normal'.
92. Shuman (1989, 2002).
93. Frances, Widiger, First, Pincus et al. (1991); Frances, Widiger, & Pincus (1989); Pincus, Frances, Davis, First, & Widiger (1992); Pincus & McQueen (2002); Widiger, Frances, Pincus, Davis et al. (1991).
94. Robins & Guze (1970). While these standards for grounding new diagnostic categories are now dated, the concept of a diagnosis being embedded in a network of patho-etiological features has persisted and reached its current elaboration in the RDoC. https://www.nimh.nih.gov/research-priorities/rdoc/index.shtml).
95. Cronbach & Meehl (1955). See also Blashfield & Livesley (1991). Chapter 3 in my *VAPD* considers the historical methods for building diagnostic categories, and interested readers can look there as well.
96. Fuller, Fuller & Blashfield (1990).
97. Knight (2010); Quinsey (2010); Thornton (2010).
98. Knight (2010).
99. Fuller, Fuller, & Blashfield (1990). See also Frances, Sreenivasan, & Weinberger (2008) and more recently Krueger et al. (2017); Longpre et al. (2020); Moser (2018).
100. Bell (2004); Bell & Dunbar (2012); Dunbar (2003, 2004); Guidon et al. (2003).
101. Dunbar (2004, pp. 99–100).
102. Both quotes ibid, p. 99.
103. Both quotes ibid, p. 99.
104. Dunbar (2004, p. 100).
105. Bell (2004).
106. Guindon, Green, & Hanna (2003).
107. ibid, p. 171.
108. Sadler (2005, Ch. 6).
109. With Donald Trump's brand of divisive populism so powerful a cultural feature since his presidency, and the trend of social media to polarize viewpoints and provide 'echo-chamber' validation, these concerns about social vice have only increased. See Sunstein (2017).
110. See http://topics.law.cornell.edu/constitution. The fate of tolerance under Trumpism is discussed Connolly (2017) and Lebow (2019).
111. Holden (2010).
112. For example, Goudriann et al. (2004).
113. Holden (2010).
114. Frances (2010).
115. Block (2008).
116. Holden (2010). For more on the ongoing development of the behavioral addiction concept, see Kuss, Griffiths, & Pontes (2017); Petry, Zajac, & Ginley (2018); Saunders (2017).
117. See Sadler (2005) for a detailed discussion.
118. Sadler (2005); Sadler & Agich (1995).
119. Frances (2010).
120. McHugh & Slavney (1998).
121. See Nestler (2014) for details.
122. White 2004.
123. ibid, p. 48.
124. ibid p. 53.
125. Swaminath (2008); http://www.reportageonline.com/2010/04/can-you-really-be-addicted-to-the-internet/. A recent history of this phenomenon is here: Dalal & Basu (2016).

126. Block (2008).
127. Here the vice-ladenness of Internet Gaming Disorder could be construed as a failure of temperance and perhaps a kind of gluttony.
128. Lenzner (2008).
129. ProPublica (2016).
130. Hill & Maughan (2001, p. 169).
131. See https://menoforder.com/blogs/blog/mental-sloth-disorder. Discusses 'sloth' as a disorder requiring assistance from the blog's product list.
132. Unger & Scherer (2010).
133. American Psychiatric Association (1987, pp. 357–358).
134. American Psychiatric Association (1994, p. 734).
135. Boerjan et al. (2010); Brown et al. (2009); Haoka et al. (2010); Prins et al. (2010).
136. Maslach, Jackson, & Leiter (1997 p. 192, internal citations omitted).
137. For example, consider Boerjan et al. (2010); Brown et al. (2009); Dobkin & Hutchinson (2010); Dyrbe et al. (2009, 2010); Eckleberry-Hunt et al. (2009); Gabbe et al. (2008); Haoka et al. (2010); Prins et al. (2010); Quinn et al. (2009); Stucky et al. (2009); West et al. (2009).
138. Leone et al. (2008); Rotenstein et al. (2018); West et al. (2020).
139. Luke 4:23.
140. Gorenstein (1992).
141. Meehl (1973).
142. Blashfield (1984); Frances, First, & Pincus (1995); Kirk & Kutchins (1992); Sadler (2005); Spitzer, Williams, & Skodol (1980) .
143. Cuthbert et al. (2013).
144. APA (2013, pp. 697–698).
145. APA (2013, pp. 99–100).
146. See Balon (2017); Galli et al. (1999); Greenberg, Bradford, & Curry (1996); Langevin (2006); Langevin & Curnoe (2008); Langevin, Curnoe, & Bain (2000); Stinson & Becker (2016); Yarvis (1995).
147. Cuesta & Perlata (2001).
148. Takahashi (2013).
149. APA (2013), pp. 685–705.
150. ibid, pp. 466–467, 476–480.
151. ibid, pp. 324–325.
152. Phillips et al. (2012).
153. See Sadler (2008, 2015) for more detailed discussions about the deficiencies of monosymptomatic disorder categories.
154. Blanchard, Kuban, Klassen et al. (2003); Ciani et al. (2019); Dyshniku et al. (2015).
155. Blanchard, Kuban, Klassen et al. (2003); Cohen et al. (2008); Seto (2012); Walter et al. (2007).
156. Eke et al. (2011).
157. Blanchard (2010).
158. See also Sadler (2015).
159. APA (2013).
160. ibid, p. 99.
161. ibid, p. 161.
162. Frances et al. (1991); Regier, Narrow, et al. (2009).
163. Frances, First, & Pincus (1995, p. 20).
164. Flor-Henry, Lang, Koles, & Frenzel (1991); Hucker, Langevin, Wortzman, Bain, Handy, Chambers, & Wright (1986); Langevin, Wortzman, Dickey, Wright, & Handy (1988); Langevin, Wortzman, Wright, & Handy (1989); Wright, Nobrega, Langevin, & Wortzman (1990).
165. Blanchard et al. (2003).
166. Blanchard et al. (2002).

167. Cohen et al. (2008).

168. Stein, Black, & Pienaar (2000).

169. Cohen, Gertmenian-King, Kunik, Weaver, London, & Galynker (2005); Cohen, McGeoch, Watras, Acker, Poznansky, Cullen, & Calynker (2002); Cohen, Nikiforov, Gans, Pozanansky, McGeoch, Weaver, King Cullen, & Galynker (2002); Grebchenko, Steinfeld, Kaleem, Cullen, Kunik, Galynker, & Cohen (2005); Raymond, Coleman, Ohlerking et al. (1999).

170. Cohen, Watras-Gans, McGeoch, Poznansky, Itskovich, Murphy, Klein, Cullne, & Calynker (2002); Galli, McElroy, Soutullo et al. (1999).

171. Cohen, Nikiforov, Gans et al. (2002); Mendez, Chow, Ringman et al. (2000); Schiltz, Witzel, Northoff et al. (2007); Stein, Hugo, Oosthuizen et al. (2000).

172. Marshall (2014); Stinson & Becker (2016).

173. Blasingame (2014); Booth (2016); Cortoni et al. (2017).

174. Cronbach & Meehl (1955); Sadler (2005).

175. Blanchard (2001).

176. Blanchard (2013).

177. Gorenstein (1992).

178. Meehl (1995).

179. See Coccaro (2004).

180. Berman & Coccaro (1998); Berman, McCloskey, Fanning, Schumacher, & Coccaro (2009); Best, Williams, & Coccaro (2002); Coccaro (2000, 2004); Coccaro & Lee (2010); Coccaro, Lee, & Kavoussi (2010a, 2010b); Coccaro, McCloskey, Fitzgerald, & Phan (2007); Coccaro, Noblett, & McCloskey (2009); Coccaro, Posternak, & Zimmerman (2005); Ferguson & Coccaro (2009); Lee & Coccaro (2001); Lee, Ferris, Van de Kar, & Coccaro (2009); Lee, Kavoussi, & Coccaro (2008); McCloskey, Berman, Noblett, & Coccaro (2006); McCloskey, Kleabir, Berman, Chen, & Coccaro (2010); McCloskey, New, Siever, Goodman, Koenigsberg, Flory, & Coccaro (2009); Murray-Close, Ostrov, Nelson, Crick, & Coccaro (2010).

181. Coccaro (2000, 2004); McCloskey, Berman, Noblett, & Coccaro (2006).

182. Coccaro (2000), p. 68.

183. ibid.

184. Barratt, Stanford, Felthous, & Kent (1997).

185. Curiously, Coccaro cites 'criminal' aggression as an example of premeditated aggression, but brief reflection makes apparent that an impulsive assault and a deliberate, planned assault can be criminal assaults in both cases, at least from the criminal justice perspective. This is to say, that what makes the assault criminal is its conformation to a legally defined offense, regardless of whether premeditated or not.

186. Coccaro (2000, 2004).

187. Dell'Osso, Altamura, Allen, Marazzitti, & Hollander (2006).

188. Coccaro (2000, p. 68).

189. Audi (1999 p. 563).

190. Sadler (2005).

191. Sadler (2008).

192. Kendler, Parnas, & Zachar (2020); Kendler & Zachar (2019); Kendler, Zachar, & Craver (2011); Zachar (2000, 2014).

193. Robins & Guze (1970).

194. See Lewis (2011) and Spence (1984) as examples.

195. See Stein et al. (2010) for an early analysis and statement of the DSM-5 definition of 'mental disorder'. As a co-author to this paper, I should say that I largely endorse this for the purposes of the DSM-5, though I also had some reservations about various points in the final product.

196. APA (2013, p. 20).

197. See Section 6.1 and 6.2 *VAPD* (pp. 204–226).

198. DSM-IV-TR definition of 'mental disorder', APA (2000, p. xxxi).
199. Sadler & Agich (1995).
200. ibid.
201. https://en.wikipedia.org/wiki/Little_Children_(film).
202. 'Moral panic' is a concept coined by criminologist and sociologist Stanley Cohen in his 1973 book. It refers to a social phenomenon where a situation, person, or group comes to be regarded widely as a social threat out of portion to the circumstances and situation.
203. American Psychiatric Association Task Force on Sexually Dangerous Offenders (1999); Winick & LaFond (2003); Wright 2014.
204. American Psychiatric Association Task Force on Sexually Dangerous Offenders (1999).
205. 'Epistemic' here simply refers to the degree of certainty of knowledge about the diagnostic category.
206. APA (2013, p. 124).
207. ibid.
208. APA (2013, p. 129).
209. Both quotations ibid.
210. Frances (2013).
211. Sadler, Jotterand, Lee, & Inrig (2009, p. 2).
212. Raine (2001, pp. 306–307).
213. Sadler (2008).
214. Orszag & Ellis (2007).
215. Angell (2009); Healy (2004); Rothman & Rothman (2011).
216. Sadler (2002, 2005).
217. APA (1980, 1987, 1994, 2000, 2013). This being said, it remains unclear just what power or influence the DSM definition of 'mental disorder' actually has on whether this or that category is included in the manual.
218. First et al. (2004); Pincus, Frances, Davis, First, & Widiger (1992).
219. Jackson (1985).
220. Szasz (1960, 1961).
221. Rissmiller & Rissmiller (2006).
222. Szasz (1960, p. 114).
223. Szasz (1963, 1991).
224. APA (2003), my editing.

4

Vice and mental illness—an ancient-to-modern iconography

Chapter outline

> The text is independent of us; it awaits us. Everyone needs his own time to come to it. The encounter occurs when the text is no longer treated as literature or artwork, but as reference point or model.
>
> —composer Arvo Pärt, liner notes to the ECM recording of Adam's Lament, 2013

4.1 Introduction—the American professional and social convergences on vice

Social deviance is a problem as old as recorded history.[1] In prehistory, archeological evidence suggests that cavemen joined into hunter-collectives to conquer and eat the woolly mammoth, setting the evolutionary stage for an ethic of cooperation. Around

Vice and Psychiatric Diagnosis. John Z. Sadler, Oxford University Press. © Oxford University Press 2024.
DOI: 10.1093/oso/9780198876830.003.0004

the same time, the discovery that grains could be stored as a winter food birthed an early concept of property, sowing the seeds (pardon the pun) for (what would be called today) an ethics of communal sharing, division of labor, and property. People who failed to play by the quite-rudimentary communal rules provoked responses from the social group, launching the earliest social deviance—the failure to adhere to collective norms, and the social response to it.[2]

In Western culture, the proper (moral) ways to control social deviance are at the core of political philosophy and civic practice and have been a focus of discussion and debate throughout recorded history. From Greek myth to the Bible, from Plato through Hobbes, Bentham, Franz Fanon, Lord Devlin, Angela Davis, H. L. A. Hart, Martha Nussbaum, John Rawls, and Cornel West, political and legal thinkers have struggled with three fundamental problems concerning vice and social deviance, determining: (1) the role of the state in regulating deviance, (2) the sources of deviance (medical, educational, maturational, religious/supernatural, and social, to name a few), and (3) the kinds of social responses that should be involved in deviance regulation.[3] Political philosophers have by necessity been metaphysicians as well, because to answer question (2) above, some kind of account of the nature of being human is required. Derivatively, such accounts of human nature then generate particular behavioral norms which reciprocally entrain sociocultural customs, mores, and traditions. This background provides the logical benchmarks for understanding social deviance, and will be discussed more directly, and contemporaneously, in the last chapters.

Social deviance can be considered the raw, undifferentiated phenomena from which contemporary vice and mental illness concepts have differentiated. Eve, after all, disobeyed God's instructions, and when she took the bite from the apple, she was deviating from the first social norm, at least from the Judeo-Christian standpoint. We may view her today as suffering gender discrimination, or Oppositional Defiant Disorder, or succumbing to temptations, or as an actor in a religious allegory, but in any case, her waywardness places her into the social deviance rubric.[4]

Having completed this topical introduction, let me share a few notes about methods.

4.1.1 Historiographic notes, qualifications, and apologies

This is the first of two historical chapters which trace the parallel developments of 'madness' on the one hand, and 'morality' on the other. This chapter considers the ancient world up to approximately the post-Enlightenment or 'modern' era. Chapter 5 will pick up the modern into the near-contemporary era, including the genesis of psychiatry as we know it today. In earlier chapters I've explained my necessity to focus on an American perspective on vice and psychiatric diagnosis. This chapter's breadth and depth will underscore this need for limiting perspective to an American one, once we get to American psychiatry, which occupies most of Chapter 5. For this Chapter 4, the focus will be almost worldwide; but as I progress through the centuries, the focus will progressively move away from a global perspective to a (primarily) Western European perspective beginning in Chapter 5, on to England and North American colonies, and ultimately 'landing' in the United States. So the arc of developments here are traced from ancient to contemporary over this and the next chapter. This funneling of the intellectual history of madness and morality from the world to the United States is practical rather than chauvinistic; ultimately, the United States is the context of my addressing the problem of the vice/mental disorder relationship (VMDR).

To aid the transition from macroscopic history to American history of psychiatry and morality, I have drawn up an online link http://www.oup.co.uk/companion/ Sadler 'timeline' which presents a two-for-one: The top timeline presents significant moments, trends, and figures in the history of madness and later, madness and psychiatry. The parallel, bottom timeline presents some significant moments, trends, and figures in the history of morality and moral ideas. The two timelines, are, more or less, synchronized (e.g., what happened in the history of madness corresponds in time with that in the history of morality, excepting the need to accommodate graphic space resulting in some inexactitude in timing the correspondences). In the first millennium and well into the second of recorded history, this history of moral ideas takes, in large part, the form of the history of sin and the supernatural, of wrongdoing and retribution; such were the forms of notions of good and evil, right and wrong, before the medieval era when the beginnings of autobiography and the interrelated notions of self, personal identity, and the individual developed in the West, and good/evil became 'psychologized' in a way we take for granted today.

A few qualifiers are indicated in reading and interpreting these timelines. First, the placement of particular events or trends on the timeline are approximate; often dates are supplied if the entry suggests an event. Other entries in the timeline indicate trends or a *Zeitgeist*, and so they appear as encompassing or spanning an approximate period. Second, as the complexity of entries (and culture) magnifies over the centuries, the timelines become jam-packed and the event's placement on the timeline becomes even more approximate. Hence the actual years of particular events are often added to add clarity to a timeline placement that is only crudely approximate. Third, from the historiographic perspective, the reader should be skeptical of any historical timeline as somehow representing the universally significant and the historically monolithic. My timeline is aimed at illustrating graphically not just significant events in these two aspects (psychiatry/madness and sin/morality), but also portraying what might be seen as historical tropes—such things as the allure of violent power, the historical and cultural contingency of moral and religious rules, and centrally, relationships between the moral and the mad. The particular focus of this book and this timeline have largely determined the entries contained—this will be an odd map indeed for people interested in kings and battles, art history, or political history![5]

A final note should address the extraordinary difficulty in portraying the context of historical trends in a timeline or in such a short summary of this chapter, especially when the history proper is not the explicit focus of this book. In preparing this book project, drafts of the proposal and early drafts of content went through a substantial amount of (grant) peer review, much of which was by historians. Reviewers' comments revealed, in my interpretation, an impossible dialectic. On the one hand, a historical background chapter which, by necessity, would be short, incomplete, and potentially, even certainly, misleading at times. On the other hand, not including a historical background chapter would impoverish and diminish any policy considerations by overlooking the lessons and ideas of history, however basic or crude. I chose to include an overview-of-history approach. My difficulty was compounded by the scarcity of secondary histories that explicitly considered the social history of mental illness, psychiatry, crime and criminal justice, intellectual impairment, and the penal system *together* as a history of Western social deviance. The works were just not out there. I had to improvise, and what follows is the result, to be taken with several grains of salt. Social historians out there, you are welcome to do this job better!

Perhaps, most importantly, I should clarify what I have retained of a parallel 'history' of madness and morality from prehistory to the near present. What is presented here is not really a proper history but rather a presentation of iconic ideas that have prevailed as important ones over the centuries. These iconic ideas, memes, or tropes are not analyzed as products of historical forces; they are introduced in a rough chronological order with little effort to establish them in the causal flow of history. I had to limit the scope of my historical effort; again, historical explanation would have been far beyond my focus and abilities, and for my later purposes simply identifying the core ideas is sufficient. I have presented a bare minimum of descriptive social context in introducing each section so that (hopefully) the iconic ideas make sense and fit into the cosmologies or worldviews of the time and culture. Moreover, within the text and especially in 'Synthesis' summaries, I attempted to establish the significance of these iconic ideas for their role in illuminating the VMDR today.

Readers will note in Chapter 5 on the post-Enlightenment birth of moral-medical psychiatry, the text transitions into a more conventional short-history style, linking social context to the emerging professional and clinical ideas. For example, one important discussion involving the problem of the meaning and sources of social deviance accompanies the development of social responses to said deviance in the American colonial days to the present. As I suggested, a history of the relationship between vice and madness is a project for a historian—and an ambitious one at that—not a philosophically oriented psychiatrist! However, an understanding of our current conundrums around the VMDR requires some historical grounding. Indeed, the fruits of these chapters will prove to be crucial to the analyses to follow in the second half of this book. In that second half, these unfolding historical tropes can be seen as the roots for the taken-for-granted cultural traditions and habits of living of the present. When I disembarked on this historical journey, I was not aiming for a particular set of conclusions that appear in the final chapters. I began as a searcher in pursuit of understanding the VMDR. This journey was very much a journey of discovery, and I hope it is for the reader too.

I introduce the VMDR[6] through the briefest sketch of a history of sin/morality and madness/psychiatry, using a variety of terms, however archaic and politically incorrect, that are more historically accurate than 'vice' and 'mental illness'. Nineteenth-century psychiatrists didn't discuss 'individuals with developmental differences', they discussed idiots and imbeciles. They didn't have 'individuals with schizophrenia or bipolar disorder', they had maniacs and lunatics. American colonial townspeople didn't have 'people experiencing homelessness'; they had paupers, vagrants, vagabonds, orphans, urchins, whores, and drunkards. So when discussing historical concepts I have used the terms of the period, however offensive and stigmatizing to contemporary sensibilities. We'll see that such old stigmatizing language is revealing in itself—and therefore worth considering.

4.1.2 Chapter organization

The following section, summarizing relationships between concepts of madness and concepts of sin, morality, and ethical ideas, warrants an introduction to chapter structure for clarity of exposition and interpretation. The aforementioned timelines, in the link, provide the 'big picture.' Summarizing recorded history for madness and morality, in one chapter, is absurdly ambitious, and to make it manageable at all I should state more clearly what kind of history this is. What I present in this chapter might be better described as a cultural iconography of morality and madness. As mentioned earlier, I'll be reviewing ideas, themes, motifs—tropes—that have arisen in history that are relevant to the issue of the VMDR. As iconic ideas they will percolate through history at various moments and eras, constituting what might be considered a collection of cultural-historical background knowledge as well as collective assumptions about morality and mental illness that persist in varying degrees in the present. What readers usually expect from a 'history' will not, and cannot, be attempted here. That is, I offer little in the way of a genealogy of ideas, their development and genesis, nor any attempt at historical explanation, nor even a smooth continuity of ideas from locale to era. While in the ideal all of these features would be desirable, as noted earlier, the focus of this work will hopefully benefit from such a historical iconography.

For the narrative discussion of these periods and relationships, I have structured subsections by historical period, themselves pragmatically drawn depending upon the richness and density of content during the particular time frame. For instance, the first section, encompassing prehistory to about 3000 BC, the Bronze Age—spans a period of millions of years, for most of which very little is known pertaining, or even vaguely relevant to, the VMDR! In contrast, the nineteenth century in the

United States alone warrants an extensive discussion because of the formative developments concerning the insane asylums, prisons, child welfare, care of the intellectual impaired, and so forth.

A second introductory note concerning structure are the subsections for each historical period. In this, I elected to organize these subsections around the timeline, including a history of 'morality' section, followed by a history of 'madness' section, with the section concluding with a 'synthesis' section that addresses relationships between the two, as well as open questions regarding such relationships—another inspiration hopefully for an intrepid social historian!

Regarding orienting the reader, perhaps of greatest importance is the clarification of the objectives of such an ambitious section as this one. In preparing this work it became evident to me what was of cardinal significance for a 'history of morality' in the context of a book about vice and mental disorders. My focus is not so much on the theory of ethics and morality but rather on images of personal morality: what it means to be a morally good person. This primary focus makes perhaps obvious sense when one is considering the relationship between mental illness and morality. So the primary focus of the morality sections is the development of a historical and cultural iconography of the morally good person, what it means to be a 'good' person, and de-emphasizing what would qualify as official or adequate intellectual history, where substantial attention to contextual factors, theory, and metaphysical assumptions would be required.

What will be shown throughout these historical discussions is the difficulty and ultimate failure to draw bright lines between vicious deviance and mad or psychiatric deviance. The VMDR has a truly ancient pedigree. Concluding comments will enumerate key ideas and relationships with contemporary concepts of the VMDR; pointing toward the later chapters and overall conclusions.

4.2 Madness and morality—the historical confounds

> *It is not easy to see any clear line of progress in human moral history.*
> —Oliver Thomson, *A History of Sin*[7]

> *Mad call I it; for, to define true madness, What is't but to be nothing else but mad?*
> —Polonius, in Shakespeare, *Hamlet*[8]

An image of the 'good' or virtuous person, in prehistory and into ancient history, was not a theoretical object, but rather emerged from revelations of a religious or spiritual nature, in parallel with the development of practical social-moral rules of conduct. Only by inference does one get a picture of the good person. As culture blossomed into the present, an increasingly theoretical and reflective account of personal goodness or virtue emerged and differentiated; with the invention of the written word, the recording of differing viewpoints about the good progressively expanded. As we'll see, theorized ethics and morality required a concept of the self, which didn't appear in the form we know it today until the early Middle Ages, perhaps best represented by St. Augustine's *Confessions*.[9] As far as what is plausible to accomplish for a psychiatrist and philosopher of psychiatry in a chapter, the metaphysical assumptions and rich detail of theory will be omitted, and instead, the focus on the 'results' of such theorizing (e.g., pictures of the morally good person) will be the primary objective. Indeed, to situate the later discussions of this book, a cultural iconography of morally good persons is all that is really needed. My role, at least for the first two-thirds of this book, is not to pass judgment on competing moral theories, but rather to describe the moral pluralism and diversity that makes up the background assumptions of patients, practitioners, and policymakers. Only in the later stages of the book will the consideration of metaphysical assumptions become required, when I rethink the received views.

Similarly, the images or cultural iconography of mental illness will be considered for the parallel history of 'madness'. The phenomenology of mental disorders is much more an established practice in social histories of psychiatry and madness; so the conceptual shifts and reformulation of disorder concepts is a focus. Needless to say that other, crucial aspects of the history of psychiatry/madness will be largely omitted here; again, considerations of metaphysical assumptions will be limited to the minimum needed to grasp the concept with a minimum of 'presentism' (the imposition of contemporary views on historical events), and discussion of treatments is entirely omitted, except as source of evidence about the relationship between vice and illness of the time period.

4.2.1 Prehistory to the Bronze Age (circa 3000 BC)

'Prehistory' is the period before history was recorded. The 'three-age' concept of prehistory encompasses the period before *Homo sapiens* first appeared (approximately 200,000 years ago) and their anthropoid predecessors, which was well into the Stone Age (beginning approximately 2.5 million years ago). The more recent Ages, the Egyptian Bronze Age (beginning circa 3000 BCE) and the Iron Age (beginning approximately 1200 BCE)[10] provide more historical traces and archeological artifacts of interest. This section addresses the section of prehistory up to the beginning of the Bronze Age, our knowledge of which is inferred from bronze tools, weapons, and other artifacts found on various continents.

4.2.1.1 Morality
Thomson[11] notes that before apes became human, the anthropoid *Homo erectus* began to share food, initiating one of the ostensibly first moral behaviors—and this was about 1.5 million years ago. Much, much later, in the Old Stone Age (about 70,000 years ago) Neanderthals built tombs, stocking them with food and tools for

the dead to use in the afterlife, making a clear sacrifice of substantive goods that could have benefitted the living at the time. Cave paintings from Cro-Magnons (circa 30,000 BC) appear to ban incest, and Stone Age humans from 15,000 years ago leave traces of stored grains in cave dwellings. Stone Age man developed the first bows and arrows, almost certainly used in hunting, but quite unclear when this weapon was turned toward one's brother. We can speculate that storing grain for the winter implies a proto-ethic of sharing, possession, and property. Such cooperation appears to not be limited to the 'gatherers' of ancient humanity, but also the hunters of the woolly mammoth as noted earlier, whose relics provide evidence of cooperative team hunting.

In the first Mesopotamian cities like Jericho (appearing approximately 9000 BCE), evidence indicates the first wine- and beer-making apparatus, and tomb-related evidence of property and inheritance. Such 'possessions' set the stage for envy, theft, imposition of rules, and likely, war. The Canaanites' building of fortifications—walls for the city—confirms a hypothesis that property and family needed protection, and that hostile others could be expected.

4.2.1.2 Madness

Evidence for prehistoric 'madness' is dependent upon physical evidence: fossil remains and early tools and other artifacts. With such little known about prehistoric life in general, and even less about prehistoric mental/behavioral life, little can be written about pre–Bronze Age mental distress. Perhaps the most significant early evidence is the finding of trephination (trepanation) in prehistoric France circa 6500 BC. Restak[12] describes one-third of 120 fossil skulls having trephination holes; many had indications of healing bone and therefore survival of the 'patient'. While uncertain if these procedures were performed to treat conditions like epilepsy or mental illness (or instead had religious or moral significance) subsequent evidence suggests that trephination was indeed used as a therapy to release evil spirits.[13]

Mesopotamia offers the first recorded religion, and religious beliefs were polytheistic, as in the later Greek and Roman world. Of relevance are two gods that were spouses—Nergal, the god of disease, plague, destruction, and war, and Ereshkigal, the goddess of the dead or netherworld. Nergal's nicknames reveal his temperament—the 'raging king', the 'furious one', and the god was portrayed as a lion.[14] Johannes Weyer, a Dutch physician and scholar who will be important in the discussion of medieval morality and madness, claimed Nergal was a demon and in cahoots with Beelzebub, Lord of the Flies, and the prince of demons in ancient Judaica.[15] In ancient Mesopotamian medicine, the first physicians treated conditions with exorcism of evil spirits or demons—but this takes us to the Bronze Age.[16]

4.2.1.3 Synthesis

The link between wrongfulness—evil—and sickness, including mental illness, is evident from these earliest artifacts and moments in recorded culture.

4.2.2 Bronze Age (circa 3000 BC) and Iron Age (circa 1500 BC)

As mentioned earlier, these Ages are part of the 'three-age system' of prehistory, and as might be expected to apply best to Mediterranean and European regions, with the dates and onset of actual metal use varying by region. Note that the time scale for these Ages has contracted substantially from the Stone Age, alluding to the expansion of culture over these centuries. The names of these Ages, of course, correspond to the development of metallurgy from bronze alloy tools and artifacts to iron alloys, blended with carbon to make steel—a harder and lighter metal than bronze. As we'll see, these Ages birthed weapons, significant in the history of morality.

4.2.2.1 Morality

The Bronze Age offers the first written evidence of moral codes or laws, along with consequences for wrongful action.

In ancient Sumeria, the Code of Ur-Nammu remains the oldest tablet of moral instruction or law known, circa 2100 BC.[17] The Code is rather harsh; declaring death sentences for murder, theft, a wife's adultery, and cuckolding a man's virgin wife. Other portions of the Code have to do with compensating wronged others through various fines of silver and provision of other goods like barley. The Code also provided for the resolution of what today we would call civil disputes involving personal injury, property rights (e.g., home and slaves), and the like.

In Babylon, King Hammurabi established, around 1700 BCE, one of the first legal or ethical codes, listing 292 laws and matching punishments on a series of clay tablets and in near-complete form as a diorite finger-shaped stele. Like the Code of Ur-Nammu, the Hammurabi Code established rules for handling both criminal wrongdoing and civil disputes and was reportedly handed down through divine authority. Theft, murder, infidelity, burglary, incest, and prostitution were all explicitly addressed. Instruction 206 from the Code of Hammurabi can be read as implying today's issues of intention, responsibility, and culpability in harming another:

> If during a quarrel one man strike another and wound him, then he shall swear, 'I did not injure him wittingly', and pay the physicians.[18]

The Egyptian Bronze Age brings us some of the earliest evidence of large-scale use of weapons-assisted aggression against other humans: war, the execution of prisoners, the conquest of territory, and slavery. Despite this explosion of bloodshed, and because the afterlife was prized and dependent upon good acts, the Egyptians coined a word, 'Maat', the first recorded term for virtue.[19] The Egyptians brought us evidence of additional early vices, among them, from Pharaoh Usertsu III, accusations of racial inferiority and rights to imperialistic conquest. Pharoah Ahmes introduced incest in Egyptian royalty by marrying his sister. A vice akin to graft could be surmised from the Pharoahs' practice of bringing gold into their tombs, to assure entrance into the afterlife.

After an earlier legacy of brutal conquest, the later Pharoah Akenaton, along with Queen Nefertiti, introduced racial equality, respect for truth, and equal rights for married women around 1350 BC. The establishment of women's rights and equality was to be short-lived.

4.2.2.2 Madness

Little is known about mental disorders in ancient Egyptian medicine, and what is known is based primarily upon the Ebers and Edwin Smith papyri[20] circa 1500 BC. These documents establish the ancient Egyptians as understanding the relationship between the brain and mental functions, and indeed Egyptian physicians incorporated an examination of consciousness in ordinary medical practice. Nasser[21] describes standard phrases in characterizing abnormalities of mental function:

- the perishing of the mind
- the mind is forgetful like one who is thinking of something else
- the fleeting mind
- his mind goes away
- it is difficult for him to hear the spoken word

Ancient Egyptian physicians treated what today would be called conversion blindness and syncope. Drunkenness, and perhaps alcoholism, is described: '. . . Beer, when it invades a man, masters his soul . . . '[22]. While not describing severe and persistent sadness as a disease, the ancients described mood changes and symptoms we would recognize as clinical depression. While no physician is identified as the specialized attendant of mental symptoms, Nasser speculates that such matters of the mind were handled by magicians or sorcerers, not physicians, given the ubiquity of supernatural explanations for mental distress.

In ancient Egyptian medicine, despite its marriage of the empirical/rational with magico-religious elements, little is found or known of 'madness' or psychotic disturbances of mental life in ancient Egyptian texts. A royal princess of the twentieth dynasty was possessed by a demon, and prayers and incantations were responsible in saving her.[23] I should note that in ancient worlds, the practice of spoken rituals like prayers and incantations often did not distinguish between invoking sacred beings and practicing supernatural magic. The differences between prayer and magical incantations were small to nonexistent.

4.2.2.3 Synthesis

The asymmetry of historical traces for mental disorders, compared to historical traces of moral developments, law, and ethical guidance, are most striking in this section. One wonders about the reasons for this. One obvious possibility is that metallurgy, a technology that defined the era for historians, resulted in artifacts whose intended purposes betray the values that inspired the design and execution of them. Weapons pose an example on the one hand, and vessels for drink or food, on the other. The design of a technological artifact, as I have discussed earlier, embodies a range of moral and nonmoral values.[24] A second reason may be that law and ethical direction presented a more demanding cultural need than the need to intervene with severe mental disorders, presuming that they indeed manifested in this era. Third, this asymmetry may depict a necessity for cultural development for mental disorder to be 'noticed'—the harsh conditions of ancient life, the potential for widespread death by plague, famine, war, or injury, may have made mental distress a *fait accompli*, the norm of the human condition, rather than a modern notion of a distinct disturbance of individual functional integrity. Finally, the metaphysical viewpoint that supernatural forces drive psychological or emotional distress may in effect remove today's 'psychopathology' from the realm of the medical and natural, and, hence, physicians may not have recognized the phenomena of mental distress as disease or injury.

4.2.3 Ancient Mesopotamia and the Hebrew Bible (Old Testament) (circa 1500–500 BCE)

This era introduces written historical traces as an access to the development of cultures.

4.2.3.1 Historiographic notes

Ancient Mesopotamian culture has left perhaps the earliest and at the time, richest traces of medical thought, mostly encoded on clay tablets in cuneiform. The oldest known Mesopotamian medical text is a Sumerian therapeutic manual from about 2000 BCE. The Sumerians, along with their neighbors the Akkadians and the Assyrians, have left a rich legacy which has recently been compiled by the scholars JoAnn Scurlock and Burton Anderson.[25] For a sense of geographic place, the Assyrians, between (1363 and 609 BCE, encompassed a territory which includes the contemporary areas of Iraq, Syria, Lebanon, Israel, Palestine, and parts of Iran and Turkey.

While the discussions that follow point toward a substantial interest and understanding of 'psychopathology', readers should keep in mind some standard historiographic limitations and barriers. To mention a few: many of the tablets were lost, damaged, or destroyed, leaving an incomplete record; the translation of ancient texts is always difficult, especially with dead languages like Sumerian; conceptual drift inevitably occurs, where the senses of a written expression are lost along with their phenomenological referents, and what appears to be a straightforward description of a recognizable phenomenon may be distorted by our contemporary concepts, linguistic filters, theoretical lenses, and common sense preconceptions.

Where on the archaeological timeline the Pentateuch (the Books of Genesis, Exodus, Leviticus, Numbers, and Deuteronomy in the Old Testament) and the 'historical books' of the Old Testament (Joshua, Judges, Ruth, Samuel, on down through Esther) fall is a source of great debate among theologians and historians.[26] In no case will I settle anything around this debate here, though the reader should recognize that what we recognize as the Bible as a historical document is a collection of manuscripts authored by a number of people, many unknown, and authored over centuries preceding the birth of Jesus Christ and extending to several centuries thereafter.[27] The comments that follow should be considered with caution, not just because of the variability of the dating, but also the colossal cultural and historical gaps between these ancient times and today. Most significantly for the discussion of *Madness* (Section 4.2.3.3), the presented evidence of 'mental illnesses' from the Biblical texts, while not mere speculation, should be read skeptically as to how and how much they apply to our contemporary notions of psychopathology. In Chapter 3 we mentioned the ontological slippage of mental disorder phenomena, that phenomena we associate with mental illness even today can merge into ordinary life experience, religious and mystical experience, existential suffering, and various extremes of human experience. With all these reservations, the following sections focus upon (mostly) morality and madness in the Old Testament era.

4.2.3.2 Morality

The times under consideration here (a) encompass the ending of the great Egyptian era and the moral importance of Mesopotamian thinkers, (b) encompass substantial portions of the Old Testament Hebrew Scriptures, and (c) introduce classical Greek thought.

In Egypt, the later Pharaoh Amenhotep IV (Akenhaton) and Queen Nefertiti introduced notions of racial equality and equal rights for married women and embraced a more modest ethic for the era, as noted earlier. A moral treatise of the time (circa 1350 BC) by Ptah Hotep urged personal and political restraint,[28] though this civilizing trend was short-lived. Ramses II, the imperialist, noted for his vanity and cruelty, built colossal statues of himself, tortured spies, and systematically killed male infants of Hebrew slaves. Ramses had 160 children, including the products of incestuous relationships with older daughters. His period was also associated with increased tolerance and use of alcoholic beverages in the population.[28] Ramses introduced the prototypical decadent tyrant.

Also in Egypt around this time, the son of Hebrew slaves, the prophet Moses (circa 1300–1220 BC) was both the deliverer of divine revelation and an original ethical thinker in his own right, though as a conduit of God's instruction. Having been summoned twice by God to Mount Sinai (the first to the 'burning bush' to receive instructions for freeing his people from slavery, and the second to receive the moral laws known today as the Ten Commandments), Moses is important to Jewish, Christian, and Islamic moral thought. In addition to delivering the Ten Commandments, Moses wrote extensively, providing guidance and instruction on

Table 4.1 The Ten Commandments (from Exodus 20.2–20.18)[30]

Then God Spoke All These Words
(1) I am the Lord Your God, who brought you out of the land of Egypt, out of the house of slavery; you shall have no other gods before me.
(2) You shall not make for yourself an idol, whether in the form of anything that is in heaven above, or that is on the earth beneath, or that is in the water under the earth. You shall not bow down to them or worship them; for I the Lord your God am a jealous God, punishing children for the iniquity of parents, to the third and the fourth generation of those who reject me, but showing steadfast love to the thousandth generation of those who love me and keep my commandments.
(3) You shall not make wrongful use of the name of the Lord your God, for the Lord will not acquit anyone who misuses his name.
(4) Remember the sabbath day, and keep it holy … the Lord blessed the sabbath day and consecrated it.
(5) Honor your father and your mother, so that your days may be long in the land that the Lord your God is giving you.
(6) You shall not murder.
(7) You shall note commit adultery.
(8) You shall not steal.
(9) You shall not bear false witness against your neighbor.
(10) You shall not covet your neighbor's house, you shall not covet your neighbor's wife, or male or female slave, or ox, or donkey, or anything that belongs to your neighbor.

Coogan (2001). Enumerations and editing mine.

domestic as well as national welfare, including particulars of sexual behavior and hygiene. Moses provided proscriptions against various aspects of personal conduct, such as public nakedness, selling one's daughters into prostitution, homosexuality, and stern warnings against worshipping idols. However, Moses described positive virtues as well, such as leaving the gleanings of the fields' and vines' harvest for the poor and left perhaps the best-known foundation of Judeo-Christian ethics: love thy neighbor as thyself.[29]

Table 4.1 reproduces the passage in Exodus that describes the 'Ten Commandments', quoted from *The New Oxford Annotated Bible*, with enumerations and minor editing for simplicity. A second version of the Commandments also appears in Deuteronomy 5.6–21, though for my purposes the differences are negligible.

The Book of Leviticus, particularly Chapters 18–20, reinforce many of the Ten Commandment teachings, but also address other areas of morality/ethics, many of which are directly pertinent to the issue of the vice-mental disorder relationship. Table 4.2 lists many of these.

Leviticus also describes rules for conduct that today appear quite idiosyncratic to modern Westerners: from regulating the trimming of beards, to regulations for the harvesting of fruit from newly planted fruit trees, to proscribing the making of clothing from two or more kinds of material. The ethical-moral significance of these, rather than the practical, is debatable.

Table 4.2 Moral-Ethical Instructions from the Book of Leviticus[31]

Instruction	Leviticus Citation
'… you shall not lie to one another …'	19.13
'… you shall not revile the deaf or put a stumbling block before the blind …'	19.14
'… with justice you shall judge your neighbor …'	19.15
'You shall not go around as a slanderer …'	19.16
'… you shall not profit from the blood of your neighbor …'	19.16
'You shall not practice augury or witchcraft …'	19.26
'Do not turn to mediums or wizards …'	19.31
'You shall rise before the aged, and defer to the old; …'	19.32
'When an alien resides with you in your land, you shall not oppress the alien.'	19.33
'You shall not cheat …'	19.35

Moses' successor, Joshua, led the Israelites into war against pagan gods of the Canaanites and other local tribes, to purge them from the Promised Land, such as in the Battle of Jericho, which followed Moses' parting of the Red Sea. Joshua's war was grim, brutal, and unforgiving, as exemplified by the Lord's guidance in Deuteronomy, '… you shall put all its males to the sword' (20.13), and 'You may, however, take as your booty the women, the children, livestock, and everything else in the town, all its spoil. You may enjoy the spoil of your enemies, which the Lord your God has given you' (20.14). Concluding, '… you must not let anything that breathes remain alive' (20.16). Such was an inspiration for holy wars to follow over millennia. The religious justification for widespread massacre, as we'll see, has coexisted as a sad counterpoint against the instruction in morals and virtue also found in the history of religions.

By 500 BC the Books of Job and Ezekiel opened the path to the afterlife being attained through the pursuit of good action and virtue, setting the stage for Christian ethics.

4.2.3.3 Madness

Ancient Mesopotamia, often called the 'cradle of civilization', provides an opportunity to examine the kinds of phenomena we would identify as psychiatric today. The cultural setting is one where disease is considered a manifestation of divine spirits, which could afflict the victim on their own, through a response to a victim's offense (often because of worshipping false gods), or through the summoning of a sorcerer. The care of the sick involved hygienic considerations, exorcisms, animal sacrifice, and incantations, as well as procedures we would recognize as 'medical' today, such as careful observation, history taking, examination of the patient's body and bodily products (urine, feces) and fluids, and making observations in all sense modalities. From this standpoint the distinction between naturalistic accounts and supernaturalistic accounts is absent for the most part, hence the equal standing of magical and 'empirical' interventions. The ancients gained knowledge of anatomy through examination of trauma victims and wounds; autopsies were believed to have been performed, and the performance of trepanation has already been discussed earlier. The multiple gods of ancient Mesopotamia ruled over particular domains and structured the conception of pathology of the time. This often took the form of diseases being linked to the 'hand of' a particular offended god, and the particularities of the illness related to that god's domain of influence. Scurlock and Andersen[32] use the 'hand of Ištar' as an example of how a patient afflicted with a sexually-transmitted disease might be explained. Evil spirits—ghosts—and animals with supernatural powers were also attributed as sources of mental distress.

The ancient Babylonian physician Esagil-kin-apli wrote the first diagnostic manual of medicine, the 'Akkadian Diagnostic Handbook', also sometimes called 'Diagnoses in Assyrian and Babylonian Medicine',[33] which included epilepsy and mental disorders. Yuste and Garrido provide some descriptions of the conditions of Babylonian patients:

> If a man is quivering all the time when lying down, shouts like the shouting of a goat, roars, is apprehensive, shouts a lot all the time, (then it is) the hand of *bennu*, the demon...

They also present an early definition of mental disorder: 'a person who is well but his behaviour is sick'.[34]

Ancient Mesopotamian texts contained an astounding amount of clinical observation and description, including description of what today would be considered mental illness. Table 4.3 lists some of the signs and symptoms of mental distress from ancient Mesopotamia, and what follows are some actual translations of clinical phenomena, both drawn from Spurlock and Anderson.[35]

Table 4.3 Some Signs/Symptoms of Mental Distress in Ancient Mesopotamia[35]

'Gnashing teeth' (bruxism)	Psychosomatic illness	Abnormal handling of body
Stress headache	Mournful/worried expression	Hallucinations
Nightmares	Altered mentation	Inappropriate emotions
Insomnia	Mumbling/unintelligibility	Antisocial behavior
Sleep talking	Excessive talking	Self-mutilation
Stress angina	Mutism	Addiction
Anxiety	Confusion	Mood disorders
Anxiety and seizures	Staring off into space	Psychosis
Anorexia	Staring at body parts	Dissociation
Love-sickness	Inappropriate use of clothing	Paranoia

Adapted from Scurlock & Anderson (2005).

Scurlock and Anderson's numerous translations of psychopathological phenomena from Sumerian, Akkadian, and Assyrian medicine cannot be reproduced here; the following are only a sample:[36]

'(The demon) who crosses the edge of my bed, frightens me and makes me roll over and over, shows me troubled dreams . . .'

'I cannot sleep at night because of worry about you.'

'If a person continually has crushing of the heart (and) day and night he has fearfulness/shuddering, his god is angry with him; in order to make his god at peace with him . . .'

'If his limbs are as still as those of a healthy person (but) he is silent and does not take any food, "hand" of a murderous ghost . . .'

'[If] his mentation is altered so that he is not in full possession of his faculties; "hand" of a roving ghost; he will die.'

'If his tongue is tied in knots and he cannot open (his) mouth [. . .], he has kissed the ēntu-priestess of his god, [he has done] something offensive [to his god].'

'If derangement seizes a person [so] that his mentation "alters" his words are unintelligible, his thinking continually fails him, and he continually talks a lot, to restore his mind to him . . .'

'If he wanders about, he does things slowly, (and) he is continually thrown down (var. falls down), he will die.'

'[If] he continually "gazes" at [his hands], he has changes of mood, he "gets up" and (has to) squat down, (and) [he is particularly affected] at the beginning of [the night . . .]'

'[If] he keeps taking off and beginning to get into his "garments", "hand" of the twin gods; he will die.'

'If he continually strikes his face and screams, the ghost of someone burned to death afflicts him.'

'If (the skin under) his headband stings him, his ears roar, the hair of his body continually (feels like) it is standing on end, his whole body crawls as if there were lice but when he brings his hand up, there is nothing to scratch, "hand" of ghost *ṣētu* . . .'

'. . . he continually opens his eyes and, when he sees the one who afflicts him, he talks with him and continually changes himself, 'hand' of *lilû,* messenger of his god'.

'If a mournful cry continually cries out to him and he continually answers it (and) when it cries out to him, he says "who are you?" a *mutillu*-bird has touched him and is bound with him (and) stands at his head; he will die.'

'"Hand" of god (is when) he curses the gods, speaks blasphemy, (and) strikes whatever he sees.'

'If a person drinks fine beer and as a result his head continually afflicts him, he continually forgets his words and slurs them when speaking, he is not in full possession of his faculties, . . .'

What is remarkable from the list of translations from Scurlock and Anderson is the prevailing picture of (see Chapter 3) nonmoral bads, excepting the blasphemous person. However, this observation may be an artifact of the authors' selection of phenomena to present, or more profoundly, the ancient's framing of illness as opposed to moral/religious phenomena.

Any discussion of the Hebrew Bible or the Old Testament's portrayals of mental disorders should immediately call attention to the broader context. While presented holistically as part of the Holy Bible today, the Old Testament is a collection of manuscripts by multiple authors from various eras, that describes the Creation, the early development of Judea, Moses and others forging God's word into moral proclamations and guidance, the early Mesopotamian societies, and the emergence of the Israelites and Jewish religious identity. In this context 'insanity' was usually judged as a manifestation of demonic forces or the punishing Hand of God; a monotheistic outgrowth of the Mesopotamian pagan beliefs discussed above. Mental distress like extreme sadness, anxiety, and suffering were similarly viewed as the existential lot of humanity after the Fall, described in the Book of Genesis. From this standpoint, what constitutes disease or disorder versus ordinary human distress and despair was perhaps more ambiguous in 500 BCE than it is today.

A good example of demonic causes of madness appears in *The Testament of Solomon*,[37] where King Solomon confronts various demons, one of whom is Obizuth:

> I am called among men Obizuth; and by night I sleep not, but go my rounds over all the world, . . . For I have no work other than the destruction of children, and the making their ears to be deaf, and the working of evil to their eyes, and the binding their mouths with a bond, and *the ruin of their minds*, and paining of their bodies.[38]

Perhaps the best known of Old Testament stories of madness is King David's escape from his enemy King Achish of Gath:[39]

> 11 The servants of Achish said to him, 'Is this not David the king of the land? Did they not sing to one another of him in dances,
>
>> "Saul has killed his thousands,
>> And David his ten thousands"?'
>
> 12 David took these words to heart and was very much afraid of King Achish of Gath. [13] So he changed his behavior before them; he pretended to be mad when in their presence. He scratched marks on the doors of the gate, and let his spittle run down his beard. [14] Achish said to his servants, 'Look, you see the man is mad; why then have you brought him to me? [15] Do I lack madmen, that you have brought this fellow to play the madman in my presence? Shall this fellow come into my house?' [22] David left there and escaped to the cave of Adullam; . . .

While acknowledging madness as a phenomenon, not much of the 'pathological' phenomena are revealed here.

Also in 1 Samuel 16 is the description of King Saul's rivalry with the upstart David, particularly piquant in the face of Saul's abandonment by God:[40]

> [14] Now the spirit of the Lord departed from Saul, and an evil spirit from the Lord tormented him.

After young David's defeat of the Philistine warrior Goliath, Saul was even more threatened by David's influence:[41]

> [10] The next day an evil spirit from God rushed upon Saul, and he raved within his house, while David was playing the lyre, as he did day by day . . .

Various physicians and scholars have attempted to describe Old Testament phenomena in terms of contemporary psychopathology. At least one author in the literature[42] argues that Saul exhibited symptoms of bipolar I disorder. Kapusta and Frank[43] present Job's torment as depression.[44] These are, of course, disputable historical claims, with all the historiographic limitations discussed at the beginning of this chapter.

The testing of Job's faith by Satan poses early descriptions of existential misery and perhaps a depressive mood disorder. (Satan has destroyed Job's prosperity and killed his children.) In describing his 'lament', Job visits many of the signposts of contemporary 'mixed anxiety/depression':[45]

> 7. [1] Do not human beings have a hard
>   service on earth,
>   and are not their days like the days
>   of a laborer?
>   [2] Like a slave who longs for the
>   shadow,
>   and like laborers who look for their
>   wages,
>   [3] so I am allotted months of emptiness,
>   and nights of misery are
>   apportioned to me.
>   [4] When I lie down I say, 'When shall I
>   rise?'
>   But the night is long,
>   and I am full of tossing until dawn.
>   [5] My flesh is clothed with worms and
>   dirt;
>   my skin hardens, then breaks out
>   again.

> ⁶ My days are swifter than a weaver's
>   shuttle,
>   and come to their end without
>   hope.

The prophets, with their mystical experiences and the accompanying idiosyncratic forms of expression, have long stimulated speculation about the question of psychopathology. Broome[46] presents a succinct albeit dated review, where authors have attributed all kinds of psychopathological experiences to Ezekiel: for example, catalepsy, catatonia, stupor, hallucinations, and dissociations. Broome concludes his review by claiming Ezekiel exhibits 'behavioristic abnormalities consistent with paranoid schizophrenia',[47] but his final sentence addresses the significance of Ezekiel's experience for the Judaic, Islamic, and Christian world:[48]

> The fact that each of these is couched in religious terminology has rallied many to the defense of the prophet's normal mentality, but his religious significance is by no means impaired by our diagnosis of a paranoic condition, as Williams James convincingly argued in the case of other great spiritual leaders.

4.2.3.4 Synthesis

The ethical and medical writings of ancient Mesopotamia encourage an interpretation of the closeness of religious experience to psychic torment, and by implication, the close connections between religious inspiration, spiritual suffering, and psychopathological phenomena—connections that persist through today. Moreover, the clash between spiritual-religious-supernatural accounts of mental distress and naturalistic medical accounts is evident from the earliest writings in Western civilization. These themes will be seen to persist when the contemporaneous Greek culture is described in the next section.

4.2.3.5 Ancient Greek culture (1500–500 BC)

This section primarily focuses on the extraordinary influence of Greek and Roman thought for both morality and mental disorder. Supporting this goal, Bennett Simon[49] offers a helpful conceptual scheme for understanding the psychology of ancient Greece and Rome, a psychology pertinent to both the moral and the medical: (1) the *poetic model*, based upon Homeric and classical Greek tragedies; (2) the *philosophical model*, based upon Plato, Aristotle, and other philosophers of the era; and (3) the *medical model*, primarily based upon the Hippocratic corpus. Granting the slippage to oversimplification, the significance of Simon's insight for a joint history of morality and madness is that contemporary discourses around morality and mental disorders echo many related themes. However, to claim a lineage of these ideas is not legitimate and can be only speculated about.

4.2.3.6 Ancient Greek psychology

Simon's *poetic model* draws upon ancient Greek oral history and writings as exemplifying a worldview where little of our contemporary sense of self, inner directedness, or self-awareness is evident, and instead the person is portrayed as a pawn of supernatural and specifically, divine forces.[50] Simon provides some succinct examples:[51]

> In Homer's *Iliad*, Agamemnon explains and exculpates his own arbitrary and tyrannical behavior against Achilles—behavior that led to the 'wrath of Achilles', by invoking *Até*, a deity of infatuation and madness, and Achilles accepts the explanation. In Greek tragedy, the gods or demons drive heroes mad, sometimes with some clear motive of divine revenge (e.g., Ajax in Sophocles; Orestes, in *Bacchae*) but sometimes more capriciously (e.g., Heracles, in Euripides, *The Madness of Heracles*). Healing comes from outside interventions, either by a divinity or another human being, and the healing of restoration is described in the language of one agency or person influencing the afflicted person.

Simon notes that while this model of external, divine influence was dismissed as superstitious by the rival philosophical and medical theorists, evidence of its ongoing influence persisted throughout the age—not the least of which was the ongoing popularity of ancient Greek theater. Robinson[52] identifies Agamemnon's and Achilles' excuses as prolegomena to the insanity defense of today.

For the *philosophical model*, Simon notes that Plato's *psyche* depicted an internal mental life characterized by conflict or struggle between internal divisions of the mind: the rational, the spiritual-affective, and the appetitive.[53] The motif of internal struggle between opposing psychic forces is relevant to the discussion of Aristotelian moral psychology and vice/virtue in Chapter 3; for efficiency's sake that discussion will not be repeated. The resonance of these cultural tropes of intrapsychic conflict, impulse, moderation, control, and reflection is obvious in contemporary psychodynamic, cognitive-behavioral, and other psychotherapeutic models of the mind.[54]

The *medical model*, not surprisingly, situates pathology, physical or mental, in bodily systems and organs. For mental disturbances, physicians in the Hippocratic tradition saw the brain and heart as the key organs.[55] Disease was a natural phenomenon, to be understood through reason and subject to the same physical laws as the rest of nature. The core of an ancient Greek medical psychology had to do with the notion of equilibrium in health and disruption and imbalance in sickness. The notion of equilibrium and balance was concretized in the humoral theory of disease, where imbalances of elemental fluids (i.e., black and yellow bile, phlegm, and blood) resulted in disease, including psychopathology. The paradigmatic example, melancholia, was characterized as an excess of black bile, and prevailed for a millennium, well into the Middle Ages.[56]

The metaphysical details of humoral theory, however fascinating, cannot be addressed here. Suffice to say that humoral theory, while 'medical' and perhaps proto-scientific, nevertheless exhibited conceptual and ontological links to moral, religious, magical, and supernatural ideas, as well as links to other traditions (e.g., Indian and Middle Eastern). Simon notes, as an example of these links, the use of emetics for both black bile–related diseases as well their use in exorcisms.[57] Moreover, and as part explanation for the 'proto-scientific' status of humoral theory, Simon notes the absence of historical traces of the ancients' interest in *evidence* of humoral excess—descriptions of black bile proper are absent, leading to speculation about what bodily products, in fact, were linked to black bile.[58] Simon notes that, despite the profundity of humoral theory, and especially the idea that black bile was a response for wide varieties of human ills, the Hippocratics offered little direct or observational evidence of 'black bile'. Its actual identity as a bodily fluid remains obscure today.[59] One should note that the mechanistic claims of hot/cold and wet/dry black bile for disease did not exclude supernatural explanations; humoral theory provided a medium in which physicians might intervene. This motif of proximal cause ('Why melancholic? Because of an excess of black bile.') from distal or perhaps 'ultimate' cause ('Why an excess of black bile? It is a punishment from the gods.') is a motif that we'll see is preserved today, that of the physician as mediator and therapist to proximate causes and faith seen as the mediator and 'therapy' for ultimate causes. As a simple example of this tension today, consider physicians and faith healers.

Perhaps Draco of Athens (circa 700 BC) as pioneer of written law, offers a peculiarly ruthless synthesis of the era. While distinguishing the difference between intentional and accidental homicide,[60] the fate of even minor offenses was death, inspiring our contemporary adjective 'draconian'. When asked why his punishments were so severe, he '. . . considered these lesser crimes to deserve it, and he had no greater punishment for more important ones'.[61]

4.2.4 Greek and Roman philosophy and the New Testament (circa 500 BC to 500 AD)

With this period morality and ethics became explicitly theorized, both in secular contexts, as with the Greek and Roman philosophers, and in the religious context, as with the moral life as embodied in Jesus Christ's teachings and actions.

4.2.4.1 Historiographic notes

As this review more fully enters the era of recorded history, and papyrus and other forms of writing replace stone and clay tablets, the historical traces might be expected to be more reliable and are. However, many historiographic difficulties persist: translation difficulties continue, and determining authorship of (particularly) the New Testament remains. For the latter, questions persist about some of the New Testament book's relationships to Jesus Christ's historical life and teachings. Raymond Martin and John Barresi, in their magisterial work *The Rise and Fall of the*

Soul and Self: An Intellectual History of Personal Identity,[62] review historian's viewpoints about the historical veracity of the New Testament, concluding:[63]

> Aside from the extreme scarcity and ambiguity of the evidence on which historians have had to rely in constructing their accounts, there are two main reasons they have been unable to agree about Jesus' message. First, they disagree about what the evidence should include. The main source of contention here has to do with whether to regard as authentic certain literary evidence that is outside of the New Testament. The most important potential evidence of this sort is the Gnostic Gospel of Thomas, a collection of sayings of Jesus apparently based in part on early sources other than the canonical Gospels. Second, virtually all academic historians, whether conservative or liberal, agree that many of the events depicted in the New Testament are fictitious and that most of the sayings attributed to Jesus are inauthentic.

I am, of course, not able to provide evidence for or against Martin and Barresi's claims, and moreover, my single chapter on this history of morality and madness is not going to straighten out the matters of the historical truth of the New Testament! However, the debate, such as it is, concerns more the substance of Jesus' religious message, as well as his moral message. What is important for my purposes, moreover, is not the historical truth of Jesus' teachings but rather the *iconic status* of the Biblical teachings of the New Testament, as a set of cultural tropes of tremendous significance for the understanding of historical and contemporary morality. That the New Testament describes various forms of psychopathology, along with some metaphysical significance of mental illness, is also of cultural importance to my work as well.

The New Testament is important in a second way, in that it introduces a new tension between religious teachings in Judaism, based on the Old Testament, with Christianity in the New Testament, and these tensions will expand further when I later consider Muhammad and the development of Islam. As will be discussed later, the Old Testament is characterized by a God and a religious morality governed by an orientation to personal holiness and adherence to Him as the Lord Thy God, while Jesus' moral message, at least as depicted in the New Testament, introduces an expanded message about compassion for others, peace, and acceptance of others.[64] As a simple example of the Hebraic emphasis, consider the Ten Commandments in Table 4.1, where four of the ten are oriented toward faithfulness and worship of God, contrasted with Jesus' Sermon on the Mount in Matthew 5.1–12 below:[65]

5. [1] When Jesus saw the crowds, he went up the mountain; and after he sat down, his
    disciples came to him. [2] Then he began to speak, and taught them, saying:
       [3] 'Blessed are the poor in spirit, for theirs is the kingdom of heaven.'
       [4] 'Blessed are those who mourn, for they will be comforted.'
       [5] 'Blessed are the meek, for they will inherit the earth.'

[6] 'Blessed are those who hunger and thirst for righteousness, for they will be filled.'

[7] 'Blessed are the merciful, for they will receive mercy.'

[8] 'Blessed are the pure in heart, for they will see God.'

[9] 'Blessed are the peacemakers, for they will be called children of God.'

[10] 'Blessed are those who are persecuted for righteousness' sake, for theirs is the kingdom of heaven.'

[11] 'Blessed are you when people revile you and persecute you and utter all kinds of evil against you falsely on my account.'

[12] 'Rejoice and be glad, for your reward is great in heaven, for in the same way they persecuted the prophets who were before you.'

However, before we get too deeply into the New Testament, the period of approximately fifth- century BC and Jesus' life is worthy of substantial attention. As culture differentiates in the Mediterranean world, a range of traditions, philosophies, and ethical and medical ideas proliferated. The period of about (1000 years to be discussed covers a lot of ground—from Platonic and early Greek philosophy, to later Hellenistic and Roman philosophy, to Persian Zoroastrianism, to the birth of Christianity, and the influence of the New Testament and the influence of early medieval religious and medical figures such as Augustine of Hippo and Galen. As before, the structure is from morality, to madness, and synthesis.

4.2.4.2 Morality

The millennial span of 500 BC to 500 AD could be characterized as the first great millennium of moral reflection and theorizing. Moral/ethical ideas, philosophies, writings, and practices were proliferating around the globe. For this section, only a small sampling of major trends is feasible, as culture as a worldwide phenomenon explosively proliferates and differentiates. For clarity's sake, I will first consider the 500 years before the birth of Christ.

This period demands a more inclusive and international treatment, partly because many of the ideas discussed in the following persist today in Western and Eastern cultures, and because of some remarkable resonances of ideas between widely separated cultures—implying something ontologically central to being human and therefore of perennial, and perhaps universal, importance.

Having neglected Asian and South Asian culture up to this point, perhaps a good place to start is by considering the ancient Hindu philosophical texts, the *Upanishads*.[66] Given that these Sanskrit texts number at least 200, and span periods from 500 BC to well into the AD period, I've relied on secondary sources to sketch relevant features of the emerging Hindu ethics. The materials were passed down via the oral tradition (*Upanishad* refers to sitting with a teacher).

Circa 500BC–1 AD: an explosion of moral reflection: Upanishad metaphysics and 'ethics'. The *Upanishads* are a collection of approximately 200 philosophical and religious Sanskrit texts in the Hindu tradition. The oldest of these, the 'main' or *mukhya* texts, were written before 500 BC, predating the Buddhist tradition and continue through several centuries following, and indeed newer texts were composed as Hinduism moved into the medieval and modern eras. The best known of the newer texts, the *Bhagavad Gita*, is estimated to have been composed between 500 and 200 BC, though the Hindu tradition is diverse in various sects or schools that differ in metaphysics and practice. The ethic or morality associated with the early Hindu tradition is derivative from their metaphysics. In one thread of this thought, the metaphysics is built around a unity of a universal, encompassing spirit (*Brahman*) and the spirit of the individual or self (*Atman*). The religious path (*bhakti*) or devotion to God involves the individual's seeking the unity of self with an encompassing God. Moral conduct is a vehicle to good *karma*, or ascension toward the highest good, which in Hindu tradition involves reincarnation—one ascends or descends from higher or lower life forms depending upon one's actions in the prior life. Ethics are secondary to the primary goal of seeking of unity of *Atman* and *Brahman* or enlightenment through yoga and related practices, with enlightenment signaling the end of reincarnation and eternal bliss.[67] In another thread of Hindu thought, ethics is driven through respecting a natural order or natural law—*dharma*.[68] In this account, enlightenment and the renunciation of social duties is only permissible at the last two stages of spiritual development. Ethical or moral development is required as a preparation for the higher stages of spiritual development toward enlightenment. The morality emphasizes duty, nonviolence, honesty, modesty, asceticism, and avoidance of social immorality like stealing. The *Bhagavad Gita* attempts to bridge the tension between spiritual withdrawal and social duty by enlisting yoga as a practice that facilitates, rather than hinders, social duty and engagement. Mahatma Gandhi summarized the *Gita* way as 'the gospel of selfless action'.[69]

Buddhist moral thought. Prince Siddhartha Gautama Buddha was born circa 500 BC, and founded a nontheistic religion and philosophy based upon a recognition of *samsāra* (the cycle of suffering and rebirth) and the renouncement of craving or desire. Buddhist practice, for following the path, leads to the renouncement of desire, and subsequently enlightenment occurs, and the individual may attain *nirvana*, or perfect enlightenment, ending the cycle of *samsāra*. Like Hinduism, Buddhism recognizes *karma* and emphasizes proper conduct in one's life as contributing to outcomes in later reincarnations. Buddhism is one of the world's largest religions by numbers of practitioners, if one counts the considerable number of variations and sects associated with it—from Zen to Shinto. The Path—or 'noble eightfold path' governs personal conduct, especially *Śīla*, Buddhist morality, which occupies three of the eightfold: *vāc* (speaking truthfully and without rancor), *karman* (acting without harm), and *Ājīvana* (earning a living honestly, peacefully, and without exploitation).[70]

Resembling Buddhism in attitude but relatively independent in development, Taoism, or 'The Way', was founded by Chinese philosopher Lao Tzu, a contemporary and probably the main rival to Confucius as the most influential ancient Chinese

thinker. Since Lao Tzu's time, Taoism has differentiated into a number of related religions and practices and influenced Chinese folk beliefs.[71] Taoist ethics emphasize
the three jewels, or treasures of the Tao: *ci* (love, compassion, mercy, kindness, and
benevolence); *jian* (moderation, economy); and *Bugan wei tianxia xian* (humility,
or literally 'not dare to be first in the world').[72] Distinctive in these Asian traditions
is the emphasis on what Thomson calls the 'submissive virtues', quoting Lao Tzu 'He
who is self-exalting does not stand high.'[73]

Confucianism. Confucius (551–479 BC), the most influential Chinese philosopher, articulated a virtue-based philosophy that addressed individual and family
conduct as well as collective or governmental thought. His interest and contribution
to the latter were no doubt related to his extensive experience in the politics of the
time. His ideas were transmitted in the oral tradition until around 221 BC, when his
ideas were recorded, leaving some question for scholars about the authenticity and
accuracy of what is now regarded as his 'standard work', the *Analects of Confucius*,
a collection of aphorisms that collectively constitute a systematic moral philosophy.[74] As a variety of virtue ethics, Confucianism emphasizes *junzi*, an aim toward
integrity and excellent conduct or, more literally, the 'superior man'. Confucius'
philosophy emphasizes the family as the core moral unit (differentiating it from
Aristotelian individualism and modern Western liberalism) and core values include
jen (humaneness), *yi* (righteousness), and *li* (rules of propriety).[75] The role of the
physician in Confucian medicine is also notably different from modern conceptions: the Confucian physician, in the pursuit of the 'the art of humanity', commands
greater moral authority in decision-making than contemporary Western egalitarian
physician-patient relationships.[76]

Ancient Greek philosophy develops and differentiates. In the centuries preceding
the birth of Christ, ancient Greek culture differentiated and flourished, despite
Assyrian and Babylonian warlords' militarism, executions, and tortures of their enemies. In so doing, a notion of 'philosophy' was articulated that frames present-day
notions of Western philosophy. The earlier Homeric virtues of courage, honor, and
pride were supplemented by other virtues. Hesiod's *Works and Days* poem (circa
700 BC) articulated a more domesticated morality and ethics, based upon honest
work, the elevation of home life, and honor. Later, however, the Spartan ethic was
to be influential in the rise of Rome.[77] Spartans promoted fecundity, the eugenic
selection of better infants, the praise of physical prowess, personal discipline, and
military sacrifice and honor, all articulated by Lycurgus. New sexual mores were explored in Sappho of Lesbos' poetry, celebrating erotic love between women (circa
600 BC), and in the articulation of *Kaloskagathos*, the unity of moral goods and aesthetic goods—the beautiful—leading to a morality of the sensual. The contemporary Thucydides, however, would have none of this and railed against the decline
of Greek morality. The period exhibited moral diversity galore, as homosexuality,
orgies, cults of Bacchus, and infanticide were tolerated in many states. The Athenian
Solon articulated an early notion of democracy in emphasizing government for the

governed, while Thales articulated a prolegomenon to the Golden Rule: 'We should never do ourselves what we blame in others.'[78] In the 'popular culture' of the time, the playwrights Aeschylus, Sophocles, and Euripides explored moral themes, including perhaps the first explicit contrast between law and morality. *Antigone*'s Creon, King of Thebes, required traitors be left unburied to rot, and Antigone, defying Creon, buries her dead brother because she believes burial is an unwritten requirement of the gods.[79] While the significance of Sophocles' *Oedipus* is obvious for all Freudians, perhaps less appreciated is Sophocles' introduction into popular recognition that one can act immorally by accident and without intention. Oedipus violates an incest taboo through the unrecognized killing of his father and marrying his mother.[80] Through drama, Greek theatregoers were introduced to 'moral ambiguity'. We've all struggled with this since.

For a history of morality and ethics, however, the fame of these thinkers, authors, and scholars—the 'Pre-Socratics'—was exceeded by the influence of Socrates (469–399 BC) and a group of five additional philosophers who were to have lasting influence on moral thought into the present day: Plato, Diogenes (the Cynic), Zeno (of Citium), Epicurus, and Aristotle.

Socrates' significance for the history of morality and for this book is through his status as the popularizer and systematizer of rationalistic, or reason-based, approaches to morality and determining the good or right action. His secularist accounts of morality, in contrast to the prevailing religious viewpoints of his day, extend into the present, where religious and secular morality still coexist as rivals, stimuli to the most important of discussions, and guides to personal conduct, law, and politics. While Socrates was not anti-religious, and not even anti-intuitionist, his approaches to truth and morality were independent from religious rule or dogma, a fact that got him into trouble.

Socrates' foremost student and documentarian of Socratic thought was Plato (circa 428–347 BC). However, historians note that Plato's work was likely written after Socrates' death and wonder about the historical accuracy of Plato's and others' depictions of Socrates in the dialogues. Indeed, none other than Aristotle himself disputes the agreement between Socrates and Plato on some issues.[81] Moreover, definitive opinion on Plato's own views, especially ethics, is in some debate as well, because of the often-inconclusive nature of the Socratic dialogues that Plato uses as a pedagogical device for his written philosophy. Indeed, the central personal feature of Socrates as depicted by Plato is of profound intellectual humility, as Socrates' critical inquiries are typically accompanied by exhortations of his own ignorance on such matters.

Key ideas identifying the moral person, explored by Socratic/Platonic ethics, have to do with exploring the idea of aretē—the notion of virtue, or personal excellences, and to accounting for wrongdoing, which for Plato involved either illness, ignorance, or compulsion by another. For Plato, 'treatment' of wrongdoing typically involved education, but may have involved medical treatment and addressing social circumstances as well. The Platonic idea that, without any of these three conditions prevailing, 'no one would choose wrongful conduct' is one that has persisted over millennia into the present day, at least in philosophy, though less so in psychiatry! My colleagues in psychiatry may well have trouble with the narrow notion of personal irrationality in Plato. Socrates' practice of rigorous definition of concepts was a crucial first step in saying anything else worthwhile about them; we must be able to define courage before we can say much more about it. Socrates confidence, however, in his and others' ability to define concepts was low, and this ambiguity provoked Plato's metaphysical interests, including his notion of Forms, which are, to quote Taylor, '*both* perfect paradigms and universals'.[82] This is to say, Forms are both the summative shared features of otherwise ambiguous concepts as well as ones that are universal and indeed immortal and eternal.[83]

Later Platonic writings considered the soul and 'moral psychology' in more detail; Plato pioneered the idea that the soul or immaterial self was characterized by conflict between three functions—reason (the rational), emotion (or spirit), and desire (appetites)—and that conflict between these three functions provided explanations for behavior.[84] Which of these parts of the soul persisted after the body's death became an ongoing concern in Plato's metaphysics[85] and needn't concern us here. However, each function may have played different roles in different virtues, so that 'wisdom' was a function of reason, while 'justice' was a function of all three parts working in harmony.[86] In the development of this moral psychology, Plato identified what came to be known as the classical virtues: wisdom, courage, fortitude, and justice. In the *Gorgias* Plato also emphasized the notion of the virtuous person; the most important aspect of these was that a 'good' necessarily involves a constraint and social restrictions. MacIntyre[87] summarizes: '. . . if anything is to be a good, and a possible object of desire, it must be specifiable in terms of some set of rules which might govern behavior'. Consequently, a bad person is one who cannot respect a limitation and the associated rules, and thereby cannot 'share [in the moral sense] a common life'.[88]

Our second philosopher could be typified well by recounting his infamous retort after being censured for masturbating in the town square: 'If only it were as easy to get rid of hunger by rubbing my stomach.'[89] Diogenes, founder of the Cynic school, argued that only the distinction between vice and virtue counted in moral discourse and action. For 'the dog' (Diogenes) all convention had no moral hold at all, and this view provides the semantic root for the contemporary misuse of 'cynicism': not that nothing matters, but conventional values and conformity are shallow.

The Stoic school, founded by Zeno of Citium but elaborated through writings by Chrysippus (circa 280–207 BC), Posidonius (circa 135–51 BC), Epictetus (55–135 AD), and in Roman thought, by Seneca (1 BC–AD 65). Stoic thought was based upon a rigid deterministic metaphysics where events, including human actions, were strictly determined by a rational order, yielding the metaphysically influential idea that the cosmos, and derivatively, Nature, were not chaotic but rather structured, and ultimately, understandable through reason. In this sense the Stoics differed from Platonic metaphysics, which depended upon the otherworldly Forms, and seem friendlier to today's scientific rationality. For Stoics, moral goods or virtues were the only good, and vice the only evil, so if a person has acted morally, misfortunes must be providential within the divine order. As Sharples[90] puts it, '. . . being perfectly virtuous the wise man will by definition have done the best he could, there is nothing for him to regret'. The pursuit of non-virtue goods such as health and wealth are secondary, merely preferential rather than essential to a good life. Emotions such as regret, pity, sadness, and anxiety were to be distrusted as misleading about what is wrongful or evil. This position lead to the familiar psychological instruction in Stoicism to avoid pathos as well as the articulation of 'natural law', the latter becoming important later in formulating Christian religious and Western political theory. 'Natural law' was also to later frame deviations from natural law, such as sexual deviations, as evils or much later, disorders. Perhaps the central paradox of Stoicism is if the divine order is Good, why is most everyone vicious to some degree?

While the Hellenistic philosopher Epicurus (341–271 BC) formulated his own distinct ethics, his area of greatest influence might be his metaphysics, summarized poetically by Lucretius circa 50 CE, 'On the Nature of Things'.[91] Developing and revising the 'atomism' of Democritus, he postulated all was either material or void (empty space) with elemental, indivisible particles called atoms making up the material, and exhibiting regular patterns or structures of motion which constitute the different forms of matter encountered in the cosmos. The resemblance to contemporary molecular and atomic science, not to overlook philosophical materialism, needn't be elaborated here, other than to say how prescient Epicurus and Lucretius were. However, I should note that Lucretius' and Epicurus' secularist ontology was an influential counterpoint to the divine metaphysics of Platonism and Stoicism, and hence a challenge to the Christian naturalism to come later.

Epicurean ethics, however, was dominated by the value of pleasure as dominant. Like Stoicism, Epicurus framed ethics within a deterministic cosmos, but this cosmos was not divine but rather secular and mechanistic. Moreover, the Epicurean seeking of pleasure was not an empty hedonism as his philosophy is commonly misunderstood today. Epicurean ethics rather endorsed the classical virtues based upon their value in assuring a pain-free life, which was believed to be superior to indulgences. A moderation of pleasure-seeking was necessary on two key fronts: (1) freedom from excessive desire, and the cultivation of tranquility were requirements for the possibility of pleasure, and (2) excessive indulgence in pleasures of the body (sex, drink, food) inevitably led to the pain of loss and deprivation.[92]

For Westerners today, perhaps virtue's greatest voice was Aristotle of Stagira (384–322 BC). A student of Plato, Aristotle is generally regarded as one of the greatest philosophers of the Western world, and his contributions extend to all the major branches of philosophy—ethics, metaphysics, logic, politics, and sesthetics, and the like, throughout history to the present. Charles[93] describes an Aristotelian Circle which situates and elegantly organizes Aristotle's key concepts on the good life, which he saw as the aim of ethics as well as politics. The first term, *eudaimonia*, commonly translated as well-being, happiness, or human flourishing, frames the ends of ethics. The second, *aretē* (virtue), mentioned earlier regarding Plato, is described as the pursuit of excellent actions, while the third, *phronesis* (practical wisdom) is the means toward the recognition of excellent actions. What is 'circular' about the Aristotelian Circle is the interdependence of each concept upon the other. Excellent actions require practical wisdom to achieve; the wise person successfully thinks through the path to well-being; well-being promotes wisdom and excellent action. These and other elements of Aristotle's ethics have remained food for debate for scholars in the ensuing centuries. The relationship of Aristotle's ethics to his political theory is also a matter of debate.[94]

In Chapter 3 I considered some elements of Aristotelian ethics and moral psychology which serve as iconic landmarks for the VMDR, and bear some reminding and elaboration here. First, the pursuit of aretaic or virtuous action requires discipline and practice. Second, and sometimes called the 'doctrine of the mean' or the 'golden' mean, many Aristotelian virtues can be placed as a mean between two vicious extremes: as a common example, courage being the moderate practice between the extremes of rash fearlessness, on the one hand, and cowardice on the other. Third, *phronesis* or practical wisdom, functions as a kind of 'metavirtue' to navigate situations that demand multiple, perhaps conflicting virtues.[95] Fourth, the pursuit of virtue is spontaneously accompanied by pleasure—a contemporary Aristotelian might say that pleasure is an 'emergent property' of the practice of virtue. Fifth, Aristotle distinguishes between depravity (pursuit of the worst wrongs or evils) and moral weakness. Depravity in his view can be 'found chiefly among foreigners,'[96] but Aristotle's cultural or racial xenophobia aside, (and significantly for the history of the VMDR) depravity is also associated with madness, diseases, and ill-formed habits. Moreover, any extremely developed vice can be a depravity. Hutchinson mentions cannibalism, ritual murder, and 'effeminate homosexuality' as examples.[97] Moral weakness (*akrasia*) a concept that has also fueled innumerable philosophical treatises and philosophy dissertations in the ensuing centuries, refers to a self-aware failure of virtue—'I know I should not have stolen the shoes, but did anyway.' The cultivation or habituation of virtue results in a release from the temptations of impulsive wrong action, hence the discipline-aspect of virtue.

Aristotle's moral psychology, we can see, is resonant with many of our common sense understandings of vice and mental illness today. For example, the doctrine of the mean implies that extremism of a character trait is problematic, and indeed the manifestation of extreme personality traits today is a prominent conceptual feature for defining personality disorders.[98] The notion of moral weakness relates to folk psychology today when we attribute bad behavior to a weakness or faultiness of character. Aristotle implies that the idea of freedom from disease or madness is associated with a spontaneous movement toward virtue, a point discussed in Chapter 3. Finally, Aristotle's moral psychology provides us one of the earliest links between madness or mental illness and wrongdoing.

Circa 1–500 AD: the rise of Christian morality and ethics. The period of Jesus Christ's teachings and the development of early Christian teachings was significant both for the history of morality, as rules of conduct, as well as with ethics as the reflective study of moral conduct and of the Good. Over the same period, important changes and diversification occurred in other traditions (such as Buddhism) as well as cultural practices apart from religions.

As always, the focus in this section is not so much on historical development but rather on understanding key cultural tropes or iconic ideas that contribute to the cultural fabric of contemporary thought. The historiographic concerns stated earlier hold profoundly, as Jesus' teachings in the Bible were authored years after the fact by a diverse group of followers. Moreover, centuries of theological reflections on the true meanings of Jesus' teachings about morality and ethics make for further diversity of opinion, not to forget the extraordinary diversification of Christian sects, all claiming correct interpretation of the Bible, adding even more complexities. Last, the application of Jesus' New Testament teachings is debated constantly today in the face of our evolving mores, historical and cultural changes, and technological achievements. As might be expected, my focus here is on the generally agreed-upon, and relatively noncontroversial, themes in Jesus' teachings.

In Section 4.2.4.1 the core content of Jesus' Sermon on the Mount was presented, which the reader might want to review again, as these themes in Jesus' teachings encapsulate many of the novel elements of Christian morality. Most centrally the role of Christian love is manifested concretely by the stories of Jesus's tending the poor, the weak, the meek, and the oppressed. How Jesus' doctrine of loving thy neighbor translates into a Christian ethics, much less a 'New Testament' ethics, is a source of ongoing debate in academia.[99]

The debates cluster around several fronts. How encompassing, in the moral realm, is Jesus' command to love God, and how does love of God and love of one's neighbor relate to each other? Is loving one's neighbor a unity with loving God, or somehow derivative? In a related vein, the meaning of Christian love (*agape*) is debated. Is *agape* simply love of God's creations? Or is it a more comprehensive love of God and all His creations? How do right moral and ethical actions emerge from *agape*?

Even the very question of Jesus' having a conventional ethics is debated among theologians. As but one example, a Presidential Address to the 1995 Annual Meeting of the Society of Biblical Literature, Leander Keck notes:[100]

... much that passes for New Testament Ethics makes into ethics what is not really ethics at all but a heterogeneous mass of imperatives, counsels, parables, narratives, and theological statements that pertain to the moral life without actually being 'ethics'.

Unlike the straight-up moral directives found in Old Testament books like Leviticus or directives like the Ten Commandments, the New Testament contains comparatively little in the way of an explicit morality or 'ethics'. When considering the ethical content of the New Testament, if one defines 'ethics' as a *reflection upon* the good and moral life, even less of an explicit ethics is apparent. Rather, the teachings of Jesus stand upon a foundation of the Old Testament and supply new directions of moral guidance, namely, the new emphasis on Christian love, concern, and charity, as well as turning one's cheek to oppressors and even loving one's enemies.

Keck[101] provides some concrete examples: noting that the word 'virtue' appears five times in the New Testament, the meaning in each case does NOT include the idea that virtue is a character trait that warrants cultivation, a la Aristotle. Rather, the importance of honor and deference to those higher in social status, which was a prevailing moral expectation in then-contemporary Greek and Roman times, was expected as 'virtue'. Stanley Hauerwas[102] reorients us to Jesus' teachings, saying that Jesus' story is a *story* of ethics, not a reflection on the Good. Jesus taught by example, model, and parable, not 'theoretically'. Despite Keck's disavowal of a contemporary, reflective ethics in the New Testament, a modicum of explicit (as well as implicit) moral guidance appears as he notes:[103]

> For instance, in 1 Thessalonians 4, after Paul grounds an exhortation in God's will for human sanctification (1 Thess 4:3), he goes on to urge his readers to live quietly, mind their own business, and work with their hands, so that they will earn the respect of outsiders and be dependent on no one (1 Thess 4:11–12). Thus he begins with a biblical-theological warrant that might have sounded odd in Gentile Thessalonian ears and moves to considerations that had become familiar through popular moral discourse . . .
>
> The defining feature of New Testament ethics is its orientation to an event, namely, the event of Jesus (including his resurrection and exaltation to God's right hand), and to the community that resulted
>
> . . . what distinguishes the ethics of the New Testament from the philosophical tradition is its appeal to the shape of Jesus' life, to what had happened through it, as well as to what happened to those who believed that this was the salvific work of God. And this is what links it to the Old Testament, where this event-oriented mode of ethics was learned.[104]

In Keck's reading, the aim of Christian ethics is redemption, in accepting Christ (Eph 1:10), entering God's presence (Heb 10:14, 12:23) and emancipating creation from death (Rom 8:21).

Faith in God then generates a divinely guided moral spontaneity, as described in 1 John 4:11–12: 'God abides in us and his love is perfected in us.' The other primary moral motivator in Jesus' teaching is the potential accountability in provoking God's wrath, here explained when Keck relates Jesus' message to slaves and masters in Colossians:[105]

> Thus, the admonition to slaves in Colossians begins by referring to the coming judgment as reward: 'Whatever your task, work heartily, as serving the Lord, not men, knowing that

from the Lord you will receive the inheritance as your reward', and then refers to the judgment as punishment, 'for the wrongdoer will be paid back for the work he has done, and there is no partiality. Masters, treat your slaves justly and fairly, knowing that you too have a Master in heaven' (Col 3:23–4:1 RSV).

Mott[106] argues against scholars who would place the New Testament outside of the domain of social ethics, or even social prescriptions. Like Keck, Mott emphasizes understanding the New Testament morality in relationship to the Old Testament—the latter a set of scriptures that held force in Jesus' day. The details of Mott's scriptural interpretation cannot be restated here, but the gist is that the Gospels' recurrent themes of empowering the weak amount to directives for social justice.

In a revealing take on the ancient meaning of 'sinner', Mott clarifies that Jesus' conduct of associating with and including sinners amounts to an ethic of social inclusion, similar to how we would understand such today:[107]

The term sinner (hamartolos) was not a moral description but a technical term. It was a title used to refer to a group of people who could be both identified and segregated. In the Gospels the 'sinners' are the tax collectors, prostitutes, and drunkards. They are characterized by an observable lifestyle or economic activity which has been ethically condemned. In the Hellenistic world a 'sinner' was the opposite of those who are right and proper ('our kind of people'). For Jewish writers it was a derogatory term of abuse. The lifestyle of the 'sinners' had cut them off from the community. No matter what other attributes Zaccfhaeus had, as a tax collector he was a 'sinner' and therefore cut off and despised.

The implied ethic of social justice and inclusion and loving thy enemy in Jesus' teaching continued in the centuries following Jesus' death and resurrection; even in the face of Roman decline, decadence, and debauchery, ultimately to the Empire's fall in the mid-400s. Such decline was addressed by the aforementioned Stoic philosophers too, including Seneca.

I now turn to the development of Christian thought proper, in the centuries following Jesus' life and teachings. The Christian reaction to Roman sexual licentiousness set the stage for St. Paul's endorsement of celibacy for clergy; ultimately becoming a Roman Catholic Church requirement. Origen, the great Christian scholar of Alexandria, became a eunuch and praised celibacy as the first virtue.[108] Mary, the Virgin, became a symbol of restraint's ideal, and St. Ambrose and St. Hecla were models of celibacy and chastity. The Church made celibacy for the priesthood a requirement in 402, in face of all the indulgences in food, drink, and sex in the Roman elite. Five years later, in 407, divorce was banned.[109]

Renouncing his misspent youth, Augustine of Hippo's *Confessions*[110] posed to many historians the first serious autobiography as a narrative form, and raised concerns regarding faith, with the consequences of heaven and hell, to new heights (or depths, as the case may be). Orthodox engagement with the Church became the primary route to salvation, over that of noble actions.[111] Key moral concepts of Augustine were derivative of his theology. Perhaps most famous is the notion of 'original sin', which for Augustine was a metaphysical condition of being human—human nature—because of Adam and Eve's fall, making all humans sinners and reenacted through concupiscence (i.e., the human's metaphysical condition of lust) as the primary source of evil. Only acceptance of God's grace can redeem original sin, not to overlook ordinary, individually perpetrated sin. Of additional interest in Augustine's work is the discussion of 'just war'—the idea that the pacifist Christian may engage in war for the purpose of restoring peace. This motif of the justifiable Holy War was to result in the loss of millions of lives over the ages.

Our timeline now in the early Middle Ages (a.k.a. the 'Dark Ages'), the Roman Empire was crumbling, and Europe was consumed by regional wars, provoking a degradation of intellectual and moral activity, with little crucial to recount here until the later medieval period (e.g., after the tenth century).

However, in other parts of the world, morally significant developments were appearing. In the third/fourth century, at least some segments of Hindu India were entering a morally permissive period, with the writing of the iconic *Kama Sutra*[112] by Mallanaga Vatsayana. While mostly known today for its guidance on sexual love between men and women, the *Kama Sutra* was intended as a general guide to aesthetic and erotic pleasure (*kama*), so its content goes beyond that of sex alone, but also general guidance on the pleasures of domestic life. Thomson[113] notes that Hindu/Indian attitudes toward sexuality were more tolerant during this period, with more accepting attitudes toward homosexual behavior, and the Gupta dynasty (320–550) with its pacifist ethics and prevailing vegetarianism enjoyed a period of peaceful flourishing.

Buddhism of the period was undergoing substantive differentiation into various sects, with perhaps the most relevant interest being the Tantric sect, also known as Vajrayana Buddhism and other names. While Tantric Buddhism seeks, as with all forms of Buddhism, the highest enlightenment of a Buddha, Tantrism differs in the methodological path to enlightenment. Rather than the practice of celibacy, Tantrism seeks enlightenment, compassion, and altruism through the body, and in particular, sexuality.[114] The differentiation of Buddhism was, as might be guessed, accompanied by more tolerant cultural attitudes in India regarding sexuality, and specifically toward homosexual relations.[115]

From this whirlwind coverage of the 500 BC–500 AD millennium of morality, the focus now turns to concepts of 'madness' and mental illness of the period.

4.2.4.3 Madness

The millennium centered by the chronology of Jesus Christ was, as the prior section illustrated, a worldwide period of great attention, reflection, and differentiation of moral thought and moral practice. Ethics as a mode of inquiry, and the differentiation of moral conduct, were developed to a degree never encountered. The same cannot be said for the attention, reflection, and differentiation of accounts of madness over this same millennium. Science as we know it today was still a centuries-away development, and the intellectuals of the period worked within prevailing religious and philosophical traditions. George Mora notes that the accounts of madness/mental illness from the Classical Greek and Roman eras changed little until about the twelfth century AD. Consider Mora's summary of the popular understandings of mental illness of the early medieval era:[116]

> Popular concepts, based on centuries-old folk beliefs, attributed abnormal psychological phenomena to magic, contagion, and sympathetic or antagonistic interactions between human beings and their surroundings. . . . the diseases themselves were mostly attributed to violations of taboos, neglect of ritual obligations, loss of vital substances from the body (mainly the soul, that is, the principle of life), introduction of foreign and harmful substances into the body (possession by spirits), and witchcraft.

Simon's earlier-described tripartite understandings of mental illness—popular notions, medical, and philosophical—persisted throughout the period, and in terms of medical therapeutics, Hippocratic humoral theory prevailed. Nevertheless, over this period, the naturalistic account—mental illness is rooted in natural occurrences rather than divine or supernatural ones—grew through the work of influential physicians and philosophers of the period.

Circa 500 BC to 1 AD: Naturalism gathers momentum. Plato, in the *Phaedrus* Socratic dialogue, presents the idea of 'madness', which can be noble or positive. Socrates identifies four kinds of madness—prophetic, involving the passions of divine gifts or insights; telestic, involving the discharge of impulses in ritualistic practices; poetic, which is involved in art and creativity; and erotic, having to do with emotional and physical love.[117] Plato's tripartite model of the mind, involving the appetite, reason, and spirit, as mentioned earlier, anticipated tripartite models of the mind to follow, including Freud's. Plato also addressed the issue of mitigating criminal offenses because of madness; nicely discussed in detail by Daniel Robinson in his *Wild Beasts & Idle Humours*.[118]

The work of Hippocrates of Cos (circa 469–399 BC) represents the strongest statement of disease naturalism to date. Summarizing Hippocrates on madness involves at least two caveats. One, Hippocrates' writings as we know them contain little in the way of actual discussion of madness proper, though psychopathological phenomena appear in the detailed clinical descriptions of patients. Secondly, details of Hippocrates' life and writings are limited, and indeed whether Hippocratic writings represent a single individual or multiple authors—the 'Hippocratics'—is an open question.[119] Nevertheless, Hippocratic thought established many of the iconic beliefs that persist today regarding the naturalistic approach to illness, whether mental or physical. These included the importance of clinical observation in inferring disease processes; the idea that illness is a natural event with discoverable causes; the brain as the seat of mentation, both normal and pathological; and the importance of sharing careful clinical description in the generation of knowledge of disease. With all these contributions to naturalistic medicine, Hippocrates articulated the humoral theory of disease as well, which reached its furthest elaboration later with Galen of Pergamum's work, which will be taken up shortly.

Of particular interest to the VMDR is the Greek scholar Posidonius (135–51 BC). As a moral philosopher he was identified with the Stoic school, but his interests were wide-ranging, including weighing in on the sciences, medicine, and what today would be called psychology. In his introduction to the surviving fragments of Posidonius' writing, Kidd[120] describes Posidonius as viewing the ordinary man as a mixture of health and illness, with illness reflected by irrational passion-driven decisions and actions. He described the person's struggle with 'beast-like' impulses[121] with the opposing forces of reason or logic. Posidonius' approach to aiding emotionally ill people involved showing them images of the consequences of their conduct; he believed that using reason to influence the unreasonable was futile.

The naturalistic orientation to mental disorders generated a greater interest in the workings of the brain. Erasistratus (304–250 BC) and Herophilus (335–280 BC) were among the first neuroanatomists, describing, between the two of them, sensory and motor nerves; convolutions of the cerebral cortex, cranial nerves, and the arachnoid and dura mater.[122] Herophilus, the older of the two, is often credited with articulating the first medical empiricism—that medical understandings should be grounded in observations, and articulated the relationship between good physical health and good mental health:[123]

> In the absence of health, Herophilus said in his treatise *Regimen*, one's wisdom cannot be demonstrated, one's scientific skill or craft remains invisible, one's strength cannot be exerted in contest, one's wealth is useless, and one's power of speech powerless.

Circa (1 to 500 AD: early Christendom and transition to the early medieval period. As we cross over into the Christian era following Jesus' life, we should not overlook what might be considered Jesus Christ and his followers' contributions to understanding of mental illness. Of course, Jesus offered no theory of mental illness, only loving concern for the stigmatized mad, and worked within the received cultural understandings of his day. Bennett Simon makes the astute point that Jesus' contribution was more as a therapist than a diagnostician or scientist:[124]

> Possession by a demonic being, with a ritual of contending with and driving out that demon, seems to come into prominence more in Hellenistic times and cuts across national and religious boundaries. The most famous ancient examples are the accounts in the Gospels of Jesus driving forth demons, especially the accounts in Mark and Luke of the man possessed by the demon, 'my name is legion, for I am many'. These accounts imply that possession as an explanation of illness was quite commonplace, and that Jesus was not unique in being able to heal by exorcism, but rather that he was especially good at it.

Jesus' iconic exorcism of demons provides a powerful image that has persisted throughout the centuries in protecting the possession account of mental illness from secularist attack, surviving, and even flourishing in some religious circles, to this day. Only later will concerns about secularist interpretations arise (e.g., that the people Jesus exorcized may have had a 'possession state') or other naturalistic psychopathology.

Aulus Cornelius Celsus, a first-century Roman scholar authored an influential treatise *De Medicina*, which articulated standards of clinical management for the mentally disturbed, some of which are recognizable today—from using lighting to calm the delirious, to emphasizing the role of proper and adequate sleep. Aretaeus of Cappadocia (circa first century A.D.) articulated the relationship between melancholia and mania and described the importance of calming and humane settings for treatment of the mad.[125] Aretaeus also articulated the idea that madness is related to excesses of ordinary capabilities.[126]

The Stoic school philosophers were not just important contributors to notions of ethics and moral conduct, but also to the theory of madness. The earlier Greek Stoics, like Posidonius, emphasized the importance of *apatheia* (moderation of strong emotions or passions) to good health. Later Roman Stoics like Seneca differentiated the passions from madness, seeing the former as normative disturbances of the soul—raising the issue that is current today regarding the distinction between ordinary emotional distress and mental disorder. Cicero, in articulating the concept of the libido, argued that excesses of the passions could lead to madness, while moderation, as with the rest of the Stoics, was crucial to mental health as well as to virtuous conduct.

The most influential medical thinker of the early Christian era, and indeed up through the Renaissance, was Claudius Galenus (Galen) of Pergamum (circa 129–201 A.D.). For the purposes of this chapter, Galen offers multiple iconic images of medicine and madness. Born into a privileged family in what is today Bergama, Turkey, Galen was encouraged by his architect father. Galen was also inspired by a provocative dream involving Asclepius, the Greek god of medicine and healing. Galen entered medical training at an early age and received an extensive education to support his goal. Galen's iconic medical status was not just practical and scientific, but also personal. He embodied the image of the egotistical, prideful physician, a familiar stereotype today. Porter[127] describes Galen as often humiliating 'lesser' physicians, waiting out the diagnostic discussion to point out the missing critical element. He was fond of name-dropping and boasting of the social status of his patients. He often held court with admiring students and patients and showcased anatomical dissections and physiological demonstrations. He wrote prolifically and immodestly presented himself as the physician who perfected Hippocratic humoral theory.[128]

That he wrote extensively and elaborated humoral theory is beyond question, composing hundreds of texts that, more than any other physician of his time, have survived to the present day. Galen posed, as the core of his etiological understanding of disease, what we would call today a four-by-four matrix of etiological factors: on one axis, the four humors: black bile, yellow bile, phlegm, and blood; on the other axis, the state factors: hot, cold, wet, and dry. These factors interacted in complex ways, yielding not just sixteen states but perhaps hundreds, given that each kind of potential imbalance in his system was graded on excesses and deficiencies for each. Galen emphasized that medicine was built upon three core disciplines:[129]

> ... logic, (the discipline of thinking), physics (the science of nature), and ethics (the science of action). Philosophy and medicine were thus counterparts: the best doctor was also a philosopher, while the unphilosophical healer (the Empiric) was like an architect without a plan.

Galenic therapy was based upon, like Hippocratic medicine, the idea of balance and equilibrium among the four humors and four states, and so interventions involved purgings, bloodlettings, heatings, coolings, and the like, as well as use of multi-ingredient salves, oral brews, slurries, and other concoctions.[130] Ingredients for these numbered in the hundreds, and included pioneering use of botanicals as well as ordinary and exotic animal ingredients like viper meat or ground lizard. Galenic herbal medicine was elaborated upon by Dioscorides (circa 40–90 AD) in a five-volume *De Materia Medica*.[131]

At the core of Galenic science was the study of anatomy and what today would be considered physiology. Though not an experimentalist in the contemporary sense, Galen put great credence in dissection and observation of function, though his anatomical and physiological observations were limited to animal studies. The study of animals leads to some serious errors and misgeneralizations from today's perspective, such as the attribution of animal anatomic details to human anatomy. The major exception to the study of animal anatomy was Galen's appointment as the physician to gladiators, where dramatic injuries afforded rare opportunities for structural observation of human tissue, bone, and organ. Galen situated the Platonic tripartite model of the soul within the heart, brain, and liver, each serving to process aspects of the soul:[132]

> Within the human body, *pneuma* (air), the life breath of the cosmos, was modified by the three principal organs, the arteries and nerves. Pneuma, modified by the liver, became the nutritive soul or natural spirits which supported the vegetative functions of the growth and nutrition; this nutritive soul was distributed by the veins. The heart and arteries were responsible for the maintenance and distribution of innate heat and pneuma or vital spirits to vivify the parts of the body. The third alteration, occurring in the brain, ennobled vital spirits into animal spirits, distributed through the nerves (which Galen thought of as empty ducts) to sustain sensation and movement.

A premier theorist and author on the significance of the pulse, Galen also brought his medical observational skills into the 'forensic' realm through describing the symptoms of anxiety and elevated pulse in lying offenders. Galenic psychopathology was not particularly innovative and included the standard concepts of the time: melancholy, delirium, phrenitis, mania, and hysteria, though his description of catatonia was novel.

St. Augustine (354–430 A.D.), while not contributing to the understanding of psychopathology in a literal sense, was important in demonstrating a kind of psychology based on the personal self-reflections in his *Confessions*.[133] Augustine articulated concepts like memory, will, and reason and used these abstract concepts to facilitate his own self-understanding in reflection. Of course, the primary source of understanding was divine revelation, but Augustine gave credence to introspection and self-consideration as secondary sources of knowledge.[134] Augustine's astute psychological observations are many, but his description of Alypius' fall into the bloodlust of the gladiatorial amphitheater captures a phenomenon closely related to what today we would call social contagion or mass hysteria:[135]

> He (Alypius) held such spectacles in aversion and detestation; but some of his friends and fellow-pupils on their way back from a dinner happened to meet him in the street, and, despite his energetic refusal and resistance, used friendly violence to take him into the amphitheater during the days of the cruel and murderous games. . . . When they arrived and had found seats where they could, the entire place seethed with the most monstrous delight in the cruelty. He kept his eyes shut and forbade his mind to think about such fearful evils. . . . A man fell in combat. A great roar from the entire crowd struck him with such vehemence that he was overcome by curiosity. Supposing himself strong enough to despise whatever he saw and to conquer it, he opened his eyes. He was struck in the soul by a wound graver than the gladiator in his body, whose fall had caused the roar. . . . Thereby it was the means of wounding and striking to the ground a mind still more bold than strong, and the weaker for the reason he presumed on himself when he ought to have relied on you. As soon as he saw the blood, he at once drank in the savagery and did not turn away. His eyes were riveted. He imbibed madness. Without any awareness of what was happening to him, he found delight in the murderous contest and was inebriated by bloodthirsty pleasure. He was not now the person who had come in, but just one of the crowd which he had joined, and a true member of the group which had brought him.

This story anticipates the power of the mob to be explored explicitly in twentieth-century psychology and sociology.

Augustine and others contributed to the Patristic Period, the period beginning roughly with the death of St. John circa 100 AD, and extending into about the fifth century. The Roman Church over this period consolidated its power and sorted through the confusion of Jesus' sudden death and resurrection, developing the early structures, orthodoxies, and practices of the Roman Catholic Church. The growth of the Church, the fall of the Roman Empire and its intellectual elite, and the resulting chaos from the spread of warring tribes across Europe, moved the primary sources of education into the Church, which could do little to address the prevailing illiteracy among the masses. Believers' resignation and faith in the afterlife, promised by Jesus, led to a uniform dependence upon the Church, and a waning of naturalistic/philosophical understandings of disease. Regarding mental illness, the subsequent rise of belief in supernatural causes segued into the Dark Ages, a long-fallow period regarding the development of new understandings of psychopathology, or indeed, many new achievements at all in natural philosophy, or the Science yet to come.

4.2.4.4 Synthesis

This millennium generates a series of very important concepts, traditions, and iconic ideas that will recur in later centuries into the present. To summarize in short-titled points:

1. *The bifurcation of accounts of disease*: The competing understandings of mental illness through rationalist/empirical/secular accounts, versus supernatural/religious understandings, consolidated the former among, largely, the educated elites. For the latter, these views settled in large part among clergy and ordinary peoples.
2. *The families of virtues*: The major religions describe a range of habitual patterns of living well, associated with religious enlightenment and/or salvation, as well as personal tranquility.
3. *The good acts/good faith tension*: Many religions exhibit disagreement, both across faiths and within faith traditions, regarding the role of good acts as leading to enlightenment/salvation versus devotion alone as leading to enlightenment/salvation.
4. *Early classifications of madness*: Ancient Greeks introduce categories of mental disturbance, and standard terms consolidate in the latter part of the millennium, terms, such as mania, melancholia, phrenitis, and delirium.
5. *Secular versus supernatural understanding of madness*: The early Greek diversity of empirical, philosophical, and magical/religious understandings of madness consolidate over the millennium into two persisting kinds of accounts of madness: rationalist/empirical/secular understandings, versus supernatural/religious understandings.
6. *Role of religion in morality and health:* The major world religions address universal human suffering and its relation to moral life and psychological health.
6. *Early moral faculties and capabilities*: Iconic ideas underwriting moral psychology are introduced: self, responsibility, guilt, reason, and will.
7. *Morality and health*: Many, perhaps most, major religions link positive moral conduct with physical and mental health or well-being.
8. *Moderation as health*: Many physicians and religious traditions identify a connection between indulging in strong emotions/passions with ill health physical and mental.

9. *Morality and health*: Many, perhaps most, major religions link positive moral conduct with physical and mental health or well-being.
10. *Moral diversity*: Moral diversity appears, as philosophers and religious leaders define widely differing norms which shift from belief system to belief system, and era to era.
11. *Sexual diversity*: Perhaps excepting the moral acceptability of war or justified killing, no area of moral regulation grew into greater diversity by geography, belief system, and era than sexual conduct.
12. *Consolidating moral proscriptions*: Nearly universal moral proscriptions were made against theft, murder, and deceit emerge across culture and era.
13. *Distinguishing law, morality, & religion*: While still overlapping in conceptual content, traditions increasingly make distinctions between law, morality, and religious directives.
14. *Illness, ignorance, and wrongfulness.* The idea that illness, impairment, or ignorance accompanies wrongdoing gathers cultural weight.
15. *Metaphysics underlie ethics*: Observing the histories of moral and philosophical ideas over this period introduces the conclusion that metaphysical assumptions or beliefs (assumptions about the nature of being human) can be closely related to ethical viewpoints and moral directives.
16. *The rise of empiricism*: The importance of empirical observation, not just reflection, upon understanding diseases and madness appears and increasingly guides medical thought.
17. *Religious healing*: Religiously guided healing, while a part of many religions, is powerfully and influentially depicted by Jesus Christ.

4.2.5 European medieval era to the early Renaissance, 500–1500 AD

The millennium spanning 500–1500 BC was one of tremendous social change, involving wars, the rise of the Christian Church and Islam as religious and political powers, and extensive travel among (particularly) warriors, generating cultural diasporas of a number and complexity that Western culture had never seen before. The period spans the so-called Dark Ages of Europe (roughly 500–1000 AD), where the generation of knowledge and cultural achievement was curtailed by warring factions that battled over the failing Roman Empire and territories beyond and surrounding. The millennium spans the eras of the Byzantine Empire, essentially the Western Roman Empire, and later, the Ottoman Empire. The power of the Roman Church expanded, and the period saw the coronation by the Church of the conquering Roman Emperor, Charlemagne, as the first Holy Roman Emperor in 800. However, throughout this millennium political instability prevailed, and the invaders of various stripes brought back the influences of their would-be conquests back to their home countries. For example, the then-superior Arab and Persian science was brought back to Western Europe by the Crusades soldiers.

4.2.5.1 Morality

Circa 500–1000 AD. As the corpulent Roman Empire declined over the fourth century, roaming tribes sought new empires as Western pieces of the old Roman Empire were carved up by invaders. Internal European strife involving Ostrogoths, Visigoths, Vandals, Sueves, Franks, and Burgundians vied for territory from Iberia (Spain) in the west to the Mediterranean territories to the east. The borders of territories were constantly redrawn, and Kingdoms, at least by the earlier standards of Rome, were small, brutish, and short-lived. Over the same period invading outsiders penetrated territories all over Europe: Vikings, Magyars, Lombards, Bulgars, Avars, and Slavs—the latter lending their name to 'slaves' in medieval England. Later, jihadist Muslim Arabs built an empire that rivaled the Roman in size and influence.[136] The times were not friendly to the development of morality, peace, and virtue, much less science and scholarship.

Nevertheless, despite the pervasive presence of war, destruction, and religious vainglory, some positive aspects of culture developed, such as the values of public service in 'chivalry'. Natural Philosophy and scholarship increasingly moved into the Church through the developing monastic sects and their corresponding monasteries and abbeys; ascetic monks spent much of their time copying manuscripts, and assimilating the knowledge of older work like Galen's, the Greek and Roman philosophers, and later, Islamic scholars and physicians. However, in the world of the peasant or commoner, outside the rarefied setting of the castle or monastery, the boundaries between religion, science, and magic eroded as artisanry, folk magic, and folk medicine developed and intermingled.

Warring barbarians and bloody knights contributed to the general decline of popular morality, and the victors indulged all manner of appetites: for example, sex, drink, and food. Viking moral culture in particular was a peculiar combination of Homeric honor/loyalty combined with decadent excess (e.g., feasting, boozing, and womanizing) was accompanied by various praises of classical virtue: 'The good name never dies of one who has done well.'[137] The Roman Church attempted to address moral decline in a variety of ways, but most notably for this book is the articulation of the Seven Deadly Sins (see Chapter 3, Section 3.2.1) and their corresponding virtues, articulated in early form by Evagrius Ponticus and (Saint) John Cassian in the fourth century, and then formalized by Pope Gregory I in 590.[138] Rampant fornication throughout Europe, resulting in a crisis of bastardy, coupled with Church scruples against infanticide, abortion, and child abandonment led to the founding of the first 'orphanage' in Milan in 787, and various, often unsuccessful, attempts to diminish prostitution.

The remains of the old Roman Empire shifted its center of gravity to Byzantium and Constantinople (now Istanbul, Turkey), and in Emperor Justinian's era

(482–565) there was some potential for reuniting the Eastern and Western Roman Empire. Justinian is relevant to this chapter because of his elaboration and formalization of Roman law, and the paradoxes of his ruthless conquests, on the one hand, and humane changes in Roman law and practice, such as reducing mutilations, 'amnesty' for homosexuals (to confess their sins[139]), and the loosening of constraints on other vices. Justinian differentiated public law (concerning government), 'natural law' ('the law which nature teaches all animals'), law of nations (international law), and civil law (laws of nations or states).[140] Regarding the latter, Justinian placed great emphasis on protecting the family, and included provisions for caring for children, the senile, and the mad. Provisions of civil law in today's sense were also developed, such as invalidating a will by an insane person.[141]

While the Church continued its missionary work in winning converts, an increasing number of priests poured more energy into identifying heretics within their own ranks, at first by censure and excommunication, and later and more grimly, violent means. These trends consolidated with the Crusades (circa 1000–1200) and the Inquisition (twelfth century), both activities that profoundly undermined a favorable historical appraisal of the period's moral achievements. The warring factions left domestic chores to women, whose investment in crafts, agriculture, and especially secular and 'magical' (often herbal) healing arts set the stage for their explicit persecution as witches in the High Middle Ages (roughly 1000–1500).[142] This to be echoed centuries later in the American Colony, Salem, Massachusetts era of witch trials.

The most significant development for the history of morality in this half-millennium may be the birth of Muhammad ibn 'Abdullāh, the prophet-founder of Islam in 570. Considered a third prophet of the monotheistic God of Judaism and Christianity, Muhammad, like Jesus Christ, taught morality by example, described through the *Sunnah*, a document of the Prophet's teachings, instructions, and actions, which added explicit religious-moral instructions for followers. *Shari'a*, Islamic law, is based upon God's revelations to Muhammad in the Quran, also gives explicit instruction, like Leviticus in the Old Testament, as regarding religious practices and common moral questions of family, sexual, and community life. Thomson[143] gives a succinct summary of Muhammad's moral principles and values:

When Mohammed (570–632) withdrew from Mecca in 622, it was a reaction against the complacent and commercial materialism of the city created by the wealth of the caravan trade. His doctrine was therefore anti-materialistic and appealed in the first instance, like Christianity, mainly to slaves and the poor. He insisted on submission to the will of God (Islam) and the five daily prayers, fasting during Ramadan, abstinence from wine, gambling, and usury. He violently protested against the Arab custom of female infanticide. Mohammed's basic programme of regular prayer, alms-giving and fasting was to bring about a tranquil, happy attitude of mind.

Sexual morality was strict—while polygamy and slave concubinage were permitted, pederasty and prostitution were punishable by death. The story of Adam's fall was especially significant for Islam in demonstrating Satanic excess. The foremost Islamic virtue is *taqwa*, a moral awareness which combines the basis for moral action and describes a morally motivated state of mind that inspires a person to be good.[144]

Classical Islam does not make a distinction between political and religious laws, hence religious disagreements have powerful political consequences and vice versa. The splitting of Islam into sects occurred early for the Sunni/Shi'ite traditions, based upon disputes about the true lineages of the *Caliphs*, the descendants of Muhammad and rulers of the Islamic state. Sufism, another Islamic sect, shares some features with Buddhism and Hinduism in emphasizing an inward, even mystical awareness and seeking of spiritual enlightenment and a more direct relationship with God.

Islam proved to be a powerful uniting force for Arab peoples, and within the century following Muhammad's death, Arab jihadist forces organized and conquered Byzantine territories occupying contemporary Egypt, Libya, Syria, as well as Persia. By the end of the seventh century, followers had spread to Spain in the west and China in the east.[145]

Circa 1000–1500 AD. This period approximates the 'High Middle Ages' and the transition to the European Renaissance. The High Middle Ages was a period, at least in Europe, where education and intellectual achievement was largely confined to the Church and its developing Monastic movement, which founded several ascetic religious orders which cherished and housed scholarship and learned manuscripts. From the economic perspective feudalism prevailed, with most property controlled by small numbers of nobility and Church officials, with a large population of peasants doing most of the labor. To the East, the Muslim Arabs developed the largest empire in history to date, with a corresponding sophistication in science and medicine which was exported to their territories of conquest. In empire and science, comparable achievements developed over this period in China, though these will not be discussed here. These achievements in medicine and science will be discussed in more detail below in the 'Madness' section.

Increasing trade between East and West had multiple implications. Islamic and Chinese science and technology, as well as material goods, found their way into Europe. The threats of heresy, Judaism, and Islam provoked the Crusades to win back Christian empire. The most profound epidemic in history to date, the Black (bubonic) Plague, or 'Black Death' spread (precisely because of the increased international commerce) via rat fleas from east to west and vice versa, peaking in the 1300s and killing approximately 100 million people, reducing the population of Europe by (disputably) half.[146]

Such grim realities led many Christians to conclude that they were suffering the wrath of God, and extreme forms of penance appeared, crystallizing into movements such as the Flagellants of the thirteenth century, who indulged in constant self-floggings and mortification of the flesh. Such practices were later to be declaimed by the Church as heretical, although severe forms of self-infliction of pain persist today, though more typically a more conservative interpretation of 'mortification of the flesh' prevails. The latter typically refers to denying oneself various pleasures and is a part of Catholic asceticism.[147]

The popular images of the High Middle Ages are of knights and chivalry, castle kingdoms, the Plague, and the Crusades. However, the period was host to what might be construed as the birth of 'philosophy' as construed in the contemporary sense, as a very specialized kind of intellectual activity, with its own rigorous methods and specialized areas of study: epistemology, ontology, ethics, and others, all pursued by scholars in universities. Indeed, the period saw the birth of universities as we know them today in large part because of the flourishing of the Scholastic movement beginning around 1000. The Scholastics, most notably for our interest Albertus Magnus, John Duns Scotus, and Thomas Aquinas, did not so much pose a 'school of thought' but rather embodied disciplines of learning and methods of inquiry. Many of the core methods of contemporary philosophy today—dialectical reasoning, conceptual analysis, and the making of philosophical distinctions—had roots in Scholasticism. The movement of ideas also concretized in political practice in 1215 when the English limited the power of the monarchy through the Magna Carta, taking an important step forward in replacing imperial whim with the rule of law.

The earlier Monastic movement with their abbeys had sought out, developed, and distributed translations of classic Greek texts into Latin, and the new avenues of travel across the continents had permitted the importation of scholarship from not just Greek sources but also Jewish scholars like Maimonides and Islamic philosophers like Ibn Rushd (Averroes) and Ibn Sina (Avicenna). The intellectual exchange across culture and language promoted the growth of the Monastic schools into larger, more research-oriented universities, which not only taught students but debated ideas and generated new ones. By the mid-thirteenth century, universities had been founded in Oxford, Paris, Poitiers, Chartres, Bologna, Coimbra, and elsewhere.[148]

The Monastic and later Scholastic movements developed settings and practices where crucial decisions on Biblical interpretation and Christian practice could be made. Sidgwick[149] associates the birth of Scholasticism with St. Anselm's 'comprehensive and profound attempt to render the dogmatic system of orthodox Christianity, so far as possible, intelligible to reason'.[150] Anselm's younger contemporary, Abelard, formulated a now-contemporary notion of sin. Each person is born into the potential for wrongful conduct, and that potential per se is not sin, nor is necessarily the wrongful action associated with this potential. Abelard notes that the notion of virtue presupposes vice, which is what virtue struggles against in its efforts to perform rightful actions. The cases of ignorant, uninformed, or mad wrongful actions are also not sin, in that culpability or responsibility cannot be assumed. What constitutes sin is, as Sidgwick summarizes it, 'contempt for God and His commands' which is 'manifested in conscious consent to vicious inclination.'[151] Sin, then, in Abelard's view, is the intent to disregard God's word in performing wrongful action. The core of true repentance for sin is not regretting just the wrongful act, but rather amending the intention to reject or ignore God's direction.

Similar concerns were characteristic of the philosophy of Abu 'Ali Al-Husayn Ibn Sina (Avicenna) perhaps the most influential Islamic philosopher-physician of his era (980–1037). Avicenna argued that human perfection (in the sense of pursuing the excellences of virtue) should be sought through rational activities and the life of the mind. Correspondingly, evil manifested from 'privations of one's capabilities'.[152] More a metaphysician and scientist than a moral philosopher, Avicenna bridged the gap between Islamic religion and his Greek philosophical predecessors by modifying Aristotelian virtue to be compatible with Platonic concerns about the hereafter. Later, Abu 'L walid Muhammad Ibn Rushd (Averroes), Avicenna's chief rival and critic as the prince of medieval Islamic philosophy, purged any Platonic elements from his own version of Aristotelianism, but nevertheless sought to preserve the relations between religion and philosophy, claiming each held its own form of truth. Influenced by many works of Aristotle, especially the Poetics, Averroes argued that poetry was closely related to rhetoric and consisted of two genres: praise and blame, thus linking poetry to moral reflection.[153]

Among the most influential thinkers in ethics, and especially medical ethics, was the Cordoban, Moses Maimonides (Rambam, Rabbi Moses ben Maimon) (1186–1237), a Jewish philosopher-physician and Talmud scholar. Like Thomas Aquinas to follow (for the Christian Bible), Maimonides believed that the teachings of the Torah were compatible with secularist ideas like Aristotle's. Maimonides' greatest work, the *Guide to the Perplexed*, aimed to reconcile reason and faith.

Maimonide's *Oath* could be contrasted with Hippocrates':[154]

> The eternal providence has appointed me to watch over the life and health of Thy creatures. May the love for my art actuate me at all time; may neither avarice nor miserliness, nor thirst for glory or for a great reputation engage my mind; for the enemies of truth and philanthropy could easily deceive me and make me forgetful of my lofty aim of doing good to Thy children.
>
> May I never see in the patient anything but a fellow creature in pain.
>
> Grant me the strength, time and opportunity always to correct what I have acquired, always to extend its domain; for knowledge is immense and the spirit of man can extend indefinitely to enrich itself daily with new requirements.
>
> Today he can discover his errors of yesterday and tomorrow he can obtain a new light on what he thinks himself sure of today. Oh, God, Thou has appointed me to watch over the life and death of Thy creatures; here am I ready for my vocation and now I turn unto my calling.

Notable for Maimonides' instructions for physicians are the warnings against the doctor's hubris and narcissism, and in contrast, the emphasis on empathic relatedness to the patient.

Maimonides could be considered a virtue ethics theorist influenced by Aristotle but also very much his own thinker. He had a more contemporary view of virtues as fluid and conceptually indistinct, requiring the use of philosophy to clarify them, and particularly a flexibility to adapt to Jewish precepts.[155] Some of his views were frankly in disagreement with both St. Thomas Aquinas (discussed below) and Aristotle. For instance, Maimonides was distrustful of strong passions; he thought anger in any measure was toxic (as in Buddhism), and that an Aristotelian mean of anger offered little virtue.[156]

The thirteenth century and the Catholic Church brought the period's greatest Christian scholar and moral theorist, St. Thomas Aquinas, whose *Summa Theologica*[157] attempted to unify Aristotelian philosophy and ethics with Christian doctrine. Aquinas' work could claim the primary responsibility for the close link between Aristotelian virtues and Catholicism today. Aquinas' extraordinary quantity of philosophical writings for his relatively short life (1225–1274) ranged from ethics to metaphysics and counted as philosophy because of his careful and still-influential systematic reasoning by argument and counterargument. Perhaps the most important set of ideas for his moral philosophy were not even explicitly moral, but rather metaphysical, in that all rational creatures were guided by teleological or goal-directed thought, including both rational and irrational thought. Aquinas' teleology directs both ordinary and spiritual aspirations. While a variety of life-aims may occupy people, only those guided by God's grace assure true happiness or satisfaction. Like Aristotle, Aquinas divided virtues into intellectual and moral ones, and endorsed many of the Aristotelian ones, as well as St. Paul's theological virtues, Faith, Love, and Hope. Aquinas was influential as a legal theorist: law being in his view the 'ordinance of reason for the common good'.[158]

Aquinas' Christian metaphysics framed his four notions of law: the first being eternal law, emerging from God's reason and embracing all of God's creations. The second, 'natural law' was a portion of eternal law that applies to rational beings, thus situating Nature within the Christian cosmos. The third, 'human law' was the specifying and situating of natural law within human cultures or communities. The fourth, 'divine law' which referred to the laws of the Old and New Testament, especially the Gospels, which were given to humans by revelation. In the latter context, two kinds of moral/law guidance are discussed, one set constitutes the absolute requirements or commands of God, while the other are recommendations or guidance for living the best life.

Of most significance for the VMDR was Aquinas' theory of natural law. Aquinas' natural law was grounded in two metaphysical aspects: the first held natural law as a part of eternal law, governed by divine providence or God's will and thereby establishing both the 'nature' of natural law, as well as conferring the (divine) status of 'law' to natural law. The second arm enabled rational beings like humans to comprehend natural law through reason; Murphy identifies this arm of natural law theory to rational beings' God-given capacity for 'practical rationality'.[159] That is, through reason humans can come to recognize natural laws. While the ethical content of natural law is not given comprehensively by St. Thomas, one can recognize common Biblical proscriptions, most pertinently for this book about vice: adultery, sodomy, murder, deceit, and blasphemy are prominent examples. Aquinas' ethics were context-sensitive; he recognized that moral situations were complex and that some natural laws could instruct contradictory actions in some situations. For example, prostitution, while wrongful, served as a hedge against greater sins.

Political concepts were influential contributions emerging from Aquinas' work. Grounding the idea of human being as social by nature (following Aristotle), and the parallel grounding of this social nature as God-given, then it was a short deduction to link the notion of the state and governance to God's intentions. These considerations, along with Aquinas' concept of natural law as God's design, then set the stage for unnatural conduct to be both an offense to the State as well as an offense against God. Aquinas' views about law as serving the common good had as a correlate that law promotes citizens to pursue their own virtue. Together, these ideas established a powerful cultural link between law and morality that persists today. For Aquinas, law is not just a practical means to help people get along together. Law is a derivative of God's moral designs for us.[160]

Finally, and perhaps of most relevance to the VMDR of today, Aquinas was influential in describing the role of criminal law and punishment. For Aquinas, criminal law does not 'micromanage' all vices from which people may indulge, but instead regulates 'particularly those vices which are damaging to others and which, if they were not prohibited, would make it impossible for human society to endure; as murder, theft, and suchlike, which are prohibited by human law'.[161] Aquinas formulated early notions of criminal rehabilitation and deterrence:

> . . . there are others, of evil disposition and prone to vice, who are not easily moved by words. These it is necessary to restrain from wrongdoing by force and fear (*per vim et metum*) so that, they ceasing to do evil, a quiet life is assured to the rest of the community; and they are themselves drawn to eventually, by force of habit, to do voluntarily what once they did only out of fear, and so to practise virtue. Such discipline which compels under fear of penalty is the discipline of law.

Not surprisingly, Aquinas also addressed criminal responsibility, viewing this as dependent upon voluntariness: '. . . the difference between involuntary and voluntary action; he who does an action involuntarily suffers the lighter penalty . . .'.[162]

While Aquinas was the prevailing theoretician of the day, perhaps the most inspiring moral 'role model' was Francis of Assisi (1181–1216), founder of the Franciscan order which emphasized a vow to poverty, service to all living things, and equal care to all, including the sick and mad. Earning a measure of controversy because of their rejection of the pomp of the increasingly decadent Roman Church, Francis and his followers were able to secure recognition by Pope Innocent III through their total loyalty to the Roman Church, including the acceptance of the Inquisition of the Albigensians.[163]

Two Franciscans, John Duns Scotus, (circa 1266–1308), one of Aquinas' chief critics, and William of Ockham (c. 1290–1347, author of medicine's 'Ockham's Razor') disagreed with Aquinas' idea that morality could be both derived through reason and received through revelation; believing that God made for the right, underscoring the idea of divine authority as the core of morality.[164] Such divine authority was concretized by divine recognition of royalty throughout Europe and the imperious power of the Church of the period. Such emphasis on deference to not just Church but royal authority was demonstrated by Dante Alighieri's (circa 1315) reservation of the ninth circle of Hell (in *The Inferno*) for treachery and treason, placing heresy, violence, and fraud as lesser sins.[165] In contradistinction to the Franciscans, it was the Dominicans who were the partners with Rome in implementing the Inquisition.[166]

Compliance with the Roman Church doctrine became a prevailing moral value of the medieval era. The Crusades, beginning at the end of the eleventh century, served multiple functions: to crush heresy, to win back lost portions of the Holy Roman Empire to Christian rulers, and to spread Christianity into territories dominated by Islam, pagan religions, and Judaism. Continuing for 3 centuries, the Crusades involved the killing of approximately 9 million people.[167] Shortly after the beginning of the Crusades, Christian sovereignties pursued their own violent means enforcing Christian orthodoxy, with Inquisitions popping up in multiple countries in Western Europe, and a formal declaration of papal Inquisitions articulated by Pope Gregory IX in the thirteenth century. Peaking during the high medieval era but persisting into the nineteenth century, several Christian sects were subject to particular prosecutor attention, the Albigensians and later the Cathars and Waldensians in southern France and Italy, with four major movements (the medieval Inquisition, the Spanish, the Portuguese, and the Roman). Non-Christian faiths were also subject to inquisitorial repression, which included transfer of heretics to the secular authorities and commonly included death by burning at the stake. The Inquisition era ushered in a persisting moral panic about witchcraft, articulated and promulgated by the *Malleus Maleficarum*,[168] the influential guide to establishing the existence of witches and instructions on how to identify and prosecute them. (More on witchcraft and its persecution in Section 4.2.5.2.)

4.2.5.2 Madness

As noted earlier section 4.2.5.1, the 500–1500 European millennial span encompassed the decay and fall of the Roman Empire, European conquests by Northern and Muslim invaders, the breaking up of Europe into short-lived kingdoms, and the associated oppressive consequences of constant war. Feudalism had divided the people into rigid social roles as fighters, laborers, and clergy. The development of mass diseases like the Black Plague and leprosy, the rise of Church power and consequent oppression of heretics and witches, and the fragmentation of culture in general made for dark times. The Dutch historian Johann Huizenga argued in his *The Waning of the Middle Ages*[169] that the mid-to-late Middle Ages amounted to an age of melancholia; exemplified by hellish images from iconic medieval artists like Albrecht Dürer and Hieronymus Bosch as well as discussion of melancholia and madness in the literature of the period.[170] The cultural preoccupation with death and torment was further expressed though Gothic architectural decorations of monstrous gargoyles (e.g., Paris' Notre Dame), thought to scare off evil spirits, as well as depictions of Biblical sufferings and torments,[171] as well as penitent cultural movements like the Flagellants, discussed earlier. Mora notes that symbolism and allegory became prominent in the iconography of the period; numbers, colors, and animals assumed metaphorical significance, and visual images in general became much more important in depicting human experience.[172] The life for women of the period was by and large not good; women's roles being primarily domestic servants in homemaking, childrearing, and crafts-making, with few rights or privileges of their own.

In general, the iconic descriptions of madness and mental distress did not change much over this millennial period; the language and theory being persistently Galenic in inspiration and detail. What was important, however, was the influence of the Monastic and later Scholastic movements, the founding of universities, and the importation and distribution of Islamic elaborations of Galenic medicine from renowned scholars like Ibn Sina (Avicenna) and Ibn Rushd (Averroes). These practices were harbingers for the intellectual renewal of the Renaissance to come, as well as the seeds for a more contemporary vision of science to follow. St. Thomas Aquinas' pioneering faculty psychology,[173] dividing up the mind into interacting components, was a germ for the later faculty psychologies taken up by philosophers and psychiatrists, while his strict distinction between the immortal soul, protected from disease, and the mortal body, the seat of disease, was to be a metaphysical orthodoxy for pioneering asylum doctors, alienists, and psychiatrists to come, through the 1800s. Albertus Magnus (Albert the Great), Aquinas' teacher and mentor, elegantly summarized the emerging rationalism as 'Natura est ratio' (Nature is reason),[174] while perhaps unintentionally raising the question of madness and unreason as unnatural, as Foucault[175] was to aver centuries later.

Mora[176] provides a very useful summary of the changes in the understanding of human nature during these Middle Ages; these changes are more important to the historical iconography of mental illness than this or that restatement of humoral theory or the redrawing of melancholia or other conditions. Mora notes that during this period our contemporary notion of a 'self'[177] did not exist; the period was in large part dominated by a fatalism about one's place in the universe; people's purposes in life were predetermined by a Great Chain of Being, and this divine order was be-lieved to work together, piece by piece, like a clock: nature, after all, was reason.

Only until the thirteenth century, with the development of crafts guilds and bourgeois notions of business, self-sufficiency, and self-efficacy, that a psychology enabling the possibility of pursuing one's own personal direction in life became con-ceivable for the ordinary person. In the latter centuries of this period people increas-ingly became defined by their jobs or work, and less by their place in a divine order or from a place of origin: a John Sadler would be a maker of saddles, not a John from Sadler, a town or region. Secular goals increasingly tended to supplant religious ones.

These early ideas of pursuing one's own fate simultaneously bred a distrust and re-sentment of the mad. Instead of being viewed as fitting into God's mysterious order, the vagabond, the orphan, the widow, and the mad came to be increasingly viewed as problems and a burden upon the common good. As Mora puts it, they came to be lumped with the 'poor, Jews, vagrants, homosexuals, heretics, foreigners, [and] lepers . . . .'[178] Insanity came to be feared and was increasingly depicted as a divine punishment in the art and literature of the period. While not described as such at the time, historians have described the era as birthing social practices involving mar-ginalizing of certain groups, along with the idea of *social deviance* lumping together ostracized, compromised, or undesirable social groups.[179]

The cultural iconography of psychopathology was evolving. The Muslim and Monastic scholars were describing psychopathological phenomena in more de-tail, while mystical experiences among Christians (e.g., Hildegard of Bingen) and Muslims (e.g., Sufism) were commonly described. Mystical experiences were not re-garded, by and large, as 'mad' but rather the embodied expressions of a theocentric, religious cosmology. Similarly, possession by demons was recognized as a personal invasion by concrete, tangible evil, and any disturbance of the mind or soul was a consequence of the demon's cruel mischief. Melancholia in particular was portrayed in multiple forms, ranging from Cassian's notion of *acedie*, a monastic vice of the time, although through our contemporary filters was more a mixture of lassitude, apathy, despondency, and depression; to Timothie Bright's (1586) more contempo-rary, major depression–like description of the melancholic condition.[180] Suicide, in particular, in the early Middle Ages was, as before, an offense against God, and rep-resented a failure in one's internal struggle between virtue and vice.[181] However, by the thirteenth century, England ended its mark of suicide as a felony—heretofore a crime where the perpetrator disappeared and thus evaded punishment in this world, but only to suffer eternal torment in the next.

Management of the uncontrollable or disruptive mad was through confinement in the early jails or in church or castle dungeons; these techniques were not considered as punishments, as the prevailing Justinian and Roman sensibility was that of '*satis furore ipsa punitur*'—madness was punishment in itself.[182] Rather, as noted earlier in considerations of Roman law, formal legal concern focused on management of the property of the lunatic.[183]

Medieval English law had begun to address mad offenders, leading to the introduction of law that marked early concerns of the forensic psychiatry and mental health law to come. Mora[184] describes elements of the 'Statute of King's Perogative' of 1255, which split incompetents into two categories: 'natural fools' who were intellectually defective from birth, presumably comparable to our recent notions of mental retardation, intellectual disabilities, and developmental disorders, and individuals who were '*non compos mentis*' (e.g., individuals whose impairments were acquired and perhaps temporary). These divisions were made to aid the Crown in deciding about property disputes and protection of the ill person's property.

Medieval Europe is believed to have developed the first hospitals caring for the mad in the twelfth century, though the dates are unclear. Islamic sultans and Roman Catholic priests in the regions of present-day Spain were particularly progressive in this regard, establishing multiple hospitals for the mad throughout the fourteenth century. However, the most common practice of the period was to lump the 'physically' ill with the 'mentally' ill, as did the legendary Bethlem in London, established in 1247 as a general hospital by the sisters of the Order of the Star of Bethlehem. Only later did its unique identity as a hospital for the mad emerge, and its further contracted nickname, Bedlam, entered our popular lexicon to describe a general state of chaos and disorder.[185]

In the thirteenth century, the Belgian town of Gheel had developed a reputation for family oriented, noninstitutional care of the mentally ill.[186] Treatment involved constructive work and exorcisms of the demons causing the madperson's torment. Gheel remained a historical signpost in the development of humane care for the mentally ill.

Perhaps the inverse of Gheel's humanitarian approach to care of the mad was the aforementioned *Malleus Maleficarum* in 1487. However, the 'Witch's Hammer' had been preceded by papal orders regarding witchcraft—the *Malleus* was only a formal statement and essay documenting what was already practiced—it was a sign of the times. In 1326, Pope John XXII issued a bulletin which equated witchcraft and magicians with heretics. Rosen notes, by 1330, more than 400 were accused of witchcraft in Toulouse and Carcassonne, with about half executed. In 1484 Pope Innocent VIII 'declared open war' on witches,[187] and the seeking, persecution, and execution of witches became a formal part of the Roman Inquisition.

What did witchcraft have to do with madness and mental disorder? This remains controversial among historians. Wallace[188] calls the *Malleus* 'a psychiatrist's casebook', while Porter describes the *Malleus* as 'viciously misogynistic' and describes the victims of witch persecution as a mixture of legitimate midwives, folk healers, and the mentally ill. In any case, the persecution of witches represented a general fear and distrust of women by the (often-scientific) men of the period:

> The standard view was that men and women shared a common physiology, but in perfect and flawed versions. Female generative organs were like those of men, but inverted

and inferior—the vagina was an inverted penis which had never fully developed. Thus, the female form was a faulty version of the male, weaker, because menstruation and tearfulness displayed a watery, oozing physicality; female flesh was moister and flabbier, men were more muscular. A woman's body was deficient in the vital heat which allowed the male to refine into semen the surplus blood which women shed in menstruation; likewise, women produced milk instead of semen. Women were leaky vessels (menstruating, crying, lactating), and menstruation was polluting.[189]

Perhaps the most notorious alleged witch was Joan of Arc (1412–1431), a teenage wonder-woman and proto-feminist who led the French Army to multiple victories during the Hundred Years' War, only to be burned at the stake as a witch at age 19 years.[190] Male ambivalence toward women had only begun to be expressed through the language of social deviance.

4.2.5.3 Synthesis

The medieval era in Europe, in terms of cultural iconic change, initiated, at least among the elites, murmurings of diverse ideas, beliefs, and practices that will grow, gain new recruits, and diversify further in the Renaissance and into the modern age. While we may be tempted to distance ourselves from the medieval era in terms of contemporary notions of democracy, equal opportunity, and universal humanity, the massive class differences between clergy, aristocrat, and serf are haunting echoes of class, racial, and economic inequities today, especially in the realms of morality and madness, as wide differences exist in the morality of ordinary citizens versus the wealthy ruling, intellectual, and business elites—no less true then as now. Similarly, the dichotomies between common beliefs about madness/mental illness then and now differ little in core content, and the proportions of popular belief to educated belief then and now would be a fine matter of debate for historians and social scientists today.

Iconic ideas for this section, in no particular order of importance:

1. *Reconciling faith and secular knowledge.* Beginning most prominently with St. Augustine, we see persistent efforts to reconcile faith and divine authority with secular knowledge in all three of the great Western monotheistic traditions: Christianity, Judaism (e.g., Maimonides), and Islam (e.g., Avicenna and Averroes). Many of these reconciliations share the belief that reason is divinely given and could, on its own, find genuine knowledge.

2. *Expanding regulation of sexual morality.* Ongoing, and differentiating, regulation of sexual morality grew both within the three monotheistic religious traditions and through the governments of the times.

3. *Madness linked to social class & role.* The 'diagnosis' of madness appears to be linked to social class or social role: different names and different conditions begin to sort along the lines of class or social role (e.g., 'hysteria' begins to be associated with midwifery, witchcraft, and peasantry). A related trend is the

beginnings of the identification of madness with deprived, degraded social classes and the beginnings of social marginality for these groups (e.g., the mad, the widow, the pauper, the racial minority immigrant, the orphan, and the criminal).

4. *Human nature undergirds morality and madness.* The expansion of philosophy beyond its Greek beginnings is associated with new metaphysical ideas, ideas which appear to shape conceptions of both morality and madness. Philosophy begins its transition to the modern era, where the concepts of morality/ethics, as well as politics and the polity, were based upon conceptions of human nature, and more deeply, the nature of existence itself.

5. *Reason, rationality, and education gain cultural power.* The educated elites increasingly invest in rationalism and reason, both improving the lot of humanity but increasingly posing rivalries with faiths and their institutions.

6. *Greater appreciation of the social nature of humanity.* Recognition grows regarding the social nature of humanity and use of government and law to solve shared problems, including those of social deviance.

7. *Academia is born.* The founding of universities ushers in a world practice of scholarship and research, in addition to education and the perpetuation of ideas across generations: culture.

8. *Travel and war increase cultural mingling.* The segregation of cultures erodes through travel and conquests, resulting in a prologue to multicultural differentiation and the blending of local ethnicities. With these multicultural influences, metaphysical viewpoints and assumptions begin to differentiate, and the seeds of fear of the 'other' are sewn.

9. *'Nature' is moralized explicitly.* The distinction between 'unnatural' and 'natural' behavior and conduct takes hold, and the view that the unnatural is against God, and, therefore, is immoral, tends to accompany this distinction, strengthening suspicions about the madperson as evil or possessed.

10. *Distinctions between law and morality are explored.* The relationships between law and morality are beginning to be explored and situated within metaphysical viewpoints.

11. *Law related more to the collective; morality to the individual.* The law begins to be linked with abstract concepts of social order and community, while morality continues to be linked with individual conduct and adherence to religious and other mores.

12. *Madness demands a bridging of law and morality.* Madness is increasingly identified as a concept and social problem that demands a bridging between law and morality.

13. *Social deviance increasingly linked with madness.* Connections between heresy, deviations from orthodoxies and conventions, and idiosyncratic individual differences, on the one hand, with madness/psychopathology on the other, develop over this period.

14. *A sociocultural Zeitgeist related to psychopathology.* Huizenga makes an early link of cultural/historical temperaments or cultural trends to the psychopathology of the day—with melancholia being the principal example for the late Middle Ages.
15. *Economic conditions shape social deviance.* The importance of economic conditions in framing social deviance is introduced.
16. *Ambiguities between madness and mysticism are introduced.* Ambiguities between mad vision versus mystical vision are introduced through the example of religious mystics.
17. *Connections between madness and punishment.* Cultural themes connecting madness with punishment (internal and external to the person) are elaborated concretely.
18. *Diversity of Church views on responsibility.* The diversity of viewpoints about what constitutes moral-personal responsibility begins to be elaborated during this period.

Many of the trends above point toward some themes of the Enlightenment, and increasingly my iconographic history of madness and morality will focus on themes pertaining to Western Europe and the American colonies, culminating in an explicit discussion of these themes in Colonial America and ultimately the United States.

4.2.6 Renaissance, Reformation, & Enlightenment, 1500–1800

With Christopher Columbus' 'discovery' of the New World in 1492, an entirely new geographic and social realm entered the morality/madness consideration, but this was only one of many dramatic transitions in the Western Hemisphere on either side of the Atlantic. Feudalism was breaking down as an economic system, and the myriad kingdoms of the medieval era were congealing into more modern nation-states. These social changes were led by England, France, and Spain, putting together large and economically powerful nation-states over the period, led most notably by the English King Henry VII and later Elizabeth I, the French Kings Louis XI and Francis I, and the merger of Aragon and Castile to make a contemporary Spain through the marriage of Ferdinand and Isabella in 1469. The new nation-states were not so impressed with the Holy Roman Empires nor the corruption and moral decay of the Catholic Church, and the new governments fueled new religious thinking as well. The Church's divided papacy was to end soon through the Reformation, which led to the proliferation of Protestant Christian denominations throughout the world, a reassertion of conservative Christian morality, the weakening of Roman Catholic authority and its persecution of heretics, and a new freedom for ordinary believers to read and interpret the Bible for themselves. In Italy, a Renaissance developed in the fourteenth century which generated an unsurpassed proliferation of the arts, sciences, and scholarship, as Italians excavated as well as critiqued the classical Greek and Roman texts and reassembled an intellectual life that had atrophied during the preceding centuries. The development of technology that had been on hold for so long, rekindled under the Renaissance, and advances in navigation, astronomy, and medicine stimulated a new secularism, a humanism, that was to usher in the Enlightenment (the Age of Reason), where confidence in secular rationality prevailed, and the questioning of older traditions, values, and customs was routine.[191]

In his rhapsodic prose, Roy Porter provides a summary of the psychological and metaphysical changes of the period:[192]

> The history of the self is commonly told as the rise of modern individualism, the maturing self-consciousness of the self-determining individual. Here lies the fulfilment of the cherished ideas first of 'knowing yourself'—the *gnothi seauton* of the Delphic oracle—and then of 'being yourself': 'this above all, to thine own self be true', as Polonius puts it in *Hamlet*, wearying his son as ever with unwanted advice. In this triumphalist telling, the secret of selfhood is located in authenticity and individuality, and the story presented is one of the surmounting of intractable obstacles in the achievement of autonomy. This great labour of inner character-building typically involves breaking free from religious persecution, political tyranny and the shackles of hidebound convention. Such ideals of self-realization, nobly voiced a century and a half ago in John Stuart Mill's *On Liberty*, still carry a strong appeal, and they square with other values—democracy, freedom of speech, equal opportunities, doing your own thing—which we all hold dear and to which the 'free world' at least pays lip-service.

For this section, I have, as has been typical, broken subsections into *Morality*, *Madness*, and *Synthesis*, but each of these subsections are further divided into *Renaissance*, *Reformation*, and *Enlightenment* subsubsections. This organization is not to suggest a strict chronology among the three; rather, this framing seemed an intuitively sensible way to organize the iconography of the period: for the *Renaissance*, the material is primarily focused on intellectual developments of the period; for the *Reformation*, the discussion focuses on religious changes, and for the *Enlightenment*, both themes are woven together as we transition to the modern era. My earlier qualifiers about chronology notwithstanding, some sort of demarcation is needed to address the transition in time from the Renaissance to the Enlightenment and, therefore, to sort the thinkers and iconic ideas of the times. For this purpose I've selected—imprecisely—1650 as a fuzzy line to separate the earlier Renaissance from the later Enlightenment. Again, for more convenience purposes than any other, the discussion of the Enlightenment as a distinct historical period ends around the turn of the nineteenth century, when 'psychiatry' proper comes into play, and the modern era more or less unfolds.

4.2.6.1 Morality

Renaissance. The European Renaissance spanned roughly the fourteenth–seventeenth centuries and is remembered today as a period of reawakening of intellectual ambitions and achievements, though this reawakening was perpetrated and enjoyed by mostly an elite few. However, the Renaissance was not all bright and shiny. For the masses, the poor, and the marginal, the Renaissance extended, and perhaps amplified, the darkness of the Middle Ages. During the Renaissance period, especially in the earlier times, war was still commonplace; the Medieval, Spanish, Roman, and Portuguese Inquisitions were still chasing down heretics, witches, and various other social deviants; while corruption and lip-smacking decadence continued to characterize the Roman Catholic Church and the Holy Roman Empire. The loosening of sexual mores was reflected in widespread prostitution and adultery (even among the royalty), increased toleration of pederasty, sexually provocative cleavage-baring dress, and tolerance, even encouragement, of wife-beating. The advances in science and technology not only brought forth benefits and conveniences, but also the invention of novel and creative devices for torture; the misery-making achievements of the period including the invention of thumb-and ankle-screws, the rack, the dunking stool, and the iron maiden, to name a few favorites of medieval torment. For the commoner, some sort of rebirth was long overdue.[193]

On the more positive side, the period was indeed one for an explosion of achievements in the arts and sciences, being the era of such notables as Leonardo da Vinci (1452–1519), Botticelli (1445–1510), Michaelangelo (1475–1564), Titian (1488–1576), Galileo Galilei (1564–1642), Nicolaus Copernicus (1473–1543), Johannes Kepler (1571–1630), and Isaac Newton (1643–1727), to name but a few. The period not only articulated our contemporary idea of science through Francis Bacon's work (1561–1626), but also framed the counterpoint of the 'humanities' as a set of scholarly endeavors, at the time embracing poetry, grammar, history, moral philosophy, and rhetoric.[194] The era ushered in modern philosophy and the development of philosophical systems that addressed, holistically, metaphysics, ethics, aesthetics, and political philosophy. Philosophical reflection had moved out of Scholasticism and the Church, and with it, the associated dogmas. Moreover, the proliferating of the new philosophical theorizing and writing was delivered, in large part, by lone, privileged scholars such as Descartes, Hobbes, Hume, Locke, and Kant, creating the trope of the academic philosopher, removed from the hurly-burly of everyday life, formulating grand ideas from the library easy chair. On the religious front, the period encompassed the Reformation and Martin Luther's provocation of Protestantism, leading to a diversification of Christianities in Europe and the New World.[195]

For the remainder of this section on Renaissance iconic contributions to the history of morality and ethics, I will present some of the iconic figures of the era, and a very brief summary of their relevant contributions.

Desiderius Erasmus (1466–1536) played important roles in contributing to the new 'humanism' movement, centering intellectual interests and values on human beings' capabilities and potential. The author of *In Praise of Folly* is primarily known for his humorous and satirical jibes directed at home and ecclesiastical life. His ends, however, were to restore moral standards to the Church and to the community. His rhetorical skills were such that he avoided the inquisitors while amusing those to whom the satire was directed. His work was included ultimately on the Church's Counter-Reformation reading list of the Council of Trent, the latter intended to re-furbish moral order in the Church. Erasmus' iconic status for our current interest consists in his literary popularization of the idea that madness and folly were not simply awful states to be avoided—punishments and internal torments—but alter-nate states of mind that offered insight, edification, and even truths that others dare not utter.[196]

Niccolo Machiavelli (1469–1527) is arguably the founder of political science through his interest in finding out how the State could use power effectively to main-tain order. His adjectivized name ('Machiavellian') today evokes the image of the ruthless, amoral tyrant, but his actual political philosophy was much more subtle. Machiavelli incorporated strong support for republicanism as well as a pragmatic approach to political morality, claiming that (only) sometimes the ends justify the means. Machiavelli introduced the idea that the pursuit of virtue by leaders could undermine political control, power, and order.[197] For Machiavelli, the security of the people and the liberty of the people were inversely related, and while Machiavelli actually favored promoting liberty, he believed that such liberty incurred deep tradeoffs against the security of the State.[198] We can see a germ here of the use of the State's power in maintaining political control through the regulation of deviance; an idea to be expounded upon centuries later by Szasz, Scheff, Foucault, and others. We can also cross-reference this view as we struggle as recently as 2024 with the regula-tion of social media misinformation and efforts to dismantle democratic institutions in favor of presumably more secure autocracies.

William Shakespeare (1564–1616), of further significance in the 'Madness' sec-tion to follow, should be mentioned as the greatest articulator of the human drama of morality and madness since Homer and the Greek tragedians. Here was a playwright who displayed madness and morality as living psychodramas, present in ordinary and exceptional living. For his audiences, Shakespeare linked the development of 'distraction'[199] to not just supernatural influences but the effluvia of human nature and an emerging sense of selfhood and individualism.

The Dutch Protestant Hugo de Groot, 'Grotius' (1583–1645), identified by Kelly[200] as the founder of international law, is significant here not so much for that, but for the idea of separating out the concept of natural law from Aquinas' grounding in God, leading the way for distinguishing secular and religious accounts of law and mo-rality. Grotius did not reject a divine order of natural law, only that 'natural law is the command of right reason' thus obviating Aquinas' requirement for a divine order.[201]

Of additional significance was the elaboration of a concept of 'rights' to preserve peace by ensuring the respect of others. Such rights included self-defense, the ability to marry, private ownership, parental authority over children, and the will of the majority over the minority. Related to his theory of rights was excluding what was not a right, and for our interest, a consideration of rights in the setting of criminal law. Grotius claimed ones' thoughts or beliefs were not subject to criminal charges nor punishment but may of course be considered in the context of criminal actions. In this sense he delegitimized 'thought crimes' and contributed to the contemporary understanding of crime requiring social, and physical, action. While Grotius acknowledged the motive of vengeance in criminal punishment, he endorsed Seneca's tripartite rationale for punishment—(1) reform, (2) deterrence and example for the populace, and (3) protecting the public. Scholars and the public have been debating the respective role of each ever since.[202] This book will pick up this crucial theme in later chapters.

Through his influence in articulating a comprehensive political philosophy, including the grounding of his moral/political views in a metaphysics (an account of human nature), Thomas Hobbes (1588–1679) is of founding relevance to the analysis of the VMDR. (Hobbes also articulated a psychology of the passions, with madness representing an excess of passions, which will be described in more detail in Section 4.2.6.2.)

For the purposes of this book, how Hobbes did philosophy was as significant as the philosophy itself. Hobbes's philosophy was concerned centrally about maintaining peace; understandable given the bloody period in which he lived. Hobbes went to great effort to discredit interpretations of the Bible and Christianity that were, in his assessment, incompatible with peace, and he devotes substantial portions of his writings to an exegesis of the Bible that was compatible with his political account and pacifist goals.[203] The significance here for the VMDR is the assumption that the Bible is an hermeneutically fluid document that can be interpreted to satisfy particular political agendas—as contemporary an idea as has been noted to date. Hobbes articulated the influential notion of a 'state of nature'—the situation of humankind without government, and the picture described of man in a state of nature was not favorable to the development and maintenance of social goods as we know them. In popular culture Hobbes is oft quoted for his memorable summary of human life in the state of nature, likening it to a state of war: 'solitary, poore, nasty, brutish, and short'.[204] This trope has never been more powerful than today, with the proliferation of dystopian fiction and fantastically popular yet doomy TV serials like *The Walking Dead* and *Game of Thrones*. Hobbes argued that deference to the government, or sovereign, should be absolute; to do otherwise inevitably compromises the maintenance of peace. (He did provide for the right of self-defense of subjects to resist when their lives were in danger.) His overriding moral precept was a convoluted inversion of the Golden Rule: to not treat others as we ourselves would not want to be treated. Hobbes's approach to political philosophy, by appealing to a social agreement of reasonable and free persons, founded what was to be known as social contract theory, with many variations to come.

The second grand metaphysician (and the first scientist) to be considered here, Rene Descartes (1596–1650), is often cited as the founder of modern philosophy. Most influential in his work on metaphysics (and not so much on ethics), Descartes' *cogito ergo sum* argument—I think therefore I am—is studied by every philosophy undergraduate as a founding moment in the history of modern philosophy, a land-mark in the effort to provide a foundation for knowledge, to answer the question How do I know anything? The ramifications of this core epistemological problem are legion and away from our interests for this book, apart from establishing 'Cartesian dualism' as a perennial problem in the history of philosophy following the seven-teenth century. Descartes believed that the soul, or mind, was immaterial, yet linked somehow to the body—the nature of this linkage the fodder for generations of philo-sophers, psychiatrists, and neuroscientists to follow. The 'mind-body' problem, or more contemporaneously—the 'mind/brain' problem, raised the question of how immaterial concepts like ideas, convictions, passions, came from, and influenced, our material bodies—and vice versa.

Though identifying ethics and morality as important 'sciences', Descartes did not pursue ethics in much detail, so his importance in the historical iconography of mo-rality[205] is less than many others discussed here. Nevertheless, the often-referenced four maxims of morality from the *Discourse on Method* offer an interesting take on the emerging morality of the times. One wonders if Descartes' maxims were a window into the everyday morality of the Renaissance/early Enlightenment elites:[206]

> The first was to obey the laws and customs of my country, adhering firmly to the Faith in which, by the grace of God, I had been educated from my childhood, and regulating my conduct in every other matter according to the most moderate opinions, and the farthest removed from extremes, which should happen to be adopted in practice with general con-sent of the most judicious of those among whom I might be living . . . My second maxim was to be as firm and resolute in my actions as I was able, and not to adhere less stead-fastly to the most doubtful opinions, when once adopted, than if they had been highly cer-tain; . . . when it is not in our power to determine what is true, we ought to act according to what is most probable; . . . My third maxim was to endeavour always to conquer myself rather than fortune, and change my desires rather than the order of the world, and in ge-neral, accustom myself to the persuasion that, except our own thoughts, there is nothing absolutely in our power; . . . In fine, to conclude this code of Morals, I thought of reviewing the different occupations of men in this life, with the view of making choice of the best. . . . devoting my whole life to the culture of my Reason, and in making the greatest progress I was able in the knowledge of truth. . . .

Obedient, steadfast, prudent, and rational—the idealized beginnings of the modern citizen?

Reformation. Earlier I briefly mentioned the 'Great Schism of Western Christianity' (1378–1416) related to the political rivalries between Roman papacy and an upstart Avignon papacy. The Avignon papacy in particular elicited disillusionment with the Church as the practices of 'simony' (selling of Church office) and the selling of 'indulgences' (credits against time in Purgatory) led many would-be believers to pagan beliefs and practices.[207] Chief among the critics of the selling of indulgences was Martin Luther, an Augustinian cleric originally associated with the University of Wittenberg.

Luther was not just concerned with simony and indulgences, he was concerned about the general dissolute state of the Church, as well as his recognition that an independent reading of the Bible could contradict papal interpretations. Aided by the newly invented printing press, a distribution of pamphlets raised these issues across the lands, best known as Luther's *Ninety-Five Theses*. Luther's written protest spread quickly throughout Christendom, leading to his excommunication. Aided by John Calvin and like-minded others, the 'Protestants' churches proliferated during the sixteenth century and into the seventeenth up to the present. The Protestant movement spread throughout Europe, associated with the separating of the (Anglican) Church of England from Rome: a Calvinist consortium of followers in Switzerland, Hungary, Scotland, Germany, and elsewhere; the Reformed Churches in France and Holland, and later, the Puritans in England and the American Colonies.[208]

Of most significance for this book, however, is Luther's rejection of the concept of free will. Luther believed that original sin and our fallen state required divine grace to predestine our lives; our good works flowed from our acceptance of God's will. Luther's account of free will inverted the Catholic practice of awarding tokens of grace by good work and payments, as well as undermining academic and papal authority.[209]

The spread of Protestantism could only provoke a Counter-Reformation within the Catholic Church, also known as the Catholic Reformation, which emphasized scholarship, the strengthening of pious religious orders like the Jesuits and Franciscans, the development of charity services, regulating the bishopric and practices like indulgences, and reaffirming the theology of Aquinas, all in effect shaping the modern Catholic Church.[210]

Enlightenment. 'The Enlightenment' or 'The Age of Reason' is an historical term, like that of the Reformation and Renaissance, which encompasses a broad set of historical events, trends, ideas, and mores that cut across geographic, and to a lesser extent, time, boundaries. Thus, the plural, Enlightenments, may well be more accurate. Characterizing the Enlightenment broadly (and very briefly), as I do here, is perhaps best done by framing the period as a blossoming change in cultural values. The earlier discussions of the Renaissance and the late Middle Ages suggested that the theocentric nature of European culture was unraveling along with the feudal economy. With the Enlightenment, the Church was nudged aside as the premier vehicle for moral and ethical thought among intellectual elites. The dogmatic reformulations of classical Greek and Latin texts by the Scholastics were replaced by an explosion of secular scientific and philosophical thought. The deference to Church authority was replaced by a deepening recognition that the individual can shape who he or she is and could be; that the powers of Reason could allow individuals, and humanity collectively, to define itself. As a concrete example, ecclesiastical justice shifted to court justice.[211] The convictions about the central importance of Reason generated both the effort and the freedom to rethink human problems anew, apart from the past. This rethinking led to a diversity of ideas and perspectives, and a still-further expansion of the universe of Western ideas. This emphasis on Reason enabled the development of social accounts of humanity that could provide a moral-ethical basis for action. Human nature, in essence, was good; and the general decency of humanity only requires the application of reason to address and counter the lure of indecency and evil. Many Enlightenment thinkers believed that humanity was perfectible.

Enlightenment values were distrustful of religion, and theistic beliefs posed differences to be tolerated; neither expounded upon nor repressed. The newly optimistic view of humanity embraced democratic ideals, and social values like equal opportunity, justice, self-government arose and gained cachet. The idea that offenders, criminal or mad, were ill, not evil, flourished, and the idea of the reform of socially deviant behavior took hold. Emotions, or passions, were largely cast as counter to reason, and were distrusted along with religion and mysticism, and blamed for wrongdoing. People, in a 'state of nature' had a relatively uniform constitution and could be understood through reason. Enlightened individuals were also skeptical of cultural customs and traditions, and regularly challenged them. Instead of the gallows, public humiliation, and forced labor as punishment for wrongdoing, the then-more humane ideas of incarceration and reform of the offender were promulgated.

In summary, the values of the Enlightenment were that of reason over passions; an elevation of the individual; a skepticism toward religion, customs, and traditions; a belief and willingness to invest in intellectual traditions like science and philosophy; and a confidence in the rational development of social institutions and governments to improve, even perfect, humanity.[212] The resemblances of these cultural values to those we identify often with 'modernity' are formative; not until the late twentieth century were these values and their associated worldviews seriously challenged within the academic world and beyond into the twenty-first century. However, Enlightenment values also concretized the cultural dichotomies between a rationalist, intellectual elite, and a religious, traditionalist common polity. In the twenty-first century the dark side of the digital/internet revolution brought humanity closer to a virtual state of nature, where an ongoing struggle between dichotomies like rationality/irrationality, tolerance/hate, truth/lies, greed/fairness, and bullying/reciprocity continue. The tensions between these general worldviews persist into the present and are especially relevant to views of morality as well as madness.

As still another historiographical note, as these discussions enter the Enlightenment and the beginnings of psychiatry emerge, I should note some particular contentions within the history of psychiatry and my own attitudes toward them. Beginning in the 1960s, a 'revisionist' thread within the history[213] of psychiatry emerged which provided a counterpoint to the prevailing (at least in the minds of these critics) historiographical Whiggishness of the extant scholarship in the field. Briefly, the history of psychiatry up to that point (with Alexander & Selesnick (1966) and Zilboorg (1967) as good examples) tended to cast the history of psychiatry as a progressive arrow toward the (authors') present day, which represented the highest level of achievement in terms of care of the mentally ill and the scientific achievements of the field. In reaction to this alleged Whig history of psychiatry, the revisionist historians were interested not just in the internal workings of the professional field but also the external workings of society's relationship to psychiatry, as well as the experience of patients. These authors, which included Michel Foucault,[214] Andrew Scull,[215] David Rothman,[216] and others were often quite critical, even severe in their claims about the self-interested nature of the new 'psychiatry', the insensitivity of the doctors and administrators to the patients' plights, and the general conclusion that psychiatry was more about the social control of deviance and self-aggrandizing doctors rather than part of a humane and moral service-tradition of medicine. To give you a sense of the withering judgments of the so-called revisionists, I reproduce this short excerpt of Andrew Scull's recent *Lancet* reflection on his career (and his discovery of the newly corrupting potential of Pharma):[217]

> . . . I began my explorations at a time when the museums of madness that were the Victorian age's response to Unreason still loomed large in our collective conscience. The massive, ramshackle piles retained their hold, not just on our imaginations, but upon thousands and thousands of people with mental illness, still confined in what had once been proclaimed as a therapeutic isolation. It is hard to forget the sense of constriction and confinement that oppressed one's spirit on crossing the threshold of one of these establishments. Above all, perhaps, I remember the smell, the fetid odour of decaying bodies and minds, of wards impregnated with decades of stale urine and faecal matter, of the slop served up for generations as food, the unsavoury mixture clinging like some foul miasma to the physical fabric of the buildings.

One extracts little in the way of ambivalence from Scull's eloquent appraisal of nineteenth-century English asylums! This revisionist trend prompted a substantial backlash from contemporary historians of psychiatry who, in their view, neither saw themselves as Whiggish nor felt that their historiographic practice was in any way inferior to the revisionists.[218] For the purposes of this chapter and this book, a critical engagement with these debates among historians is neither productive nor particularly relevant; the tensions between social control, organized psychiatry, and humane therapeutics, between exploitation, neglect, and advocacy, are persistent throughout this book. All these threads of history are relevant in providing iconic ideas about the VMDR and framing the complex morality of mental health care and criminal justice today.

My own view is that both groups (with all their distinctive and diverse viewpoints intact) are right. Abundant evidence exists about the well-meaning efforts of psychiatrists and related reformers, as well as the appropriation of psychiatrists by larger social forces in service to social control or other interests, as well as their giving-in to venal motives. Such is human nature, as repetitively illustrated in the preceding content of this chapter. As the arguments in this book will make apparent, the history of psychiatry, as well as the history of humankind, is a complex amalgam of goods, middling moralities, and evils; selfishness, self-engagement, and selflessness; altruism, compromise, and corruption; as are the histories of the cultures and politics that encompass it. Concluding this brief historiographic digression, I return to Enlightenment thinkers.

Like Hobbes, John Locke (1632–1704) cast his influential political philosophy in the context of a (limited) metaphysics and human psychology, as well as his own variety of social contract theory. Locke's political philosophy has been a richly contested domain in academic philosophy,[219] debates which will not be addressed here as our focus is on influential ideas and not systems. Profoundly influential to America's founding fathers, Locke's philosophy supported (1) the idea of human rights as entitlements which all people should possess; (2) religious tolerance; (3) separation of church and civic/governmental function—that religious authority should not substitute for governmental authority; (4) states, or governments, exist for the sake of advancing the people's interests (civil interests I call life, liberty, health, and indolency of body, and the possessions of outward things, such as money, lands, houses, furniture, and the like.');[220] (5) the idea of personal identity, the individual as unique, is central to governmental interests, and perhaps most importantly, (6) the idea that government should be conducted through the consent of the governed. The irony and tragedy of Locke's work was his persistent racism.[221]

Baruch Spinoza (1632–1677) cut a controversial path in doing his philosophy and ethics, ultimately excommunicated by Jewish leaders because of his alleged atheism and deviance from Jewish doctrine. Rather than an atheist, many interpreters consider him a pantheist.[222]

Spinoza's *Ethics*[223] cast metaphysics, psychology, and ethics in terms of a stepwise logical system which resists summary, much less a brief one. What is significant about Spinoza's ethics, for current purposes, is nicely stated by MacIntyre:[224]

> . . . Spinoza did not simply dismiss the theological vocabulary; he treated it, as he treated ordinary language, as a set of expressions which needed reinterpretation to be made rational. He is thus the ancestor of all those skeptics who have treated religion not as simply false, but as expressing important truths in a misleading way. Religion needs not so much to be refuted as decoded. . . . the counterpart of understanding God as identical with Nature is understanding ethics as the study not of divine precepts but of our own nature and of what necessarily moves us.

Psychiatric historians Alexander and Selesnick[225] cast Spinoza as a predecessor to modern psychology, both through the above suggestion that religious phenomena are worthy of study and understanding not as divine truths but as anthropological artifacts (to use more contemporary language), but also that moral/ethical behavior and conduct could also be distinguished and studied apart from their moral-normative implications: that is, moral behavior is just another kind of behavior. The latter insight seems particularly relevant to the VMDR.

Gottfried Leibniz (1646–1716) is known today as a metaphysician and logician, and inventor, along with Isaac Newton, of calculus. He articulated the most optimistic of Enlightenment philosophies, providing a detailed account of cosmological harmony: even apparent evils figured into a positive and divine Plan. His ethics appealed to natural law theory, virtue, and the instruction to model one's own behavior after divine behavior.[226] Leibnizian optimism was to be lampooned later by Voltaire (see below).

Charles-Louis de Secondat Baron de Montesquieu (1689–1755) deserves mention not so much as an innovator in ethics and political philosophy but as a popularizer of ideas. His articulation of three forms of government—republican, monarchy, and despotism—with the latter two distinguished by rule of law in monarchies, and the absence of rule of law with the despot.[227] Montesquieu's warnings about the corrupting potential of the spirits of 'inequality' and 'equality' have a contemporary ring as described by Hilary Bok:[228]

> The spirit of inequality arises when citizens no longer identify their interests with the interests of their country, and therefore seek both to advance their own private interests at the expense of their fellow citizens, and to acquire political power over them. The spirit of extreme equality arises when the people are no longer content to be equal as citizens, but want to be equal in every respect. In a functioning democracy, the people choose magistrates to exercise executive power, and they respect and obey the magistrates they have chosen. If those magistrates forfeit their respect, they replace them. When the spirit of extreme equality takes root, however, the citizens neither respect nor obey any magistrate. They 'want to manage everything themselves, to debate for the senate, to execute for the magistrate, and to decide for the judges'. Eventually the government will cease to function, the last remnants of virtue will disappear, and democracy will be replaced by despotism. [internal citations omitted]

Montesquieu's worries deserve reconsidering in a twenty-first century characterized by social media echo chambers, distrust of expertise, alternative facts, greed, my rights over yours, and 'post-truth'.

While he was generally not considered an original philosophical thinker, Francois-Marie Arouet Voltaire, or just Voltaire (1694–1778) should be mentioned here as a very important popularizer of the Enlightenment mythos, and perhaps one of the most influential exporters of Enlightenment values to popular culture. In his early adult years he advocated for civil liberties, religious tolerance, and free trade, becoming an influential figure in the American Revolution and the design of US democracy. As a man of letters he wrote philosophy, history, poetry, essays, plays, and fiction in various forms, often with satirical elements. He believed strongly in practical reason, and in midlife he was influenced by Leibniz's optimism, using the phrase that later became iconic for Enlightenment naivete, that we lived in the 'best of all possible worlds'. Voltaire's satirical pen garnered him trouble and threats of prison on several occasions, leading him to a more pessimistic worldview with age. His best-known novella, *Candide*, could be read as an allegory of the rise and fall of Enlightenment rationalism and optimism, in some ways ushering in motifs of existentialism and cynical nihilism that were to gain cachet in the twentieth century. *Candide*'s appeal to contemporary sensibilities is evidenced by Leonard Bernstein's very successful adaptation as a comic operetta in 1956. Through this work, the Leibnizian optimist of the book entered his name into popular discourse as an adjective describing a naive belief in the power of Reason: 'panglossian'.

The contributions of David Hume (1711–1776), however, are among the most substantial in the history of ethics as well as modern philosophy in general. As still another metaphysician often lumped with Locke and Berkeley as a 'British Empiricist', Hume's ethics were based upon his theory of mind, which unfortunately cannot be discussed here, nor his contributions to the philosophy of science. Cohon[229] identifies four key theses to Hume's ethics, admitting that the interpretation of each has been subject to intense debate among Hume scholars:

> (1) Reason alone cannot be a motive to the will, but rather is the 'slave of the passions'.
> (2) Moral distinctions are not derived from reason. (3) Moral distinctions are derived from the moral sentiments: feelings of approval (esteem, praise) and disapproval (blame) felt by spectators who contemplate a character trait or action. (4) While some virtues and vices are natural, others, including justice, are artificial.

The idea that morality is not derived from reason but from emotion, desires, or feelings is an idea that was radical at the time and is still provocative today. For Hume, we are linguistic animals, and language dresses up and modulates the passions. Moreover, Hume introduced the now-popular idea in psychology, from neuroscience to psychoanalysis, that emotion provides the motivational mojo that powers reason to action. Consistent with this view is Hume's account of virtue and vices, where sentiment (emotion) evaluates character traits as either pleasurable/approvable, or painful/disapprovable. As will be discussed in section 4.2.6.2 on *Madness*, the mental links between passion and reason are associations, which make him important not just in moral theory but in scientific theory of the mind. Interpersonally, we comprehend others' moral intentions through 'sympathy', which we understand today as empathy, the ability to view the world from the perspective and feeling-states of another person. Hume categorized some virtues as 'natural'—eliciting instinctual positive responses in self and others, while other virtues, like justice, were 'artificial' (e.g., created to advance social or collective interests).

To conclude this briefest sketch of Hume's moral tropes, some attention should be given to the so-called is-ought distinction. The basic idea is that moral prescriptions, or things we ought to do in a moral sense, cannot be inferred or deduced from fact statements (expressed through 'is' statements), leading to the motto 'no ought from an is'. In other words, no factual state of affairs, in itself, necessitates a particular moral or ethical evaluation. While the is-ought distinction remains one of the most intense areas of debate for Hume scholars, what is significant for our purposes here is Hume's inspiration for the fact-value distinction, that facts possess different kinds of logical properties than values. Facts and values, in large part, are not translatable one into another.[230]

Perhaps the best-known social contract theorist in the Western world is Jean-Jacques Rousseau (1712–1778). Though he must be considered a philosopher through his writings and thought, Rousseau was withering in his opinion of philosophers in general, finding them to be conniving *post-hoc* justifiers of any manner of cruelty and injustice *du jour*. His moral psychology was built around a tension between *amour de soi* or self-love, and *pitie* or compassion. Behavior for Rousseau is conditioned upon the modulation and balance between the self-interested behavior of *amour de soi* and the more altruistic vector of *pitie*. In his best-known work of political philosophy, *The Social Contract*, Rousseau advocated for the citizenry to rule over itself through expression of a 'general will' but whether this represents a consensus of intentions by the polity or is a derived and abstract expression of the citizenry's common interests, has been a source of debate. Rousseau's expression of support for liberty and equality was, and has been, appropriated by revolutionaries of many stripes, inspired by the oft-quoted first sentence from *The Social Contract*: 'Man is born free but everywhere he is in chains.'[231] Rousseau saw human beings as being good-overall in nature, but society was corrupting and so required people's collective consent and constraint. The particulars of how this social contract was to be implemented, however, were vague, leading to its appropriation by groups of quite divergent ideological loyalties, as exemplified today by Rousseauian ideas appearing on conservative-democratic websites as well as Marxist ones.[232]

Immanuel Kant (1724–1804), as opposed to Hume, argued from a fundament in ethics that was rational, not as a 'slave to the passions'. In introducing the categorical imperative, Kant wanted to establish moral action on a rational basis, and in so doing, introduced related concepts that are still-powerful today. The categorical imperative, as an imperative, is a (rational) command. The 'categorical' part means that this command is not dependent upon some set of additional conditions; so a categorical imperative is an unconditional command to moral action. (Kant contrasted the categorical to hypothetical imperatives—a command dependent upon one or more conditions—such as 'If you want to earn the praise of your teacher, you should actively participate in class.') Kant offered several formulations of the categorical imperative (CI) as a first ethical rule. His first formulation emphasized that one should 'act only in accordance with that maxim through which you can at the same time will that it become a universal law'.[233] Kant thought that a justified moral action must be universalizable; that is, the action could be converted into a maxim, or guiding principle, that could be applied by reasonable persons similarly in every situation.[234] Another formulation of the CI focuses on how one should treat humanity as a whole, that humanity broadly conceived, should be treated as an end and not as a means. Here, 'end' means that humanity, with its unique capabilities and potentials, should be realized through a dedication or commitment. This regard engenders a respect for humanity, and this moral respect described by Kant has been important for later thinking in the modern/contemporary bioethics era. Kant provides still another formulation of the CI, that is a variation of the first one, but this round he suggests that the maxim implied by one's moral action should represent a universal law for others—that is, would your moral action be one that you would legislate and impose on others? Finally, what is sometimes called the 'kingdom of ends' formulation of the CI in some ways encompasses the others—that one should act as if 'only on principles which could earn acceptance by a community of fully rational agents each of whom have an equal share in legislating these principles for their community' as Robert Johnson puts it.[235]

The close linkage between morality and reason in Kant's and others' philosophy maintains a vestige of the idea that rationality is conceptually linked to irrationality; perhaps a leftover from earlier medieval thought, and relevant to understanding the VMDR.

4.2.6.2 Madness

In considering the Renaissance/Reformation/Enlightenment period regarding madness and folly, one can often find many of the same minds making contributions to understanding of madness as to understanding of morality. Keeping my earlier framing of the period in mind, we can resume discussions of the ideas organized around these three themes, followed by influential thinkers and their iconic contributions.

Renaissance. I start again with consideration of Desiderius Erasmus (1466–1536), an early humanist and influential reformer, not just of the Church but of popular thinking about madness and mental distress:[236]

> But there are two sorts of madness, the one that which the revengeful Furies send privily from hell, as often as they let loose their snakes and put into men's breasts either the desire of war, or an insatiate thirst after gold, or some dishonest love, or parricide, or incest, or sacrilege, or the like plagues, or when they terrify some guilty soul with the conscience of his crimes; the other, but nothing like this, that which comes from me and is of all other things the most desirable; which happens as often as some pleasing dotage not only clears the mind of its troublesome cares but renders it more jocund. And this was that which, as a special blessing of the gods, Cicero, writing to his friend Atticus, wished to himself, that he might be the less sensible of those miseries that then hung over the commonwealth.

For Erasmus, madness could be the punishment and torture symbolic of medieval darkness but could also be a feature of us that grounds our humanity, opens up new ideas and insights, spares us painful truths, and even amuses. Such latter romanticizing of madness is imbricated into contemporary popular culture through using the word 'crazy' to depict not a state of mental illness, but a desirable state of unconventional belief, attitude, and resilient spirit. For examples, pop musician Paul Simon titles a record album 'Still Crazy After All These Years', and when I travel to Austin, Texas, bumper stickers implore me to 'Keep Austin Weird'. We'll see that this positive notion of 'crazy' persists today in the recovery, Mad Pride, and user/survivor movements in mental health, though often in a more refined form that madness has positive, even indispensable, aspects for individuals as well as cultures.

Relatively unknown in contemporary times, Juan-Luis Vives (1492–1540) a Valencian cleric and restless intellectual, presented substantial and prophetic ideas in the areas of education, what today would be called social justice or social welfare, and medical approaches to madness. While deeply religious, Vives rejected, and crusaded against, the reigning ideas of the supernatural in causing madness, and argued that not only were the mentally ill not possessed by demons, but indeed were products of social deprivation and poverty. A critic of the almsgiving approach of his own Catholic Church of the time, Vives believed that simply providing relief was not enough. Education toward self-care and independence was crucial, and mental and physical health barriers to these goals should be addressed by hospitals and doctors, not priests. His contributions to psychology anticipated much better known theories and theorists to follow. We can see in Vives an anticipation not just of a medicalized mental illness, but a germ for the practices of social work and rehabilitation. Consider for example his discussion of associationist psychology, a hundred years before Hobbes and centuries before Pavlov: 'When an animal enjoys something at the sounding of a tone, then when the tone is heard again, it will expect to experience the object it enjoyed previously.'[237] Vives' formulation of the range of medical care for the ill brightly anticipates the biopsychosocial approach to medicine:[238]

> Remedies suited to the individual patients should be used. Some need medical care and attention to their mode of life; others need gentle and friendly treatment, so that like wild animals they may gradually grow gentle; still others need instructions. There will be some who will require force and chains, but these must be so used that the patients are not made more violent. Above all, as far as possible, tranquility must be introduced in their minds, for it is through this that reason and sanity return.

Perhaps more suitable as a case study in Renaissance narcissism rather than as an influential theorist, Paracelsus (1493–1541) presents a strikingly flamboyant character as mystic, alchemist, astrologer, and medic. His assumed name, Paracelsus ('beyond Celsus') and his self-elaborated given name Philippus Aureolus Theophrastus Bombastus von Hohenheim, says it all: Paracelsus intended to toot his own horn, and did so loudly. Derivative of his interests in alchemy, Paracelsus argued that madness was neither demonic nor divine in nature, believing that madness was caused by natural derangements in the body, and over his lifetime devised various chemical treatment interventions—though none were to survive the test of time. These 'treatments' could be conceived as representing elements of magic as well as proto-science. Paracelsus devised his own classification of disorders—*lunatici* were mad reactions to phases of the moon; *insani* were congenital and likely heritable disorders; *vesani* were poisonings, intoxications, or other invasions by outside pollutants; *melancholici* were emotionally-related incapacities of reason; while *obsessi* involved preoccupation about the devil.[239] At least one historian of psychiatry, Gregory Zilboorg, argues that Paracelsus first described the unconscious motivation of symptoms.[240]

A bundle of paradoxes, in his person as well as his work, Girolamo Cardano (1501–1576) was a mathematician as well as numerologist, a demonologist who crusaded against the persecution of witches, an astronomer and astrologist, as well as a philosopher and professor of medicine at the University of Pavia. He is of primary interest here as an influential physician who restimulated debate around his view on criminal responsibility and the mentally ill, averring that the latter could not be held responsible for criminal misconduct.[241]

Cardano was likely influenced by Heinrich Cornelius Agrippa von Nettesheim (1486–1535), an earlier physician, theologian, and likely sorcerer whose work, including *De Occulta Philosophia* and *On the Variety and Uncertainty of the Arts and Sciences*, attempted to frame occult practices as a kind of natural magic.[242] Typical of the time, Paracelsus, Cardano, and Agrippa practiced a mixture of knowledge-seeking practices we would today describe as magic, as well as recognizable 'science'. These figures depict the murky transition between supernatural/magical knowledge practices, and the emerging rational-empirical knowledge practices which became modern science.

Agrippa also influenced Johann Weyer (1515–1588), better known as the critic of the *Malleus Maleficarum* and crusader for medical treatment of the mentally ill, as well as the liberation of witches from persecution, documented in his 1563 book, *De praestigiis daemonum et incantationibus ac veneficiis* (On the Deceptions of the Devils, On Enchantments and on Poisonings). Weyer did not deny the existence of demonic influence, only was skeptical of the alleged power and prevalence of witchcraft. Pioneering what we might today describe as psychological management of somatoform symptoms, Weyer was both kind and resourceful.[243]

Juan Huarte (1530–1588) pioneered the idea that people vary in their aptitudes to different psychological functions. Huarte described congenital, characterological, and environmental factors in determining the capacities of individuals, and described three kinds of 'wits'—psychological faculties—memory, imagination, and intellectual, each of which demanding different kinds of educational development to flourish fully.[244]

Earlier I mentioned Francis Bacon (1561–1626), arguably the founder of modern science, then called 'natural philosophy', as the branch of philosophy which addressed natural phenomena. Bacon criticized Aristotle's reliance on deductive logic and the Scholastics' deference to authority, promoting a scientific attitude 'free from idols' and received dogmas. Bacon is best known today for the *Novum Organum* (1620), which he aimed to be a general theory of science. Always discerning in scientific reasoning, Bacon cautioned against the four 'idols'—(1) the idols of the tribe, which were illusions or perceptual miscontruals; (2) idols of the cave, which were assumptions or beliefs to which individuals dogmatically cling; (3) idols of the marketplace, which identify how taken-for-granted words and expressions can mislead us; and (4) idols of the theatre, which involved entrapment within dogmatic philosophical systems. Bacon advocated empiricism, the observation of phenomena. For many he introduced the use of inductive reasoning as a scientific method for identifying commonalities and differences between phenomena, which when recursively performed, could derive greater and deeper understanding of a given phenomenon. Findings that disconfirmed or refuted hypothetical generalizations were of equal value to Bacon (and anticipated Karl Popper's falsificationism), because identifying falsehoods is as essential as finding true knowledge. The use of observation and inductive reasoning was to be later picked up by Thomas Sydenham among others in developing a scientific medicine, leading to the development of 'syndromes' and continuing into the present modes of empirical reasoning about disease presentation.[245]

Though not philosophers, scientists, or physicians, William Shakespeare (1564–1616) and Miguel Cervantes (1547–1616) produced literary works that explored psychopathology in rich detail. Shakespeare has already been noted for his (literal) setting of the stage for public discourse about personal ethics and morality. The same could be said for Shakespeare's and Cervantes' (*Don Quixote*) depictions of psychopathology in their literary works, where Erasmus's foresight in viewing psychopathology as a part of being human was dramatized and brought into Renaissance popular culture.[246]

If a sixteenth-century scholar could ever qualify as a pop psychology icon, Robert Burton (1577–1640) would. Radden[247] notes the compelling interest of his 1621 *Anatomy of Melancholy*, having gone through several editions and its contemporary readings. His detailed descriptions of foul and desperate moods, as well as emotional states in general, may well have prefigured the modern-day mental illness confessional or madness memoir, centuries before Clifford Beers's *The Mind that Found Itself* (see the next chapter).

While primarily known for his description of the heart's function and the circulation of blood, William Harvey (1578–1657) is significant for his description of the powerful influence psychological and emotional phenomena could have on bodily functions. This work combined with his interest and description of hysteria, pseudocyesis, and sexual disorders has made him one of the fathers of psychoso-matic medicine.[248]

Influential in his work on legal aspects of psychopathology, Paolo Zacchia (1584–1659) a Roman physician and personal doctor to Pope Innocent X, asserted that only physicians were qualified to assess the mental state of a person. He intro-duced rules to address, from a clinical perspective, whether an individual could marry, execute a will, enter a religious order, testify in legal proceedings, and con-sidered criminal responsibility for several conditions from mania to alcoholism to epilepsy. His *Quaestiones Medico-Legales* (1621) addressed a wide range of legal-medicine issues, provoking many to view him as a founder of forensic medicine, and he wrote one of the first medical discussions of sodomy and child abuse. He believed that alcoholic individuals should be treated rather than punished; the court should give special dispensation for crimes committed in the heat of pas-sion; and malingering should be evaluated from the standpoint about symptoms that can, and cannot, be elicited from intent alone.[249]

As a metaphysician and psychologist, Thomas Hobbes (1588–1679) is of interest to the iconic history of madness not so much because of his proto-empiricism (e.g., belief that sensations are the building blocks of thought), but because of his contributions to understanding the role of the passions in human conduct. Hobbes described the passions, or emotions, as motivating internal motions to-ward or away from external objects. Hobbes is described as offering a materi-alist psychology, believing that internal bodily motion of various kinds created the passions. Hobbes offered simple taxonomies of passions, where some (ap-petite or desire, aversion) are hierarchically more powerful, and others combine to make more complex phenomena in mental life. Like Aristotelian virtues and vices, Hobbesian passions had their own antinomies, but Hobbes's were often antinomies of motivation (e.g., 'admiration', 'contempt'). Schmitter[250] iden-tifies 30-some passions in Hobbes's writings, though his passion-taxonomies vary somewhat from source to source. In *Leviathan*, Hobbes identifies six pas-sions: appetite/desire, love, aversion, hate, joy, and grief, which are then mod-ified into more complex ones through combination with other passions and 'opinion'. Table 4.4 presents a sample of Hobbes's passions described in Chapter 6 of *Leviathan*.[251]

Hobbes's accounts of the passions describes their expression as exhibiting sub-stantial individual variation, which was, in Hobbes's account, opposed to the more universal Reason. However, as Schmitter argues, Hobbes's apparent polarity of reason against passions is not Aristotelian, or even Freudian, but rather analo-gous to his picture of the state's interests relative to individual interests: 'The dif-ference between passions and reason is analogous to that between the natural state of liberty, particularly the liberty of acting on idiosyncratic preferences, and the civil state where there exists a common measure.'[252] In Schmitter's interpretation, reason is opposed to the passions in the way the state must restrain individual

Table 4.4 A Sample of Hobbes's Passions

Simple	Complex
Appetite/desire	Hope
Love	Despair
Aversion	Fear
Hate	Courage
Joy	Anger
Grief	Confidence
	Diffidence
	Indignation
	Benevolence
	Covetousness
	Ambition
	Pusillanimity
	Magnanimity
	Valor
	Liberality
	Miserableness
	Kindness
	Lust
	Luxury
	Jealousy
	[Others]

interests in service to the collective. In this view, Hobbesian psychology is a microcosm of the control of individual motion by the State.

What then of madness? Roy Porter quotes Hobbes in saying, 'Madness is nothing else but too much appearing passion.'[253] Porter continues a variation on Schmitter's take, and its elaboration into political discourse:[254]

> Thus the state was ordered, and the psyche likewise organically made up of parts; sanity was rational government of the parts, madness the appetites' insurrection. No wonder, then, metaphors of madness formed a malignant rhetoric of cursing. Political opponents, heretics, critics were dubbed 'lunatic', 'whimsy-headed', 'witless'.

Attributing madness to one's political opponents apparently has a long history continuing into the present moment.

The significance of Rene Descartes (1596–1650) and his mind-body dualism for psychiatric epistemology is ongoing and was described in the *Morality* section 4.2.6.1.

Reformation. The relevance of the Reformation for this book is primarily in the moral, not medical realm. However, in reviewing Reformation thought, the use of 'madness' to describe an objectionable, irrational, wrongful, or otherwise undesirable situation is more common, so that as early as the 1500s to make a disagreeable statement would be metaphorically described as 'madness'. For example, consider this passage of John Calvin's (1509–1564) critique of the Anabaptists:[255]

> Some Anabaptists fantasize about some crazy excess instead of the spiritual regeneration of the faithful. It seems to them that, after the children of God are brought back to a state of innocence, they do not need to worry about restraining the concupiscence of their flesh but must follow the Spirit as their guide, under whose direction they cannot err. It would be unbelievable that human understanding could fall into such a madness except that they arrogantly publicize this teaching.

The Reformation contributed to rhetoric through appropriation of madness as a critical tool in dismissing contrary ideas.

The historian Norman Dain characterizes the traditional Christian/Protestant view of madness as the wages of sin, while acknowledging many Christian sects of the New World, such as the Quakers, were forgiving of mental illness and even designed services for the afflicted.[256]

Two influential Puritan ministers, Increase (1639–1723) and Cotton (1663–1728) Mather's attitudes toward mental illness perhaps represent many people's attitudes today. Increase Mather was not just a prominent Puritan theologian but also a later president of Harvard University, who believed in the existence and power of witchcraft, though was highly critical of the methods used in the detection and 'prosecution' of witches.[257] His son Cotton, another prolific Puritan theologian and author, participated in the now-notorious Salem witch trials, though like his father, was critical of the feeble evidence presented as well as the general conduct of the trials. Cotton Mather was also an influential commentator on slavery and alleged violent criminal propensities, as well as the widespread idiocy of Blacks, thus contributing to racist tropes pervasive into the twenty-first century. Deutsch[258] describes the worldview of Puritan New England as generally suspicious of deviations from the natural norm in all spheres—bad weather, for instance, was interpreted as a sign from either God or the Devil. Deviations in personal behavior, as well, were suspect; not just the behavior of psychopathology was provocative, but the practices of any pagan religion we also suspicious. We see here a contribution from fundamentalist Christendom to the stigma of mental illness persisting into the present.

Enlightenment. In earlier portions of this section, I noted the general characteristics of the Enlightenment, and the refurbishing of natural philosophy into empirical science, more or less, as we know it today. The Enlightenment period was one of extraordinary change in medicine, as the influence of Galen and Hippocrates' humoral theory of medicine was supplanted by alternative metaphysics from the philosophers and the new hypotheses and observations of physician-scientists. These general intellectual trends could only differentiate the understanding of madness still further. Moreover, the Enlightenment also brought novel ways of handling criminal offenders. Moving away from the punishments of the stocks, the scaffold, and various public humiliations, English criminal justice founded workhouses for debtors to work off debt, offenders to pay debt to society, and the public to be protected from at-large deviants. By the turn of the nineteenth century, debate about the establishment, as well as reform, of the prison and the asylum had taken hold. These themes will be taken up in more detail below and in Chapter 6.

Oxford physician Thomas Willis (1621–1675), while best known to medical students as the describer of the Circle of Willis (the circular collection of arteries at the base of the brain that interconnects the brain's main arteries), made numerous contributions to medicine and what was to be psychiatry. His dissections and descriptions of brain anatomy were unparalleled at the time, articulated in his *Cerebri Anatome* (1664), accompanied by detailed renderings of brain structure by Sir Christopher Wren. Wren was distinguished in his own right, one of England's greatest architects, the builder of St. Paul's Cathedral in London and the designer of the regal Hampton Court and its gardens. Willis described syndromes such as mania, hysteria, epilepsy, and dementia in detail. Hunter and MacAlpine attributed the contemporary folk expression 'nerves' to Willis, to denote a general psychosomatic arousal state.[259] Willis articulated the term 'Neurologie' for specialists of the nervous system, and 'Psycheology' for specialists in the afflictions of the soul.[260]

Thomas Sydenham (1624–1689), one of fourteen children of an English Puritan family, is considered the English Hippocrates. As a contemporary and friend of John Locke, he emphasized the observables in medicine and dismissed the search for causes of disease as premature and perhaps ill-founded altogether. Sydenham was, above all, a taxonomist of disease: 'It is necessary that all diseases be reduced to definite and certain species, and that, with the same care which we see exhibited by botanists in their phytologies.'[261] His emphasis on description and longitudinal course of illness, along with groupings of signs and symptoms into syndromes, provided the core of the modern description of disease, still practiced today in the *Diagnostic and Statistical Manual of Mental Disorders* (DSMs) and International Classification of Diseases (ICDs). He believed that one-sixth of his patients had hysterical disorders, and agreed with Thomas Willis that hypochondriasis was a 'male hysteria',[262] in effect inserting the proto-idea that psychopathology could be gendered based on symptoms, not bodily organs.

The philosophy of John Locke (1632–1704) became quite influential to British physicians, particularly those interested in psychopathology. Locke's psychology was based upon the idea that human minds are born as a blank slate (*tabula rasa*) without innate ideas, knowledge, and values. Development, history, and experience then form the mind and thought from two basic sources. These sources, sensation and reflection, provide the raw experience to form into ideas and ultimately knowledge. Locke's psychology was dependent upon the idea of associations, that knowledge is formed through the linkage of one idea to others, making more complex ideas and ultimately the plethora of mental contents. If the linkages between sensation and reflection, or one set of ideas to another set of ideas were disrupted, this would disrupt the relation between ideas and external reality, resulting in madness. For Porter[263] Locke's psychology made for a rather tenuous grasp on reality:

Locke's philosophy of experience left mind in the balance. Rational certainty was a chi-
mera; yet there might be progressive paths to reliable-enough knowledge. Our senses
were deceptive, indeed they often lied; yet experience could be consolidated by regular
habits of thinking.

That Locke's psychology was motivationally fueled by the passions[264] made the potential disruption of associations even more likely. Nevertheless, Locke's philosophy
of mind made for a convenient instrument for later physicians to appropriate in explaining mental illness.

The significance of Baruch Spinoza's (1632–1677) *Ethics* for this book resides in
his description of unconscious motivation for behavior, as well as the strength of his
argument that psychological or mental processes could have causal power in determining behavior, setting the stage for Freud 200 years later and providing an alternative perspective on understanding behavior.[265]

The idea of mental disorders being caused by psychological influences, rather
than somatic ones, is a legacy of Georg Stahl (1660–1734). Stahl also was critical of
the distinction between body and mind, believing that they were much more interdependent than that described by contemporaries. Importantly, Stahl argued that
the outward manifestation of a patient's disorder is of only limited value when determining if the cause is somatic or psychological.[266]

A significant development from the social perspective in England during
the Enlightenment was the development of asylums and a for-profit market for
madhouses. The most well-known of the early English madhouses was Bethlem
Hospital, a.k.a. 'Bedlam', about which much has been written, both positive and
negative. The therapeutic intent of seclusion in Bethlem was questionable at best,
and the institution served as a permanent prison for the violent mentally ill, dramatically initiated by Margaret (Peg) Nicholson's and James Hatfield's attempts to
assassinate King George III in 1786 and 1800, respectively.[267] Large institutions
like Bethlem were more the exception rather than the rule in the early 1700s and
the so-called trade in lunacy was dominated by smaller, for-profit private madhouses, converted residences of variable quality. However, as Weiner[268] notes,
their reputation fell as quickly as they were founded. By 1774 in England, the asylums were regulated, but reforms were slow in developing, even with legislated
'encouragement'.

Perhaps the foremost British reformer of asylums and madhouses was William
Battie (1703–1776), whose scathing criticism in his *Treatise on Madness* (1758)
of Bethlem and its then-superintendent James Monro provoked the Regulating
Madhouses Act of 1774. Battie founded his own hospital, St. Luke's, in response to the
therapeutic nihilism of the day, claiming that patients with 'original insanity' (akin
to the idea of an endogenous, constitutional madness) were indeed incurable, but
that 'consequential insanity' was indeed curable with management and education
in coping. Close personal intervention could reduce or eliminate acute delusional

states and other forms of insanity. Battie's philosophy and techniques were to be developed and elaborated by Thomas Arnold, Joseph Cox, and Francis Willis as 'moral management' which gathered further steam later as 'moral treatment' by the Tukes and others.[269]

William 'Old Spasm' Cullen (1710–1790), inspired by the botanical classifications of Linnaeus and Boissier de Sauvages' massive classification of disease, sought to simplify nosology into four general categories: pyrexias, cachexias, local diseases, and neuroses. Cullen's explanation of physiology placed the nervous system as the center of his account. The organism's interaction with the environment set up various kinds of nervous excitement; deranged irritation of nervous tissue, dubbed 'spasm' by Cullen, inspiring his student's nickname.[270] Of note, Cullen's use of the 'neurosis' term was of limited applicability to our contemporary sense of the term; with the category of neuroses, Cullen included four subcategories: *comata*, which were disturbances of voluntary movements; *adynamiae*, disturbances of involuntary movements; *spasmi*, abnormal muscle movement; and *vésanies*, disorders of judgment, in which insanity was placed.[271] Porter relates Cullen's work to Locke's associationism, placing it within Cullen's physiology of nervous excitation:[272]

> Delirium may depend . . . upon some inequality in the excitement of the brain . . . for . . . our reasoning or intellectual operations always require the orderly and exact recollection or memory of associated ideas; so, if any part of the brain is not excited, or not excitable, that recollection cannot properly take place, while at the same time other parts of the brain, more excited and excitable, may give false perceptions, associations, and judgments . . .

Though David Hume (1711–1776) did not make any direct contribution to the understanding of mental illness, his psychology of association also was relevant and influential. He presented three ways perceptions and sensations are associated: through similarity, through closeness in place or time, and through causal mechanisms. Despite his general skepticism, Hume's observations were such that the contiguity of space and time between psychological motive and voluntary action were as profound as any other space/time contiguity in nature. Wallace[273] argues that this insight situates psychological causation on the same basis as physical causation.

Of the new generation of Enlightenment philosophers, perhaps Immanuel Kant (1724–1804) is the most important in terms of influencing the conceptual framing of psychopathology. Though not a physician, Kant had a particular interest in mental illness, and especially hypochondriasis, from which he is reported to have suffered.[274] The substance of his work on mental illness appears in the *Anthropology from a Pragmatic Point of View*.[275] Radden[276] notes that Kantian faculty psychology, distinguishing reason/cognition from passion/emotion/affection, and again the third faculty, from conation or the 'will', is one of the mainstays of clinical psychiatric classification today.[277] Kant agreed with some of his contemporaries that physicians are needed in considering the competence of a criminal offender, noting that somatic causes might have provoked the crime; and that philosophers are needed in addressing the psychology of the alleged offender.[278]

Perhaps most influential in Kant's work is the role of 'common sense' or *sensus communis* in madness, a version of which has been elaborated for schizophrenia today by philosophers of psychiatry.[279] Kant describes common sense disturbances in the *Anthropology*:[280]

> The only universal characteristic of madness is the loss of common sense (*sensus communis*) and its replacement with logical private sense (*sensus privatus*); for example, a human being in broad daylight sees a light burning on his table which, however, another person standing nearby does not see, or hears a voice that no one else hears. For it is a subjectively necessary touchstone of the correctness of our judgments generally, and consequently also of the soundness of our understanding, that we also restrain our understanding by the *understanding of others*, instead of *isolating* ourselves with our own understanding and judging *publicly* with our private representations, so to speak.

The significance of Cesare Beccaria (1738–1794) for the VMDR lies in his contributions to the Enlightenment's reform of criminal justice and the founding of what today criminologists call classical criminology.[281] Beccaria's notion of human nature centered on humans seeking pleasure and avoiding pain; criminals must derive pleasure from offenses; therefore, punishment is necessary to counterbalance the crime-related pleasure. In this framework, the purpose for punishment was deterrence, not retribution or revenge. Beccaria, however, strongly rejected capital punishment, on the basis that the state had no basis to take lives, and the death penalty was not effective as a deterrent to crime. He described the relationship between poor social conditions and crime; believing that improvement in social conditions would diminish criminal offending. With Voltaire, he argued that only offenses against humans should be punishable by law, offenses to God were sins, and handled, so to speak, in another domain.[282] He anticipated the observations of Skinnerian behaviorism by asserting that punishment, to be maximally effective, should be immediate, not delayed; and the certainty of punishment was a more effective deterrent than severity of punishment.[283] Along with Jeremy Bentham (see below) Beccaria advocated that punishments should be proportionate to the crime committed; agreeing with Bentham's principle of utility (utilitarianism), the idea that social justice is meted through seeking out the greatest happiness for the greatest number. As we'll see in Chapter 6, Beccaria coined major concepts in criminal justice and framed issues in the field which are relevant into the present.

Perhaps the figure of greatest fame as a proto-psychiatrist of the Enlightenment, Phillipe Pinel (1745–1826) is known as the liberator of the maniacs of the Bicêtre in 1796 during the Reign of Terror. Pinel removed the fetters from the madpersons, believing that humane therapy was possible. Weiner,[284] among others, challenged this account, citing documents that indicate that a Bicêtre ward supervisor, Jean Baptiste

Pussin, was the actual remover of the manacles. Nevertheless, Pinel is deserving of his fame for his popularization of a Cullen-inspired nosography, his articulation of 'moral therapy', and his early framing of what came to be known as monomanias, which will be elaborated in more detail later in this chapter.[285] Importantly, the choice of 'moral' in 'moral therapy' may have been misleading for English-speaking audiences. Pinel's sense intends psychological treatment, not treatment that is concerned exclusively with rightness and wrongness. Nevertheless, moral therapy was intended to be humane, at least more humane that the prior treatment characteristic of the Bicêtre and later Saltpêtrière patients, and was quickly adopted and elaborated in England, Italy, and the United States through William Tuke (1732–1822), Vincenzo Chiarugi (1759–1820), and Benjamin Rush (1746–1813), respectively. While generally recognized by historians as a relative humanistic advance for the mad, appraisals of Pinel's work and moral therapy for critics such as Michel Foucault[286] propose that these changes reflected a more sophisticated and subtle repression of social deviance and 'unreason'. For reasons that will not be elaborated here, but in later chapters, I believe that both readings are compatible; regulation of deviance will become a core theme of my later analyses. Finally, Weiner notes the influence of Pinel's concept of *aliénation mentale*. In Weiner's translation, the term 'implies that the mental patient feels foreign to the "normal" world, a stranger (alienus) to the land of sanity'.[287] The term stuck, and nineteenth-century physician-specialists in madness became 'alienists'.

One of the notables in British jurisprudence, Sir William Blackstone (1723–1780) was a judge, professor of law at Oxford, and a Parliament member. His significance for the discussions here resides in his distinction between 'idiots' (those intellectually disabled at birth) and 'lunatics' (the mad) in terms of legal responsibility and their capacity to handle their civic affairs. In 1765 Blackstone distinguished between idiots *a nativitate* and lunatics *non compos mentis*; the former had deficiencies in intellect at birth, while the latter was 'one who hath had understanding, but by disease, grief, or other accident hath lost the use of his reason'.[288] Notable also is the separate determination by the Court of the status of the individual in question; physicians had not yet been involved in forensic cases, and Blackstone describes how the determination of *non compos mentis* is made:[289]

> The lord chancellor, to whom, by special authority from the king, the custody of idiots and lunatics is intrusted, upon petition or information, grants a commission in nature of the writ *de idiota inquirendo*, to enquire into the party's state of mind; and if he be found *non compos*, he usually commits the care of his person, with a suitable allowance for his maintenance, to some friend, who is then called his committee. However, to prevent sinister practices, the next heir is never permitted to be this committee of the person; because it is his interest that the party should die. But, it hath been said, there lies not the same objection against his next of kin, provided he is not his heir; for it is his interest to preserve the lunatic's life, in order to increase the personal estate by savings, which he or his family may

hereafter be entitled to enjoy. The heir is generally made the manager or committee of the estate, it being clearly his interest by good management to keep it in condition; accountable however to the court of chancery, and to the *non compos* himself, if he recovers; or otherwise, to his administrators.

Blackstone further specified the conditions where a criminal act could be excused due to 'want or defect of will'. These were three. (1)[290]

[A] . . . defect in understanding. For where there is no discernment, there is no choice; and where there is no choice, there can be no act of the will, which is nothing else but a determination of one's choice, to do or to abstain from a particular action: he therefore, that has no understanding, can have no will to guide his conduct.

(2) A second criterion involved a deficiency in will, which could include an impairment to (in today's terms) participate in his defense: if 'he becomes mad, he ought not to be arraigned for it; because he is not able to plead to it with that advice and caution that he ought'. If the lunatic has lucid intervals, his responsibility returns for those acts he commits in said state. Blackstone provided for 'confinement' until such time the lunatic's reason returned. Finally, (3) the third criterion involved 'voluntary contracted madness', involving drunkenness or other intoxications. For this criterion, the 'law looks upon this as an aggravation of the offence, rather than as an excuse for any criminal misbehaviour'. These criteria and concepts have been revisited and rethought many times up to the present day.

Two writers, one eighteenth-century and one nineteenth-century, warrant some discussion as literary influences on, and perhaps cultural promoters of, 'deviant' sexual practices. Donatien Alphonse François (a.k.a. the Marquis de Sade, 1740–1814) is perhaps the most notorious of the two. As a French nobleman, sexual libertine, and far-left political figure whose fictional and philosophical writings celebrating sexual pain, even torture of others, his work earned him persecution in his time and ongoing controversy into the present. No less a figure than Napoleon himself ordered de Sade arrested as the then-anonymous author of *Justine* and *Juliette*. His appraisal from literary critics over the past 2 centuries have both praised him as a liberator and condemned him as a misogynist pornographer. Of significance for psychiatry and morality, de Sade and his later counterpart, Leopold von Sacher-Masoch (author of *Venus in Furs* (1870), were the prime influences for the alienist Richard von Krafft-Ebing's adding 'sadism' and 'masochism' into his catalogue of 'perversions'—to be discussed in more detail later.[291] Thus de Sade and Sacher-Masoch were nominal contributors to the VMDR.

Thomas Arnold (1742–1816) was one of the early private madhouse owners of his time, but also a theorist of lunacy. Disagreeing with his mentor William Cullen, Arnold proposed a classification of insanity based upon two distinctions or superordinate groups of psychopathology: 'ideal insanity' and 'notional insanity'. 'Ideal insanity' was described as a pervasive hallucinosis without fever. 'Notional insanity' excludes hallucinosis but involves what we might identify today as delusional states and various sorts of overvalued ideas: '. . . yet conceives such notions of the powers, properties, designs, state, destination, importance, manner of existence, or the like, of things and persons, of himself and others, as appear obviously, and often grossly erroneous or unreasonable, to the common sense of the sober and judicious part of mankind'.[292] Under the category of Notional Insanity, Arnold listed Delusive, Fanciful, Whimsical, Impulsive, Scheming, Vain Self-Important), Hypochondriacal, Pathetic, and Appetitive. Arnold organized these categories, it seems, around semantic content of the patient's preoccupations or actions. Of these, the 'impulsive' is of interest as anticipating impulse-control disorders, as the patient does what is 'imprudent, improper, unreasonable, impertinent, ridiculous, or absurd . . .' and the 'appetitive' describes 'immoderate, and ungovernable, desire. [sometimes called] Satyriasis . . . [and] Nymphomania'.[293]

The name, and visage, of Benjamin Rush (1745–1862) will be familiar to many American psychiatrists, as one of the founders of the American Psychiatric Association (APA), whose portrait, until recently, constituted the APA seal/logo, and as one of the signers of the American Declaration of Independence in 1776. (Rush was removed from the APA logo in 2015 in part because of his racist belief that slavery made Black people inferior.) Both progressive in his advocacy of careful clinical observation and recording of clinical data, and old-fashioned in his clinging to Galenic humoral theory with its bloodlettings and purgings, Rush's contribution to the VMDR will be considered in more detail in later sections.[294]

The British philosopher Jeremy Bentham (1748–1832) appears here in the 'Madness' subsection not because of his theorizing on mental illness per se, but because of his various contributions to matters pertinent to this book and the VMDR. Perhaps most fundamentally, Bentham's metaphysics[295] contribute to a framing of one of the fundamental assumptions of this book, that language and terms are important framers of social and political discourse. Bentham scholar Emmanuelle de Champs summarizes Bentham's view on the role of language in social discourse: 'A reform in language is necessary because language, as a symbolic system, sets the framework in which law and politics work.'[296] As one of the founders of utilitarianism, Bentham broke away from Kantianism and natural law theory, arguing that only the consequences of actions counted in morality and the law, that rightness was extrinsic not intrinsic.[297]

Of interest to the theory of stigma in mental illness, Bentham argued against relying upon 'antipathy' in guiding moral or political judgment; that a personal disgust response was no justification for legislating against an action, using homosexuality as an explicit example.[298] If punishment was to be based upon matters of taste, Bentham reasoned, what would be the limit to them? Right actions are judged against how robustly they favor the prevailing of pleasure over pain; the parameters of assessment include intensity (strength of pleasure/pain), proximity (of the pleasure/pain to the action), duration (of the pleasure/pain), purity (the proportions of the pleasure/pain mix), certainty (the probability that pleasure/pain will result from the action), fecundity (the probability of the action to lead to future pleasure/pain), and finally, extent (the number of people involved by the action).[299]

As a final note on Bentham, a mention of the 'Panopticon' is warranted.[300] The panopticon was an architectural design for 'prisons, houses of industry, work-houses, poor-houses, manufactories, mad-houses, lazarettos, hospitals, and schools' which was semicircular or circular in floor plan, with a central observation-station, surrounded by individual rooms or cells on the periphery. The idea was to have a central location where the staff of the institution could observe the inmates without being observed themselves; thus assuring a more efficient economy of desirable inmate behavior. The panopticon was to be considered later by Foucault as a symbol of the totalizing function of the State in regulating and 'normalizing' the population.[301]

The Scottish physician John Reid (1776–1822) has the honor of presenting the earliest discussion of 'institutionalization' to my review. Reid's 1816 description of institutionalization is remarkably similar to those promulgated by Erving Goffman[302] and others in the 1960s. Reid was concerned that confinement of patients in the asylum was itself a contributor to disability and impairment. The reasons included a potential contagion effect of the patient's mad surroundings, the 'coarse and humiliating treatment' provided that diminished resilience and spirit, and the top-down regimentation of hospital rules and order. Reid concludes his essay on institutionalization with a stern warning:[303]

> Many of the depots for the captivity of intellectual invalids may be regarded only as nurseries for and manufactories of madness; magazines or reservoirs of lunacy, from which is issued, from time to time, a sufficient supply for perpetuating and extending this formidable disease,—a disease which is not to be remedied by stripes or strait-waistcoats, by imprisonment or impoverishment, but by an unwearied tenderness, and by an unceasing and anxious superintendance.

Alexander and Selesnick are laudatory in their treatment of Johann C. Reil (1759–1813), the great German physician, anatomist, and, it turns out, methodologist of proto-psychiatry.[304] Reil argued that empirical science would bear out his belief that not just a physical/somatic approach is crucial, but an explicitly psychological approach to treating both the mentally and physically ill was to be the most effective. Reil's advocacy was not accompanied by sophisticated psychology and psychological treatments; his theories involved commonsensical notions of reward and punishment and appeals to reason. In any case, Reil may have been the first 'eclectic' proto-psychiatrist, at least as Nassir Ghaemi[305] describes the practice. Reil simply combined common sense psychology with the physiological interventions of the time, figuring combination treatments were better than single treatments.[306] Perhaps of significance for the VMDR is Reil's pragmatic dualism; the parallel comprehensibility and explanatory power of psychology and biology is still discussed today, from the standpoint of clinical practice. In the moral realm, Reil's complicated ethics of painful treatment is reminiscent of risk-benefit arguments of today. For instance, while Reil was comfortable with torture of various types[307] to reshape the behavior of troublesome patients, administration of pain to patients who could not understand their wrongdoing was unacceptable.

A roving author, physician, and scholar, Sir Alexander Crichton (1763–1856) deserves mention for his writings synthesizing Locke, Kant, and the Scottish philosophers' philosophical psychologies with Baconian observational science and physiological correlation. Crichton absorbed a wide range of influences throughout his European travels, and his gift for observation and detailed description, along with a rejection of the old humoral theory in favor of a combination of Locke's associationism and Kantian faculty psychology, make him a key transitional figure in the emerging 'psychiatry'.[308]

As the medical officer of London's Bethlem asylum in the early nineteenth century, John Haslam (1764–1844) presided over both ordinary and 'criminal lunatics', but also Bedlam's decline as a result of abuses and scandal, shrinking its population from approximately 300 to 122 by 1815.[309] Ironically, Haslam was to serve on an 1815 House of Commons' Committee On Madhouses, which was to provide oversight and humanistic reform of these early institutions for the insane. Haslam also provided an early discussion of the presentation of psychiatric testimony to the court. Haslam discussed many still-current issues in what came to be known as forensic psychiatry. Haslam lamented his frequent experience of medical testimonies contradicting each other, addressed the issue of criminal responsibility, yet resisted requests of the court to opine about the defendant's ability to distinguish right from wrong:[310]

> ... And having gauged his insanity he has performed his duty. If it should be presumed that any medical practitioner is able to penetrate into the recesses of a lunatic's mind, at the moment he committed an outrage; to view the internal play of obtruding thoughts, and contending motives—to commit, it must be confessed that such knowledge is beyond the limits of our attainment. It is sufficient for the medical practitioner to know that his mind is deranged, and that such state of insanity will be sufficient to account for the irregularity of his actions; and that in a sound mind, the same conduct would be deemed criminal.

As Enlightenment ideas gathered steam, by the end of the seventeenth century, the public and scholarly opinion toward the medicalization of madness had so prevailed that no less a literary personage as Daniel Defoe advocated for both hospitals for the intellectually impaired—'natural fools'—but also called for public regulation of madhouses:[311]

. . . . I wonder how it came to pass, that in the Settlement of that Hospital [Bedlam] they made no Provision for Persons born without the use of their Reason, such as we call Fools, or more properly, Naturals. . . .

. . . . if they are not mad when they go into these cursed Houses, they are soon made so by the barbarous Usage they there suffer, and any Woman of Spirit who has the least Love for her Husband, or Concern for her Family, cannot sit down tamely under a Confinement and Separation the most unaccountable and unreasonable. Is it not enough to make any one mad to be suddenly clap'd up, stripp'd, whipp'd, ill fed, and worse us'd? . . .

A pioneer in speech therapy for stammering and other impairments, John Thelwall (1764–1834) was influential in the treatment of idiocy and 'cretinism', afflictions of intellectual faculties. Thelwall described a form of acquired idiocy where the child's intellect was 'contracted in its sphere of activity by physical privation',[312] and he believed that proper childcare and focused education could improve the functioning of the intellectually impaired.

Jean Etienne Dominique Esquirol (1772–1840), student, rival, and successor to Phillipe Pinel, will be discussed in more detail in the next chapter because of his core contributions to the concept of monomania, an early psychiatric concept of importance to the VMDR. Weiner[313] describes Esquirol's pronouncements of Pinel's liberation of the Bicêtre inmates as a distraction away from Pinel's scientific contributions, so that Esquirol might seek greater scientific fame. Regardless of Esquirol's ambitions and scientific rivalries, the alienist cut a dashing figure as psychopathologist, facile politician, and pioneer of forensic psychiatry. Esquirol contributed to the French Law of 1838, which developed new governmental policy about the internment or confinement of the mentally ill in France. Rather than lunatics being subject to the Court and judges, Esquirol advocated that their confinements should be initiated and regulated by physicians through a nationwide network of custodial institutions. The superintendents of such institutions should be appointed by the government and accountable to the government. Esquirol wanted to move declarations of patients as *non compos mentis* (see Blackstone, above) from judges to physicians which, he argued, because of medical need and the opportunity for treatment. In a prescient pushback from the judges, the Law of 1838 was threatened to fail because lawyer-judges wanted to retain the internment authority. Weiner notes: 'Esquirol's counterargument was clever indeed: the doctor prescribed *isolation*, for medical and therapeutic reasons, and supervision was *administrative*, not judicial. And as for *non compos mentis* judgments, they only concerned financial matters and wealthy heirs (which was true).'[314] Esquirol was persuasive, the law passed, the beginnings of contemporary 'involuntary commitments' established, and psychiatry's unique seclusion powers initiated.

The influential German physician Johann Christian August Heinroth is often credited as coining the term 'psychiatry' to refer to medical treatment of the mind,[315] is of primary interest here for his contributions to the crime-mental illness relationship, contributing two influential texts of forensic medicine. Believing that crime and criminality was due to sin, Heinroth, bucking the prevailing secular view of the day, argued against the idea that severe criminal acts were products of psychopathology. While working to limit the applicability of the insanity defense, Heinroth also distinguished between guilt and punishment, arguing that the guilty mentally ill should be spared punishment, as mental illness was all the punishment the offender deserved. While Heinroth's contrary views limited his influence during his lifetime, his standards for forensic examination were important even after his time.

While not contributing explicitly to the VMDR, William Tuke (1732–1822), along with his grandson, Samuel Tuke (1784–1857), implemented English innovations in care of the mentally ill, based on Pinel's example of moral treatment. The Tukes began their efforts to reform asylum treatment after the death of a fellow Quaker girl at the York Asylum, a death likely because of mistreatment. The Tukes wished to establish a care center for the mentally ill that would be based on humanistic principles, and after some substantial fund-raising, established The Retreat in 1796, the name reflecting the safe haven they wished to establish. Of significance for my iconic history is the Tukes's relegation of physicians to a secondary role for their Retreat. The Tukes were wealthy merchants and philanthropists, not medical men; their approach to care of the mentally ill was commonsensical and humane:[316]

> Experience . . . has happily shown, in the Institution whose practices we are attempting to describe, that much may be done towards the cure and alleviation of insanity, by judicious modes of management, and moral treatment . . . The moral treatment of the insane, seems to divide itself into three parts . . . 1. By what means the power of the patient to control the disorder, is strengthened and assisted. 2. What modes of coercion are employed, when restraint is absolutely necessary. 3. By what means the general comfort of the insane is promoted . . .

While not rejecting of medical treatments, and the Retreat indeed made use of, for example, opium for assisting the sleep of 'maniacs', as well as seclusion and restraint, the therapeutic core was of lay therapists using psychological and humane persuasion, classwork, honest work, and respect. Hunter and MacAlpine, in their introductory annotation, note that the practice of moral treatment was not at all easy, and required substantial ethical discipline from all staff:[317]

> Not that Samuel Tuke did not realise that 'contradictory features in their [madness] character frequently render it exceedingly difficult to carry out this mode of treatment' as so much depended on the attendants: 'To consider them at the time both as brothers and as mere automata [that is not responsible]; to applaud all they do right and pity without censoring whatever they do wrong, requires such a habit of philosophical reflections, and Christian charity, as is certainly difficult to attain.'

Erica Lilleleht[318] has compared the Tuke Retreat to contemporary psychiatric re-habilitation, and the tension reflected in these short excerpts between medical and 'psychosocial' treatment, as well as the psychiatrist/alienist as central or peripheral to care of the mentally ill, is still present today in public sector mental health settings where psychiatrists are often dispensers of medications but otherwise not leading the treatment efforts.

Asylums were only a few decades old at the time the early nineteenth-century reform movements were already mounting. The spirit of reform was not limited to just asylums, but to the neglect of other socially marginal groups who had not even an asylum as refuge. Samuel Gridley Howe (1801–1876) was a Yankee physi-cian, reformer, and abolitionist who is primarily known for his advocacy and de-velopment of education for the blind. Influenced by the development of education programs for 'idiots' by Eduard Séguin (1812–1880) at France's Bicêtre, as well as Hervey Wilbur's (1820–1883) founding of the first school for the intellectually im-paired in his home in 1848, Howe was positioned politically to develop the first publicly funded school for idiots in Massachusetts in 1851, appointing Wilbur as its Superintendent.[319] Prior to the humane leadership of Séguin, Wilbur, and Howe, the intellectually impaired were commonly regarded as hopeless and were typically neglected and abused, as industrialization set in and the neighborhood tolerance and support of the 'village idiot' became unfeasible and the person who heretofore was simply part of humankind became a burden and even a threat.[320] The full story of the development of education and services for the intellectually impaired follows in Chapter 5.

4.2.6.3 Synthesis

The period encompassing the Renaissance/Reformation/Enlightenment, as the length of this section betrays, is a rich one for understanding the burgeoning rela-tionships between vice and mental disorder. As before, I list a series of iconic points, in no particular order of importance:

1. *Secular reason grows in influence.* Philosophical and scientific secularism comes to dominate intellectual/academic life; its influence upon the broader culture is felt as well.
2. *A bourgeois (middle) class arises* in Western Europe as nation-states develop; a Protestant 'work ethic' becomes normative; and these two social develop-ments fuse to view social deviance as (at minimum) a burden and, at worst, a threat to bourgeois flourishing.
3. *Secular morality grows in influence.* Morality and ethics are increasingly sep-arated from religion and natural law; new reflections upon the right and the good are often secular.
4. *From collectivism to individualism.* The economic shifts from agriculture to trades- and crafts-persons, bourgeois business, the rise of professions and

manufacturing, Protestantism, the secularization of law, and the growth of democratic governments shift social and moral responsibility away from local collectives to individual selves.

5. *Many intellectuals endeavor to mend the religion-secular rift.* Intellectuals identify a rift between rational (science, philosophy) and religious accounts of humanity, and many try to address and manage this rivalry and disagreement.

6. *The naturalizing of deviance.* Social deviance is increasingly naturalized; poverty, idiocy, insanity, and criminality are progressively viewed as social and medical problems correctable through science, reason, and sociopolitical action.

7. *Distinctive circumstances of the American colonies.* The social conditions of the American colonies (e.g., few universities, sparse populations, untamed land, economic dependency, and the Atlantic ocean as a travel barrier) cause American medicine to fall behind its European counterparts. Humoral theory reigns, and local, informal care of the socially deviant persists into the nineteenth century.

8. *The rise of 'psychology'.* Intellectual and scientific interest in individual psychology influences both the shaping of the understanding of morality as well as the description and classification of psychopathology.

9. *Intellectual culture both proliferates and segregates.* As well as emerging socioeconomic class distinctions, parallel paths between popular or lay belief systems and the intelligentsia or elite subculture of the educated and highly educated set up growing divides between popular beliefs about morality and madness and scientific/philosophical understandings of morality and madness.

10. *Institutionalizing punishment.* The legacy of late medieval and Renaissance witch hunting, Inquisitions, torture, heresy, and the development of jails and prisons establish a norm of corporal punishment and incarceration for wrongdoing and deviance from social norms.

11. *Mental illness as part of human nature.* Humanist thought frames mental illness as not just divine punishment, nor demon possession, nor (simply) a mechanistic concatenation of biological failure, but as a revealing of facets of human nature within all people. Subsequently mental illness increasingly becomes a phenomenon that teaches us about what it means to be human.

12. *Psychological forces multiply and interact within individuals.* Hobbes, Locke, Machiavelli, Shakespeare, and others describe a human nature that is not simply a dialectic between good and evil, but rather a psychological admixture of rational and irrational forces and capabilities within the self. These psychological forces interact in complex ways, turning old moral dichotomies between black and white into contemporary shades of gray, and muddling the previously clear distinctions between sanity and insanity. Physicians and,

later, alienists, respond in kind by describing partial insanities, monomanias, and neuroses as the global insanity concept became recognized as insufficient for understanding milder forms of psychopathology.

13. *Secularized law prevails.* Law becomes progressively more secular; the notion of natural law loses traction; and talk of the separation of church and state increases.

14. *Civil affairs become more complicated.* Bourgeois economic change demands more nuanced legal handlings of the domestic, criminal, and legal affairs of the mentally ill.

15. *Diversification of Christianity.* The printing press, the Reformation, Protestantism, and an emerging individualism provide ordinary citizens the opportunity to interpret Scripture and other religious documents and develop their own religious-moral vocabularies and ideologies. The pre-Reformation corruption of the Roman Catholic Church and the Holy Roman Empire tarnish the image of the Church as divine resource and temple of virtue, provoking rebellion, and a shift of moral responsibility away from divine or supernatural inspiration and more upon individual virtue, reason, and resolve.

16. *The individual as civic and moral unit.* The elaboration of human rights by Grotius and others further concretizes the individual person as a civic and moral unit; democratic theory and the U.S. Declaration of Independence later engrave the individual as a fundament of governmental structure and reference. However, who counts as 'an individual' is still in development as racism, classism, and sexism, as known today, marginalize various groups as full citizens.

17. *Theories of the mind emerge, influencing psychopathology.* Metaphysicians and philosophical psychologists like Locke, Hume, Kant, and Spinoza articulate both psychological structures of the mind, as well as psychological mechanisms that provide novel and medically influential explanations for behavior.

18. *Medical science, as recognized today, emerges.* The British Empiricists, Francis Bacon, Thomas Sydenham, William Harvey, and many others, shift the inquiries of 'natural philosophy' away from introspection and speculative thought into the realm of experiment, systematic observation, and inference; thereby birthing scientific medicine.

19. *The science of society emerges.* The beginnings of social science, exemplified by Spinoza, suggest that all human social phenomena, including religion, are subject to study, independent of their metaphysical status or moral power.

20. *Psychology's tools for psychopathology.* Associationism and the psychological faculties of cognition (intellect/reason), affection (passions/emotions), and conation (will/motivation) become the most influential psychological reference points for the emerging alienists'/psychiatrists' description of, classification of, and theorizing about psychopathology.

21. *Democratic theory and practice takes hold.* Divine monarchies weaken their grip on the emerging European and New World nation-states; the ideas of

government by consent of the governed, rule of law, social contracts, and civil liberties/rights take hold and proliferate, at least in the West.

22. *Moral-ethical theory differentiates into novel aspects.* The premodern and modern philosophers develop independent modes of reasoning about moral problems; making it possible, even likely, that different moral problems could generate distinctive moral analyses and judgments, depending upon what ethical theory one was using. The diversity of ethical theory sets the stage for nihilism, existentialism, and postmodernism to come later.

23. *Supernaturalism out, dualism in.* Renaissance physicians like Vives, Paracelsus, Weyer, and Cardano, along with many later Enlightenment physicians, progressively reject divine and supernatural accounts of mental illness. The dualistic distinction between somatic/bodily and psychological causes of insanity emerges and influences theorizing about mental illness.

24. *Narratives of mental illness proliferate.* A popular literature on mental illness emerges, through fiction authors like Shakespeare and Cervantes, as well as nonfiction writers like Robert Burton, enabling a demystification and greater understanding of psychopathology among the literate public.

25. *Movement of madness from courts to physicians.* Influential physicians in the Renaissance and Enlightenment argue that the assessment and management of the mad should be handled by physicians, not the courts.

26. *Church responses to the mentally ill differentiate.* Humanistic Protestant groups like the Quakers advocate compassionate care for the mentally ill, and design influential services for them, symbolizing the emerging humanistic role of churches in the care of the ill. The early Puritan leaders, Increase and Cotton Mather, embodied the ambivalent feelings and even stigmatizing attitudes toward the mentally ill that persist for many fundamentalist religious groups today.

27. *Madhouses and asylums appear and reform themselves.* Private madhouses and public asylums—institutions to house, care for, and treat the mentally ill, are established in Europe during the late Enlightenment era. While intentions were often, even usually, humane, the early madhouses and asylums were quick to fall into neglect and be subject to calls for reform. The madhouse/asylum movement had not yet taken hold in the American colonies and early United States by the end of the eighteenth century.

28. *The mad and bad are lumped together.* Of the early English asylums, Bethlem perhaps best symbolizes the exploitation of the hospitalized mentally ill for public entertainment (through exhibitions of the lunatics), as well as the blurring of social regulation roles, through the internment of 'criminal lunatics'.

29. *The theory of penology emerges and influences the handling of crime and punishment.* Jeremy Bentham and Cesare Beccaria emerge as influential theorists in what would become penology and criminology, raising philosophical and scientific questions of the function and efficacy of criminal punishment,

arguing that punishment must be prompt to be effective, and be proportionate to the crime committed.

30. *Idiocy-insanity distinction.* For the courts, Blackstone and others distinguish between intellectually impaired individuals from birth, and individuals with acquired mental illness later in life, spelling out differential legal proceedings for each.

31. *Moral treatments spread.* Pinel, Chiarugi, and the Tukes articulate a more human vision for asylums and care for the insane; founding institutions based upon the principles of moral treatment, a psychological approach involving fair and humane treatment, counseling and education, work scheduling, and the soothing structural order of the institution.

32. *Distinction of fact from value.* Hume's is/ought distinction provided a philosophical basis for distinguishing facts from values; and introduced an issue in moral philosophy directly relevant to the VMDR.

33. *Forensic medicine.* The Enlightenment era develops a self-aware forensic medicine, including alienists, which identifies and elaborates on the issue of criminal responsibility, what became the insanity defense, and what are reasonable consequences for mentally ill offenders.

34. *Madness as unreason appears in rhetoric.* Metaphors of insanity and madness appear frequently in philosophical, literary, religious, and legal writings, to indicating not a literal condition of insanity, but used with negative connotations to portray beliefs, reasons, or actions that are fallacious, foolish, or specious.

35. *New theory and classification.* Humoral theory of disease falls into disrepute on the Continent and England; new theories of disease are offered, and new, non-Galenic classifications of disease and insanity appear.

36. *Moral treatment as psychosocial.* The *Zeitgeist* of moral treatment spreads, providing a 'psychosocial' alternative to medicalized diagnosis, science, and treatment of mental disorder.

37. *Bio- versus psycho-.* Rivalries emerge between psychological theory of psychopathology versus somatic theory of psychopathology.

38. *Psychiatry and Neurology.* The medical specialties of psychiatry and neurology are founded and grow, in large part, separately.

Notes

1. My use of 'social deviance' is intended as a generic reference to the failure of an individual to conform to social norms. Such norms may be local, but more typically cultural, typical of the country or tribe. In the digital contemporary world, recognizing an individual's practice or behavior as socially deviant becomes more problematic; our identities have become both more complex and diffuse.

2. Thomson (1993).

3. Connolly (1987); Hampsher-Monk (1992); Kymlicka (1990).
4. Eve here is a kind of gendered icon about social deviance.
5. One's resources in this context tends to come from the history of medicine, psychiatry, religion, and more narrowly, sin, and later, histories of the prison and criminal justice.
6. Throughout this book I abbreviate the 'vice/mental disorder relationship' as VMDR.
7. Thomson (1993).
8. Shakespeare (2005).
9. St. Augustine (2009, 1876).
10. Teeple (2006).
11. Thomson (1993).
12. Restak (2000).
13. Porter (2002).
14. Chisholm (1911).
15. ibid.
16. Sigerist (1951).
17. Roth, Hoffner, & Michalowski (1997).
18. Code of Hammurabi: http://avalon.law.yale.edu/subject_menus/hammenu.asp.
19. Thomson (1993).
20. Nasser (1987).
21. Nasser (1987, p. 420).
22. Nasser (1987, p. 420).
23. Citing Zilboorg (1941), see Weckowicz & Liebel-Weckowicz (1990, p.10).
24. Sadler (2005).
25. Scurlock & Anderson (2005).
26. See for instance Thompson ([1974] 2002).
27. Coogan (2001).
28. Thomson (1993).
29. Leviticus (19.18); see also Holy Bible, Exodus 20:2, 2–17; Deuteronomy 5:6–21; Leviticus (18–20 [Coogan 2001]).
30. Coogan (2001).
31. ibid.
32. Scurlock & Anderson (2005).
33. Quotation following this citation was from Yuste & Garrido (2010, p. 78).
34. Yuste & Garrido (2010, p. 80).
35. Scurlock & Anderson (2005, pp. 367–385).
36. Adapted from Scurlock & Anderson 2005, Chapter 16, pp. 367–385.
37. Conybeare (1898).
38. Conybeare (1898, p. 30), italics added.
39. Coogan (2001, 1 Samuel 11–22, p. 433).
40. Coogan (2001, 1 Samuel 15.14, p. 424).
41. Coogan (2001, 1 Samuel 18.10, p. 428).
42. Ben-Noun (2003, pp. 270–282).
43. Kapusta & Frank (1977, pp. 667–672).
44. See also Covey (2005, pp. 107–114).
45. Coogan (2001, p. 734); see also Kutz (2000).
46. Broome (1946, pp. 277–292).
47. ibid, p. 291.
48. ibid, p. 292.
49. Simon (1980, 2008).

50. See also Martin & Barresi (2006); Rosen (1968).
51. Simon (2008, p. 176).
52. Robinson (1996).
53. Simon (1980, 2008).
54. See also Martin & Collesi (2006).
55. Simon (1980, 2008); Pilgrim (2007); Rosen (1968).
56. Porter (1999, 2002); Radden (2002).
57. Simon (2008, p. 182).
58. ibid, p. 183.
59. ibid, p. 183.
60. Robinson (1996).
61. Plutarch, Plutarch's Lives, tr Aubrey Stewart and George Long Vol. 1, Life of Solon, XVII, available online: http://www.gutenberg.org/files/14033/14033-h/14033-h.htm#LIFE_OF_SOLON.
62. Martin & Barresi (2006); see also Martin (2018).
63. Martin & Barresi (2006, p. 44). Professor Martin provides a nice review of the scholarship around the historical accuracy of the Bible in his 2018 book.
64. Thomson (1993).
65. Coogan (2001, p. 13co).
66. McKenzie (1922); Sircar (1933a, 1933b).
67. Hopkins (1924); Sircar (1933a, 1933b).
68. Dhand (2002).
69. Gandhi (1933); see the following wikilivres citation: http://www.wikilivres.info/wiki/The_Gita_According_to_Gandhi/Introduction.
70. Macy (1979); Prebish (1996).
71. Jensen (1987).
72. For quotation see: https://en.wikipedia.org/w/index.php?title=Three_Treasures_(Taoism)&oldid=1025960510.
73. Thomson (1993, pp. 88–89).
74. Confucius (1971).
75. Fan (2002); Tsai (2005).
76. Fan (2002).
77. Mora (2008); Sigerist (1961); Thomson (1993).
78. Wattles (1996, p. 29).
79. Sophocles (2009).
80. Sophocles (2009); see also Thomson (1993).
81. MacIntyre (1998); Taylor (2005).
82. Taylor (2005, p. 721).
83. Plato (2009).
84. Plato (1991).
85. Martin & Barresi (2006).
86. Taylor (2005).
87. MacIntyre (1998, Kindle edition, location 797).
88. ibid.
89. Denyer (1995, p. 202); see also MacIntyre (1998); Sidgwick (1888).
90. Sharples (1995, p. 853); see also MacIntyre (1998); Sidgwick (1888).
91. Lucretius, 'On the Nature of Things'. available online: http://classics.mit.edu/Carus/nature_things.html). Around the time of this writing, Stephen Greenblatt's popular book, *The Swerve: How the World Became Modern* brought contemporary attention to the prescience of Lucretius' metaphysical thought.
92. MacIntyre (1998).

93. Charles (1984, p. 55).
94. See also Hutchinson (1995); MacIntyre (1998); Sidgwick (1888).
95. See Radden & Sadler (2010).
96. Hutchinson (1995, p. 214).
97. ibid.
98. Clark (2002).
99. Frankena (1973); Harrelson (1951); Keck (1996); Mott (1987); Meeks (1986); Ramsey (1950).
100. Keck (1996, pp. 3–4).
101. Keck (1996).
102. Hauerwas (1991).
103. Keck (1996, p. 8).
104. ibid, p. 10.
105. ibid, p. 14.
106. Mott (1987).
107. ibid, p. 235.
108. Thomson (1993).
109. ibid.
110. Chadwick (1992).
111. Thomson (1993), Chadwick 2010.
112. Danielou (1994).
113. Thomson (1993).
114. For more details, see Hopkins (1990); Lawrence (1996); Saunders (1923, 1924).
115. Thomson (1993). In Section 4.9.7 of this chapter, a discussion is provided of the genesis of the concept of 'sexuality' in the Western world, marking the transition in the West from sex as a behavior to sexuality as part of personal identity and lifestyle.
116. Mora (2008, p. 199).
117. Plato, Phaedrus, not dated, See also Mora (2008).
118. Robinson (1996).
119. Simon (1980, 2008); Wallace (1994).
120. Kidd (1999).
121. ibid, p. 23.
122. Mora (2008); van Staden (1989).
123. Mora (2008, p. 398).
124. Simon (2008, p. 184, internal citation omitted); see also Gilbert (1901); Hollenbach (1981).
125. Mora (2008).
126. Millon et al. (2004).
127. Porter (1999).
128. See Porter (1999) for extensive discussion, as well as Gonzalez de Pablo (1994); Mora (2008).
129. Porter (1999, p. 74).
130. Porter (1999, 2003).
131. Porter (1999).
132. ibid, p. 77.
133. Chadwick (1992); see also Porter (2003).
134. Millon et al. (2004).
135. Augustine, tr. Chadwick (1992, p. 101).
136. Teeple (2006).
137. Thomson (1993, p. 126).
138. Chapter 3 provides a discussion of the seven deadly sins and their relationship to psychopathology.
139. Thomson (1993).

140. See an annotated Justinian Code: https://www.uwyo.edu/lawlib/blume-justinian/ajc-edition-2/books/book1/index.html.

141. ibid; Robinson (1996).

142. Thomson (1993).

143. ibid, p. 197.

144. Nanji (1993).

145. Teeple (2006).

146. Teeple (2006); Thomson (1993).

147. Thomson (1993).

148. McDonald & Kretzmann (2000, pp. 552–560).

149. Sidgwick (1888,).

150. ibid, p. 137.

151. ibid, p. 138.

152. McGinnis (2010, p. 223).

153. Copeland (1994).

154. Maimonides: https://www.jewishvirtuallibrary.org/oath-of-maimonides.

155. Weiss (1991).

156. Seeksin (2021): https://plato.stanford.edu/archives/spr2021/entries/maimonides/.

157. Aquinas (1981).

158. Sidgwick (1888, p. 144).

159. Murphy (2019). 'The natural law tradition in ethics' in Stanford Encyclopedia of Philosophy: https://plato.stanford.edu/archives/sum2019/entries/natural-law-ethics/.

160. Kelly (1992).

161. Aquinas in the *Summa Theologica*, quoted by Kelly (1992, p. 155).

162. Both quotations ibid, pp. 155–156.

163. Thomson (1993); also see discussion in following paragraph in main text.

164. Kelly (1992).

165. Kelly (1992); Thomson (1993).

166. Gonzalez (2010a).

167. Thomson (1993).

168. Kramer & Sprenger 1487, Mackay Translation 2009.

169. Huizenga (1954); see also Mora (2008).

170. Radden (2002).

171. Mora (2008).

172. Gilman (1998); Mora (2008).

173. Butera (2010).

174. Sighart (1876).

175. Foucault (1965).

176. Mora (2008).

177. Sadler (2007).

178. Mora (2008, p. 216).

179. Mora (2008).

180. Radden (2000).

181. Mora (2008).

182. Nedopil (2009).

183. Kelly (1992).

184. Mora (2008 p. 218); see also Robinson (1996).

185. Thomson (1993).

186. Goldstein & Godemont (2003).

187. Rosen (1968, p. 11). I should note that this era is also associated with the development of the distinction between religious prayer and the incantations of white and black magic, enabling the demonizing of women who practiced pagan magic. See Kieckhefer 2022.
188. Wallace (1994, p. 57).
189. Porter (1997, p. 130); see also Laqueur (1990).
190. Thomson (1993).
191. Porter (2004).
192. ibid, p. 3.
193. Thomson (1993).
194. Monfasani (2000).
195. Gonzalez (2010a, b).
196. Thomson (1993).
197. Machiavelli, *The Prince*, tr. W. K. Marriott, on Project Gutenberg website: https://www.gutenberg.org/cache/epub/1232/pg1232.txt.
198. Nederman (2009). Niccolo Machiavelli, in the *Stanford Encyclopedia of Philosophy*, available online https://plato.stanford.edu/archives/sum2019/entries/machiavelli/.
199. Neely (2004).
200. Kelly (1992).
201. ibid, p. 226.
202. Kelly (1992).
203. Gert (2005).
204. Hobbes (1651). Leviathan, Chapter XIII, Of the Natural Condition of Mankind, as Concerning Their Felicity, and Misery, section 'The Incommodites Of Such A War' [no page numbers] available online through Project Gutenberg, http://www.gutenberg.org/cache/epub/3207/pg3207.txt. Hobbes' vision of the chaotic State of Nature has been vigorously challenged recently by the archeologist/anthropologist team of David Graeber & David Wengrow (2021).
205. Rutherford (2008). Rutherford, Donald, 'Descartes' Ethics', *The Stanford Encyclopedia of Philosophy* (Winter 2019 Edition), Edward N. Zalta (ed.), https://plato.stanford.edu/archives/win2019/entries/descartes-ethics/.
206. Descartes, ([1909–1914] 2001).
207. Gonzalez (2010a.b).
208. ibid.
209. ibid.
210. ibid.
211. Spierenburg (1995).
212. Inwood (2005); Porter (2003).
213. See Grob (1977, 1983); Scull (1991a, 1991b).
214. Foucault (1965, 1978, 2003, 2008).
215. Scull (1977, 1979, 1981, 1989, 1991, 1996, 1999, 2000, 2004, 2005, 2015, 2018, 2021).
216. Rothman (2002a, 2002b).
217. Scull (2010, p. 1246).
218. See Grob (1977, 1983); Micale & Porter (1994).
219. Tuckness, Alex, 'Locke's Political Philosophy', *The Stanford Encyclopedia of Philosophy* (Winter 2020 Edition), Edward N. Zalta (ed.), <https://plato.stanford.edu/archives/win2020/entries/locke-political/.
220. Locke ([1689] 1812). (11th edition. A Letter Concerning Toleration, available online: https://oll.libertyfund.org/title/locke-the-works-vol-5-four-letters-concerning-toleration.
221. Locke ([1689] 1764, 1690). See also Kendi (2016); Tuckness, Alex, see note 219; Woolhouse (2005).

222. See for instance Alexander & Selesnick (1966); MacIntyre (1998); Nadler, Steven, 'Baruch Spinoza', The Stanford Encyclopedia of Philosophy (Summer 2020 Edition), Edward N. Zalta (ed.), https://plato.stanford.edu/archives/sum2020/entries/spinoza/.

223. Spinoza (1883).

224. MacIntyre (1998, Chapter 10, Kindle Edition, location 2564–2577).

225. Alexander & Selesnick (1966).

226. Youpa, Andrew, 'Leibniz's Ethics', The Stanford Encyclopedia of Philosophy (Winter 2016 Edition), Edward N. Zalta (ed.), https://plato.stanford.edu/archives/win2016/entries/leibniz-ethics/.

227. Montesquieu (1748, tr. T. Nugent 1752).

228. Bok, Hilary. 'Baron de Montesquieu, Charles-Louis de Secondat', The Stanford Encyclopedia of Philosophy (Winter 2018 Edition), Edward N. Zalta (ed.), URL = https://plato.stanford.edu/archives/win2018/entries/montesquieu/.

229. Cohon Rachel, 'Hume's Moral Philosophy', The Stanford Encyclopedia of Philosophy (Fall 2018 Edition), Edward N. Zalta (ed.), <https://plato.stanford.edu/archives/fall2018/entries/hume-moral/ . Internal citations omitted.

230. ibid; see also Broakes (2005); Hume (1605). Also, Tom Beauchamp's edition of *David Hume, An Enquiry Concerning the Principles of Morals* (1998). My own work has been influenced by Hume if primarily through his interest in the fact-value distinction, which has been a cornerstone for me (Sadler 1997, 2005).

231. Rousseau (1913): The Social Contract and Discourses, tr. GDH Cole, London/Toronto: JM Dent & Sons, (1923, p. 35). https://oll.libertyfund.org/title/cole-the-social-contract-and-discourses.

232. See also Bertram, Christopher, 'Jean Jacques Rousseau', The Stanford Encyclopedia of Philosophy (Winter 2020 Edition), Edward N. Zalta (ed.), https://plato.stanford.edu/archives/win2020/entries/rousseau/.

233. Kant (1998, p. 31).

234. Kant's first formulation of the CI was based upon the requirement that one's actions be in accord with guidance which can be made into a universal law. Later scholars spelled this out in terms of four conditions: (1) formulate a maxim that encompasses your reason(s) for action; (2) cast this maxim as a universal law of nature for all rational agents; (3) critique your maxim for its applicability as a law of nature; and (4) ask oneself if you could, or would, intend to act on your maxim within such a world of nature. If so, the action is morally permitted. See Johnson, Robert and Cureton, Adam, 'Kant's Moral Philosophy', The Stanford Encyclopedia of Philosophy (Spring 2018 Edition), Edward N. Zalta (ed.), <https://plato.stanford.edu/archives/spr2018/entries/kant-moral/>.

235. Johnson, Robert, 'Kant's Moral Philosophy', The Stanford Encyclopedia of Philosophy (Spring 2018 Edition), Edward N. Zalta (ed.), <https://plato.stanford.edu/archives/spr2018/entries/kant-moral/>. Rohlf, Michael, 'Immanuel Kant', The Stanford Encyclopedia of Philosophy (Fall 2020 Edition), Edward N. Zalta (ed.), https://plato.stanford.edu/archives/fall2020/entries/kant/.

236. Erasmus (1958).

237. Vives, quoted in Millon (2004, p. 89).

238. Vives, quoted in Zilboorg (1941, p. 188).

239. Alexander & Selesnick (1966); Millon (2004); Mora (2008); Zilboorg (1941).

240. Zilboorg (1941); see also Mora (2008).

241. Alexander & Selesnick (1966); Mora (2008).

242. Mora (2008). See also Bever & Styers (2018) for a fascinating series of essays about magic and science in modernity.

243. Mora (2008); Porter (2002, 2004).

244. Millon (2004).

245. Klein, Jürgen, 'Francis Bacon', The Stanford Encyclopedia of Philosophy (Fall 2020 Edition), Edward N. Zalta (ed.), https://plato.stanford.edu/archives/fall2020/entries/francis-bacon/.
246. See for instance Neely (1991); Overholser (1959); Truskinovsky (2002).
247. Radden (2000).
248. Henry (2007).
249. Allan, Louw, & Verschoor (1995); Mora (2008).
250. Schmitter, Amy M., '17th and 18th Century Theories of Emotions', The Stanford Encyclopedia of Philosophy (Summer 2021 Edition), Edward N. Zalta (ed.), https://plato.stanford.edu/archives/sum2021/entries/emotions-17th18th/.
251. Adapted from Hobbes, *Leviathan*, Chapter VI, 'of the Interiour Beginnings of Voluntary Motions Commonly Called the Passions, and the Speeches by Which They are Expressed'. (No page numbers): http://www.gutenberg.org/ebooks/3207.
252. Schmitter (2021, Section 6. Passions and Reason).
253. Porter (1983, p. 36).
254. ibid.
255. Calvin ([1541] 2009, p. 92).
256. Dain (1992).
257. Gonzalez (2010a, b); see also Kendi (2016).
258. Deutsch (1949).
259. Hunter & MacAlpine (1963).
260. Hunter & MacAlpine (1963); Weiner (2008a).
261. Sydenham, quoted in Lawrence (2007, p. 1210).
262. Hunter & MacAlpine (1963, p. 221); Koutouvidis, Marketos, & Beveridge (1995).
263. Porter (2004, p. 191).
264. Wallace (2008a).
265. Alexander & Selesnick (1966); Wallace (2008a).
266. Alexander & Selesnick (1966); Millon (2004).
267. Alldridge (1974).
268. Weiner (2008a).
269. Porter (2002, 2004).
270. Porter (1999).
271. Alexander & Selesnick (1966); Porter (2004); Weiner (2008a).
272. Cullen, quoted in Porter (2004, p. 183), editing is Porter's.
273. Wallace (2008b).
274. Mooij (1998).
275. Kant ([1798] 2006).
276. Radden (1996).
277. See also Berrios (1996).
278. Mooij (1998).
279. Chung, Fulford, & Graham (2007); Lysaker & Lysaker (2008); Stanghellini (2004).
280. Kant ([1798] 2006, p. 113).
281. Siegel (2006).
282. Kelly (1992).
283. Beccaria (1767).
284. Weiner (2008b).
285. Weiner (2007, pp. 1008–1013). See also Weiner (2008b).
286. Foucault (1965, 1980, 2003, 2006); Gutting (2001).
287. Weiner (2008b, p. 284).
288. Blackstone, quoted in Hunter & MacAlpine (1963, p. 435).
289. Blackstone (1765–1769), quoted in Hunter & MacAlpine (1963, pp. 435–436).

290. All quotations from Blackstone in this paragraph are ibid, p. 437.

291. Garton (2004); Porter & Teich (1994).

292. Arnold (1782–1786), quoted in Hunter & MacAlpine (1963, p. 469).

293. ibid, p. 471, editing and bracketing mine.

294. McCullough (2007, pp. 1092–1094). Regarding Benjamin Rush and racism, see Kendi (2016).

295. Ogden (1932).

296. de Champs (1999, p. 15).

297. Driver, Julia, "The History of Utilitarianism", The Stanford Encyclopedia of Philosophy (Winter 2014 Edition), Edward N. Zalta (ed.), <https://plato.stanford.edu/archives/win2014/entries/utilitarianism-history/.

298. Bentham (1907); Driver (1999).

299. Driver (1999).

300. Bentham (1787).

301. Foucault (1977, 2008). 'Normalizing' here refers to the socializing of the population into group conventions and, therefore, conformity to a group norm.

302. Goffman (1961).

303. Hunter & MacAlpine (1963, pp. 723–725).

304. Alexander & Selesnick (1966).

305. Ghaemi (2010).

306. Marx (2008).

307. As apparently the rest of Europe was, as noted earlier.

308. Berrios (2006); Charland (2008); Weiner (2008a).

309. Hunter & MacAlpine (1963).

310. ibid, p. 637.

311. ibid, pp. 265–267.

312. ibid, p. 657.

313. Weiner (2008b).

314. Weiner (2008b, p. 310).

315. Marx (2008).

316. Tuke (1813), quoted in Hunter & MacAlpine (1963, p. 689).

317. Hunter & MacAlpine (1963, p. 687).

318. Lilleleht (2002); see also Charland (2002).

319. Obituary of Hervey B. Wilbur, M.D. 1883; Rafter (1997a, b); Trent, (1994).

320. Rafter (1997a, b); Trent (1994).

5

Building a moral-medical psychiatry

The voice of intelligence is drowned out by the roar of fear. It is ignored by the voice of desire. It is contradicted by the voice of shame. It is biased by hate and extinguished by anger. Most of all it is silenced by ignorance.

—Karl A. Menninger, The Progressive, 1955

Vice and Psychiatric Diagnosis. John Z. Sadler, Oxford University Press. © Oxford University Press 2024.
DOI: 10.1093/oso/9780198876830.003.0005

5.1 Psychiatry, morality, and mental illness—transition to the nineteenth and twentieth centuries

With this chapter springing from the legacy of Enlightenment thought for morality and mental illness, the style of this chapter should transition accordingly. The prior chapter consisted of an iconographic history of morality and mental disorder, with some effort to synthesize these parallel histories of ideas. With this transition away from the Enlightenment period around the turn of the nineteenth century, we have many of the key elements toward understanding the roots of the VMDR. First, we have an emerging psychiatric identity for asylum physicians, as well as the preliminaries in place for an expansion of the psychiatrist's role beyond the asylum. These include, among others: (1) The development of finer-grained concepts of psychopathology, such as neurosis, partial insanities, and newly fashionable conditions like hypochondriasis and hysteria which provoked an extension of psychiatry's bounds outside of the walls of the asylum and the needs of the severely ill and the globally incapacitated. (2) The establishment of alternative institutions for other kinds of social deviance: schools for the intellectually impaired, the penal/criminal justice system for criminal offenders (and to arrive later, a juvenile justice system for offending youth), the development of orphanages, almshouses, and other social-community resources for the poor and disadvantaged. (3) Evolving governmental models and special legislation for civil issues and criminal offenses recognizing the particular challenges posed by the mentally ill in these domains. (4) The appearance of nonmedical approaches to aiding the mentally ill, from psychological approaches to religious charity. (5) The development of what were to be called 'professions' which required extensive education, training, and knowledge in service to humanity, scholars of mostly noble intent who were also subject to the human frailties of self-interest and self-promotion. (6) The evolution of a bourgeois citizenry and democratic governmental principles, which empowered those governed to have input upon policies that affect them. (7) The birth of the practice of social reform, where conscientious citizens organized, often independent of, or otherwise in collaboration with, governments, which addressed shared concerns or problems in the community.

These ingredients make up the social forces that now can be considered in a more conventional narrative voice, one that addresses historical causes and effects, providing a narrative background to the vice-mental disorder relationship.

5.2 Social-historical threads in America's response to vice and mental illness

As discussed earlier, the handling of social deviance in Western Europe was different from that of the American colonies' softer approach. Which was better is debatable.

At this stage of our discussion, the end of the eighteenth and the turn of the nine-teenth century, some context-setting is needed regarding the control of social devi-ance in the American colonies, and later, the United States.

5.2.1 Social deviance in the early American colonies

The early American colonists were essentially small groups of pioneers, religious in-dependents and rebels, struggling to establish themselves as settlers in a new and often-hostile environment. They had little opportunity or inclination to develop pol-icies to assist or control populations which didn't, and often couldn't, follow local norms and social expectations. They faced a rugged landscape already occupied by native peoples.

A variety of existential inevitables created the colonial poor: (1) time and infir-mity generated the aged sick; (2) a harsh living environment provided for ample op-portunities for injuries and ultimately a short adult life span; (3) subsequent widows and orphans; (4) the absence of prenatal health care along with the limitations and availability of midwives resulted in physically and mentally handicapped children; and (5) the lure of demon alcohol and other vicious temptations which threatened families. These existential inevitables (as well as ordinary misery) did not generate coordinated social policy and intervention but rather generated reflexive, practical, local, and neighborly responses and solutions. The American colonists couldn't rely upon the more formal English legal or social approaches because the colonies were sparsely populated, rural, or frontier endeavors. Moreover, the specialized schools (law, medicine, and ministry) for preparing civic professionals were only in the earliest stages of development. David Rothman neatly summarizes the colonial handling of deviance:[1]

> Eighteenth-century Americans did not define either poverty or crime as a critical social problem. They did not interpret the presence of the poor as symptomatic of a basic flaw in the citizen or the society, an indicator of personal or communal failing. Compared to their successors, the colonists accepted the existence of poverty with great equanimity. They devoted very little energy to devising and enacting programs to reform offenders and had no expectations of eradicating crime. Nor did they systematically attempt to isolate the de-viant or the dependent.

We can recognize that the social order we take for granted today was yet to be de-veloped, even while a social order regulating crime, illness, and poverty was being developed in Europe.

5.2.1.1 Dealing with madness in the American colonies
Regarding the care of the mentally ill in the American colonies, madpersons posed social and economic problems to their communities, much like the poor, the sick,

the injured, and the widowed. When possible, the problems posed by the deviant were handled within the confines of the family, and often through the Church. Stigma, while present, was not much of a barrier to recovered madpersons regaining work because of the great community/social need for all to contribute. People found ways to contribute in spite of disabilities. Persistent troublemakers, criminal or mad, may have found themselves run out of town, or subject to the stocks or other forms of public humiliation. The purpose of punishment was deterrence, and expulsions of troublemakers from the community were pragmatic decisions. The colonists' social ethos was heavily influenced by the mores of Western Europe and particularly England, which cast the responsibility for care to the family and local community,[2] especially in the absence of the resources of European cities. Every community larger than a handful of citizens had one or more drunkards. The drunkard slept off benders in the stables and eked out a meager existence based on the generosity of neighbors, who knew his community history, furnished him with odd jobs, and tolerated him. Intellectually impaired and/or physically handicapped children were the responsibility of the family, and their treatment varied widely.[3] While British, Charles Dickens's Tiny Tim and the story of *A Christmas Carol* illustrates the grim possibilities for handicapped English youth of the era. Handicapped youth in the colonies likely fared far worse. Severely impaired children were simply fated to die; today's ideas of 'allowing' to die were yet to be conceived of.

The colonial era was a period of great transition in the understanding of the mad. Over the course of the seventeenth century, modern science was born, and scholars struggled over the meaning of madness. Consider Cambridge theologian William Perkin's (1602) refutation of the madness theory of witchcraft in an essay entitled 'Devils not Humors':[4]

> Witches of our times (say they) are aged persons, of weake braines, and troubled with abundance of melancholie, and the devill taketh advauntage of the humor, and so deludes them, perswading that they have made a league with him, when they have not, and consequently mooving them to imagine, that they doe, and may doe strange things, which indeed are done by himself, and not by them.
>
> This reason is a meere melancholy like conceit, without ground. And the contrarie is a manifest truth, that they are not so, as is affirmed, parties deceived by reason of their humors. For first, our Witches are as wise and politike, yea as craftie and cunning in all other matters, as other men be; whereas brainsike persons troubled with melancholy, if their undeerstanding be distempered in one action, it will be faultie likewise in others, more or lesse. Agine, our Witches know that they sinne in their practises of Witchcraft, and therefore they use subtill meanes to cover them, and he that would convict them, must have great dexteritie to goe beyond them. Now if they were persons deluded, through coruption of any humors; looke what humour caused them to doe a thing, the same would urge them to disclose it. Thirdly, they are also of the same stamp, they take the same courses in all their practises, their consent in word and action is universall. . . . Fourthly, our Witches are wont to communicate their skill to others by tradition, to teach

and instruct their children and posteritie, and to initiate them in the grounds and prac-
tises of their owne trade, while they live, as may appear by the confessions recorded
in the Courts of all countries. But if they were persons troubled with melancholie, their
conceipts would die with them. . . . [sic]

The wariness of supernatural causes of misbehavior, as well as religious reservations about madness existed not just in England but in the colonies; though this wariness was not to manifest in widespread stigmatizing behavior by the citizenry until
the next century.

Strong interest in the classification of mental illnesses had not yet developed,
partly because the diffuse population and local care provided by the colonial neighbors posed no practical need for classifying mental disorders, either on the basis
of disease characteristics, disease etiology, or allocation of resources. However, as
asylums developed for housing larger numbers of madpeople, the young alienists
argued for a classification of mental disease—while the practical demands for a
nosology had yet to materialize, the scientific merits of nosology were debated.
Nevertheless, as early as 1886, Pliny Earle, President of the Association of Medical
Superintendents of American Institutions for the Insane (later the American
Psychiatric Association), assessed the need for a medical-scientific classification
system this way:[5]

In the present state of our knowledge, no classification of insanity can be erected upon a
pathological basis, for the simple reason that, with but slight exceptions, the pathology
of the disease is unknown . . . Hence, for the most apparent, the most clearly defined, and
the best understood foundation for a nosological scheme for insanity, we are forced to fall
back upon the symptomatology of the disease—*the apparent mental condition*, as judged
from the outward manifestations.

With the exception of the archaic 'insanity' language, Earle's viewpoint could easily
dovetail into the *Diagnostic and Statistical Manual of Mental Disorders* (DSM)-III
discussion in the late 1970s.

5.2.1.2 Dealing with criminal offenders in the American colonies

The social conditions that structured the colonial response to mental illness also
framed the sixteenth- and seventeenth-century responses to criminality. The small
colonial communities had to be self-reliant and handle criminal deviance locally—
militias were one resource, but those were only called in for major rioting.[6] Police
forces had not yet been conceived—not until a century later in the 1800s. The colonial repertoire of crimes included some obvious ones: thievery, arson, murder,
inebriation. On the other hand, the uniquely religious and staid nature of many
American colonists (e.g., Pennsylvania's Quakers, Massachusetts' Puritans) added
Christian sins to the list of criminal offenses (e.g., idolatry, blasphemy, and witchcraft),[7] making colonial criminal law more explicitly religious compared to the more

secular English law of the time.[8] For many American colonists, the wrong ideas and the wrong speech could be crimes.

The insular nature of colonial communities likely made transients—then called 'rogues' and 'vagabonds' worthy of suspicion, harassment, and eviction. Newly arriving widows with children and unwed mothers with bastard children might be warned by community leaders and encouraged to move on. Newcomers were expected to bring letters of reference with them from prior communities or have evidence of property or means to earn respectability.[9] Evictions were common and hence drifters could run into more serious trouble by returning to an offended community.

Criminal offenses, correspondingly, were handled differently depending upon one's familiarity. For locals, less serious offenses were almost exclusively handled by fines, and less commonly upon public humiliation, like being locked up in the stocks or cages in the town square. More serious crimes generated floggings and hangings. The threshold for more severe punishments, with the addition of expulsions, was lower for undocumented immigrant newcomers, such as the Irish, not to overlook the grim discipline of African slaves. Capital sentencing was applied liberally, often common for offenses like horse-stealing, picking pockets, and counterfeiting, as well as for murder and grand larceny. Repeat offenders were even more likely to be sentenced to death by hanging.[10]

5.2.1.3 Orphaned children in colonial America

Little appears to be known of the history of orphaned children in colonial America. The history of orphans and orphanages in America appears to begin in the nineteenth century and will be discussed in a later section. Hacsi briefly discusses the care of colonial children by 'adults other than their own parents.'[11] Prior to the founding of orphanages and other modes of assuring child welfare in the 1800s, Hacsi notes that orphaned children often earned their keep prior to 1800 by being indentured to families, learning trades so they could both contribute to the supporting family and also develop skills to assure their independence in adulthood. In the eighteenth century, community officials often had the authority to send orphaned children (as well as children of poor families) to such indentured service. Some parents entered into indenture agreements independent of the government. Education was not a priority in these indentured arrangements, and the motivation was largely economic, as again, there was more than enough work for each family member to do.

5.2.1.4 Slavery and racism in colonial and antebellum America

As I transition to the 1800s and the antebellum United States forward, my discussion would be incomplete without considering the legacy of slavery in the colonies and United States forward. As Ibram X. Kendi describes in his intellectual history of racism in the United States, discussion by White scholars, as well as politicians, physicians, and slaveowners, during this period was remarkable for its persistent mix of double-talk and self-contradiction about race and Africans and later African Americans.[12] For example, empowered Whites embraced claims of Black inferiority when the discussion concerned racial equity, voting rights, and even counting Blacks for the Census, while claims of Black, and particularly *enslaved* Black, constitutional superiority were made when the necessity of slavery was questioned, when a defense of unreasonable, inhumane work demands was needed. The self-serving discourse of Whites, whether pro- or antislavery could be manifested in any region of the United States. Consider this excerpt from the 1842 *Boston Medical & Surgical Journal* where the Yankee Edward Jarvis discusses the dramatically low rate of insanity in the 1840 US Census, in Southern Blacks compared to Northern Blacks:[13]

> . . . Second, the very great disproportion of the insane among the colored population, at the north and at the south. In the free States there is one lunatic or idiot among every 162.4 of the colored inhabitants. While, in the slave States, there is only one in every 1558 of the colored people. This shows almost a ten-fold proportion of colored insane in the free, above that of the slave States. . . . . There is a vast difference between the condition of the colored men in the free States and that in the slave States. Slavery has a wonderful influence on the development of moral faculties and the intellectual powers; and refusing man many of the hopes and responsibilities which the free, self-thinking and self-acting enjoy and sustain, of course it saves him from some of the liabilities and dangers of active self-direction. If the mental powers and propensities are kept comparatively dormant, certainly they must suffer much less from mis-direction or over-action. So far as this goes, it proves the common notion, that in the highest state of civilization and mental activity there is the greatest danger of mental derangement; for here, where there is the greatest mental torpor, we find the least insanity.

Compare this with Samuel Cartwright's title of his now-familiar 'drapetomania' condition:

> Drapetomania, or the Disease Causing Negroes to Run Away: Dysaethesia Aethiopios, or Hebetude of the Mind and Obtuse Sensibility of Body—A Disease Peculiar to Negroes—Called by Overseers Rascality.[14]

The title alone summarizes the racist fervor in the Southern White community of the time.

Perhaps the tragic ironies of enslavement racism is encapsulated most vividly by Wendy Gonaver's *The Peculiar Institution and the Making of Modern Psychiatry, 1840–1880*.[15] Gonaver describes the journey of John M. Galt II, the White superintendent of the Eastern Lunatic Asylum, who was the first superintendent to accept both White and Black patients, as well as employed attendants of both races—including both free and enslaved Blacks as staff. While racial tensions between residents and staff were present, Gonaver describes a by-and-large harmonious institution providing moral treatment. Yet Galt was proslavery, ambivalent at best about abolitionism, yet was commonly decried by colleagues, ultimately contributing to his suicide at age 42 in 1862.

Summers[16] frames the historical arc of White psychiatry and treatment of slaves and freedmen in nineteenth-century America as part of a larger context of Anglo attitudes, assumptions, and fears of African primitivism, violence, and animism. These racist assumptions play out into the present day through the legacy of disproportionately diagnosing Blacks with poorer-prognostic conditions and criminalizing blackness through three-strikes laws and similar legislation, now documented through video-recordings of police shootings of unarmed Black citizens. These sorrowful motifs will reappear in later chapters.

5.2.2 The need to differentiate social responses to social deviance and the needy

By the time of the American Revolution, the colonies had expanded, and the coastal towns had expanded into cities, rural villages proliferated, and the frontier pushed westward. The local, neighborly quality of community management of the needy and deviant moved west with the frontier-seekers, as the values of cooperation and mutual protection were just as necessary in the new Northwest Territory (now Ohio, Indiana, and Illinois) as they were in early Massachusetts.

On the Atlantic coast, unprecedented immigration ensued from Western Europe, for those seeking religious freedom and the promise of cheap, even free, land. The resulting urbanization of early colonial towns was driven by the growth of populations from the hundreds to the thousands and tens of thousands by the mid-eighteenth century.[17] The 'poor' of the mid-eighteenth century consisted of the aforementioned motley crew of the needy and the different: the handicapped, the widowed, the orphaned, the mentally ill, the criminal, and increasingly, the immigrant. As urbanization developed, the initial 'institutional' response was to imitate England and develop almshouses, or poorhouses. These should be distinguished from the English model of the workhouse, which was based upon the idea of paying for one's keep through daily, usually hard, labor. The British workhouse was an institution both for relief of the poor needy, as well as a site for serving one's criminal sentence, making the workhouse a sordid, dangerous, and arduous place, especially for widows and orphaned children.[18]

In contrast, the American colonial almshouses were at least aimed toward more consistently charitable intentions and tried to aid the poor. David Rothman notes that the Boston almshouse of 1735, one of the first of its kind in the colonies, was one of the costliest items on the Boston city budget.[19] In more rural areas, churches provided assistance to the poor, often among the costliest of church endeavors yet fueled by the then-powerful charitable values of groups like the Quakers. Most of all, families, neighbors, and relatives were encouraged and expected to care for their own, and even provide relief assistance for nonrelatives.

However, midcentury laws about regulation of the poor initially had more to do with protecting communities from outsiders than rendering aid to the poor. With urbanization of the cities, and the growing complexity of a differentiating economy, the colonists' suspicious gaze upon strangers waned as migration from community to community became the norm by the end of the century. Around the same time the English example of the workhouse was implemented in colonial cities as a way to punish vagabonds, idlers, and petty criminals, while providing cheap labor for community work that residents avoided or rejected. Often the boundaries between the role, activities, and admission requirements of almshouses and workhouses were blurred.

At this stage in the eighteenth century, we can now recognize two kinds of institutions intended to regulate two loosely defined (and evidently overlapping) groups of the socially marginal: the poor, consisting of widows, orphans, the mentally ill, drunkards, and the handicapped, and the rogue-vagabond, the transient opportunists who manifested in the form of drifters, traveling salespersons, carnies, fortune tellers, wagon peddlers, con artists, actors, stage magicians, and quack doctors. Needless to say the distinctions between those qualified for the almshouse versus the workhouse were not always clear, and, as an example, Rothman describes a Middlesex County, New Jersey law that provided for some residents of poorhouses to labor in the workhouse. The placement of the socially marginal individual was an issue from the very beginning of the institution-building for the needy and deviant.[20]

Grob[21] lists several factors which provoked the differentiation of the almshouse/workhouse/community care into what we recognize today as four social care institutions: the mental health system, the penal/criminal justice system, the juvenile welfare and justice system, and systems for education and care of people with intellectual/developmental impairments. While Grob's main focus is the development of the asylum (nee the mental health care system), the social forces he describes, as we'll see, will be verified by other historians addressing the other three systems.[22]

What were these factors? The aforementioned urbanization of the cities was one. Grob notes that the colonial arrangement of labor into farmers and artisans/craftspersons transitioned into a mercantile model where home and workplace were separate, with barter and sales income replaced by wage arrangements. The role of the family as nurturer, teacher, and work-center dissolved into differentiated social roles (e.g., work, parenting, and education) generating the need for additional public services like schools. The family was no longer the self-sufficient entity it once was. A second factor was related to population growth. Greater immigration and a more crowded community meant more visibility and provocation by the mad. They were no longer familiar neighbors, but weird strangers. Such change in attitudes led to a diminished 'social cohesion'[23] that enfeebled the old-style community welfare approach of the colonial era. Urban crowding also led to public-health issues like cholera outbreaks and problems with sewage, waste disposal, and adequate housing, generating a lower socioeconomic class who lived in the poorly serviced areas and were more subject to illness and disability. These conditions introduced the now-familiar trope of poverty predisposing to more poverty.

While the colonists viewed the poor as an existential inevitability and the responsibility of neighbors, the emerging mercantile, industrial, and capitalistic social structure generated a new kind of poverty, one that was impersonal and arising from social factors and the blameworthiness of 'individuals'. These economic changes were paralleled by the spread of Enlightenment values, where reason and science created, as Grob puts it, a 'secular faith'[24] that social problems were explainable, manipulable, and correctable by the human sciences, engineering, and social policy endeavors. These factors, considered together, set the stage for the differentiation of institutions for the needy and socially deviant, as well as the differentiation of public attitudes toward the needy and deviant. In the ensuing sections, the development of each of these four institutions will be considered, with some effort to indicate their relationships to each other as well.

5.3 The asylums and mental health services

As sketched earlier in Chapter 5, Section 4.2, 'Morality and Madness', the pre-Enlightenment understandings of madness or mental illness tended to be dominated by what Wallace describes as 'magicoreligious frameworks'.[25] Western culture in the pre-Enlightenment centuries was populated by supernatural beings—demons, gods, monsters, hybrid beings, magi, and mythic creatures like three-headed dogs—wielding powerful, often definitive, supernatural capabilities. Madness could be divine or mystical in origin or represent supernatural evil or demonic forces. While secular or naturalistic formulations of madness did exist prior to the Enlightenment (as in the prior discussion of Hippocrates, Avicenna, and Galen among others), the flux in accounting for madness in the pre-Enlightenment era featured much more prevalent magicoreligious accounts, especially for ordinary people, than after the Enlightenment transformation in Euro-American culture. Indeed, it was the formulation of madness as a naturalistic phenomenon explained by the new sciences that contributed to the development of asylums (to be discussed in more detail below). The social, psychological, religious, and philosophical changes of the Enlightenment betray a particular *Zeitgeist* that set the stage for a progressive naturalizing of insanity. For this reason, each of these sections will primarily focus on changes in the late eighteenth- and nineteenth- and ultimately twentieth centuries.

As suggested earlier, by the end of the 1700s the major cities of the new United States had begun to develop more formal community responses to the issue of the poor, the sick, and the mad. The establishment of the influential almshouses in Boston and New York collected together the poor along with the mad, orphans, and petty criminals, and the other new states followed suit.[26] Lunatics who were disruptive enough to warrant isolation from others were secluded; placed in a metaphorical attic *a la* Mrs. Rochester in Charlotte Brontë's *Jane Eyre*. Not surprisingly, with continued growth and immigration, these institutions quickly became unmanageable.

General hospitals, unlike in Western Europe, had not yet made significant appearances in the United States.

5.3.1 Development of the asylums in the American colonies

The first hospital focused on the care of the (physically) sick as well as the mentally ill in the colonies, the Pennsylvania Hospital in 1751, arose out of Quaker political disenfranchisement in Philadelphia, with their subsequent compensatory commitment to charity care.[27] The insane patients were initially secluded from other patients in the damp basements of the building, and for a while, like in Bethlem, public curiosity about the lunatics was so strong, a fee was charged for viewing the patients. The differential benefit of care for the insane in the Pennsylvania Hospital, compared to the almshouses, was arguable at best.[28]

During the experiment with mentally ill patients in Philadelphia, other states were expressing the need for separate facilities to house and treat the mentally ill. In the earliest years of the nineteenth century, private individuals and religious groups founded the first private asylums for the mentally ill at McLean Asylum near Boston in 1818, the Friends Asylum in 1817, and the Hartford Retreat in 1824. By 1821 the New York Hospital had modified its policies and facilities so that it had its own asylum facilities. These institutions, often founded by religious and community leaders, as well as physicians, were heavily influenced by the moral therapy of Pinel and the Tukes and initiated these hospital-community models alongside more conventional medical treatments. The goals of the private asylums were therapeutic, not custodial, so a spontaneous selection process emerged, where more acute patients with a better prognosis tended to be admitted. The institutions were self-consciously small in scale in order to preserve the personnel-dense moral therapy approach. While the initial humanitarian goals of these institutions included a substantial portion of low-paying or nonpaying patients, over time the ongoing maintenance and care expenses filtered away poor patients, and increasingly these asylums catered to the wealthy.

5.3.2 The development of state-supported asylums

The social historians Deutsch, Grob, and Rothman describe a number of features in the United States in the early 1800s that contributed to the development of state-supported institutions for the insane.[29] One of these is implied in the prior paragraph, where increasingly the private institutions were skimming off the paying patients, as well as the most acute and treatable patients (a motif that was to re-emerge in the late-twentieth century into the present, with the growth of for-profit psychiatric hospitals and later, cost-controls for healthcare). This left the more severely ill and chronically ill in need, and the expected overloading of existing almshouses and other community resources for the needy dependent. A second factor was immigration into the United States, leading to a swelling of the cities' populations, as well as psychosocially marginal lower-class immigrants and freedmen, who were stereotypically presumed to be more prone to psychopathology. A third factor was the increasing awareness of the treatment innovations from Western Europe and the infiltration of European humanistic ideas about treatment of the insane. A fourth factor would be what today we would call urbanization. Increasingly, economic opportunities in cities came to exceed those from rural agriculture; families and individuals lost their rootedness in smaller, intimate communities; the sense of obligation to fellow townspeople dissipated; and subsequently social deviance of any kind—crime, intellectual disability, orphans, poverty, handicap, and mental illness came to be viewed as burdensome social problems. Accompanying this reframing of social deviance as social problem was the arising of conscientious social reformers like Dorothea Dix (1802–1887), as well as wealthy bourgeois activists, exemplified by Samuel Gridley Howe, who became America's first social reformers, many of whom I have already mentioned. Of particular, if less tangible, importance was the development of a particular American sensibility regarding social welfare. This emerging welfarism rejected the punitive approaches of (particularly) England in dealing with social deviance, distrusted central authority, recognized the intrinsic value of the individual citizen, and embraced a diverse religious community who shared, more than anything, a mutual commitment to caring for the needy.

All these factors led to the development of not just asylums for the mentally ill, but jails and reformatories (i.e., prisons aimed at rehabilitating the criminal), and state schools for those with intellectual disabilities. As a concrete example of this nineteenth-century proliferation of social institutions of care, Grob notes that in 1820, only one state mental hospital existed, by the end of the Civil War every state had at least one,[30] all the more remarkable in considering the expense, devastation, and turmoil of the Civil War period.

5.3.3 The symbiotic growth of asylums and psychiatry

The development of US asylums and the development of the medical specialty of psychiatry were interdependent. The institution and the doctor legitimated each other's existence and social role. The 'asylum doctors' became 'medical superintendents' and 'alienists'(from Pinel's description of the patients' existential alienation) and ultimately 'psychiatrists.' The first American medical association was founded by Samuel B. Woodward, then-superintendent of the Worchester asylum, along with Francis Stribling, Thomas Kirkbride, and others, forming the Association of Medical Superintendents of American Institutions for the Insane on October 16, 1844.[31] Shortly thereafter Amariah Brigham and others founded the *American Journal of Insanity*. Later, the organization was to be renamed the American Psychiatric

Association and the journal renamed the *American Journal of Psychiatry*. The early days of American psychiatry were exclusively oriented toward asylum-based care and the diagnosis and treatment of more seriously ill patients requiring such care. Outpatient psychiatry was to come later.

5.3.4 Conceptual background of early American psychiatry

The conceptual assumptions, values, and commitments of the early asylum doctors provide clues to today's VMDRs. The strong religious culture of the young United States prompted most of the superintendents to be committed to a Thomistic metaphysics of soul and body. The early psychiatrists needed, for religious reasons, to view mental illness as reflecting a sick body/brain which was independent from an immaterial, immortal, eternal soul. Where the 'mind' fit into these beliefs became one of the foremost conceptual problems in early American psychiatry. Indeed, the relations of soul/mind/brain/body had ramifications which radiated into contemporary times. The very idea of psychiatry's focus on diseases of the mind challenged fundamentalist Christian commitments to an eternal, immutable soul. You might remember from Chapter 4 that only bodies can become diseased in this view. Etiological theories of psychiatric illness of this era viewed mental illness as based upon bodily disease, and provoked by moralistic environmental causes, such as urban crowding, various kinds of immoral conduct (e.g., prostitution, gambling, masturbation, intemperance, pederasty, nonprocreative sex, infidelity, sex outside of marriage) and the deficiency of virtue (e.g., pride, excessive ambition, lust, and jealousy) . Mental illness was caused by physical and moral (i.e., psychological and conduct-related) thoughts and behaviors. Classification of psychopathology became and remained challenging, and by the mid-nineteenth century congealed around the standbys of mania, melancholia, monomania, dementia, and idiocy.[32]

5.3.5 Early American psychiatric treatment

Treatment approaches were derivative upon these etiological and metaphysical assumptions. Home treatments were viewed as self-defeating, as the corrupting home environment was to blame; institutionalization was the alternative, where moral treatment principles and other compensatory treatments could be initiated in open air settings. The conceptual legacy of humoral theory persisted, somatic treatments were guided by Galenic principles (which by this time had been largely abandoned by contemporary Western Europeans), and perhaps iconically symbolized by Benjamin Rush's fondness for bloodletting as a treatment for most conditions. Grob[33] notes that outcomes of moral treatment of the time may have been better than we might expect, even better than results today in some cases. He cites a late-nineteenth-century study by a superintendent who followed up on a cohort of 1000 asylum patients, ascertaining the fate of the patients 10–12 years later, identifying data on 984 of them: 58% were relapse-free.

5.3.6 Population growth, cultural shifts, and institutional change

The population dynamics of the asylums in the early decades of institutional growth and proliferation were to shift in the later nineteenth century and turn of the twentieth. The population algebra, in retrospect, (and with our contemporary experience) is not complicated. One has a set of institutions with a limited number of beds. New patients are continually admitted. Existing patients either improve to be discharged, or do not, and stay in the hospital. Assuming the base admissions rate of chronic patients is relatively stable, only time is required before the proportions of chronic patients increase within the hospitals, ultimately to fill up the hospital completely. Chronic patients stay, acute patients leave. Soon no room remains for acute patients.[34] Moreover, with the innovations of the new biomedical science, chronic patients were living longer, and the numbers of demented elderly in the asylums began to rise as a distinct custodial population. These factors alone could precipitate an overcrowding crisis, and the superintendents' public boasting about their successes were to later haunt them as their recovery rates plummeted.[35] As just one indicative statistic, 'In 1904, 27.8 percent of the total patient population in the United States had been confined for less than twelve months. By 1910 this had fallen to 12.7 percent. . . .'[36] Nursing homes, and 'long-term care' by the way, had not yet been invented.

These hospital population dynamics, coupled with the slow abandonment of almshouses as undifferentiated welfare institutions, contributed to the shift of the asylums from therapeutic institutions to custodial ones, and quickly became not-very-humane custodial ones at that. With aged and aging mentally ill, medical comorbidities and injuries further complicated the asylum populations because patients had both serious mental illness as well as multiple physical illnesses and disabilities. What had begun as an American humanistic social experiment borne of idealism, increasingly became a nightmare of abuse and neglect, prompting public outrage and calls for reform.

In the meantime, late-nineteenth-century mainstream medicine was changing. Koch and Pasteur introduced the microbial theory of disease. Rudimentary statistics were now being applied to disease populations and epidemiology was developing as a science. Alfred Binet was researching intelligence in children and developing tests to measure it. Empirical psychology and biology were flourishing, and contemporary biomedicine was germinating. The alienists, who had been proud US medical leaders and innovators in the first three-quarters of the nineteenth century, were now being left behind by scientific advances in other fields of medicine. The American Medical Association, founded in 1847, was a feeble rival for several decades, but by the end of the century it had exceeded the Medical Superintendents' association in size and public esteem.[37]

As will be described later in their own sections, the young United States was developing a number of social welfare institutions that competed with the asylums for public funds and obviated the need for the old almshouses, which shrank continuously to the end of the century. Instead, the development of local jails to hold criminal offenders before trial, prisons for convicted criminal offenders to serve sentences, schools for idiocy, and orphanages proliferated. The neglected group in terms of the development of special welfare institutions were the sick aged, and they ended up increasingly in the asylums, as discussed above. Grob[38] notes a policy motif familiar today: as the states' obligations to care of the mentally ill grew over the period, local communities had strong financial incentives to define the senile elderly as a psychiatric problem, thus cost-shifting their care from local budgets to state ones.[39]

5.3.7 A first cycle of reform

The increasing overcrowding, the dissolution of the asylum's mission, the feeble therapeutics, and the competition for state and philanthropic funds led to increasingly deplorable conditions in the institutions, and a public outcry was inevitable. A storied example of this outcry is embodied by Elizabeth P. W. Packard, a late-nineteenth-century proto-feminist and crusader for patients' rights. Packard was committed to the Illinois State Hospital for the Insane in 1860 at the behest of her husband and the superintendent, remained there for 3 years, and upon release pursued legislative reforms to limit commitment proceedings, which, in her view, institutionalized the subordination of women to their husbands.[40] She provoked reforms requiring jury trials for commitment hearings, beginning in Illinois in 1867. She also promulgated legislation to permit patients free privileges in letter-writing, thus helping patients maintain contacts with family and community. Grob notes that the response from superintendents, including the newly influential 'forensic' doctors like Isaac Ray, was largely negative. The male superintendents viewed this as a challenge to their professional authority and autonomy; the rhetoric involving strong paternalistic themes about doctors knowing better than patients about what's good for them.

Psychiatrists found their practices under scrutiny by their rivals in neurology as well, some of whom argued for assimilating psychiatry into neurology. E. C. Séguin, the neurologist who was to be so influential in the care of idiocy, assailed the asylums as little more than prisons for the insane. The distinguished American neurologist S. Weir Mitchell, in an invited address on the occasion of the American Psychiatric Association's fiftieth anniversary in 1894, criticized the psychiatrists as medical separatists, insufficiently scientific, lacking accountability, lacking in effective therapies, and neglectful of the social and political ramifications of their work. Rather than being offended, the psychiatrists recognized the deep problems in their field, and in his response, Walter Channing acknowledged that Mitchell's points were commonly recognized by their colleagues.[41] Indeed, the superintendent's organization had changed its name already in 1892 to the American Medico-Psychological Association. By 1921 the consolidation of a new formal identity for psychiatrists was imbricated by changing the name of the organization again to the American Psychiatric Association.

American psychiatry's reconsideration of its patient-service identity, its conceptual assumptions, and its scientific basis provoked a number of parallel developments within the field in the first half of the twentieth century. With these changes came the differentiation of psychiatric theory, practice, and therapy that characterize the mental health field today. Just a few of these developments will be mentioned here. (a) One strand of psychiatrists pursued a 'dynamic' school of thought that conceived mental health not on a strict either/or disease model, but rather a continuum of psychological health and psychopathology. This group would be influenced by figures such as Adolph Meyer and Sigmund Freud; but not until the mid-twentieth century would the influx of post–WWII European Jewish psychoanalyst/psychiatrists develop psychodynamic psychiatry into the dominant 'orientation' to the field. (b) A school of 'neuropsychiatry' evolved, with an invigorated medical-scientific orientation. The new neuropsychiatrists were inspired by European colleagues who were developing new somatic treatments. For example, Julius Wagner-Jauregg's development of pyrotherapy (fever therapy) was based upon the observation that patients with neurosyphilis who suffered high fevers could be cured. Wagner-Jauregg's work was to earn psychiatry its first Nobel Prize, though his use of castration to attenuate masturbation-induced schizophrenia, as well as his Nazi sympathies, are seldom mentioned alongside his Nobel accomplishment.[42] (c) A renewed interest in early intervention, acute care psychiatry, and hospital-based research led to the development of 'psychopathic' hospitals, spearheaded by Adolf Meyer with the New York Institute (now the New York State Psychiatric Institute), Boston Psychopathic Hospital, and the Henry Phipps Clinic at Johns Hopkins. (d) Led initially by Clifford Beers, a patient, the Mental Hygiene movement was originally intended to reform the still-ailing asylums into more humane, effective institutions, but Beers' strategic alliances with influential psychiatrists of the time, like Adolph Meyer and Thomas Salmon, backfired, and led to the latter's appropriation of the movement and the affiliated National Committee on Mental Hygiene. The doctors' agenda was to expand the scope of psychiatry to primary prevention as a public mental health process, and the promotion of good mental health habits, as well as support the emerging psychopathic hospitals.[43] Notable in this reform effort was the meager impact these changes had on the overcrowding of the asylums; prevention and the creation of acute care hospitals simply left the asylums behind as second-class institutions, a stain that often persists today in so-called public sector psychiatry.

5.3.8 A second cycle of reform

The aforementioned psychiatric version of the mental hygiene movement sought to expand the domain of psychiatric influence through the prevention of mental illness, care of idiocy, the development of a eugenics program, the treatment of criminals, the prevention of crime, intemperance, prostitution, and care of children with birth defects and other congenital diseases. Psychiatry's domain was now expanded to its peak. These interests arose in the context of a larger early twentieth-century 'Progressive' movement within the United States. The Progressives, which we identify today with American presidents like Teddy Roosevelt, Woodrow Wilson, Franklin Roosevelt, and later, John F. Kennedy and Lyndon Baines Johnson, as well as influential philanthropists, were influenced by the new social sciences of sociology, economics, and anthropology, which were yielding new insights into the causes of social problems[44]. The Progressives believed that the initiation of social-based programs of prevention, early detection, and early intervention could diminish broad social problems like crime and poverty, as well as social deviance like mental illness, intellectual impairment, and juvenile delinquency. One example of the Progressive spirit was the development of the Child Guidance movement, which in turn spawned the subspecialty of child and adolescent psychiatry. One of the important legacies of the Progressive movement was reform of psychiatric hospitals, and the refinement of the penal/criminal justice system, which will be taken up in more detail in section 4.5 below.

The successes of World War II psychiatrists in treating 'shell-shock', as well as the US military's recruitment of huge numbers of military psychiatrists was influenced by the ideas of local (in this sense, behind the battle lines), not secluded, treatment of mental illness, as well as drug-augmented psychodynamic interviewing—'narcoanalysis'—using new sedative compounds like sodium amobarbital. Psychiatry's relative successes in this regard are memorialized on film in John Huston's *Let There Be Light* (1946) documentary, demonstrating these techniques for conditions like 'shell-shock', a precursor to today's Acute Stress Disorder.[45] The return of these doctors to civilian medicine, along with the influx of the aforementioned psychoanalysts into the United States in the postwar period, increasingly dominated the American medical schools' departments of psychiatry, and doubled the membership in the American Psychiatric Association (APA) from 1940 to 1945. The psychodynamic psychiatrists were entirely comfortable with Progressive views about the socio-environmental etiology of mental disorders, and the two trends significantly influenced the mid-twentieth-century psychiatric *Zeitgeist*. These trends toward psychological, and limited medical interventions and outpatient treatment further differentiated psychiatry and moved the psychiatric mainstream away from the state hospital, asylum psychiatry, and psychiatric superintendents.

The founding of the Group for the Advancement of Psychiatry in 1946 was an important landmark in the expansion of psychiatry's purview. At the time of the Group for the Advancement of Psychiatry's (GAP) founding, the APA's activities were limited to their annual meeting and publication of the *American Journal of*

Psychiatry.[46] A group of so-called young Turk postwar psychiatrists led by William Menninger were concerned about the poor state of 'civilian psychiatry' in the United States, and intended to improve clinical service but also proffer psychiatrists as public intellectuals who could contribute to social, cultural, and political debate and, therefore, contribute to the general social welfare, expanding psychiatrists' role beyond the research, diagnosis and treatment of mental illnesses. This broad social agenda for psychiatry was to address such generic social problems as crime, poverty, war, and unemployment,[47] expanding the moral charge of the field . GAP's influence provoked controversy within the APA about the proper role of psychiatry and the organization's functions. Ultimately the GAP and like-minded psychiatrists prevailed in expanding the professional scope of APA activity—and, therefore, psychiatry's—through the development of the 'Mental Hospital Institutes',[48] which grew into the 'Hospital and Community Psychiatry' meetings and still later, the autumn 'Psychiatric Services' meeting still ongoing under APA today. APA became involved in assessing institutional care, developed outreach to smaller communities of psychiatrists, and began an ongoing series of official statements and Task Force reports about mental health policy issues which are ongoing at this writing.[49] In effect, the asylum doctors were reinvented as 'public sector' psychiatrists and were welcomed back to the APA. The APA developed the first DSM-I in 1952, based upon an early War Department—supported effort led by then-Brigadier General William C. Menninger. The document was primarily for administrative purposes at the time and had yet to be developed into a scientific classification of mental disorders.

A new, more politically active psychiatry began to lobby for legislation to support the expanded mission. Lawrence Kolb, Robert H. Felix, and others, both lay and professional, lobbied Congress to establish federal resources to support the emerging social model of mental disorder. After some stumbles, The National Mental Health Act of 1946 was passed, which founded the National Institute of Mental Health and promoted research into the prevention, understanding, and treatment of mental illnesses. In the ensuing decades, the differentiation and side-developments of federal institutional structure appeared, yielding the complex array of specialized institutes, intramural and extramural research programs, and subspecialized foci of interest that make up today's broader National Institutes of Health.

As this section enters into the second half of the twentieth century, much of the history here will be familiar, or at least less novel, to many of my readers. Moreover, by mid-twentieth century, the United States had spread from coast to coast and beyond, and each of the 50 states had developed their own approaches to mental health public policy and law. Mental health and psychiatry were more complicated than ever.

5.3.9 A third cycle of reform

Howard H. Goldman and Joseph P. Morrissey[50] have described significant changes in mental health service provision in terms of 'cycles of reform', a rubric I have borrowed for the last three subsection headers—an apt way of conceiving the history as well as casting the 'big picture' of late-twentieth-century psychiatry. The changes associated with reform of mental health care, as well as changes less significant under a 'reform' lens, will be addressed in this section on mid-to-late-twentieth-century psychiatry.

Several significant changes characterized this period, which set the stage for our twenty-first-century, contemporary psychiatric scene. (1) Deinstitutionalization and community mental health, (2) the rise of psychopharmacology and a 'mental health industrial complex', (3) the shifts in NIMH research funding, and (4) the development of new payment systems for mental health care.

5.3.9.1 Deinstitutionalization and community mental health

As can be recognized from the preceding overview, the problem of funding mental health care has been recurrent throughout the history of psychiatry. By the later stages of the Progressive era, the problems of overcrowding and ballooning costs stimulated still more innovation about how to deliver good care for less money. The Social Security Act of 1935 founded financial support for care of the elderly; enabling the differentiation of the old almshouses and asylums into boarding homes, nursing homes, and related services—'long-term care'.[51] Discussions about how to address mental health care costs were ongoing, and at the time the majority of mental health care was still delivered in the state hospital setting. The state hospitals started to differentiate their services, offering crisis care, partial hospitalization, and outpatient care in efforts to reduce costs.

However, pressures from within and outside psychiatry were powerful in shaping a national movement to 'deinstitutionalize' the mentally ill,[52] raising questions about the moral mission of mental health care. Among the participants in these changes were the previously discussed postwar psychiatrist-leaders with a social and psychodynamic orientation, who offered therapeutic optimism about the idea of treating even severely ill patients in the community. As a second factor in deinstitutionalization, beginning in the 1950s and crystallizing in the 1960s, criticisms of the inhumanity and abuses of institutional care arose within the academic as well as public sphere. In the 1960s these concerns contributed to a so-called anti-psychiatry movement,[53] which was not just critical of the asylum but (allegedly) of the entire psychiatric project, represented by Thomas Szasz, R. D. Laing, Thomas Scheff, Michel Foucault, Theodore Sarbin, and others, although few of these thinkers accepted the 'anti-psychiatry' label.[54] New concerns about the legacy of institutional treatment, encapsulated by Erving Goffman's *Asylums: Essays on the Social Situation of Mental Patients and Other Inmates* (1961), and celebrated in popular culture through such books and feature films as *One Flew Over the Cuckoo's Nest*, raised concerns that the institutionalization of patients compounded their disabilities rather than alleviated them. Ethical concerns about the fate of patients were prominent themes throughout the anti-psychiatry movement.

The passing of bills establishing Medicare and Medicaid in 1965 accomplished two objectives that contributed to reducing the state hospital populations: one,

Medicare and Medicaid provided for movement of the demented or incapacitated elderly out of the state hospitals and into the then-new 'nursing homes', and later, 'skilled nursing facilities'—long-term, chronic care institutions. Now the states had fiscal motivations to offload this population from their state hospitals and into private institutions funded by federal dollars.[55] Medicaid and Social Security Disability Insurance (SSDI) also provided possibilities for indigent, nongeriatric adults to pay for outpatient care.[56] The proliferation of private health insurance provided increased access of employed patients to care; providing a cottage industry for private, for-profit psychiatric hospitals to proliferate in the late-twentieth century, as well as nonprofit general hospitals to fund a full range of psychiatric services. Still later, private insurance funding for 'long-term care' emerged to privatize and, thereby, expand, nursing home care.

Finally, the development of a new and promising psychopharmacology raised the possibility that even the most severely ill patients could be treated and maintained in the community, closer to home, work, and family (see discussion below). As the remaining threads of the Progressive movement faded away, the Kennedy administration passed the Community Mental Health Centers Act in 1963.[57] The resulting growth (over 700 were created since the mid-1960s[58]) developed big budgets for 'public sector' outpatient psychiatry with the idea that over time, the states would take over, maintain, even expand, the services. The orientation of many of the community mental health centers was prevention and dealing with acute illness, and, once again, the needs of the chronic mentally ill were often neglected. While treatment was available to patients discharged from hospitals, little in the way of vocational/work support and housing opportunities accompanied the appearance of the outpatient clinics. Moreover, the response of the states to sustaining high-quality outpatient care and support services was inconsistent at best, resulting in the wide disparities of state spending on public sector mental health care in recent decades on up to the present.[59] These feeble commitments to the chronic mentally ill led to the growth of homeless mentally ill people as an urban problem.

The new population of 'individuals experiencing homelessness' were often reinstitutionalized as chronic mentally ill patients, but for briefer treatments and briefer stays, leading to the 'revolving door' phenomenon, where patients were admitted, treated, and discharged, only to relapse again in the community to be readmitted again, perpetuating a cycle. Moreover, and perhaps most tragically, the chronically ill ended up 'reinstitutionalized' in prisons and jails in the United States, perhaps never in greater proportions since Pinel's day. The midcentury social psychiatrists and preventionists had failed; the public distrust of social approaches to mental illness grew along with the political climate of free-market economics, fiscal conservatism, and views of 'social programs' as examples of governmental waste and excess.[60]

5.3.9.2   The rise of psychopharmacology

By the mid-twentieth century, in an era free of formal regulation of human subjects in (clinical) research,[61] physicians in the Western world, inspired by the 'magic bullets' of antibiotic treatment for bacterial infections and the growth of the chemical industry, had increasingly experimented with various compounds for treating all kinds of human disease. Psychiatrists were no exception and sought new drug treatments. The development of the first psychoactive therapeutic compounds was accomplished by varying mixtures of serendipity, increased research funding, and what was, in retrospect, an open (unregulated) research environment, along with a substantial investment by the then-new pharmaceutical industry.

While Healy[62] provides careful documentation that 'psychopharmacology' as a practice had been with the alienists and psychiatrists for a long time (the use of bromides, amphetamines, botanical anticholinergics, and even lithium salts, the latter going back to the 1880s, are a few examples he provides), the development of the first 'antipsychotic', chlorpromazine (Thorazine), and the so-called antidepressant and antianxiety drugs ushered in the era of psychopharmacology. The midcentury experimentation with new compounds was performed by physicians doing self-experimentation as well as experimentation on inpatients, as well as pharmaceutical company experiments on animals. The stories of the discovery of major categories of psychoactive agents during this era make for compelling reading, but space does not permit a retelling here, though a few examples can be very briefly mentioned.

The rediscovery of lithium use in psychiatry by John Cade in 1945 was based upon anticonvulsant experiments on animals. The discovery of chlorpromazine grew out of petrochemical dye production and the discovery of the hormone histamine and pharmaceutical experimentation with antihistaminic analogues. The clinical experiments in Germany that led to the discovery of imipramine as an antidepressant were accomplished by administering the drug to inpatients of all diagnostic varieties, in what today would be decried as an indiscriminate, 'fishing expedition' approach to clinical research. (Research ethics and informed consent were yet to be commonly discussed and practiced.) However, these small, local approaches to psychiatric drug research from the midcentury came to be replaced over the remainder of the twentieth century by 'big science' and a colossal economic agenda—an agenda which increasingly crowded out the primacy of patient care in favor of a business-commodity model for US health care as well as research.

5.3.10 An American medical-industrial complex

The development and refinement of clinical trials, the burgeoning of the pharmaceutical industry in developing new drug treatments, and the development of research infrastructures in the universities and later 'academic medical centers' in the latter half of the twentieth century contributed to the development of what Joel Kovel[63] called the 'American Mental Health Industry'. Later, the first woman director of the National Institutes of Health, Bernardine Healy, articulated a 'medical-industrial complex' (MIC) in the United States.[64] The medical-industrial complex, a term borrowed from President Dwight D. Eisenhower's concern about a military-industrial complex taking over public policy through economic domination, exhibited several features that mattered then and even more into the present day.[65]

The MIC was and is made up of a mutually interdependent and commanding network of economic factors. In no particular order, the elements are (a) a wealthy, competitive, and expanding private, for-profit product industry, (in our case, the pharmaceutical and later the medical device industry); (b) a captive, needy market for the products offered (in our case, untold masses of sick people); (c) a for-profit service industry whose relationship with the product industry is mutually beneficial (in our case, health care insurance and the later managed care organizations); (d) a political structure which permits powerful influence by special interests and well-financed lobbying in shaping federal and state budgets as well as law and policy (e.g., US politics with its unregulated campaign spending and open lobbying policies); and (e) well-financed propaganda mechanisms to sway public opinion and frame issues in favor of the industry (e.g., American advertising and mass media).[66] These economic forces converge and mutually benefit to dominate social policy in advancing their common fiscal interests.

The MIC was to transform US health care, including mental health care, by redefining the terms of engagement for the medical encounter. Rather than a private, patient-to-physician encounter, the MIC redefined health care in terms of a commercial business transaction between customer, provider, and a network of related, for-profit services. Health care became a commodity to be bought and sold by large corporate entities; subject to market forces. Even institutions marginal to the complex proper, (e.g., nonprofits and public sector psychiatry) had to participate, and increasingly so over the remainder of the century. (As an example, the transition from state-supported care in public sector psychiatry to the states' contracting with managed care organizations to provide care at the end of the twentieth century served to ensnare state-supported public sector psychiatry into the MIC by the turn of the twenty-first century).

The ramifications were profound. The private pharmaceutical industry came to dominate clinical trials of new therapeutic agents, while National Institutes of Health (NIH) and NIMH were to do the more exploratory (and unprofitable) basic and 'translational' science to complement the pharmaceutical industry's R&D.[67] The Bayh-Dole Act of 1980 gave, for the first time, the right of academic centers to profit-share in intellectual property developed on their campus, formalizing the subsidy of pharmaceutical companies with taxpayer and university funds by enabling university-industry formal partnerships. Psychosocial and preventive research was progressively marginalized as the quest for magic bullets and miracle cures expanded, and academic medical centers jumped into unprecedented profit-seeking.[68]

The immersion of academia into profit-making did not stop with Bayh-Dole. Academic medical centers were already increasingly providing patients for clinical trials, and their faculty came to be dependent upon pharmaceutical industry research funding to support faculty salaries and institutional growth. The practitioner-researcher of the mid-twentieth century became the researcher-entrepreneur by late century.[69] The public, through widespread media marketing and advertising, came to expect and demand 'magic bullets' from industry, cures requiring little to no patient effort beyond the taking of pills.

This passive therapeutic approach came to dominate healthcare social practice, contrasting with the active engagement models of moral therapy in the prior century, and prevention and mental hygiene from midcentury, and the emerging, and contrarian, 'recovery' model at the end of the twentieth century.[70] The orientation on prevention, social care, and psychological treatments from the postwar psychiatrists in the 1950s came to be replaced by a psychiatric identity increasingly dominated by the prescribing of pills and waiting for them to work. Psychiatric diagnosis that was reliable and reproducible became important; psychiatry needed specific disease entities to evaluate, test, and market new medications.[71] Psychiatric treatment plans increasingly depended upon, and came to be dominated by, medications. Psychosocial treatments were no longer affordable because they were too labor-intensive, even when the scientific evidence for efficacy was sound. The research-design difficulties in testing the efficacy of psychosocial treatments (compared to controlled clinical trials of medications), along with the lack of industry capital and political lobbying, caused them to fall behind in the mounting 'evidence base' of medical treatment in the late-twentieth century. The new 'evidence-based medicine'[72] in psychiatry became a movement that defaulted to selling the pharmaceutical solution. The public and Congressional demand for magic bullets reshaped the funding priorities of NIMH; from a social-intervention strategy in the early 1950s to a basic neuroscience, developmental neuroscience, and genetics agenda by the turn of the twenty-first century.[73]

Not surprisingly, a minority-voice backlash literature appeared, lamenting the unrealistic confidence in medicine by American patients, the latter too-often believing that lifestyle changes were unnecessary, and that medical technology would rescue them from any ills resulting from poor habits or needs for lifestyle changes.[74] The progressive erosion of patient engagement and personal responsibility in caring for oneself was a corollary.[75] By the turn of the twenty-first century, a backlash alleging the convenience-medicating of children for dubious psychiatric illnesses had crystallized.[76] Psychiatry increasingly became viewed as social control made for profit.

These changes within psychiatry and outside the field are important to the background of the VMDR because of a single interesting observation. Throughout the billions of dollars of investment, and several decades of research in biological treatments in psychiatry, the treatment advances within the core of vice-laden DSM categories have yet to appear, and as a group, constitute a set of disorders situated among the worst treatment outcomes in the field.[77] Antisocial and other personality disorders in the various iterations of the DSMs, and psychopathy remain treatment riddles altogether[78] and typically acknowledged as hopeless or prohibitively expensive; effective somatic treatments for paraphilias remain feeble in terms of effect size or specificity of treatment.[79] Effective treatments for Conduct Disorder and other disruptive behavior disorders remain a deep challenge.[80] The reasons behind these mysteries will be taken up in later chapters of this book.

5.4 Penal and criminal justice systems

From the briefest tour of the development of psychiatry and mental health in the past two centuries, this section takes up a sketch of the development of the penal and criminal justice systems. Considering the penal/criminal justice system and its history is essential to understanding the VMDR, as this system is the 'interface' with the forms of social deviance that have variously fit, and not fit, into the mental health system. My discussion will take up two subsections. The first considers the distinctive iconic history of American prisons and penology from the turn of the nineteenth century to present. A second subsection will consider the development of legal handling of mentally ill offenders, and the development and impact of forensic psychiatry. Following this, two other social welfare systems must be considered to understand the scope and fuzzy boundaries of the vice/mental disorder relationship (VMDR). The history of the development of care for the intellectually and developmentally impaired, and the need for and development of a juvenile justice system for child and adolescent criminal offenders will have their own sections following this one.

5.4.1 American prisons and the new penology

> *It is to the defects of our social organization, to the multiplied and multiplying temptations to crime that we chiefly owe the increase of evil doers.*
> —Dorothea Dix, *Remarks on Prisons and Prison Discipline in the United States* (1845)[81]

Earlier I discussed the American colonists' attitudes and handling of social deviance, with some mention of criminal deviance. This section directs our full attention to the development of prisons and criminal justice in the colonies and early United States.

To briefly review, David Rothman[82] noted that the 1700s colonists' original attitudes toward crime tended to the fatalistic: Crime, because of its derivative link to sin, was a fact of human life and an immutable part of human nature; the elimination of crime was not a consideration any more than the elimination of sin would be. As a consequence of this social mind set, the colonists' response to criminal conduct was pragmatic, limited, and focused on discouraging criminal misconduct—the latter being referred to as 'deterrence' today. However, reforming or rehabilitating the criminal offender, in the sense of remolding the offender into a 'law-abiding citizen' was not considered, and likely not even conceived, given the metaphysical assumptions about humanity's fate as sinners. Jails, when there were any, mainly served to hold alleged offenders for trial, and prisons as yet had not appeared. The convicted offender might find himself in the stocks or in a public cage for varying periods of time; subject to shame and humiliation by the populace, which was thought to be an effective deterrent. Recognized community members of means would more likely be fined. The use of the lash, as well as banishment from the community, were additional options. The possibility of the criminal reoffending in another community seemed abstract and literally remote from local concern. For persistent offenders of property crimes, as well as more serious violent crimes, hangings from the gallows were also used, but infrequently. Preying upon Western frontier families by outlaws was a continual challenge and has borne many legends. Escaped slaves were often recaptured and brutally disciplined.

As the colonies developed into a new republic, the spirit of freedom, participatory democracy, and human rights that had informed the American Revolution, alongside the growing problem of crime in US cities, prompted the leaders of the new United States to rethink their approach to crime and criminals. The new Americans were very much Enlightenment thinkers when it came to crime theory, they were influenced by Cesare Beccaria's reforms regarding punishment and saw the latter as often propagating, not dissolving, crime. Many having been recipients of the harsh punishments meted out in Britain and in America under British rule, the colonists and early Americans were dedicated to not doing justice the British way and made fair-minded criminal justice among the top priorities in the new states. Religious tolerance was a cherished value, one not easily given up in a return to British-style persecution of religious minorities. Punishment by death came to be identified as a British social vice; by the turn of nineteenth century most all the states had revoked the death sentence.[83]

If not death for serious crimes, then what? Incarceration in a prison seemed a humane alternative, in keeping with Beccarian (as well as the less-appreciated Benthamian) principles: having offenders serve time in prison was humane, immediate in punishment, and proportionate to the severity of the crime through assigning longer and shorter sentences. As the opening quotation from Dorothea Dix implies that the worldview on crime was also changing; crime was due to repressive monarchical social systems like Britain's, combined with inadequate social support structures as illustrated in the novels of Charles Dickens and callous, greedy characters like Ebenezer Scrooge. Moreover, social thinking was becoming less bound by religion and more elaborated by secular reason. Prisons and social theory could change, even reform, criminal conduct.

Following the development of state prisons around the turn of the nineteenth century, not much time was needed for the wardens and prisoners to realize that more was needed than simple incarceration, if the ideal of reforming criminals was to prevail. Rothman[84] notes that over the 1820–1850 period, the Americans began to develop a more contemporary view of crime and criminals: they were a threat to society. The transition of the perception of crime as a benign inevitability, to crime as a threat to social structure and individual citizens, emerged as industrialization, bourgeois trades, and mercantilism increasingly became the economic backbone of the new society. Crime in these economic settings was a threat to an emerging middle class rather than to the poor or wealthy. A decline in morality and moral education was attributed to these social changes. The family was declining in influence as fathers increasingly spent time away from home, working 'jobs' in support of their families. Increased mobility of families looking for better opportunities eroded the Church's power as well as the moral stability of Church and community membership. Childrearing shifted from being completely delivered in the home, to teachers in their increasingly important role in the new schools.

By the mid-nineteenth century, these social changes had stimulated an interest in childrearing as a discipline into itself. The teaching of morality had moved from the chapel and the dinner table into the classroom. Education reformers like John Dewey believed that education was the ground for social change. The new confidence in education was applied to the prison, where educational engineering could reform, or rehabilitate, offenders, turning them into productive citizens.

These elements—the aversion to capital punishment, and proliferation of bricks and mortar to segregate and house offenders, and the belief in rehabilitation education; all contributed to a midcentury prison reform movement, itself hotly debated within the field between rival theories. One model, (the 'Auburn' model) had prisoners isolated from each other in individual cells, coming together only to eat and work, and even then, with little to no conversation permitted. The rehabilitation was to occur through the routine of discipline, obedience, and work. The rival plan, exemplified by the 'Pennsylvania system'[85] was essentially the same except the prisoners did everything in solitary confinement: work, eat, and rest. As an economist might predict, the Auburn plan prevailed because it was cheaper and more productive in terms of work and economic output.

In practice over these decades, the distinction between punishment and discipline became blurred. With no conversation permitted, strict uniforms required, work limited only by daylight and sustenance, and the use of the lash and other physical methods for 'discipline', the commitment to humane rehabilitation was too often a facile motto rather than a consistent practice. Nevertheless, the American prisons were quite innovative for their era; visitors from around the world came to visit them and see how they worked.

What was the appeal of the prison to the new Americans? Many reasons contributed to the rise of the prison, and its persistence today. One, with the diminished power of the family and the Church, society needed an alternative force in maintaining order. Second, the American juries had been conviction-averse in the colonial days because the standard punishments for offenses under British law were seen as cruel and excessive. The prison allowed a more humane alternative and permitted juries to feel better about making convictions. Prisons, then as now, provided jobs in communities. Finally, as already mentioned, the new Americans wanted to be protected from criminal offenders as the old colonial mechanisms for law and order increasingly failed. What is distinctive and somewhat foreign to our contemporary sensibility here is that the colonists and new Americans developed policy from a fresher perspective, familiar as they were with hardship and desperation that could breed crime. They had a kinder, gentler disposition to offenders than we typically have today.

Part of the penology of the era involved forced silence for convicts, arduous work hours, and obedience to rules. In contemporary views, these seem feeble, even counterproductive rehabilitative efforts, but at the time these rules were believed to inculcate the habits of social participation in the convict, and perhaps model Christian modesty and personal restraint. That said, and as one might imagine, such demands of discipline required consequences for failure to adhere to the program—and inevitably, as prison populations increased and discipline became harder to enforce, the use of harsh punishments proliferated, undermining the original humane intentions of the prison model. The rehabilitation ideal faded, and prisons became more custodial and more punitive in practice.

While Europeans showed great curiosity over the American experiment in penology, increasingly they criticized the American approach.[86] Alexis de Tocqueville, the admirer of American democracy and the French author of *Democracy in America* (1835–1840) believed that the prison undermined the very American freedom the United States had worked so hard to secure. Charles Dickens, the British novelist and describer of nineteenth-century British poverty amidst social change, believed American prisons led the convict to '... pass into society again, morally unhealthy and diseased.'[87]

The ideals of the American prison from the first half of the nineteenth century, however compromised they may have been from the beginning, were rapidly lost in the post–Civil War era. After decades of state prison admissions and discharges, the motif of overcrowding became dominant. In parallel with developments in the asylums, a sorting algebra served to both overpopulate the prisons as well as shift their inmate demographics progressively toward more severe and violent offenders. Just as the asylums progressively filled their institutions with chronic patients, so did the prisons fill their cells progressively with more violent or hardened offenders with longer sentences. The acute patients and the reformed, less severe criminals left; the chronic and severe remained while new inmates continued to be admitted. Today's American legacy of the longest prison terms and highest incarceration rates in the Western world[88] began in the late-nineteenth century. Moreover, the continuing influx of new immigrants compounded the overcrowding. The values of law, order, and convenience for prison employees supplanted the humane ideals of the early founders. Individual cell design became dominated not by reform ideals, but how to pack more inmates in the smallest space for the least amount of money.[89] Rotman notes that while prisons were deteriorating as humane institutions in the post–Civil War period, the jails had fallen into even worse shape—even dirtier, more crowded, and more custodial than ever.[90] The failure to sort prisoners into types left juvenile offenders and women mixed in with violent adult male offenders, to horrific effect. These circumstances were to contribute to the founding of child welfare and juvenile justice reforms that will be discussed shortly.

The public outcry was inevitable. In 1867, the prison reformers Enoch Wines and Theodore Dwight, published the substantial *Report on the Prisons and Reformatories of the United States and Canada*, commissioned by the New York Prison Association.[91] The report detailed a litany of deficiencies from inadequate facilities to indiscriminate physical punishment to a complete abandonment of any detectable reform effort. They proposed a number of reforms, including reemphasizing the effort to rehabilitate the criminal using the newly described program of earned privileges, leading the cooperative convict into increasingly greater levels of freedom, as they earned their way to freedom. The National Congress of Penitentiary and Reformatory Discipline of 1870 described this procedure as '. . . through his own exertions to continually better his own condition, a regulated self-interest should be brought into play'.[92] A second substantive reform was the introduction of 'indeterminate sentencing', which removed the fixed determination of length of sentence from the convicting judge and jury, and placed it into an independent sentencing body which would consider the offender's response to positive incentives in advancing toward a release date. Indeterminate sentencing was a substantial contributor to the institutionalizing of psychiatry and clinical psychology into the correctional system, as their expertise in assessment of behavioral reform earned the new doctors special seats on the new parole boards. Around the same time, the American Prison Association (now the American Correctional Association) was founded in 1870, as a self-regulatory arm of the penal system.[93]

Other experiments in prison reform followed. Reformatories like Elmira tried adding formal curricula and trained educators into the program mix; literally training convicts for success in the outside world. How effective such reforms were to be, however, were never demonstrated in the face of inexorable new admissions and overcrowding.[94] Even these institutions devolved into the common denominator of repressive discipline and the dissipation of reform programming. Nevertheless, these education-minded reforms left behind a legacy of positives such as prison libraries, some educational efforts, and prison chaplains, all of which persist into the present.

Some states, like those in the Deep South, distinguished themselves through slave-like work conditions and harsh discipline for the predominantly Negro inmates; later memorialized in hundreds of blues songs about chain gangs, ball-and-chain shackles, prison life, and even particular institutions, like Parchmann Farm, also known as the Mississippi State Penitentiary:

> We go to work in the mo'nin
> Just a-dawn of day
> We go to work in the mo'nin
> Just a-dawn of day
> Just at the settin' of the sun
> That's when da work is done, yeah

—Booker T. Washington 'Bukka' White, Parchman [sic]
Farm Blues, Roots RTS 33055, 1940

A rise in federal offenders needing incarceration, as well as increasing reluctance of state penitentiaries to house federal convicts led Congress to pass the Three Prisons Act in 1891 to establish a Federal prison system, with the first established in Leavenworth, Kentucky in 1897. The establishment of the federal prison system led to the promulgation of several innovations of relevance to the VMDR. Some of these were humane reforms and addressed the prevention of prison corruption, including criteria for selection of wardens, limitations on guard duty, and the like. After some failed attempts by individual states to develop an effective classification system for prisoners, the federal system inaugurated a more successful system by segregating prisoners by categories of low-risk, serious offenders, inmates that could benefit from agricultural education, and physically/mentally ill inmates. The growth of Federal prisons was likely assisted by the increase of federal offenses after passing of the eighteenth Amendment to the US Constitution, establishing 'Prohibition' of the production, transportation, and sale of alcohol in 1919. Having 'raised the bar' for prison conditions around the United States, substandard conditions (e.g., crowding, abuse, lack of sanitation and adequate food) become once again intolerable, though this time for the inmates, leading to a series of high-profile rioting within several prisons in the 1950s, involving multiple states: New Jersey, Michigan, Ohio, Illinois, California, Oregon, New Mexico, Massachusetts, Washington, and Minnesota.[95] The American Prison Association identified the usual institutional and community offenses leading to poor prison care in a report of 1953: inadequate funding, programming and staffing deficiencies, overcrowding, personnel not meeting their professional standards—this list was now too familiar.

Postwar psychiatrists and psychologists, riding the crest of their wave of success in the WWII era, and eager to take on the psychologization of crime and criminality, made inroads toward a renewed rehabilitative focus for postwar prisons—no doubt gathering a boost from the prison riots that were becoming frequent headlines in the 1950s. Psychoanalytically oriented psychiatrists of the postwar era approached crime as a result of trauma or developmental arrest, while the new social and behavioral psychologists contributed new psychological profiling with tests as well as reward/punishment management contingencies from the new behaviorist psychology. The prisoner was recast from social reprobate to a psychologically or emotionally disturbed patient; from 'bad' to 'mad'; from morally deficient to psychologically handicapped. Rehabilitative approaches to the convict were tailored, like Meyerian therapy outside the prison, to unique individuals with detailed case files, multidisciplinary assessments (e.g., psychiatry, psychology, social work, and vocational counseling). Erving Goffman's influential sociological work on the toxic effects of institutionalization led to experiments in less restrictive and autonomy-promoting institutions like the California Chino State prison.[96] Inmates, among other innovations, were given increased input in decision-making and prison policy. These innovations and therapeutic orientation resonated with a formal prisoner's rights movement which took hold nationally midcentury. A prisoner's use of the *writ of habeas corpus* challenged the legitimacy of warden authority, and some of the worst abuses in prisons of the time were successfully litigated as cruel and unusual punishment in 1910. The *writ of habeas corpus* guarantees citizens a right to a court hearing addressing the legitimacy of that citizen's confinement.

By the 1960s the times were one of general liberal reform, with the appointment of Earl Warren as the Chief Justice of the Supreme Court; the passing of the US Civil Rights Act of 1964, prohibiting discrimination for racial, gender, color, religion, and national origin. The Black Muslims achieved a significant victory for prisoners' rights in securing freedom of religion for prisoners in the early 1960s. These trends among others furthered the restoration of civil liberties to prisoners as more comparable to that of citizens.[97]

By the latter half of the twentieth century, while some progress had been made in terms of prisoner's rights, and legal oversight of prison services, the problem of overcrowding and the associated custodial/punitive orientation persisted and continued into the present day. Morris[98] notes that from 1970 to 1980 the prison population in the United States doubled and doubled again from 1981 to 1995. Today the United States has the highest incarceration rate in the world, representing 5% of the world's population though with 25% of the world's prisoners,[99] and in 2009, one out of 31 Americans are in prison, in jail, on probation or parole.[100] Over the comparable period, Federal Bureau of Investigation statistics showed that violent crime fell by 25% in the past 20 years.[101] In comparison, in 2002, other Western countries average between 50 and 100 residents per 100,000 people in prison on an average day, while 700 Americans are in prison on an average day.[102]

The reasons are complex for this disproportion of American prisoners. One of them is the proliferation of nonviolent offenders in US prisons. For example, in Texas in 2008, 5500 prisoners were driving-while-intoxicated offenders.[103] The dynamics of contemporary prison economics provide another clue. The sentencing judge determines who pays for the offender's sentence: if sentenced as a federal or state felon, the Feds or the state pay for the imprisonment, offenders convicted of misdemeanors go to (local) jail or pay fines; offenders who are diverted into treatment programs are paid locally or by the state, depending upon the program. Local politics and economics then favor sending the offender out of town to serve his sentence and may well drive tougher sentences. Another reason is that US sentencing is longer; life sentences, including those without the possibility of parole, are common. In Europe, murderers with life sentences are commonly offered parole or pardons; and are typically released after 8 to 12 years.[104] In many European countries, the longest sentences that can be served do not exceed 14 years. A tragic irony of these facts is the per capita violent crime rate in these countries is lower than the United States rate.[105]

The distinguished American criminologist Michael Tonry[106] provides a detailed analysis of the reasons for our current expansive prisoner situation, the details of which cannot be presented here. Tonry debunks the hypothesis that we have more prisoners because we have more crime. Indeed, he presents data that indicate the irrelevance of crime rates to incarceration rates. Late twentieth-century public opinion about being 'tough on crime' is also complex and can be misleading. Research indicates that public opinion is swayed by political posturing about crime and that public opinion is driven by politician and media coverage rather than the reverse.[107] A third factor is the proliferation of 'wedge issues' used in political campaigning beginning in the 1970s. Wedge issues—issues that are intended to drive a 'wedge' between voters—were not limited to issues around crime, but since the 1970s being 'tough on crime' is a survival requirement for any self-respecting politician, and any policy that releases offenders, or diverts them from prison, is assumed to be inherently flawed and 'political suicide'. Use of the wedge issue provides for poor policy, as Tonry puts it:[108]

> A broadly defined sexual psychopathy law, three-strikes law, or mandatory minimum sentence law may be ineffective or cruel or unduly costly, but none of that may matter. If the law's proponents, and voters, view it as an expression of revulsion with crime and outrage toward criminals, whether it will work or achieve just results in individual cases is often politically irrelevant.

The historian of penology Norval Morris calls this state of affairs the 'Humpty-Dumpty' principle—if all the kings horses and all the king's men couldn't put Humpty together again, then it makes no sense to add more horses and men (punishments) in order to suppress crime.[109] If imprisonment is ineffective in diminishing the crime rate, as the evidence shows, then imprisoning more and more offenders isn't the solution. Tonry's analysis features much more relevant to this book; his work will be employed later in the book in understanding the VMDR.

In the face of this proliferation of prisoners, the penal system has accordingly differentiated itself across the 50 states in providing a wide variety of mechanisms intended to both improve penal outcomes as well as reduce prison demand. These need not be presented in detail here, but include (1) increased use of parole and probation procedures; (2) a differentiation of prison services and settings from minimal security institutions for low-risk nonviolent offenders (e.g., 'white collar criminals') to maximum security settings for dangerous repeat offenders, to hospitals for the 'criminally insane'; (3) developing alternatives to incarceration proper, such as 'house arrest' where the convict is confined to home, to use of tracking technologies such as ankle bracelets to track or limit a convicts' movements; (4) a variety of education and vocational rehabilitation programs to enhance the convict's chances of not reoffending; and (5) use of 'intermediate punishments',[110] such as providing community service or even participating in drug or alcohol treatment.

From this very brief overview of American penal policy and practice, we turn to history of care of the intellectually impaired, as well as the nineteenth-century criminalization of this group.

5.5 Criminalization of and care for the intellectually impaired

The wealth of English words for 'intellectually disabled people' betrays the history of its stigma: 'simpleton', 'idiot', 'imbecile', 'fool', 'moron', 'cretin', 'half-wit', 'retard', and 'degenerate'—to name a few. These terms in use today are not tolerated in polite, educated, and moral company. However, their medical origins in the eighteenth and nineteenth centuries were descriptive terms for referring to those of limited intellectual ability, and with time and common usage they have deepened whatever negative connotation accompanied their original coinage. In ordinary use today they more often are hurled as insults to mistake-making others instead of used to describe a group of people with limited learning ability.

Perhaps the premier social historian of mental retardation, James Trent,[111] uses the somewhat tamer, and historically apropos term 'feebleminded' in describing what today refers to as mental retardation or intellectual/developmental disability. As with our other examples of the Colonial and early American socially marginal (i.e., orphans, criminals, lunatics, and widows) the feebleminded also found varying degrees of tolerance and sustenance in their local communities, churches, and families. What today would qualify as the most severely impaired, including those with severe chromosomal and genetic disorders, were not a social burden as they didn't survive long in an era that neither had conceived of behavioral management and education, nor much to offer in the way of corrective medical care. Those of moderate to mild intellectual impairment were cared for as best as possible by the family and community.

5.5.1 From local care to specific care

With the building of almshouses, the feebleminded who could not be managed or cared for locally were sent to these early institutions. The early orphanages rejected the feebleminded.[112] Trent notes that in the immediate postrevolutionary period the mad and criminal may have been feared, but the feebleminded were by and large, not feared, but rather the butt of jokes and humor. For the kinder Christian townspeople, the feebleminded were a symbol of charity. For the reasons described earlier, in the post-Jacksonian, post–Civil War era, social changes of urbanization, crowding, and bourgeois business and professions, tended to reframe the socially marginal into two general categories: 'worthy dependents', including widows, orphans, and disabled people, and 'unworthy dependents', including criminals and the unemployed vagrants, drifters, and prostitutes.[113] The place of the feebleminded (and the mad) in this dichotomy was an ambiguity then, one that has both persisted and metamorphosed over the two centuries into the present.

The so-called Jacksonian era (Andrew Jackson was President from 1829 to 1837) was a period of great social change—growth of the US territories, the expansion of immigration, and the aforementioned growth of cities and the transition from an agrarian to a capital economy. Following Jackson's presidential term into the Civil War era (1861–1865) economic downturns heightened the need for a social response to dependents either unworthy or worthy, and these changes provided the social background for the emergence of humanitarian reform of care for many dependents, including the feebleminded.

Samuel Gridley Howe (1801–1876), a Boston physician and prominent abolitionist, deserves some specific mention in this regard, as an individual but also through his family, which included his wife Julia Ward (Howe), famous as a women's suffrage advocate and the lyricist of the Union's Civil War anthem 'Battle Hymn of the Republic'. In addition to his key role as founder of the first state institution for 'idiocy', Howe established schools for the blind and established relief for Polish political refugees along with author James Fenimore Cooper and code smith Samuel F. B. Morse.

Howe is credited for founding the Massachusetts Asylum for the Blind in 1847, and at the same time, another physician, Hervey Wilbur (1820–1883), was admitting his first idiot pupil into his home in Barre, Massachusetts. Both men were influenced by the pioneering work of Edouard Séguin, a French pioneer of educating the feebleminded. Both Howe and Wilbur were to import Séguin's methods into the United States, and ultimately, import Séguin himself to lead efforts in establishing schools to educate the feebleminded. Remarkably, many of Séguin's methods are still practiced today.[114]

5.5.2 Educating and classifying the feebleminded

A student of Esquirol,[115] Séguin called his method 'physiological education'. His theory of idiocy was built upon the disconnection of the will, or motivational processes, from the senses:[116]

> Idiocy is a disorder of the nervous system in which the organs and faculties of the child are separated from the normal control of the will leaving him controlled by his instincts and separated from the moral world. The typical idiot is one who knows nothing, thinks nothing, wills nothing, and can do nothing, and every idiot approaches more or less this *summum* of incapacity.

Séguin's methods were intended to reconnect the will to the senses, and in this regard his methods were influenced by moral therapy and involved individually tailored physical activity—exercises in the gym and exercises in stimulating the five senses, beginning with touch. In a theory reminiscent of John Locke's associationist psychology, the idiot, for Séguin, would begin to link these experiences to 'notions'—the names for things, experiences, and feelings, and the reflective linking of notions together was the birth of ideas, which the training would cultivate. Other methods for cultivating notions and ideas included mimicry, music, comparisons, drawing, and ultimately, writing and reading. Séguin had his own interpretation of moral treatment, defining it in terms of a benign authority—the teacher- directing the student toward the goal of socialization. However, pity played no role in Séguin's theory—to pity the idiot was to transform him into an animal.[117] Séguin, however, along with his students Howe and Wilbur, was not naive nor grandiose; his overall goal was, as Trent puts it, a 'respectable mediocrity'.[118]

Classification of idiocy became increasingly important to establishing a prediction for improvement, or prognosis, and the history of idiocy involves a substantive flux and argument about the terms of classification. The era identified several potentially confounding conditions, which classification was intended to tease apart: one example was abused children. Howe recognized the distinction between the idiot and the child frozen in fear of adults. A second confounding population was the adult with intellectual impairment—conditions common to the asylums, like tertiary syphilis and what was to be identified as dementia praecox by Kraepelin later, were difficult to discern from congenital idiocy, especially without family informants. Amariah Brigham, head of the Utica Lunatic Asylum describes the distinguishing of idiots from the insane:[119]

> Strictly speaking, idiocy is not like insanity, a disease, or the result of disease, but the consequence of the malformation of the brain, and exists from birth or from very early life. This distinction, however, is not generally made, as those who, from long continued insanity, have become demented and exhibit but little mind are considered, though incorrectly, to have become idiots.

Howe, in disagreement with his colleague Hervey Wilbur, thought the term 'idiocy' was too hopeless a term, in connoting a state, and preferred 'feebleminded' as a term implying a weakness capable of being corrected. Howe classified the feebleminded in terms of degree of capability, with 'simpleton' identifying those of highest ability, 'fool' intermediate, and 'idiots' proper, the lowest level of capability. By 1910, the American Association for the Study of the Feeble-Minded classified idiocy into three classes, making the reference point for intellect that of a normal child:[120]

A. Idiots: Those so deeply defective that their mental development does not exceed that of a normal child of about 2 years.
B. Imbeciles: Those whose mental development is higher than that of an idiot but does not exceed that of a normal child of about 7 years.
C. Morons: Those whose mental development is above that of an imbecile but does not exceed that of a child of about 12 years.

The classification of idiocy not only considered the severity of intellectual deficit but also introduced special subtypes of idiots that were directed to particular clinical and social concerns, as will be discussed shortly.

5.5.3 Reforming services for the feebleminded

By the second half of the nineteenth century, social reformers like Dorothea Dix became increasingly distressed over the inappropriate and degrading conditions and placement of idiots in almshouses, alongside all other—adult—paupers. The reformers showed little interest in medicalizing idiocy, even though the leaders of the movement for schools and idiot education, individuals like Howe, Wilbur, and Séguin, were physicians. Rather, the reformers emphasized the humanitarian need of the population as well as the social benefits in educating this group.[121] The social advocates for idiocy reform overstated their case—as Albert Deutsch put it, they participated in the 'cult of curability'.[122] Like the asylum superintendents before, the advocates for education of idiots overstated the schools ability to educate idiots, in an effort to overcome the widespread fatalism about care of idiocy. Nevertheless, this overstatement and excessive optimism set the stage, once again, for crashing disappointment. The advocates, however, were largely successful in spreading the growth of schools for idiocy, likely facilitated by the parallel development of public education and the general expansion of state-supported services for the socially needy.[123]

5.5.4 Turf wars over the feebleminded

The development of state schools for the intellectually impaired in the second half of the nineteenth century was accompanied by sometimes bitter disputes over jurisdiction (who was 'in charge' of the population) as well as institutional philosophy. If anything, Hervey Wilbur, in the last years of his life, and as a founding father of the idiocy education movement, polarized the rivalries between the asylum superintendents and the school superintendents. Highly critical of the increasingly custodial asylums, Wilbur was vehement in his rejection of the philosophy of custodialism, and advocated for education, training, and ultimately discharge of the insane into the community. The new psychiatrists, in response, thought Wilbur was a respectable but ultimately misinformed critic, inappropriately applying the model of the state school to the asylum. History was to demonstrate that both groups were right; the expense and limitations of education and treatment were too often condemn both sets of services to a custodial minimum.

From midcentury through the turn of the twentieth century, a 'turf war' characterized much of the discourse about idiocy care—the educational and custodial advocates battled for supremacy in the field. Many asylum psychiatrists wished to assimilate idiots into their disciplinary domain, to justify state support for custodialism, while many members of the newly formed (1876) Association of Medical Officers of American Institutions for Idiotic and Feeble-Minded Persons (AMOAIIFMP) were critical of custodialism and wished to pursue an educational, not medical model.[124]

However, these turf battles were both internal to each organization, as well as external. Within the AMOAIIFMP Hervey Wilbur, as an 'educationist', argued bitterly with Isaac Kerlin, a 'custodialist'.[125] The differences in approach were profound for the students/patients/inmates of these institutions. Educationists valued individuality and active engagement with their pupils; custodialists instead valued passivity and conformity to rules and regulations. The growth of the institutionalized feebleminded (from a few hundred in 1875 to 10,000 at the turn of the century),[126] coupled with the increasing demands and waiting lists, effected the predominance of the custodial model. A strong public argument for custodial care of the feebleminded was provided by eugenics and degeneration theory, which promised control of the alleged proliferation of depraved, licentious, and criminal idiots and imbeciles. Rafter notes that the superintendents of the mentally retarded needed an intellectual basis to prop up their competing claims as professionals (compared to the more-established asylum doctors), and eugenics and degeneracy theory were the solution to this crisis in professional development.

5.5.5 From needy innocents to social threats

By the Civil War era and afterwards, these social factors congealed to effect a transition in public and professional perception of the feebleminded from needy innocents to social burdens and threats. Two of the crucial influences were Benedict Morel's degeneracy theory (to be discussed in detail below) and the complementary 'atavism' theory of the Italian 'criminal anthropologist' Cesare Lombroso. In the case of degeneracy theory, the core idea was that immoral practices—prostitution, crime, gluttony, sexual or alcoholic profligacy—degraded the 'germ plasm' (the hereditary vector in this pre-DNA era). The degraded individual with tainted germ plasm could pass on a Lamarckian potential for additional degradation in succeeding generations. Such processes then contributed to de-evolution and 'degeneracy' of the family line. Lombroso built his theory of constitutional criminality around this idea of atavism (lapsing into more devolved forms in succeeding generations) and believed that criminals could be sorted into atavistic types based on the analysis of (primarily) facial morphology.[127]

The often-open display of sexuality on the part of students in the schools for idiocy were long an embarrassment to the superintendents, and as the state schools proliferated, public awareness increased. The sexuality of idiots increasingly posed not just an embarrassment but led to concerns about proliferation of needy idiots and moral depravity among them. Related concerns revolved around the increasingly observed pattern of multiple childbearing in idiot women. This along with degeneracy theory fed the fears of highly influential philanthropists in the United States like Josephine Shaw Lowell, whose Newark Custodial Asylum for Feeble-Minded Women (founded 1878) became the first eugenic institution in the United States.[128] Public fear of degenerates was expanded by widely read exposés of degenerate families such as Richard Dugdale's *'The Jukes': A Study in Crime, Pauperism, Disease, and Heredity* (1877), which described wanton generations of inbred criminals, prostitutes, and drunkards, establishing a callous stereotype of the poor for generations to come. These public images came to blend the image of poverty, feeblemindedness, and criminality, linking them together in the public mind. 'Custodials' were developed as specialized institutions for idiocy which essentially imprisoned feebleminded women for the purposes of isolating them from copulation and childbearing. Rafter as well as Noll and Trent[129] suggest that the *Zeitgeist* of the day, involving progress in women's independence and social power, was accompanied by the counterpoint of 'purity crusades' (see below) to control women's sexuality, into which the concerns about feebleminded women so clearly played a role.

These concerns about the moral conduct of the feebleminded found their way into the classification of the population, and the notion of the 'moral imbecile' gained traction, particularly with the asylum superintendents and the burgeoning psychiatrists. The discussion of the moral imbecile paralleled that of the notion of 'moral insanity,' the latter to be discussed below. The founding father of American forensic psychiatry, Isaac Ray, in his influential (1838) *A Treatise on the Medical Jurisprudence of Insanity*, when describing moral imbecility, compares and contrasts moral lunacy (insanity) with moral imbecility. Ray admits to the difficulty in distinguishing between 'extreme moral depravity and insanity,'[130] but clearly establishes the morally insane in the sphere of contemporary moral misconduct—vice—in the following example of patient ES:[131]

> He appears, however, so totally callous with regard to every moral principle and feeling— so thoroughly unconscious of ever having done any thing wrong—and has proved himself utterly incorrigible throughout life, that it is almost certain that any jury before whom he might be brought would satisfy their doubts by returning him insane, which in such a case, is the most humane line to pursue. He as dismissed several times from the asylum, and sent there the last time for attempting to poison his father; and it seems fit he should be kept there for life as a *moral lunatic*; but there has never been the least symptom of diseased action of the brain, which is the general concomitant of what is usually understood as *insanity*.

Ray was but one example of physician theorists in the mid- to late-nineteenth century concerned with the links between vice, idiocy, and insanity. (A more detailed discussion of moral insanity follows in its own subsection below.)

Of special significance for this section on the care of the feebleminded, is the gathering interest on the concept of 'moral imbecility' among members of the AMOAIIFMP in the last quarter of the nineteenth century. Rafter[132] lists a series of papers from the AMOAIIFMP exploring the idea of the intellectually, as well as a morally, impaired criminal, or would-be criminal. By this time, at least in the United States, the notion of 'moral' in this usage had differentiated from the era of Tukian moral therapy—at that time 'moral' meant an amalgam of humanistic and psychological propensities—to the latter nineteenth-century sense, articulated much earlier by Benjamin Rush in his 'An Inquiry into the Influences of Physical Causes upon the Moral Faculty', a paper delivered to the American Philosophical Society in 1786.[133]

> By the moral faculty I mean a capacity in the human mind of distinguishing and choosing good and evil, or, in other words, virtue and vice.... The moral faculty is to the conscience, what taste is to the judgment, and sensation to perception. It is quick in its operations, and like the sensitive plant, acts without reflection, while conscience follows with deliberate steps, and measures all her actions by the unerring square of right and wrong.

Moral imbeciles, framed in contemporary language, were moderately intellectually disabled individuals who had additional, and specific, defects in their moral faculty, allegedly leading them to criminality, prostitution, and poverty. Some theorists, like Ray, tended to believe that all idiots/imbeciles exhibited deficits in the moral faculty, while others, notably Rush, tended to encounter intellectual deficit and moral deficits as often interrelated, but also encountered cases where the moral deficits were independent phenomena. In any case, by centuries' close, the trope of the dangerous idiot/imbecile had provoked a first wave of eugenics programs and permitted Lombroso's idea of the 'born criminal' to gain traction in US institutions.[134] The horrors of eugenic intervention in intellectually disabled persons, including involuntary sterilization, are not a crucial part of the story for the purposes of this book, though are thoroughly and compellingly documented by Rafter, Noll and Trent, and Trent.[135]

Through the turn to the twentieth century, other trends emerged involving the curious combination of care, custody, and persecution of the mentally retarded. The advent of the Binet-Simon intelligence test in 1908 was intended by Alfred Binet to be used in identifying children who needed extra assistance in school. Nevertheless, the Binet-Simon and the later Stanford-Binet Intelligence Scales were popularized in the United States by psychologist Henry Goddard, who introduced IQ testing to his colleagues in their renamed professional organization American Association for the Study of the Feeble-Minded (AASFM).[136] IQ testing provided a formal basis for classifying the intellectually impaired, and as noted early, by 1910 had influenced the AASFM's classification, adding a new category of 'moron' which represented a more subtle determination of children who appeared normal, but were substandard in intellectual capacity. IQ testing in the feebleminded arena also provided for professional legitimation for psychologists, who at the time were asserting themselves increasingly into the institutional care of the mentally retarded. IQ testing was a core component in classifying mental retardation up through DSM-IV-TR.

Walter Fernald, another influential leader in the emerging field, believed that testing would also facilitate the early diagnosis of children with 'criminal propensities'[137] and through providing the proper environment such propensities might be prevented. Goddard contributed to the degeneracy literature himself, with his own 'Jukes'-style book, *The Kallikak Family: A Study in the Heredity of Feeble-Mindedness*

(1812), which traced the decline of the fictitiously named Kallikak family over multiple generations and '143 feebleminded protégées, along with dozens of epileptics, alcoholics, prostitutes, and common criminals'[138] not to overlook the bastardy and redolent poverty. Goddard's prognosis was poor for improving the Kallikak families and their like, and he remarked upon their propensity to reproduce: 'There are Kallikak families all about us. They are multiplying at twice the rate of the general population, and not until we recognize this fact, and work on this basis, will we begin to solve social problems.'[139]

Over the first decade of the twentieth century, both private and public institutions for the feebleminded proliferated. Trent notes that by 1924 there were 58 public institutions for the feebleminded, and private institutions had proliferated even faster, with 80 nationwide at that time. Deutsch notes that by 1923, the population of 'mental defectives' in institutions had grown to 43,000.[140] Institutions took advantage of poor farmers selling land, and the institutions put the able feebleminded to work to help defray costs of care. The increasing reliance of American families on institutions led to spiraling growth, as well as costs for care, and superintendents responded by instituting sterilization as a longer-term strategy for limiting new admissions. Isaac Kerlin among others advocated use of sterilization to maintain order, to remove the sexual interests which were 'an offense to the community'.[141] By 1910, sterilization by vasectomy and tubal ligation were widespread practices, with Indiana passing the first sterilization law in 1907.

However, some brutal cases of castration of men in institutions contributed to the rising backlash against sterilization practices at large, albeit US eugenics for the feebleminded had always been controversial. Over the decade from 1910–1920 the resistance to eugenics gathered momentum. Contributing to these changes included superintendent ambivalence and frank opposition to the procedure, as well as legislative and public criticism leading to the repeal of many of the state sterilization laws. Some superintendents simply refused to recognize the laws, even when maintained.[142]

Nevertheless, the triad of factors driving sterilization practices—population control, eugenic intent, and sexual behavior control—continued. Oliver Wendell Holmes, in a 1927 US Supreme Court opinion supporting the constitutionality of sterilization, provided no abatement of the practice. Indeed, the use of sterilization provided only limited help in controlling institutional overpopulation. Contemporaneously, the superintendents considered use of parole, or temporary release to address the problem.

By the mid-1930s in Europe, Hitler's new Nazis were influenced by American, as well as German eugenic theory, and began their own eugenic programs in 1934, targeting mental defectives, individuals with schizophrenia and other severe mental disorders, and Jews and other religious minorities, intending to build a 'master race'. The same year (1934) Leon F. Whitney, then the Executive Secretary of the American Eugenics Society, introduced voluntary sterilization, partly in response to the negative public linkage of sterilization with German National Socialism.

Viewpoints on eugenic and sterilization issues in the United States were always complex. Distinguished psychiatrists like Adolph Meyer, William Healy, and even Walter Fernald began to question the value of eugenic controls, challenging the relationship between vices and mental retardation. Fernald's studies found that paroled/discharged patients did relatively well in the community.[143] The developing community psychiatry, mental hygiene movement, and focus on outpatient psychiatry also contributed to the disillusionment with eugenic practices.

Amid these midcentury controversies, a promising model of feebleminded care arose. Charles Bernstein's 'farm colony' model proliferated and gained positive attention because of his successes in implementing a parole and discharge program with good outcomes for less disabled inmates. To state legislators and advocates Bernstein could show both the ability to diminish or recover care costs while preparing inmates for independent and assisted living in the community. Sterilizations became reserved for those prognosticated to be dischargeable from the institution. Momentum toward more tolerant attitudes toward the mentally deficient was aided by the appearance of writings and letters of discharged inmates, sharing their experiences on the inside the institution as well as the outside in the community. Despite these changes, through the war years and midcentury, voluntary and involuntary sterilizations among the mentally deficient were common.

The farm colony model, however, was to face worse times by midcentury, as the military draft for World War II decimated the staff for the institutions, and the Great Depression took its toll on the economy and jobs. Even otherwise salutary legislation, such as F. D. Roosevelt's 8-hour workday legislation posed serious problems to institutions, as shifts limited to 8 hours compounded their staff demands beyond feasibility. Discharge of even the most able of the inmates was not possible because there were no jobs to discharge the inmate to. The only place to turn was to put the inmates of greater ability (e.g., morons) to work as aides within the institution.[144]

As might be expected as hard times supervened, the institutions for mental deficiency decayed literally and figuratively. Letchworth Village in Haverstraw, NY, in mid-twentieth century enjoyed a reputation as one of the very best of institutions for mental deficiency. However, it transitioned from being as symbol of humanistic care to the symbol of what scandal journalist Geraldo Rivera called in 1972 'the last great disgrace'. Thus were the decades following WW II to be marked as an era of outrage over the care of the mentally deficient. In addition to deteriorated facilities, neglect of residents, abusive treatment, impoverishment of stimulation, the patients themselves were enlisted to maintain order, often by cruelty.

5.5.6 Public outrage and advocacy

A raft of public outrage and exposés in media and magazines erupted in the 1950s concerning the care of the mentally deficient. The popular novelist Pearl S. Buck took these problems as her mission, publishing a series of exposé articles in *Ladies Home*

Journal, Reader's Digest, and other popular publications of the time. Through these articles, Buck revealed her 'twenty-five-year-old secret',[145] that her daughter Carol was mentally deficient and had been a student at the Vineland Training School. In researching the opportunities for assistance for her mentally deficient child, Buck in effect developed the basis for her bestselling book, *The Child Who Never Grew* (1949), both contributing to the new literary genre of the mental health confessional and providing a jump-start for public awareness of the challenges posed to families with mentally deficient members.

Numerous other parents of mentally deficient children stepped forward and wrote their own accounts. One of the most important of these was Dale Evans (Rogers), spouse of Roy Rogers, who together were one of America's most popular 'cowboy celebrities' in television, movies, and publications. Evans's own confessional, based upon her and Roy's biological daughter with Down syndrome, *Angel Unaware* (1952), became a spectacular best-seller and likely was instrumental in sensitizing the public to the conditions of care for the mentally deficient.[146] Royalties from Evans's book became the first major infusion of support for the emerging National Association for Retarded Children, which was to become the premier US advocacy organization for mentally retarded people. These trends transformed a social problem seemingly limited to the lower classes to a social problem affecting all groups, including middle- and upper-class families. New scientific findings rejecting degenerationism and presenting new hereditarian understandings of mental deficiency were promulgated, and while not eliminating stigma from affected children and families, likely diminished it and permitted the transition from moving intellectual disability from a shameful secret into an open community of stakeholders and advocates.

Legislation favorable to mental retardation care accompanied related social reforms, from the growth of the Civil Rights movement, the founding (1946) and development of the National Institute of Mental Health, and the passage of the Mental Health Study Act (1955), which boosted funding by 700%.[147] Civil rights reforms of the Kennedy era likely contributed to the continued transformation of public perception and legislative action, and Kennedy directly contributed to reform through his appointment in 1961 of a presidential commission on mental retardation. JFK's sister, Eunice Kennedy Shriver, became a transformational leader in rights and care of the intellectually disabled.[148] By this time nonphysician membership in the American Association on Mental Deficiency had grown to 60%, marking a transition toward psychologists, social workers, and educators dominating the field. The positive trends in these areas provoked a reinvestment by the states in institutions for the retarded in the 1960s and 1970s. However, these too were to be short-lived as the growth of the institutions again strained state budgets.

Other changes in the care and regard of the intellectually disabled occurred in parallel with other social trends.[149] Samuel A. Kirk, an 'educationist', differentiated the concept of learning disability from mental retardation. Learning disabilities were focal deficits in learning particular topics, though his advocacy had the consequence of further stigmatizing mental retardation.[150] The advent of Medicare

and Medicaid funding in 1965 opened new opportunities for funding of intellectually disabled people, and different states developed different pathways to care
and education, from continued institutional care to placement in community settings, to nursing home placements and beyond. The states were eager to close costly
institutions and shift costs to the new federal dollars. Increasing support for assistance and education moved many children home, and development of special
education and related programs in public schools intended to move intellectually
disabled children closer to the mainstream of education. Charismatic psychologists like Wolf Wolfensberger and Gunnar Dybwad assumed leadership roles and
advocated for 'normalization', under the philosophy that effective and ethical care
required acceptance of the intellectually disabled into the community, and the community had a responsibility to adapt itself to the differences of the intellectually
disabled. (Interestingly, this movement was reminiscent of the previously discussed
American colonial approach to social welfare.) These leaders provided a moral rationale for deinstitutionalization. However, as Trent[151] argues, the actual reduction
in institutionalization was not as large as expected. What happened was many retarded persons were moved from large state institutions to smaller local ones, such
as nursing homes, local schools, and smaller for-profit and not-for-profit institutions. Then and now, such services and facilities are quite vulnerable to economic
contingencies and suffered similar underfunding fates as the community mental
health movement.

5.5.7 More classification changes

Over the last 50 years of the twentieth century, research generated new knowledge
that differentiated the realm of intellectual deficiency considerably, though not always have institutions and services followed the distinctions of science. Recognition
of perinatal injuries like cerebral palsy generated the distinction between birth-
related cortical injury and mental retardation. Research expanded into 'developmental disorders' after Leo Kanner's description of 'early infantile autism' in 1943
and Hans Asperger's description of his syndrome in 1944. These discoveries served
to differentiate developmental differences in interpersonal engagement and social
relationships from intellectual disability. Other 'pervasive developmental disorders'
(as the DSM-IV-TR called them) were to follow, as well as specific learning disorders
such as dyslexia. The description of DNA structure and function, the development of
karyotyping and recognition of chromosomal abnormalities, along with the identification of genetically related inborn errors of metabolism, enabled the development
of preventive and therapeutic interventions. In terms of the genetic contributions,
these changes continue to raise questions about the role of genetics in contributing
to human flourishing, the question of whether, as cell biologist and philosopher of
science Fred Grinnell[152] puts it, whether genetics should 'make people better' or
'make better people'.

As modern medicine sharpened its etiological understanding of what used to be called idiocy, so had the scientific explanation of the classified populations of people now considered intellectually disabled.

In 1952, the American Psychiatric Association published its first edition of the DSM. At that time, the DSM-I distinguished 'mental deficiency' as either idiopathic (cause unknown) or hereditary, and included stages of severity by IQ score:[153]

325.0 Idiocy: IQ Under 20
325.1 Imbecility: IQ under 50
325.2 Moron: IQ between 50 and 69
325.3 Borderline Intelligence: IQ from 70 to 85
325.4 Mongolism (Down syndrome)
        Staged by IQ: Mild: (70–85), Moderate (50–69), Severe (under 50)

In 1961, the rival American Association on Mental Deficiency (AAMD) abandoned the idiocy/imbecility/moron language and classified mental deficiency at five Stanford-Binet IQ-defined levels of severity:[154]

Borderline: 83–67
Mild: 66–50
Moderate: 49–33
Severe: 32–16
Profound: 16

In 1968, DSM-II classified 'Mental Retardation' similarly, but not identically:[155]

Borderline: 68–83
Mild: 52–67
Moderate: 36–51
Severe: 20–35
Profound: under 20

The APA included subcategories by etiology as well (e.g., various infections, trauma, and metabolic/nutritional), suitable to its medical orientation. One must remark upon the insubstantial differences between the language and wonder about the confusion in application of competing cutpoints in various clinical, administrative, and educational settings. The quotations are exact in that AAMD presents their ranges from higher to lower, and APA the reverse. At least the two organizations could agree on the general levels of severity!

During these and later years, the AAMD had internal disagreements about whether the definition of mental deficiency should include a note about 'incurability'.[156] By the time of the 1973 revision, the optimists prevailed, and the new definition of mental retardation explicitly omitted a comment on prognosis, focusing only on behavior in the present. Accordingly, the new classification removed the 'Borderline' category, leaving:[157]

Mild: 67–52
Moderate: 51–36
Severe: 35–20
Profound: 19 and below

The AAMD's 1977 revision left this structure and scoring intact, with the manual's editor, Herbert Grossman, noting the difficulties with classification of mental retardation (MR). These concerns are familiar to DSM readers: MR represents multiple diseases, syndromes and causes; individuals scoring similarly, even with the same causes of the condition, function at different levels; and discriminating MR from other conditions, notably 'autism, emotional disturbance, and learning disability' is difficult.[158]

For APA's DSM-III (1980), a special note was made establishing that the DSM-III levels of severity were 'written in accordance with the terminology and classification of the American Association on Mental Deficiency'.[159] This time the ranges were once again tweaked:

Mild: 50–70
Moderate: 35–49
Severe: 20–24
Profound: below 20

In keeping with its 'atheoretical' orientation, DSM-III dropped DSM-II's specific subtyping on the basis of medical etiology, albeit readily acknowledging that medical causes were important. Indeed, the causes for MR were relocated to the new Axis III 'for physical disorders and conditions'.[160]

Mild: 50–70
Moderate: 35–49
Severe: 20–24
Profound: below 20

By the time DSM-IIIR arrived in 1987, the explicit acknowledgment of AAMD compatibility (now the American Association for Mental Retardation) was omitted. Still more tweaking of the IQ ranges occurred:[161]

Mild: 50–55 to approx. 70
Moderate: 35–40 to 50–55
Severe: 20–25 to 35–40
Profound: below 20 or 25

For DSM-IV,[162] the DSM-IIIR ranges were maintained, as they were in DSM-IV-TR.[163] One wonders about the social effect of these fluctuations in the definition of 'MR' in terms of people qualifying, or not qualifying, for services. The 2 decades of consistency within American psychiatry may have been a blessing for families seeking services, but the American Association on Mental Retardation (AAMR) was seeking a different path by the early 1990s.

In the last decade of the twentieth century, the AAMR made a 'paradigm shift' in its approach to 'classifying' MR or intellectual disability. The authors of the tenth edition of the *Mental Retardation: Definition, Classification, and Systems of Supports* briefly summarize the 'paradigm shift' of the ninth edition of the manual:[164]

> The ninth edition (Luckasson et al., 1992) of the manual retained some aspects of the 1983 definition and classification system (e.g., the IQ guidelines of approximately 70 to 75 or below), but departed from the previous definitions and classifications systems in four important ways: (a) it expressed the changing understanding that mental retardation is a state of functioning; (b) it reformulated what ought to be classified (intensities of supports) as well as how to describe the systems of supports that people with mental retardation require; (c) it represented a paradigm shift, from a view of mental retardation as an absolute trait expressed solely by an individual to an expression of the interaction between the person with limited intellectual functioning and the environment; and (d) it extended the concept of adaptive behavior another step, from a global description to specification of particular adaptive skills.

As the historian of disability Kim Nielsen notes, the shifts away from the medical model of disability (of any kind) were contemporary with these changes in thinking about intellectual disability, and currently, DSM-5 has largely followed suit with a subtyping of intellectual disability based upon descriptive conceptual/social/practical domains.[165] The AAMR had shifted away from an individual psychopathology/deficit model. Instead, they favored a social demand model focusing on the kinds of responses social care should offer to the differently abled. Disability was no longer simply a medical problem, but rather a civil rights issue embedded in institutional structures which provided barriers to functioning and discriminatory political structures to diverse individuals. While these authors describe this as a paradigm shift, readers of the history will recognize this disposition as a (perhaps) more realistic elaboration of 'normalization' described decades earlier by Wolfensberger and promulgated by Dybwad. Only the future will reveal the ongoing fate of disability reform.

5.6 Child welfare and juvenile justice

Popular culture has long recognized delinquency. Between Stephen Sondheim's comprehensive portrayal of New York delinquent gangs in *West Side Story* (c.f.,

'Officer Krupke') and the black-leather jacket sociology of Ur-punk rockers the Ramones (c.f., 'We're a Happy Family'), we have a concise iconography of not only public/professional attitudes toward juvenile offenders, but iconic statements of the VMDR for minors.[166]

From the foregoing discussion of the history of social responses to the socially marginal and deviant in nineteenth-century America, we turn to the interrelated themes of child welfare, the development of the juvenile justice system, and considerations of 'juvenile delinquency'. We have seen the tripartite motif of need-burden-threat in reference to public attitudes toward the intellectually impaired; early American attitudes toward 'dependent children' will be found to share some of these motifs. The case of orphaned and delinquent children, like the case for the intellectually disabled, is distinct in that children are more profoundly dependent both upon parents/family and the state, unlike the deviant adult madperson or criminal offender. Children also have unique vulnerabilities, as people who are smaller, weaker, less informed, economically dependent, and in the midst of development. As such, children are more subject to environmental and interpersonal adversities than adults. Finally, children have virtually no political power as individuals or as a social group, and, subsequently, they are too often caught in the political crossfire of the adult world, too often treated as means to political ends rather than treated as ends in themselves. The emergence of orphanages for children in need of effective parenting was discussed earlier; the transition from local, community, neighborly care in the eighteenth century to more formal, institutional care for needy children in the nineteenth century follows a similar history. The emergence of policy and social attitudes toward, as historian Michael Grossberg puts it, 'dependent and disorderly' children in the eighteenth century into the present is the main focus of this section.[167]

5.6.1 The birth of child welfare in the United States

When we consider the concept of 'child welfare' in the United States, the term addresses a range of child-focused policies and services which were, and are, intended to protect and nurture children. The emerging repertoire of child welfare was to include (1) the development of child welfare agencies that addressed problems like abuse, neglect, and poverty; (2) the juvenile court and justice system to both protect youthful offenders from adult offenders, as well as provide 'diversion' from incarceration and punishment into programs promoting prosocial behavior; and (3) the development of child and adolescent psychiatry, psychology, and social work, which were to contribute both the scientific study of the problems of youth dependency and delinquency as well as provide the prevention and therapeutics to address these problems.

Grossberg[168] traces the historical foundation of the nineteenth-century response to dependent children to the English Elizabethan 'Poor Law' of 1601. The bounds established by the Poor Law were influential in early America up to the present day, which, with a few but important exceptions, treated the family as a political unit within which the state infrequently intrudes.[169] Grossberg explains:[170]

> It established three fundamental features of Anglo-American welfare policy: local control; family responsibility; and a distinction between deserving and undeserving poor, tied to notions of work, gender, and age. The poor laws made parents legally liable for the support of their children and grandchildren, and children responsible for the care of their needy parents and grandparents. Embedded in the Elizabethan acts as well was a determination to limit demands on taxpayers' purses and to find alternative means of supporting the poor than public funding. These commitments expressed the continuing welfare reality that while parents might be willing to make financial sacrifices to give their own children an advantageous start in life, providing generously for children in need has never been a popular public policy.

According to Grossberg, the Poor Law set the stage for Anglo-American policy such that those of means could draw upon substantial resources to address their children's needs, while the children of the poor were awarded much more limited support from the state, in accordance with the aforementioned Poor Law philosophy and whatever meager financial support could be mustered from other sources, such as charities or religious institutions. In that sense, child welfare policy has been consistently a discussion where socioeconomic status differences are relevant.

Nevertheless, the State in Europe and the United States provided the ultimate responsibility for dependents in its *parens patriae* doctrine, in which the state holds an interest in children's welfare and may act like a parent if the family is unable to deliver upon their responsibilities.[171] The United States addressed the social demand of needy dependents (mentally ill, widows, orphans, and handicapped)—just not very generously. As discussed earlier, the eighteenth-century almshouses admitted all needy dependents, including children. As orphanages and other resources for needy children were developed in response to reform, the lot of dependent children improved, with the exception of slave children in the South, whose welfare was totally dependent upon the generosity of their owners; establishing powerful and lingering disparities between needy White and Black children.

With the post–Revolutionary War changes in American society, from the family oriented agrarian society to bourgeois urban and industrial growth, mothers became increasingly responsible for the care and rearing of children, as fathers were out of the home in the workplace.

These emerging changes in the first decades of the 1800s challenged what Elizabeth Pleck has characterized as 'the Family Ideal'.[172] Prior to the 1800s, family life was treated as a private realm for which the state had little to no rights to interfere. The transition to 'child welfare' and *parens patriae* was heralded by early efforts of the state to aid neglected or abused children when the parents failed in their responsibilities. The problem of conflict between states' interests and family interests in children was compounded by the ongoing growth of immigration. The differing values, customs, and religious traditions of immigrants imported a diverse set of childrearing practices, not all of which were acceptable to the emerging state vision of good parenting. As might be expected, the potential for conflict between families and the state was ongoing, between the private realm of the family and the public realm of government intervention; conflicts which resonate today not just for juvenile justice but for issues such as contraception, elective abortion, home schooling, care of transgender children, and family violence, to name a few.

The humanitarian reforms of the first decades of the 1800s, discussed earlier in this section, also included activism to address child welfare and the handling of juveniles in the developing criminal justice system. Later, the formation of the Society for the Prevention of Cruelty to Children in 1875 was a US landmark in promoting children's rights to make claims against their parents. An outgrowth of the child abuse awareness was the development of public/private hybrid agencies, such as New York's innovative Children's Aid Society, which were privately held institutions authorized by governments to address issues relevant to the public welfare—like child abuse and neglect. However, in the case of child abuse, the public was ambivalent about the development of regulatory agencies. Then, as today, different parents hold different values, attitudes, and practices in childrearing, and as noted earlier the nineteenth century many new immigrants felt harassed by child welfare agencies.

The founding of the Children's Bureau in 1912, at the behest of President Theodore Roosevelt, was intended to provide federal monitoring of children's needs nationwide. By this time the distinction between needy dependents and juvenile delinquents had been established in the discourse of the time, and both were under the purview of the Children's Bureau. The monitoring by the Bureau ranged from infant mortality statistics, orphan status, juvenile criminal offending, and childhood employment, among others. The Children's Bureau nationalized the need for child welfare policy.[173]

Over the period of the mid-1800s to the early twentieth century, compulsory education laws were passed by individual states; institutions for truancy developed, and ultimately juvenile courts established to address persistent truancy and juvenile crime or 'delinquency'.[174] As might be suspected with their newly captive audience, the schools became the platform and instrument for many child welfare policies and reforms. They indirectly reformed child labor abuses, by getting children out of the workplace to go to school, as well as stimulated public awareness of inappropriate child labor, and therefore contributed to the passage of child labor laws. Compulsory education also cemented the role of the state in childrearing practices; the old colonial model of the family as school, worksite, and domestic hub no longer applied, as parental authority was now shared with the schoolteacher. Many parents pushed back, resenting the intrusion of government into family/work practices, particularly farm and agricultural work.

In 1921 the Sheppard-Towner Act was passed by Congress, which provided federal funds to aid mother and child health, establishing a series of child/maternal clinics nationwide. American physicians, including the American Medical Association (AMA), however, resented the intrusion of the Feds into their turf, and attacked the law and the clinics, criticizing the latter as inferior socialized medicine. The physicians prevailed and the Act was repealed in 1929.[175] Nevertheless, the model of child/maternal clinics was set, and likely contributed to the consolidation of the medical specialties of pediatrics and obstetrics, as well as today's specialized family services like Planned Parenthood.

Child welfare reform stimulated many controversies. Reformers addressed the problem of 'illegitimate' children, or 'bastardy' by raising concerns about the rights of children born out of wedlock. Horror stories of neglect, abandonment, abuse, and even sale of these children prompted involvement from the rising profession of social work to address the needs of these children. Foster parenting programs developed to aid the placement of orphaned, abandoned, or abused children. These trends, however familiar today, were not monolithic in their development from state to state.[176] However, despite the greater awareness of children's needs, state governments were hesitant to pass laws intruding into the sanctity of the home. The development of state bureaus of charities was intended oversee both private and public institutions providing charitable support for needy dependents, but the extent of their power was limited by the local political equilibrium between constituencies favoring family autonomy and those favoring state intervention. The concept of the hybrid public/private charity was to prove influential not just in the realm of child welfare, but extending to other areas as well, including contemporary entities addressing other social needs, such as today's United Network for Organ Sharing.[177]

5.6.2 Juvenile courts and the juvenile justice system

As suggested in earlier sections, the differentiation of eighteenth-century almshouses to nineteenth-century asylums, prisons, and schools for idiocy also gathered momentum for a recognition of, and social action for, the unique status of children as criminal offenders. The Jacksonian-era realization that almshouses and prisons were awful places for children led to the concept of 'Houses of Refuge', which originally were substitutes for adult jails used for presentencing, and later the 'reform school' or reformatory—an institution that wavered between the extremes of a rehabilitative home for youthful offenders and a custodial prison for minors, depending on the time, political conditions, leadership, funding, and jurisdiction.

The development of the juvenile court and justice system accompanied these developments, but the early attempts at juvenile justice systems were a far cry from the elements we recognize today. Tanenhaus[178] presents the founding of the Cook County Juvenile Court (also known as the Chicago Juvenile Court) as the first US juvenile court in 1899, developed through the efforts of two social-activist friends, Julia Clifford Lathrop, a social worker, and Lucy Flower, a philanthropist. The initial court hearings were open to the public, as well as the newspapers, illustrating that one of the main elements of juvenile courts to be established later—privacy—had not yet been conceived or implemented. Such features as confidential records, a robust probation system, and detention homes or centers were other features yet to be developed. Nevertheless, the Chicago innovation was a landmark, and the development of an independent oversight body, the Juvenile Court Committee, by Flowers and Lathrop the same year, contributed to the refinement of the Chicago Juvenile Court. A place to put young offenders and intractably unruly children—a detention home—was recognized early and ultimately funds were raised for this institution in Chicago. Moreover, while probation services seemed essential, infrastructure was needed (probation officers, due processes for supervision, inspection, and intervention, organizational and administrative support). The probation officers (POs) in particular were viewed as crucial, as endpoint service-givers to the children and families. The POs were to serve the basic function of diverting children out of the adult criminal justice system.

Chicago juvenile justice pioneers like Judge Julian Mack and Timothy Hurley disagreed about the degree of power the POs should have. Mack supported an interventionist viewpoint, while Hurley was worried about the intrusion of the state into homes, and the imposition of uniform childrearing standards on the public. Mack and colleagues, on the other hand, were worried about the widespread recidivism that their early statistics had identified. This tension between familial intrusion and domestic security was one that was not going to go away, despite the proliferation of juvenile courts and probation models across the country.

The problem posed by vigorous interventionism, however, was resolved not so much by intent but by the rapid overload of cases encountered by the POs within the first 10 years of the Court. Tanenhaus[179] notes that in the first 3 years alone, Judge Mack had heard no less than 14,000 juvenile cases! These difficulties were mirrored in other states and jurisdictions as the juvenile court idea gained momentum. Mack's response to the case-number problem was developing a 'complaint system', which was a mechanism where members of the public could file a complaint about a disruptive youth, but POs would investigate the complaint and determine whether a formal court hearing was warranted. The complaint system thus shrank the courts' dockets, and also buffered the 'intrusionism' of the probation model.

The issue of state intrusion upon private family matters posed other problems. The development of private juvenile court hearings, which ultimately prevailed, was opposed by many who opposed aggressive interventionist POs policy. The idea that state judgments about the liberty of juveniles were made in closed-door hearings worried some members of the public, given the potential for abuse of civil liberties. Even Progressive advocates of juvenile justice were ambivalent; closed hearings served to obscure the problem of juvenile dependency and delinquency and prevented the public from being aware of the seriousness and size of the problem. Keeping the public ignorant of their court proceedings seemed likely to undercut the potential for sustaining, much less expanding, public support for the courts. One proffered solution was anonymized case histories that were released for public discussion, and likely stoked several generations of crime genre books, articles, and movies portraying the problem of juvenile misconduct—consider the aforementioned *West Side Story* or Nicholas Ray's iconic film *Rebel Without a Cause* (1955). A figure who will be discussed below in reference to the development of child and adolescent psychiatry, Judge Harvey H. Baker of Boston, published an influential 1910 paper[180] which provided an evenhanded analysis of the pros and cons of such a policy of private hearings, acknowledging that even as an advocate of private hearings, he believed that the insufficient evidence available could not establish their safety and fairness.

The development of 'mother's pensions' arose, perhaps surprisingly, in the wave of juvenile court reforms in the first decades of the twentieth century. The early twentieth-century Progressive reformers, however, saw strong linkages between dependency, on the one hand, and delinquency, on the other, so financial assistance to widowed and single mothers seemed an important adjunct to both the prevention of juvenile crime as well as a humane approach to the juvenile offender. Public ambivalence about 'welfare mothers,' while present in the Progressive era, was to grow in later decades of the twentieth century and lead to new reforms for dependents' aid.

The Social Security Act of 1935 established federal support for dependent youth. Originally called Aid to Dependent Children and later modified to Aid to Families with Dependent Children (AFDC), this program was intended to help poor families through financial assistance for their children. However, with the gender role expectations, as well as the common conditions of single parenthood of the time, the program mostly addressed poor mothers and their children. Concerns about AFDC's incentivizing women to have children instead of working led to the eventual severe reworking of AFDC through the Clinton Administration's passage of 1996's Personal Responsibility and Work Opportunity Act. AFDC was transformed into the Temporary Assistance for Needy Families (TANF). TANF imposed a 5-year limit to its assistance. The relative successes of these reforms are too contemporary to assess from a historical perspective.

The early child welfare considerations were gendered, class-bound and racial—and inequitable. The aforementioned mother's pensions were one example, the relative excusing of fathers from actual caring for children was recognized by the state, though federal requirements for states to have child support policies was not to appear until 1974's Social Services Amendments.[181] The historian Kathleen Jones describes the gender frame of how the Progressive reformers saw children's needs:[182]

> For the Progressive social activists who founded child guidance, class defined who was troublesome; gender described how they were trouble. Boys were truants and thieves; girls were 'sex delinquents' and shoplifters.

The aforementioned immigrant families, as well as African American families with their legacy of slavery, disparities in education, and post–Civil War racism, contributed to the overrepresentation of the poor and minorities in the emerging juvenile justice system.[183] Later in the twentieth century, after the influence of feminism and civil rights as cultural trends, and the increasing expectation that motherhood was not an excuse for unemployment, sympathy for the poor unemployed diminished, leading to the aforementioned reform of social welfare programs like AFDC.

The aforementioned concerns about recidivism—the limitations of the probation, detention, and juvenile court interventions—led Progressive reformers to consider the last element of the early twentieth-century juvenile justice reforms: a therapeutic approach to youth offenders. This innovation, of course, was to be a key element in the development of the VMDR in the case of children's mental disorders.

5.6.3 The child guidance movement and the birth of child/adolescent psychiatry

Deutsch,[184] writing from a nearly contemporary perspective at the time (1949), links the development of the 'Child Guidance movement' as a component of the larger Mental Hygiene movement described earlier. Prompted by other Progressive reforms, as well as the emerging social science of criminology, the idea that crime and criminality were rooted in social conditions took hold, and derivatively the idea that prevention was crucial, that[185]

> In a very real sense, it was recognized, the child is the father to the man.

The National Committee on Mental Hygiene conducted surveys among schoolchildren that identified two trends: that many 'normal' appearing children exhibited behavioral problems, and that schools had no resources, infrastructure, or personnel to address these problems.[186] Thomas Salmon MD, a psychiatrist leader within the National Committee led the effort to address these issues. Funded by the Commonwealth Fund and sanctioned by the National Committee on Mental Hygiene, a national conference on prevention of juvenile delinquency was held in 1921. The conference articulated the vision of the child guidance clinic:[187]

> . . . a psychiatric clinic designed to diagnose and treat the behavior and personality problems of childhood. These problems are made manifest by disorders of behavior, such as tantrums, stealing, seclusiveness, truancy, cruelty, sensitiveness, restlessness, and fears. The clinic treats these problems by treating not only the child through whom they become overt but treating as well the family, school, recreational, and other involved factors and persons which contribute to the problem, and whose disorder the problem may really reflect.

The child guidance clinic, reflecting the emerging multidisciplinarity of psychiatric outpatient clinics, was to include three core disciplines: psychiatry, psychology, and social work. Resonating with Progressive reforms elsewhere, the child guidance clinic trend spread across the country and by 1946, about 285 clinics were established nationwide.[188] The clinics, especially in the early years, flourished as a referral resource for the juvenile court and emerging juvenile justice system. As they and the field of psychiatry developed in the first half of the twentieth century, school referrals and family self-referrals became frequent. As will be discussed below, child guidance and the rise of child psychiatry contributed to a remarkably influential cultural transformation in the United States.

The child guidance clinic in its early manifestations was largely psychoanalytic in orientation and tended to view the etiology of childhood behavioral and emotional disturbances in terms of developmental/parental irregularities. Moreover, the focus of child guidance was not so much on children with major medical or developmental disorders, but rather on 'normal' children, who through environmental challenge or incompetent parenting, were deviating into a dangerous path toward other more overt psychopathology or criminal misconduct. While this psychoanalytic orientation held as a theoretical base for the clinics, in practice the child guidance clinic was equally Meyerian in its emphasis on biosocial influences, addressing heredity, as well as social conditions like poverty, making the child guidance clinic practice 'psychobiological' in the Meyerian sense, contributing to the constellation of a 'social psychiatry' wing of the field, and anticipating the biopsychosocial orientation articulated and popularized by George Engel later in the century. The interest in family functioning in the clinics likely contributed to the development of family therapy as a new psychotherapy approach. While child guidance in name, parental guidance was a prominent practice, to be lionized later by figures such as Benjamin Spock and Fitzhugh Dodson, whose updated editions on effective childrearing are often studied by parents today.

For many, the dark underbelly of the child guidance clinics was mother-blaming. Mothers tended to be portrayed as either neglectful, incompetent in parenting skills, or overinvolved and smothering, so treatment was directed toward mothers in multiple ways. Not yet liberated by feminism nor off the hook because of biological psychiatry's 'chemical imbalances' in the brain, abandoned by the presumed-competent and breadwinning father, mothers were often, perhaps usually, held responsible for their children's ills.[189] This motif persists today in multiple ways; from normative developmental psychology to the sociology of mothers in the workplace.[190]

The inspiration for child guidance clinics was juvenile delinquency, and the early core referrals were from the new juvenile courts. Two Chicago Progressives, William Healy and Ethel Sturges Dummer, founded the first research and treatment center for juvenile offenders, the Juvenile Psychopathic Institute in 1909. Dr. Healy, as the clinician-director of the Institute, was to write a major text in criminology, *The Individual Delinquent* (1915), based on meticulous chart reviews of the clinic's patients. Dummer was the philanthropic core of the Institute. Dubbed 'child savers' because of their concerns, the Progressives that promoted child guidance were most urgently concerned about juvenile offenders, and particularly those who were children of poor immigrants who might not have shared the emerging moral standards of childrearing that were being formulated. The clashes between childrearing values of the psychiatric experts and traditional, ethnic childrearing values of the immigrants has already been mentioned and persists today. For example, then as now, the practice of corporal punishment for children, generally disapproved by child psychiatrists and psychologists, with extensive scientific data in support, is still practiced by large numbers of the American parental public.[191]

Healy's *The Individual Delinquent* was important in several ways. First, in its study of approximately 800 juvenile recidivists, it possessed an authority and scope that was unique for the time. Healy's findings then, and to follow, also refuted many of his colleagues' received views about delinquency. Healy was contrarian to many of his colleagues who had jumped on the bandwagon of hereditarian etiologies for crime discussed earlier, such as degeneracy theory. Healy became increasingly skeptical of degeneracy theory in general, and Lombroso's atavistic criminals in particular, noting the feebleness of hereditary influences in his studies. Moreover, the idea that juvenile offenders were driven universally by mental disorders was also not sustained by his studies. Most offenders were phenotypically normal children who were responding to environmental circumstances. Similarly, he refuted the idea promulgated from Henry Goddard and like-minded mental deficiency theorists that delinquency was generally associated with feeblemindedness. Healy found that while feeblemindedness was common in his population, it was rarely the 'single causative factor of criminalism'.[192] As a final example of Healy's innovations, he articulated the view that delinquency was (in today's terms) multifactorial; identifying dozens of causative factors that contributed to a network of causal vectors in shaping juvenile offending. Before the reader concludes that Healy's formulation of juvenile crime was completely contemporary, take note of some of Healy's specific causal vectors listed below in Table 5.1:[193]

Healy's analysis was flawed by an informal approach to interpreting the causal power or weights to these factors; some factors are tabulated in case studies, others are claimed as self-evident, and as a descriptive study, Healy's causal attributions remain conjectural by contemporary standards. Other investigators came to more definitive conclusions, such as Breckinridge and Abbott's *The Delinquent Child and the Home*, which was an outgrowth of a survey of cases from Chicago's new juvenile court.[194] They concluded:[195]

> But the great and memorable fact must remain that all children need for successful rearing the same conditions: homes of physical and moral decency, fresh air, education, recreation, the found care of wise fathers and mothers. These essentials curtailed at any moment, the degree of human wastage grows with the curtailment.

Jones[196] notes that Breckinridge and Abbott's conclusions were important in passing the aforementioned mothers' pension laws, under the idea that a mother at home is a mother providing fewer curtailments of these essentials.

Healy was recruited to Boston in 1917 to develop a child guidance clinic for the Judge Baker Foundation, a model for service that was to be promulgated by the

Table 5.1 Selected Causative Factors for Delinquency from Healy's *The Individual Delinquent*

Heredity
Excessive energy, irritable temper, hypersexual tendencies; feeblemindedness, insanity

Developmental conditions
Disease during pregnancy, physical abuse during pregnancy, alcoholism during pregnancy, morphinism during pregnancy, mother working during pregnancy, congenital syphilis, mother mentally troubled; premature birth

Physical conditions
Eye strain, strabismus, large tonsils, *dental abscesses*, stuttering, deaf-mutism, enuresis, undernourishment, syphilis, menstruation, headaches, head injuries

Developmental physical abnormalities
Poor general physical development, delayed puberty, over-development, combinations of the previous factors

Habits
Masturbation, *excessive sexual activity*, idleness, vagrancy

Stimulants and narcotics: alcohol, morphine, cocaine, tea and coffee, tobacco

Environmental factors
Parental alcoholism, immoral home environment, quarrelsomeness, harsh discipline, *incompetent discipline*, parental separation, crowded housing, poverty, homelessness, parental neglect, bad companions, theatres, dance halls, *impoverished mental stimulation*, pernicious stories (*crime fiction/nonfiction*), incarceration

---

Note: Healy (1915). Items in plainface are Healy's terms; items in italics are Sadler's paraphrasing.

Commonwealth Fund through demonstration projects to disseminate the child guidance model nationwide. Judge Harvey Baker was a Boston leader in the juvenile justice movement, and Baker provided a hub of interest in extending the juvenile justice reforms to include a therapeutic component. Healy was, in a few years (1923), to spearhead the effort to organize psychiatrists, psychologists, and social workers into a professional organization, the American Orthopsychiatric Association (AOA) to promote a 'simple but revolutionary idea: The mental health of individuals depends on their social context'.[197] Healy's portrait provided the image of 'Ortho's' seal, as it was with Benjamin Rush's visage for APA's. AOA was multidisciplinary in its constituency. The emerging subspecialty of child psychiatry was not to have its own exclusive organization until 1952; the American Academy of Child (and Adolescent) Psychiatry (AACAP). The splitting off of AACAP from AOA was to mark the transition of many child psychiatrists from being members of a multidisciplinary team in public settings, to being autonomous, and often private, medical subspecialists. This transformation also marked a transition away from dynamic and Meyerian psychiatry to the new biological psychiatry embraced by the AACAP. Increasingly, the multidisciplinary ethos of 'Ortho' did not fit with the medical identity of the emerging child and adolescent psychiatry subspecialty. By 2018, AOA changed its name to the Global Alliance for

Behavioral Health and Social Justice, while retaining the original values and vision of its parent organization.[198]

Jones[199] provides a quotation from a 1907 Illinois juvenile court law which defines the juvenile delinquent:

> any male child who while under the age of seventeen years or any female child who while under the age of eighteen years, violates any law of this State; or is incorrigible, or knowingly associates with thieves, vicious or immoral persons; or who, without just cause and without the consent of its parents, guardian or custodian, absents itself from its home or place of abode, or is growing up in idleness or crime; or knowingly frequents a house of ill-repute; or knowingly frequents any policy shop or place where any gaming device is operated; or frequents any saloon or dram shop where intoxicating liquors are sold; or patronizes or visits any public pool room or bucket shop; or wanders about the streets in the night time without being on any lawful business or lawful occupation; or habitually wanders about any railroad yards or tracks of jumps or attempts to jump onto any moving train; or enters any car or engine without lawful authority; or habitually uses vile, obscene, vulgar, profane, or indecent language in any public place or about any school house; or is guilty of indecent or lascivious conduct.

Regarding the relevance to the VMDR, one can check off diagnostic criteria for current DSM-5 Conduct Disorder from within this century-old law. As has too often been the case with innovative mental health programs, long-term outcome studies of delinquents with child guidance interventions were few, and those that were done, showed little positive long-term effects.[200] By midcentury the child guidance clinic as defined entity had dissolved into the emerging diversity of mental health services nationwide: private outpatient practice, community mental health, general hospital psychiatry, freestanding psychiatric institutes, forensic psychiatry, and residential treatment facilities. Child guidance was to suffer the same pressures that the rest of the forensic mental health agenda was to face: too many patients, too few resources, and an ambivalent public.

The feeble outcomes for treatment interventions, however, didn't necessarily summarize the impact of the child guidance movement. Jones[201] makes a strong case (while never really declaring it as such) that the Progressive leaders of the movement had significant success in changing the way Americans think about parenting and misbehaving children. Jones identifies two core tropes that popularized child guidance, thus solidifying a public ideology of childrearing. One was that a state of 'predelinquency' existed, related to what today we would identify as 'at-risk' children. The other was the related idea that ordinary misconduct, if managed inappropriately, could result in more severe forms of offending and psychopathology. These tropes required the expertise of child guidance clinicians to guide parents, legitimizing the field, while presenting a broad-based sociocultural intervention in addressing a significant public problem of delinquency.

How were these tropes promulgated and how did they take hold? Jones provides several general explanations, but her text should be read for the complete story. First, the prevention mission of child guidance clinicians harmonized with the prevention mission of the then-contemporary Mental Hygiene movement as well as the Children's Bureau; publications, pamphlets, and outreach from one assimilated the goals of the other. Second, the child savers were part of the larger Progressive reform mission, and the *Zeitgeist* was on their side. Third, the child guidance movement developed at a time when American media was expanding; this was the golden age of periodicals; newspapers and magazines were an explosive industry in their own right. Indeed, the child savers' messages not only appeared in print media and radio, but also inspired new content for old magazines like the *Saturday Evening Post* and new magazines altogether, such as the founding of *Parent's* magazine in 1926. The American magazine empire, in expansionist mode, identified stay-at-home moms as an open market share; magazines like *Good Housekeeping, Better Homes and Gardens*, and *Ladies Home Journal* needed material for young mothers and housewives. What could be more enticing to moms than expert advice on common childhood behavior problems? Consonant with these changes, the new American advertising industry intended to create desire and conspicuous consumption; advertisements of the time suggested that childrearing using Grandma's wisdom was as old-fashioned as horse-and-buggy transportation. The period also witnessed the birth of the book genre of parenting advice; Dr. Spock being the benchmark,[202] but countless other publications appeared and were eagerly purchased and read. Moreover, the child savers conducted a substantial community outreach campaign; the issues of childcare and rearing were brought into the schools, and organizations like the Parent-Teacher's Association (PTA)[203] gained new momentum by disseminating child guidance wisdom.

Finally, the emerging forensic aspects of child guidance psychiatry gained a media boost from the sensational murder case of Leopold and Loeb, two wealthy Chicago college students who abducted and murdered a 14-year-old neighbor in 1924. Clarence Darrow, the now-famous defense attorney did not develop an insanity defense but sought to inspire leniency (e.g., not the death sentence) by using psychiatric testimony to generate jury sympathy for the unfortunate circumstances of the defendants' childhood and upbringing. William Alanson White and William Healy provided the expert testimony. Their explanation of the duo's psychology and circumstances was heavily covered in the media and was ultimately successful in getting the youths' sentences reduced to life in prison. Cinema buffs will recognize the Leopold and Loeb case as inspiration for Alfred Hitchcock's 1948 film *Rope*, and Meyer Levin's 1959 film *Compulsion*, still more signposts for the *Zeitgeist*.

5.7 The development of forensic psychiatry

The appearance of forensic psychiatry as a function or activity within the field preceded its development as a formal subspecialty of psychiatry. The utility of physician opinion in law/court settings had been introduced in ancient Roman law, but the prolegomena of contemporary forensic and 'correctional' psychiatry did not appear until the early modern period, through three emerging trends: (1) the use of physician testimony to address criminal responsibility, excuse, and sentencing; (2) the adaptation of prison and asylum settings to accommodate mentally ill offenders (as well as the development of psychiatric hospital forensic units); and later, (3) the use of forensic psychiatric experts in civil or tort settings to address matters such as child custody and malpractice. The review here will focus on the first two as they are most pertinent to the VMDR.

A crucial part of the story regarding the development of forensic psychiatry has to do with the taxonomy of mental disorder, and most specifically the notion of partial insanity, which will be discussed more in the subsections on monomania and homicidal insanity to follow. Prior to the late 1700s in England and France, the notion of a mad individual having limited responsibility for his or her acts was determined by the jury. Madness, or 'total' insanity, was a holistic phenomenon that would be apparent to any ordinary citizen. Specifically, lunacy was recognizable by any juror.

However, the straightforward lay recognition of madness was about to end. In 1798 the French alienist Phillipe Pinel described a phenomenon which he proclaimed *manie sans délire*, being a kind of madness where the intellect, or rational capacity was preserved, but the (often violent) behavior of the patient was mad:[204]

> . . . who present no trouble or disorder in their ideas, no extravagant deviation of the imagination; these madmen (*insensés*) respond in the most correct and precise manner to questions put to them, but they are dominated by the most impetuous furor and by a sanguinary instinct of which they themselves sense all the *horror but which they cannot master*.

This group of violent offenders, despite appearances with superficial examination, couldn't help themselves. Pinel's novel notion of a 'partial insanity' proved to be important to the emerging French (and later, American) forensic psychiatric mission—one his students and later rival Esquirol initially scoffed at, only to be latter appropriated and transformed into the concept of monomania. Pinel's findings of partially insane individuals posed a Kuhnian anomaly of sorts, given that the then-prevailing associationist psychology of Locke and Condillac (much less moral psychology going back to Plato), would have predicted that such a fracture of coherent thought and inconceivable act would be impossible. One can also see the description of *manie sans délire* as the birth of contemporary impulse control disorders: where the patient knows a particular act is inappropriate or wrongful, but finds oneself doing such acts nonetheless. A third significance of partial insanity was its demand to move some kinds of insanity out of the sphere of the layperson's assessment, and into the sphere of the discerning expert—thus cementing the professional role of the forensic psychiatrist, a shift Esquirol was to exploit later (see Section 5.8.3) as his thought spread to the United States.

5.7.1 Responsibility, excuse, and sentencing

The distinction between the total loss of reason in (total) insanity and the partial insanities, (which were later to be discerned variously as delimited irrationalities, as well as impairments of the faculties of emotion (affection) or will (conation)), had tremendous forensic implications regarding the question of whether an acknowledged offender could be held responsible for his offense. Prosono[205] notes that the English jurist Matthew Hale (1609–1676) may have been the first to use the term 'partial insanity', with melancholia being an important example of such, appearing in Hale's *History of the Pleas of the Crown* (1736).[206]

Sir Edward Coke's *The First Part of the Institutes of the Laws of England or, a Commentary upon Littleton* (1628)[207] may be the fundamental text of English common law, and certainly influential in US law, being frequently cited by the US Supreme Court.[208] In the context of indexing a wide range of English cases, Coke elaborated upon his predecessor Littleton's considerations of criminal responsibility:[209]

> Here *Littleton* explaineth a man of no sound memorie to be *non compos mentis [of unsound mind]*. Many times (as here it appeareth) the Latin word explaineth the true sense, and calleth him not *amens [demented]*, *demens [mad]*, *furiosus [frenzied, raving]*, *lunaticus [lunacy, total madness]*, *fatuus [foolish]*, *stultus [unwise, stupid]*, or the like, for *non compos mentis* is the most sure and legall . . . 1. *Ideota [idiocy]*, which from his nativitie, by a perpetuall infirmitie, is *non compos mentis*. 2. Hee that by sicknesse, griefe, or other accident, wholly loseth his memorie and understanding. 3. A lunatique that hath sometime his understanding and sometime not, *aliquando gaudet lucidis intervallis [intermittent lucid intervals]*, and therefore he is called *non compos mentis*, so long as he hath not understanding. Lastly, hee that by his owne vitious act for a time depriveth himself of his memorie and understanding, as he that is drunken. But that kinde of *non compos mentis* shall give no privilege or benefit to him or to his heires.

Some interpretive elaboration might be helpful here, for those puzzled by old English style as well as for international readers. Coke is laying out the conditions for excusing criminal conduct, with the encompassing expression being *non compos mentis*, usually translated as being of unsound mind. Under the rubric of *non compos mentis* are the varieties of more-or-less conventional madness. He describes four conditions in more detail: the first, idiocy or intellectual disability, is specified as a static, chronic condition ('perpetuall infirmitie'). The second, more transitory, is an impairment of memory or understanding due to medical illness, grief or other 'accident', a condition we would liken to transient impairments like DSM-5 Delirium or stress-related conditions like Acute Stress Disorder. The third, perhaps best exemplified today by Bipolar Disorder in a euthymic state—between manic and depressive episodes—Coke describes as conditions with lucid intervals and suggests that responsibility is limited only in the periods of active symptoms. The fourth and final condition, likened to drunkenness, is a volitional impaired state—which is specified as *not* excusing conduct, even under the impaired period of time. The reference to 'heires' refers to the common, even prevailing, practice of the time, where the common law became involved in the affairs of the mad when the inheritance of the madperson's estate, or the validity of a will, was in question.

Coke's conditions bear relevance today in that an encompassing mental disorder which disrupts the patient's sense of reality generates an excuse consideration. Similarly, intellectual impairment may pose an excuse for wrongful conduct. Interestingly, the individual under overwhelming personal circumstances or stressors may be excused as 'crimes of passion'. Periodic illness is recognized, and the state of the offender's mind *at the time of the offense* is implicated. Finally, individuals who impair their judgment and understanding through personal choice may not be excused for wrongful conduct committed while impaired. These motifs (incapacitating or total insanity, limited intellect, duress, and incapacitating choice) recur throughout the history of mental health law into the present.

The recognition in common law that certain conditions may constrain or excuse criminal responsibility is ancient, going back to the Romans and the still-relevant distinction between the Latin expressions *mens rea* and *actus reus*. *Mens rea* is commonly translated as 'guilty mind' or 'criminal intent'. Such criminal intent is referred often as an offender acting 'knowingly', 'willingly', 'intentionally', and 'purposefully' in performing a criminal action. Note that *mens rea* is a state of mind, bound by the fact of human subjectivity and only indirectly accessible (through confession or other observable evidence). *Actus reus* is commonly translated as 'guilty act' or 'criminal deed'.[209] In contrast to *mens rea*, *actus reus* is an *event* involving observable behaviors which are potentially verifiable by witnesses. However, the *actus reus* is not equivalent to those behaviors, but rather, the criminal context of human behaviors (e.g., murder, theft, and arson). Taken together, *mens rea* and *actus reus* form the core of a criminal offense.[210]

The issue of criminal responsibility depends upon both elements in common law. The role of the law is to determine that a criminal act occurred—*actus reus*—and that the defendant committed the criminal act. The second role is to determine if the defendant intended—had criminal intent—to commit the act. In the case of mentally ill defendants, the question regarding *actus reus* is the same as with non-mentally ill defendants—did the criminal event occur, and who perpetrated it? However, *mens rea* is the element where determinations of mentally ill defendants become relevant—did this defendant have criminal intent in the face of his mental circumstances?

During the modern period a number of tests or criteria have been formulated to address this and related questions. The question of 'mental disease or defect' in law is not just limited to today's 'insanity defense' in the criminal setting, but also other areas of common law, such as the validity of one's will, the suitability to parent one's children, the validity of a contract, and the ability to participate in one's legal defense ('competency to stand trial'), to name a few. However, for the purposes of the analysis of the VMDR, the issue of criminal responsibility is the most relevant and the one which will be focused on in these pages, and more thoroughly elaborated in Chapter 6.

Prior to the seventeenth century, the question of *mens rea* was rarely complicated in legal hearings, as the determination of the pervasively obvious conditions of idiocy and insanity needed no experts. The ordinary citizen was quite familiar with madness and idiocy from everyday community experience.[211] While the development of forensic medicine had preceded the use of proto-psychiatrists in the criminal setting, the asylum doctors had little to offer in the bald assessment of *mens rea* in criminal settings—either defendants were obvious lunatics or were not.[212]

This state of affairs began to change in the 1600s when Thomas Willis, the physician-anatomist (and describer of the Circle of Willis brain vasculature) distinguished two kinds of melancholia—one (universal type) which was a pervasive disorder, and the other (particular type) which was limited to one or two functional areas of mentation.[213] Willis's distinction contributed to the partial insanity concept. The notion of partial insanity was one which was to be elaborated over the next 2 centuries by such luminaries as Pinel (*manie sans délire*), James Prichard (moral insanity), and Esquirol (monomanias).[214] The significance of partial insanities to the emerging subspecialty of forensic psychiatry, as Jan Goldstein[215] has pointed out, is related to the subtler findings in partial insanities; subtleties that required the expertise of the alienist to elicit. As Esquirol established, the common knowledge approach of the lay jury was not adequate for discerning partial insanity.

As can be recognized in retrospect, the development of partial insanities—psychopathologies that were not pervasive but limited to particular domains of ideas and/or mental faculties—introduced difficult conceptual problems that persist into the present day. One aspect was the aforementioned status of *mens rea* as situated in the person's subjective experience, a mental state not directly accessible to examiners, judges, and juries. By adding the idea of partial psychopathology, the determination of *mens rea* became even more difficult. The court had to address the question of a link between the defendant's delimited psychopathology and the *actus reus*. That is, judge and jury had to figure out if the defendant committed the criminal act as a result of the delimited mental disorder or committed it in spite of the delimited mental disorder—that is, committed it for the usual reasons crimes are committed. The third conceptual issue that is posed, then and now, encompasses both of these prior considerations. Under the old view of total, encompassing insanity, the court needed to establish only how long the madperson had been affected, and if it preceded the crime, the link between madness and the crime was established. However, this was not so easy in the setting of partial insanity. The jury had to consider whether the defendant's limited psychopathology was relevant to a crime that had occurred in the past. Today this problem is called the problem of 'retrospective mental states' in the criminal setting.[216] The question becomes: "Was the defendant under the influence of mental disease or defect at the time of the offense?"

As might be expected in the history that followed, the determination of whether the defendant was acting under the influence of mental disease or defect has been subject to various tests or criteria of determination. What is remarkable about these tests, and how they reflect legal tradition, is that they all are modeled upon three key assumptions about human nature: (1) an explicit moral formulation of criminality: evil drives criminality. (2) Unimpaired people have free choice or 'free will.' (3) The human capacity for reason is required for prosocial, as well as criminal, responsible conduct. (All of these assumptions are under challenge by science today, as will be discussed in later chapters.) Table 5.2 lists the major legal decisions about responsibility briefly.

5.7.2 The insanity defense

The conceptual ambiguities in the tests for what became the 'insanity defense' in popular parlance can be elaborated from Table 5.2. Judge Tracy's 1724 description of the so-called wild beast test emphasizes that the defendant must be 'totally deprived' of understanding and memory, underscoring the early and commonsensical notion of insanity as an encompassing disturbance of mental functioning—a total deprivation of reason. Moreover, Tracy's model as quoted in Table 5.2 implies that the court sees insanity as forgiving punishment, not so much the *actus reus*.[217]

By 1800 we see that the test articulated by the distinguished British jurist Thomas Erskine (1750–1823) had already assimilated the notion of partial insanity through its emphasis on 'delusion' as the measure of madness. The associated case, *Rex v. Hadfield*, concerned the attempt on King George III's life by James Hadfield, a soldier with head injuries and subsequent grandiose delusions, whose attempt on George III's life was, in Hadfield's formulation, to abort the end of the world. However, Hadfield's urgent passion unsteadied his aim, and the gunshot only grazed the King. Prosono[218] notes that Erskine's successful defense of Hadfield shifted terms of the insanity defense away from assessments of the defendant's cognitive state of mind and instead to the presence of psychopathological symptoms and the diagnosis of a particular disorder. This shift was a boon to alienists in that this distinction was another element in moving the determination of criminal responsibility out of the jury's direct and commonsense-based judgment and promoted a need for the expert witness, who could make the requisite determinations and diagnosis. Moreover, Erskine's approach established the role of psychiatric diagnosis in the courts (for better or for worse). The significance of diagnosis for criminal responsibility was to become a major source of debate within psychiatry and law into the present day.

The McNaughton rule was to become perhaps the most influential legal test of insanity in Anglo-American history, simply because 26 of 50 US state jurisdictions use it today.[219] An influential American general practitioner, Isaac Ray, contributed *A Treatise on the Medical Jurisprudence of Insanity*,[220] which was significant for the history of psychiatry not only because of Ray's across-the-Atlantic influence on the McNaughton case, but also the signal that American psychiatry, after decades of lagging behind the progress of Western European alienists, was beginning to stand on

Table 5.2 Influential Legal Tests of Criminal Responsibility

Name	Date	Description
Wild beast test	1724	'. . . it must be a man totally deprived of his understanding and memory, and doth not know what he is doing, no more than an infant, than a brute, or a wild beast; such a one is never the object of punishment.' Judge Tracy, *Rex v. Arnold* 16 How. St. Tr. 695 (1724)[a]
Erskine test	1800	'*Delusion*, therefore, where there is no frenzy or raving madness, is the true character of insanity; and where it cannot be predicated of a man standing for life or death for a crime, he ought not, in my opinion, to be acquitted . . . .to deliver a lunatic from responsibility to criminal justice, above all, in a case of such atrocity as the present, the relation between the disease and the act should be apparent. Where the connexion is doubtful, the judgment should certainly be most indulgent, for the great difficulty of diving into the secret sources of a disordered mind; . . .' *Rex v. Hadfield* 27 St. Tr. 1281 (1800)[b]
McNaughton Rules (also spelled M'Naghten, McNaughtan)	1843	'. . . to establish a defence of on the ground of insanity, it must be clearly proved that, at the time of committing of the act, the party accused was labouring under such a defect of reason, from disease of the mind, as not to know the nature and quality of the act he was doing, or if he did know it, that he did not know he was doing what was wrong'. *House of Lords v. M'Naghten* 1 C. and K. 130, 1843[c]
'Irresistible Impulse' test	1844	'. . . mental disease as causing a loss of power to choose between right and wrong, destroying free agency at the time of the alleged criminal act'. *Commonwealth v. Rogers*, 48 Mass. 500 (Massachusetts 1844)[d]
Durham (Product) rule	1954	'A test of insanity ought to determine if the act in question was a "product" of a mental disease or defect . . .' *Durham v. United States*, 214 F.2d 862 (D.C. Cir 1954)[e]
American Law Institute (ALI) Model Penal Code	1962	'(1) A person is not responsible for criminal conduct if at the time of such conduct as a result of mental disease or defect he lacks substantial capacity either to appreciate the criminality of his conduct or to conform his conduct to the requirements of the law. (2) As used in this Article, the terms 'mental disease or defect' do not include an abnormality manifested only by repeated criminal or otherwise antisocial conduct/' [f]

[a] Quoted in Robinson, DN. *Wild Beasts and Idle Humours: The Insanity Defense from Antiquity to the Present.* Cambridge, MA: Harvard University Press, 1996, p. 134.

[b] Quoted in Hunter & MacAlpine, *Three Hundred Years of Psychiatry, 1535–1860.* London: Oxford University Press, 1963, p. 571.

[c] Quoted in Hunter & MacAlpine, *Three Hundred Years of Psychiatry, 1535–1860.* London: Oxford University Press, 1963, p. 921. See also Daniel M'Naghten's Case, United Kingdom House of Lords Decisions http://www.bailii.org/uk/cases/UKHL/1843/J16.html.

[d] Quoted in Prosono (2003 p. 21).

[e] Quoted in Prosono (2003 p. 21).

[f] Quoted in Gutheil & Appelbaum (2000 p. 276).

its own two feet. Acknowledging his influences—Pinel, Prichard, Esquirol, Rush, and others—in his elaboration of moral insanity, which he preferred to call 'moral mania', Ray's *Treatise* was a compendium of analyses of his forensic cases based upon his practice and legal testimony in New England.

In reviewing Pinel's *manie sans délire*, Ray noted that '. . . there were many maniacs who betrayed no lesion whatever of the understanding, but were under the dominion of instinctive and abstract fury, as if the affective faculties alone had sustained injury.'[221] Citing the contemporary *Cyclopedia of Practical Medicine* article on 'Insanity', Ray describes in detail the presentation of 'general' moral mania:[222]

> Among the varieties of maniacs met with in medical pactice [sic], there is one, which, though, by no means rare, has been little noticed by writers on this subject: I refer to those cases in which the individuals perform most of the common duties of life with propriety, and some of them, indeed, with scrupulous exactness, who exhibit no strong marked features of either temperament, no traits of superior or defective mental endowment, but yet take violent antipathies, harbor unjust suspicions, indulge strong propensities, affect singularity in dress, gait, and phraseology; are proud, conceited, and ostentatious; easily excited and with difficulty appeased; dead to sensibility, delicacy, and refinement, obstinately riveted to the most absurd opinions, prone to controversy, and yet incapable of reasoning; always the hero of their own tale, using hyperbolic, high-flown language to express the most simple ideas, accompanied by unnatural gesticulation, inordinate action, and frequently by the most alarming expression of countenance. On some occasions they suspect sinister intentions on the most trivial grounds; on others are a prey to fear and dread from the most ridiculous and imaginary sources; now embracing every opportunity of exhibiting romantic courage and feats of hardihood, then indulging themselves in all manner of excesses.

What was significant in these cases for Ray and his European colleagues was the preservation of reason excepting those areas driven by affection, or the heightened emotional states he described.[223]

In considering 'partial moral mania' Ray focuses in on the commission of crime in his affected patients:[224]

> In this form of insanity, the derangement is confined to one or a few of the affective faculties, the rest of the moral and intellectual constitution preserving its ordinary integrity. An exaltation of the vital forces in any part of the cerebral organism, must necessarily be followed by increased activity and energy in the manifestations of the faculty connected with it, and which may even be carried to such a pitch as to be beyond the control of any other power, like the working of a blind, instinctive impulse. Accordingly, we see the faculty thus affected, promoting the individual to action by a kind of instinctive irresistibility, and while he retains the most perfect consciousness of the impropriety and even enormity of his conduct, he deliberately and perseveringly pursues it. With no extraordinary temptation to sin, but on the contrary, with every inducement to refrain from it, and apparently in the full possession of his reason, he commits a crime whose motives are equally inexplicable to himself and to others.

Ray then goes on to detail a series of cases of partial moral mania focusing on particular kinds of crime or misconduct: theft, (repeated, perhaps compulsive) lying, sexual misconduct ('erotic mania'), 'incendiarism' (pyromania), and homicidal mania/insanity, the latter including classic cases of Esquirol in France.[225]

The aforementioned discussion of Ray's influence suggests a discussion of the McNaughton case in the UK.

Daniel McNaughton was a Scottish craftsman who shot and killed Edward Drummond, who was the personal secretary to then-British Prime Minister Robert Peel. McNaughton misidentified Drummond for Peel, and while the wound was not immediately mortal for Drummond, surgeons had not yet discovered antiseptic care, and their bloodlettings and dirty fingers probably hastened the patient's septic death. In his mid-to-late 20s, McNaughton began to have suspicions of the Tories spying on him, and at trial, briefly elaborated upon the torment the Tory spies had perpetrated upon him. Despite this paranoid delusion, McNaughton presented himself otherwise in a rational manner. His defense attorney, Alexander Cockburn, based much of his defense on Isaac Ray's account of partial insanity, saying that the insanity defense should be exculpatory on the basis of relatively isolated psychopathologies of intellect and emotion. The medical consultants for the defense argued that his delusions of persecution denied McNaughton of his ability to restrain his actions.[226] Ultimately the jury agreed, and McNaughton was acquitted by reason of insanity, and the McNaughton standard quoted in Table 5.2 became and remained a common formulation of the insanity defense in the UK and in many US states today.

Nevertheless, then and now the McNaughton standard was controversial. In 1881 in the United States, Charles Guiteau was another delusional assassin, this time for US President James Garfield. Once again the victim had a nonlethal wound which festered as a result of repeated probing by pus- and excrement-besmirched fingers of his doctors, leading to Garfield's septic death about 11 weeks later.[227] Guiteau articulately decried his lawyers' attempt at an insanity defense, and the deliberate plan Guiteau described did no good to acquit him. He was convicted and the next year was executed by hanging.

Ray's interest in the insanity defense and the role of alienists in expert testimony led to an extended correspondence with one of the New Hampshire Supreme Court justices, Judge Doe, leading to the influential 'New Hampshire Rule' based upon the *State v. Pike* case[228] (also known as the Durham Rule when adopted by the District of Columbia), and ultimately the Product Rule in legal history. The Product Rule made the determination of criminal responsibility dependent upon whether the criminal act was a 'product' of a mental disease or disability.

US Courts struggled with the application of the McNaughton rule's cognitive test, as well as determining the causal relationship between the defendant's mental state and the criminal act. A third approach appeared in Massachusetts in 1844 through *Commonwealth v. Rogers*.[229] Abner Rogers believed Charlestown State Prison Warden Charles Lincoln was the leader of a conspiracy to persecute Rogers, and in his delusional state, he believed his only chance of survival was to murder (Charles) Lincoln. Isaac Ray argued for the defense that Rogers was driven by an 'irresistible impulse' to murder Lincoln, believing it was justified self-defense.[230] A common restatement of the irresistible impulse test is the 'policeman at the elbow test', which asks if the defendant would have committed the criminal act if a policeman was standing at the offender's elbow.[231]

Criticisms of various tests or standards for the insanity defense continued, while jurisdiction after jurisdiction applied this or that standard. In fairness, the problem of the insanity defense was a sign of a larger problem in US common law, that individual states and jurisdictions within those states had divergent practices in multiple areas of common law. Different states had different criminal statutes, as well as differing jurisdictional interpretations of the law, leading to divergent treatment of the same offense from jurisdiction to jurisdiction.

In response to the chaotic diversity of US common law among the states, the American Law Institute (ALI) was founded in 1923 to provide a central clearing-house of legal policy, to improve and consolidate knowledge and policy concerning the law.[232] In 1962 ALI promulgated its own 'two pronged' approach to testing for the insanity defense, one prong being a cognitive test *a la* McNaughton and the second prong being a 'volitional' test appealing to willpower or motivational control:[233]

> (1) A person is not responsible for criminal conduct if at the time of such conduct as a result of mental disease or defect he lacks substantial capacity either to appreciate the criminality of his conduct or to conform his conduct to the requirements of the law. (2) As used in this Article, the terms 'mental disease or defect' do not include an abnormality manifested only by repeated criminal or otherwise antisocial conduct.

The effect of the ALI test was complex and is being played out to the present day and is discussed in more detail in Chapter 6. By including two prongs, the test is more inclusive. A mentally disordered offender may qualify for the insanity defense if he cannot 'appreciate the criminality of his conduct' (e.g., lacks criminal intent) OR can cannot 'conform his conduct to the requirements of the law' (e.g., could not control himself—thereby including a volitional component reminiscent of the irresistible impulse test).

By making either condition—cognitive or volitional—sufficient to qualify for the insanity defense, the ALI test in effect made it easier to qualify for the not guilty by reason of insanity (NGRI) verdict. Initially the ALI standard enjoyed wide appeal, but over the years has also encountered strong opposition.[234] The ALI test's appeal is largely based upon its liberality—it is generous in its 'forgiveness' of mentally ill offenders. On the other hand, its liberality is what makes it offensive to those who value strict law-and-order approaches to civic welfare, as well as skeptics about mental illness. Perhaps most illustrative of the public opposition to the ALI standard is the trial of John Hinckley, Jr., the young Texan who attempted to assassinate President Ronald Reagan in 1982. Under the District of Columbia standards, the insanity defense uses an 'appreciation' standard, akin to the ability to conform ones conduct to the law under the ALI test. Hinckley was acquitted under NGRI under this interpretation. The trial was well-publicized by the popular media, in that Hinckley was obsessed with celebrity actress Jodie Foster and was at least partly inspired by Martin Scorsese's grimly prophetic film *Taxi Driver*. Hinckley did not qualify for the cognitive component of the ALI test as he was open about his deliberations in preparing for the assassination, which he recognized as illegal. Instead, he was acquitted on the volitional prong of the ALI test, on the basis he could not conform his behavior to the law.[235] The public outrage at his acquittal was palpable and contributed to the issuing of new statements from the American Psychiatric Association, as well as the American Bar Association, recommending movements back to a cognitive-only, McNaughton-based standard, which many states did.[236]

The ALI test is also notable in its disqualifying certain mental conditions involving only criminal misconduct. This in effect bifurcated the universe of psychiatrically defined mental disorders into two legal kinds—those that qualify as NGRI-eligible conditions, and those that do not—most notably, psychopathy and antisocial disorders, and often the paraphilias, need not apply for NGRI. This effect was to narrow the field to those disorders which, to use my language, were vice-laden to be ineligible for the insanity defense. As will be discussed in later chapters, what qualifies as a mental disorder under legal, not clinical, grounds, still varies among the US states.

Slovenko[237] estimates that about one-third of the states today have developed a diminished capacity concept to address criminal misconduct. The idea is a bundle of confusion, defined in subtly different ways in different jurisdictions, and placed within a stew of other, related concepts like 'partial *mens rea*' and 'diminished responsibility'. The precise definition of diminished capacity is elusive; Slovenko argues that it refers to whether the offender had a 'specific intent' to commit the crime. The general idea of diminished capacity/responsibility can perhaps be conveyed most simply by saying that these concepts render the 'old' insanity defense from an either/or distinction (the defendant either is, or is not, culpable) to a graded, dimensional judgment (culpability extends across a continuum; the defendant could have limited or partial responsibility). As might be suspected, these 'diminished' concepts are not only used for determination of guilt, but also in sentencing considerations as well. In addition to jurisdictional variability, these criminal excuses open the door for all kinds of potential abuses, where any stressor, however trivial or idiosyncratic, could be used to excuse a defendant.

An important historical effect of these variations on criminal excuse has been to widen the gap between courtroom determinations of mental disorder and clinical determinations of mental disorder. Psychiatrists such as Bernard Diamond labored throughout their careers to establish psychiatrists as the determinants of criminal excuse, viewing *mens rea* as a continuum concept requiring psychiatric expertise to place a particular defendant on the scale.[238] Defense lawyers in response have contrived strategically formulated mental conditions or defects; ranging from 'rotten social background' to 'Black rage' as criminal excuses.[239] The issue of criminal excuse became symptomatic of a larger conflict within society, whether offenders should be held responsible for their individual behavior, or whether their health, social situation, cultural context, and environmental privations (e.g., the consequences of imperfect societies) should be 'blamed' instead. Or, if 'blame' is an appropriate response to the problem of crime at all.

5.8 The role of classification and early psychiatric diagnostic concepts

As noted earlier, the developing United States had to contend with sorting out different stripes of the socially marginal and deviant, and with the breakdown of family and small-community care, the need arose to develop institutions that provided containment and care.

5.8.1 Early classification and the parsing of services for social deviance

The classification of mental disorders or 'insanity', at least at the beginning of the modern era, is linked with the development of biological taxonomy and the general medical attempts at systematization of kinds of disease.[240] Only a few examples are feasible to mention here. Early nosologists like Thomas Sydenham (1624–1689) were wary of speculative theorizing about diseases, and instead, prophetically for the DSMs, relied upon close observation of symptom clusters—syndromes—and tracked their courses over time, building a case for commonalities of related syndromes with uniform courses. The physician and biologist Boissier de Sauvages pursued the classification of diseases as species-like taxons, as in biology, and Wallace[241] notes that while mental disorder-like syndromes were scattered throughout Boissier's (1731) 2400 diseases, melancholia alone exhibited 14 species by itself! Inspired by Boissier, Linnaeus expanded the former's 10 classes and 295 genera to the latter's 11 classes and 325 genera. The lure of taxonomic proliferation has been discussed in previous sections, and will be again, explicitly in the section on the 'monomanias' below.

5.8.2 Moral insanity

The notion of moral insanity seems to have hatched more or less within a few decades on both sides of the Atlantic, at least considering the slow timescale of international communications of the day. The concept seems to have developed in a series of successive approximations, while ultimately presenting more of a Wittgensteinian family resemblance concept than a sharply defined taxon. William Cullen, the Scottish Professor of Medicine at Glasgow, articulated his idea of a 'partial insanity' in his *Nosology* of 1772, with melancholia his paradigm for an insanity which primarily affected the emotions.[242] Another Scot, Thomas Arnold, articulated an early formal classification of madness in 1782, *Observations on the Nature, Kinds, Causes, and Prevention of Insanity, Lunacy, or Madness*, which divided insanity into two broad categories: Ideal Insanity, a hallucinatory psychosis, and Notional Insanity, as a condition characterized by irrational beliefs (at least including delusions, and perhaps *idee fixe* as well), in the presence of a reality-based sensorium and perceptual abilities. Notional insanities were subdivided into Fanciful, Whimsical, Impulsive, Scheming, Vain, Hypochondriacal, Pathetic, and Appetitive, reflective of their various prevailing clinical pictures,[243] with Impulsive and Appetitive being the most 'vice-laden' of them. As mentioned earlier, Pinel in 1798 articulated his own version of a partial insanity, *manie sans délire*, a concept to be at first rejected and later reformulated and expanded into 'monomania(s)' by his student Esquirol.

Operating at the time in relative isolation from colleagues in Europe, but certainly influenced by Pinel and Cullen, Benjamin Rush presented his lecture, *An Inquiry into the Influence of Physical Causes Upon the Moral Faculty* to the American Philosophical Society in 1786, which clearly redefined the older and broader psycho-emotional concept of 'moral' into its more contemporary meaning, mentioned earlier in Chapter 4:[244]

> By the moral faculty I mean a capacity in the human mind of distinguishing and choosing good and evil, or, in other words, virtue and vice. It is a native principle, and though it be capable of improvement by experience and reflection, it is not derived from either of them.

Rush's brief work discusses the medical, religious, and political aspects of 'the moral faculty' as well as elements of a moral psychology; a fascinating paper by a man who earned his place in American history as an alienist, as well as a political and religious leader. Rush sketches out the clinical contexts where the moral faculty is disrupted, ranging from the swearings of a clergyman in a fit of feverish delirium, to a condition suggestive of contemporary Kleptomania:[245]

> Do we ever observe a partial insanity, or false perception on one subject, while the judgment is sound and correct, upon all others? We perceive, in some instances, a similar defect in the moral faculty. There are persons who are moral in the highest degree as to certain duties, who nevertheless live under the influence of some one vice. I knew an instance of a woman, who was exemplary in her obedience to every command of the moral law, except one. She could not refrain from stealing. What made this vice the more remarkable was, that she was in easy circumstances, and not addicted to extravagance in any thing. Such was her propensity to this vice, that when she could lay her hands upon nothing more valuable, she would often, at the table of a friend, fill her pockets secretly with bread. As a proof that her judgment was not affected by this defect in her moral faculty, she would both confess and lament her crime, when detected in it.

Rush reiterates the distinction between partial and perfect or ideal insanity, in that the former judgment and understanding are preserved, while approximating the Freudian version of the neurosis concept—repetitive maladaptive acts recognized as such, yet are experienced as beyond the person's control. (See section below on disorders of the 'will.') From the beginnings of American psychiatry, Dr. Rush declared the moral faculty as under the domain of medical science.

His concluding oratory describes a vision of moral improvement approaching perfection, based upon the sciences and humanities, and at least a partial medicalization of morality:[246]

> Witness the many hundred people who have lately been brought back to life, by the successful efforts of the humane societies, which are now established in many parts of Europe, and in some parts of America. Should the same industry and ingenuity, which have produced these triumphs of medicine over disease and death, be applied to the moral science, it is highly probable, that most of those baneful vices, which deform the human breast, and convulse the nations of the earth, might be banished from the world. I am not so sanguine as to suppose, that it is possible for man to acquire so much perfection from science, religion, liberty, and good government, as to cease to be mortal; but I am fully persuaded, that from the combined action of causes, which operate once upon the reason, the moral faculty, the passions, the senses, the brain, the nerves, the blood and the heart, it is possible to produce such a change in his moral character, as shall raise him to a resemblance of angels—nay more, to the likeness of God himself.

The resemblance of this vision to contemporary 'transhumanism' is striking, except for Rush's implication that such an approximation of human perfection requires a unified effort among science, religion, and a politically good society. Apparently, science alone was not enough.

The moral insanity idea was also influential to the phrenologists Gall and Spurzheim (*Observations of the Deranged Manifestations of the Mind or Insanity* (1817)[247]). While the notion of cranial bumps as locators of brain functions is laughable today, their core idea of brain localization of function has endured, albeit in a more complex and sophisticated way. They divided the brain into (ultimately) 35 organs with their associated functions, fashioning an 'organology' which included vice-laden functions such as 'destructiveness', influencing degenerationists and Cesare Lombroso's later 'criminal anthropology'.

With the conceptual stage set by partial insanity, monomanias (discussed below), and Western psychopathology converging around concepts of mental faculties—cognition, affection (emotions), Rushian moral, and conation (will, motivation), someone in the English-speaking world needed to elaborate and differentiate the concept of moral insanity. This task was taken up by James Cowles Prichard (1786–1848), an English physician whose influential taxonomy *A Treatise on Insanity* (1835) popularized the moral insanity group of disorders for an Anglo-American audience. Hunter and MacAlpine[248] remark that Prichard resisted the reformulation of moral insanity into a perhaps equally vague and mutating concept—psychopathy—but Prichard probably didn't live long enough to resist the latter's prevailing success.

Moreover, Hunter and MacAlpine remark upon early forensic concepts of partial responsibility and irresistible impulse in Prichard's work.

The core of Prichard's concept is described as:

> This form of mental derangement has been described as consisting in a morbid perversion of the feelings, affections, and active powers, without any illusion on erroneous conviction impressed upon the understanding: it sometimes co-exists with an apparently unimpaired state of the intellectual faculties.[249]

For Prichard moral insanity was a polymorphous phenomenon: 'In fact, the varieties of moral insanity are perhaps as numerous as the modifications of feeling or passion in the human mind.'[250] Melancholia was clearly the most common form of moral insanity, and his inclusion of a variety of emotional states returns Prichard's notion of 'moral' to the broader psycho-emotional sense, in contrast to Rush's more contemporary sense. Nevertheless, Prichard certainly includes vice-laden disorders under the moral insanity umbrella:[251]

> One of the most striking of these forms is distinguished by an unusual prevalence of angry and malicious feelings; which arise without provocation or any of the ordinary incitements. All the examples of madness without delirium reported by Pinel belong to this class of disorders. . . . There are instances of insanity in which the whole disease, or at least the whole of its manifestations, has consisted in a liability to violent fits of anger breaking out without cause. . . . When the morbid phenomena include merely the expressions of intense malevolence, without ground or provocation actual or supposed, the case is strictly one of the nature above described.

This variety of moral insanity is suggestive of 'homicidal insanity' to be discussed below, and points toward contemporary notions of psychopathy as well as DSM-5 Intermittent Explosive Disorder. Isaac Ray's notion of moral mania has already been discussed as his version of moral insanity.

By mid-nineteenth century, the encompassing and ill-defined qualities of the moral insanity concept led to its abandonment by the Brits, to new formulations and differentiation, despite influential advocates like Henry Maudsley.[252] In their concluding comments about the fate of moral insanity, Hunter and MacAlpine saddle Prichard with some of the blame for founding one of psychiatry's perennial problems, that of imprecise disorder concepts used differently by different clinicians: 'To some extent therefore Prichard was also responsible for rendering acute psychiatry's besetting problem of semantics which allows the same terms to be used with different meanings by some, while others use different ones to mean the same.'[253] The elaborations of moral insanity provided in France by Esquirol will be covered in more detail in the section on monomanias below. However, the fall of the moral insanity concept was delayed in the United States. Norman Dain[254] argues that the monomania concept was widely accepted by pre–Civil War psychiatrists, including such leaders as Amariah Brigham, Pliny Earle, and Samuel B. Woodward.

One of the derivatives of the moral insanity concept was the concept of 'psychopathy', which, while probably equally guilty of the sins of the moral insanity concept, has managed to survive, and even enjoy a renaissance of research interest into the present day.

Millon et al.[255] trace the development of the psychopathy concept. Leaving the British and Americans to their squabbles about morality, the empirically oriented German psychiatrists such as J. L. Koch rejected the term 'moral insanity' preferring the perhaps less vice-laden but no less value-laden concept 'psychopathic inferiority'. Koch's concept, however, was more etiological than clinically descriptive; it largely referred to constitutional failures of biological function and had an equally diverse phenomenological range. The psychopathic inferiority term was imported into the United States by Adolf Meyer at the turn of the twentieth century, where Meyer ultimately dropped the 'inferiority' portion as too judgmental, and rejected the explicit constitutional etiological implications, favoring more psychosocial connotations for the resulting term, 'psychopathy' and 'psychopathic'. Readers will recall that Meyer's term for the new outpatient-oriented clinics and hospitals used 'psychopathic' as their general descriptors for what today we would term 'psychopathological' (e.g., having to do with mental disorders in general). Millon and colleagues attribute the development of the more contemporary sense of psychopathy to Emil Kraepelin's use and redefinition of the term over the many editions of his textbooks of psychiatry. They note by 1904 Kraepelin had four categories of antisocial, vice-laden conditions: morbid liars and swindlers, criminals by impulse, professional criminals, and morbid vagabonds. Kraepelin continued to revise his vice-laden conditions into the 8th edition of his text. Millon et al summarize these categories:[256]

> He separated them into two broad varieties: those of morbid disposition, consisting of obsessives, impulsives, and sexual deviants; and those exhibiting personality peculiarities. The latter group was differentiated into seven classes: the excitable (*Erregbaren*), the unstable (*Haltlosen*), the impulsive (*Triebmenschen*), the eccentric (*Verschobenen*), the liars and swindlers (*Luegner unde Schwindler*), the antisocial (*Gesellschaftsfeinde*), and the quarrelsome (*Streitsuechtige*). Only the latter three possessed features similar to current notions of the antisocial.

The authors link the antisocial concept in youth to the later development of Conduct Disorder in DSM-III. Indeed, given Millon's influential role in DSM-III through IV, and the open 'Neo- Kraepelinian' orientation of many of the DSM-III architects,[257] one can suspect a number of proto-DSM, vice-laden categories from this short passage. They attribute the genesis of the term 'sociopathic' to Birnbaum in the early twentieth century, which challenged the constitutionalism of prior terms, suggesting that social/environmental factors could be important—influencing American psychiatry through such authors as our previously mentioned William Healy and

A. Bronner[258] and G. E. Partridge.[259] They note that the early twentieth-century German psychiatrist Kurt Schneider distinguished two kinds of psychopathic youth, one more constitutional and incorrigible, the other more acquired and potentially more manageable; also suggesting the taxonomic relevance of an aggressive/nonaggressive distinction. Multiple psychoanalytic theorists, including Freud, consider antisocial/psychopathic conduct, with Franz Alexander distinguishing antisocial 'neurotic character' from 'true criminality' in the early 1930s.[260] Hervey Cleckley, however, through his detailed clinical description of a vice-laden psychopathy concept, through multiple editions of his book *The Mask of Sanity*, popularized the more contemporary psychopathy concept. Cleckley influenced psychologist Robert Hare in the late-twentieth century to develop his theory and empirical measurement of psychopathy, the Psychopathy Check List, into perhaps the most scientifically robust construct for psychopathy today.[261] Cleckley in his Fifth Edition identified 16 core clinical features for his description of psychopathy:[262]

1. Superficial charm and good 'intelligence'.
2. Absence of delusions and other signs of irrational thinking.
3. Absence of 'nervousness' or psychoneurotic manifestations.
4. Unreliability.
5. Untruthfulness and insincerity.
6. Lack of remorse or shame.
7. Inadequately motivated antisocial behavior.
8. Poor judgment and failure to learn by experience.
9. Pathologic egocentricity and incapacity for love.
10. General poverty in major affective reactions.
11. Specific loss of insight.
12. Unresponsiveness in general interpersonal relations.
13. Fantastic and uninviting behavior with drink and sometimes without.
14. Suicide rarely carried out.
15. Sex life impersonal, trivial, and poorly integrated.
16. Failure to follow any life plan.

The split between 'psychopathy' and 'sociopathy', however, was to linger into the present with various versions of Antisocial Personality Disorder appearing in the late-vintage DSMs,[263] a matter discussed in earlier chapters and to be discussed again in later ones.

5.8.3 Monomanias

The role of Jean Etienne Dominique Esquirol (1772–1840) has been discussed earlier in the context of the development of psychopathology-as-science, as well as the development of French (as well as Anglo-American) forensic psychiatry. A clinical contribution for which he is noted, and of particular interest to the VMDR, is the concept of monomania. Noted earlier was Esquirol's insight that monomania was a partial insanity that was based upon a single defect in intellect, emotion, or will.[264] Monomania was differentiated from 'lypemania' for Esquirol; the latter being his preferred term for melancholia. For the intellectual form of monomania, Esquirol describes it as:[265]

> ... confined to a single object, or a limited number of objects. The patients seize upon a false principle, which they pursue without deviating from logical reasonings, and from which they deduce legitimate consequences, which modify their affections, and the acts of their will.

For the emotional or 'affective' form:[266]

> ... the monomaniacal are not deprived of the use of their reason, but their affections and dispositions are perverted. By plausible motives, by very reasonable explanations, they justify the actual condition of their sentiments, and excuse the strangeness and inconsistency of their conduct.

For the form based upon a disorder of will:[267]

> In a third class of cases, a lesion of the will exists. The patient is drawn away from his accustomed course, to the commission of acts, to which neither reason nor sentiment determine, which conscience rebukes, and which the will has no longer the power to restrain. The actions are involuntary, instinctive, irresistible. This is monomania without delirium, or instinctive monomania.

These superordinate classes of monomania then generated subcategorized disorders built around the prevailing phenomenological themes encountered. In his *Mental Maladies: A Treatise on Insanity* textbook, Esquirol gives special attention to Erotic Monomania (which was to be distinguished from nymphomania and satyriasis); Reasoning Monomania; Monomania from Drunkenness; Incendiary Monomania (pyromania); and finally Homicidal Monomania. Esquirol's students and elaborators were to create countless other categories.

Some brief discussion of Esquirol's categories is warranted. In the case of Erotic Monomania, or 'erotomania',[268] the condition is described as a disorder of the 'imagination', where not lust but 'chaste and honorable' desire of the heart characterizes the patient's imagined ardor for a person little known to the patient. For Reasoning Monomania, a previously amiable and socially integrated individual becomes irascible, contrary, hostile, even violent to others. Sunny dispositions turn sour, and fastidiousness converts into slovenliness, all with no defect in reasoning. 'The signs of reasoning monomania, consist in the change and perversion of the habits, disposition and affections.'[269] These monomaniacs have only a limited disturbance of the understanding, 'since it assists in the acts of the insane person'.[270] For Monomania Resulting from Drunkenness, Esquirol describes the ubiquity of use of alcoholic beverages, but notes a minority of individuals develop 'strong desires' for drink such that irrational and self-destructive acts will be involved in securing them. He notes episodes of drunkenness characterizing this behavior, suggesting today's 'binges', and the preservation of reason between episodes. For the last, Homicidal Monomania, more discussion follows in the later section, but for Esquirol's part, he linked this disorder to Pinel's *manie sans délire*, and specified it as an instinctual, involuntary fury, essentially unpredictable and unjustifiable through reason. The social historian Patrick Singy emphasizes the role of instinct in the Homicidal Monomania (and paraphilic) disorders,[271] as does Michel Foucault in *Abnormal*.[272] Esquirol writes:[273]

> These maniacs perceived, compare, and judge correctly; but they are drawn aside, from the slightest cause, and even without an object, to the commission of acts of violence and fury. They are irresistibly impelled, they assure us, to lacerate and injure themselves, and destroy their fellow-beings. These wretched persons have a consciousness of their condition, deplore their situation, warn their friends to protect themselves against their fury, or place them where they can do no harm.

Goldstein[274] describes in detail the crucial role that Esquirol's monomania concept had on the development of French forensic psychiatry. As mentioned earlier in the section on the development of the insanity defense, prior to Esquirol, alienist testimony was rarely needed in the courts; insanity was recognized by public and professionals alike as a global phenomenon affecting all mental functions—'total insanity' or 'delirium'. Recognizing the lunatic as such was not a subtle determination, but well within the ken of the public; indeed, most anyone could recognize, and had recognized in life experience, the mad. With the introduction of monomanias, Esquirol presented a persuasive argument that alienist expertise was required to discern criminal offenders who were in thrall to disorders that preserved reason yet were associated with all manner of bizarre beliefs and antisocial conduct. The monomanias were crucial to the historical development of psychiatric testimony because they shifted the center of forensic gravity away from public appraisals of madness to professional ones.

Esquirol's ideas spread quickly to both sides of the Atlantic; probably facilitated by others' formulations of partial insanity and moral insanity. Hunter and MacAlpine[275] alone link nine different English-speaking-world authors (Gall, Spurzheim, Esquirol (in translation), Morison, Combe, Prichard, Millingen, Henry Johnson, and Robertson) to the monomania concept. Isaac Ray's *Treatise on the Medical Jurisprudence of Insanity* draws extensively from Esquirol's writings; making them crucial to the understanding of formative American notions of the VMDR.

Ray provides an extensive discussion of monomanias in his *Treatise*. Some in-stances of monomania strike the contemporary reader as instances of somatic delusions:[276]

> The most simple form of this disorder is that in which the patient has imbibed some single notion contradictory to common sense and to his own experience, and which seems, and sometimes no doubt really is, dependent on errors of sensation. Thus, thousands have be-lieved their legs were made of glass, or that snakes, fish, or eels had taken up their abode in their stomach or bowels. In many such cases the hallucination is excited by and main-tained by impressions propagated from diseased parts, the presence of which has been revealed by dissection after death.

Another type resembles a contemporary systematized delusion:[277]

> . . . The patient imbibes some notion connected with the various relations of persons, events, time, space, resistance &c. of the most absurd and unfounded nature, and en-deavors, in some measure to regulate his conduct accordingly . . . and [Rush] speaks of a judge who was rational on the bench, but constantly insane when off it.

A key feature for Ray was the preservation of the 'understanding':[278]

> The operations of the understanding, even on subjects connected with the insane belief, are sometimes not impaired in an appreciable degree; on the contrary, we are occasionally struck with the acuteness of the reasoning power displayed by monomaniacs.

Ray notes more complex cases exist, requiring clinical skills to detect and elucidate:[279]

> . . . that although the patient may reason on many subjects unconnected with the partic-ular illusion on which the insanity turns, the understanding is more extensively deranged, than is generally suspected . . . it is not necessary to insist on the importance of this fact in estimating the degree of criminal responsibility remaining in monomaniacs.

Historians Lynn Gamwell and Nancy Tomes note the importance of moral insanity and monomania to mid-nineteenth-century American psychiatrists, linking mono-mania to the Melville's literary classic *Moby Dick*, where the master sailor Ahab loses his reason in face of the white whale.[280] Gamwell and Tomes provide powerful evi-dence of the early politicization of monomania in antebellum America, noting that the White abolitionist John Brown was considered a monomaniac by none other than Henry A. Wise, then Governor of Virginia.[281]

The politicization of monomania in the United States is perhaps best illustrated by a perennial favorite example of philosophers of medicine, 'draepetomania', a dis-order described by Louisiana physician Samuel Cartwright in 1851.[282] This brand of monomania described slaves who persistently tried to flee their masters. This case serves as benchmark in the role of shifting social values in defining psychopathology, and the abuse of diagnostic categories to perpetuate political concerns—in this case, slavery and White supremacy.

By the mid-nineteenth century the French enthusiasm for monomania faded, and outright efforts to reject the term proliferated.[283] An important lesson for the VMDR is understanding the reasons why monomania fell out of favor. We earlier noted that by midcentury Esquirol's mission to legitimize forensic psychiatry had largely been accomplished; monomania was no longer needed by the profession to legitimize psychiatric forensic expertise.[284] The courts in Europe and the United States persistently had difficulty accepting the concept, seeing it as too generous in excusing criminals. Emerging French nosologists such as Falret and Morel were reformulating their own concepts of moral disorders—the latter popularizing the notion of 'degeneration' to be discussed shortly. Psychiatrists on both sides of the Atlantic complained about the imprecision and vagueness of the monomania concept, and began to refute the preservation of reason, finding that careful and sustained examination revealed loopholes and gaps in the reasoning process.[285] Clinicians reformulated single-symptom disorders in reference to their particular phenomenologies, as will be highlighted below in the discussion of Krafft-Ebing's sexual perversions (paraphilias). The nineteenth-century nosological master, at least in contemporary American eyes, Emil Kraepelin, by his 1901 edition only mentioned monomania in passing, in reference to 'progressive systematized insanity', a concept preserved today in the form of DSM Delusional Disorder.[286]

By the end of the Civil War era in the United States, enthusiasm in the United States and UK had faded as well.[287] By 1916 Bernard Glueck's *Studies in Forensic Psychiatry*[288] only mentions monomania in the context of quoting a patient; signaling the emergence of the term in popular language, where it resides today.

Why have kleptomania, trichotillomania, and pyromania persisted in contemporary diagnosis? The literature that addresses this question is quite limited. One reason may involve how the diagnosis served one or more social functions. In the case of kleptomania, historians have noted its importance in the gender politics of the time; late-nineteenth and early twentieth-century notions about the inferiority of women prevailed in the context of repressive Victorian sexuality and 'hysteria'. Moreover, the new bourgeois role of women as shoppers for the household provided a context for neurotic psychopathology to manifest.[289] O'Brien[290] notes that kleptomania served as an explanation for the incomprehensible needless shoplifting that too many middle-class women indulged in; the social mores of the time would not permit well-bred middle-class women to be simple criminals, at least on the scale that was witnessed. O'Brien also notes that the target symptom of shoplifting disguised the shame of the Dickensian domestic problems (alcoholism, domestic violence) that were the dirty secret of the *fin de siécle* middle class. The 16 January

1897 issue of the *British Medical Journal* remarks upon the ubiquity of shoplifting.[291] Abelson[292] summarized these points neatly:

> Had shoplifting, defined as a form of female delinquency, not been interpreted as illness, it would have to have been understood as crime, and the possibility that respectable, middle-class women could 'sink into such a moral cesspool and forefeit [sic] the esteem and love of their best friends for a bottle of cosmetic' was unthinkable.

In the case of pyromania, Geller, Erlen, and Pinkus[293] locate the concept's American debut with the previously discussed *Treatise on the Medical Jurisprudence of Insanity* (1844) by Isaac Ray. They detail how pyromania became wrapped up in the disputes over the validity of monomania in mid-nineteenth century. They note that the influential nineteenth-century American psychiatrist John Gray was especially critical of the concept, in that he wanted to reject the notion of diseases of the mind altogether, a wish that Hunter and MacAlpine[294] note was likely due to his firm Christian beliefs in the immortality of the soul/mind. Geller et al. link criticism of pyromania to the general backlash against the insanity defense prompted by Charles Guiteau's assassination of President Garfield. For Guiteau, the insanity defense failed despite clear-cut, crime-relevant delusions in the defendant. The anti-pyromania tide began to turn after the turn of the century when Kraepelin included pyromania in his later textbooks. From the psychoanalytic front, Stekel wrote an influential paper on the 'sexual root' of pyromania,[295] not to overlook interest by Freud himself.[296] Debate about the legitimacy of the disorder, however, persisted well into mid-twentieth century. As a counterpoint to kleptomania, Geller and colleagues note the prevailing prevalence of pyromania in boys. The authors note that pyromania is absent as a unique condition in DSM-I and II; only by DSM-III does the name and disorder re-emerge. The reasons for this reappearance of pyromania in DSM-III is curiously absent in this otherwise excellent review. They conclude by suggesting that pyromania has persisted, despite significant nosological and phenomenological confounders, because it is emblematic of 'each generation's struggle with the definition of personal accountability'.[297]

5.8.4 Degeneracy theory and criminal anthropology

The mid-nineteenth and early twentieth centuries saw the influence of two scientific movements which profoundly contributed to the merging of the medical, the moral, and the criminal. Both resonate into the present. The earlier trend, variously referred to as degeneration theory or degeneracy, was pioneered by Benedict-Augustin Morel, a nineteenth-century French alienist whose views on the origins of such conditions as dementia praecox, prostitution, and criminality bridged the old worldview of religion and the new worldview of science. The idea of degeneration was that moral misbehavior, or indulgence in sins such as adultery, inebriation, crime, and masturbation, damaged the 'germ plasm'—the stuff of heredity—contributing to further impairment and misconduct in later generations, deteriorating into madness, idiocy, and depravity. Liégeois[298] notes that Morel's ideas emerged both from the notion of original sin and the emerging idea of a primitive man created by God that faith and good moral conduct had elevated over the centuries. Degeneration, however, represented both the consequences of sin and their biological sequelae, leading to compromised, 'primitive' families such as the Jukes discussed earlier in this chapter. However, there was hope for families afflicted with degeneracy. Moral, righteous conduct could diminish the degenerate traits and families could be made whole again over only a few generations. Degeneracy theory dovetailed nicely with the eugenic theories gaining hold in Europe and the United States, and as noted earlier in the section on idiocy, the theory provided a basis for understanding, as well as segregating, idiots from each other for fear of continuing a downhill hereditary course.

Degeneracy theory fed into medical theories of idiocy in the United States, contributing to the idea of the moral imbecile within the scope of today's 'intellectual disability' concept. Criminological historian Nicole Rafter notes that degeneracy provided the theoretical basis for the idea of 'born criminals' which could be discriminated from law-abiding citizens on a biological basis.[299] Already noted in Isaac Ray's work, degeneracy theory proved influential in the emerging American prisons, promulgated by leaders such as Zebulon Brockway, superintendent of the Elmira Reformatory; Isaac Kerlin, founder of the Pennsylvania Institution for the Feeble-Minded, and Richard Dugdale, author of *The Jukes: A Study in Crime, Pauperism, Disease and Heredity*. Rather than condemning degenerates to hopelessness, degeneracy theory provided support for reform efforts through the idea of passing on positive traits to the next generation, indeed, suggesting that crime could be eliminated by reformatory, moral discipline, and good breeding.[300] These mid-nineteenth-century psychiatrists were very much in the mode of 'medicalizing' criminality.

The other trend, criminal anthropology, is associated with the work of Italian physician Cesare Lombroso, whose 'Criminal Anthropology' is often attributed as the founding of criminology as a distinctive domain in science.[301] Lombroso's work was radical in the sense that it moved the understanding of crime out of the realm of the moral-religious, and into the realm of observational science, data collection, and analysis, even using control groups (albeit without randomization!). Lombroso authored monographs on male and female criminal types, partly inspired by phrenology, but associated with collections of facial and body metrics of criminals. These included the size of the cranial vault, the proportionate length of arms, facial asymmetry, the shape of the jaw, and the sloping forehead, as examples of criminal morphology. Lombroso referred to these changes as 'atavisms' and considered these as physical traces of the effects of degeneracy, traces which could be captured and quantified by science. Today we can recognize the derivatives of his vision, such as criminal profiling (as well as a morally corrupt racial profiling) and biocriminological techniques such as fingerprinting and DNA analysis. However, Lombroso's science was primitive by today's standards, and his influence was less evident in Europe than it was in the United States, where he and his student, Enrico Ferri,[302] collected numerous and influential adherents who elaborated their theories.[303] The combination of criminal types with degeneration then had implications for the emerging penal systems, concerns about moral imbecility, heredity, and eugenics. Lombroso himself viewed both biological/constitutional factors and social factors as important in the genesis of crime; the 'criminaloid' was an occasional offender particularly susceptible to adverse social conditions as well as reform.[304]

In a fascinating paper published posthumously by his daughter Gina Lombroso-Ferrero in 1912, Cesare Lombroso speculated upon 'Crime and Insanity in the Twenty-First Century'. Noting that insanity was proliferating at the time in Europe, Lombroso predicted that insanity will only increase in the next (twenty-first) century. He identifies the disproportionate increases in insanity to worsening of the world-wide drug abuse problem, and notably, the collusion of the medical profession:[305]

> This [increase in insanity] is bound to happen everywhere, for the causes responsible for the plague are increasing in number and intensity. South America exports mate and cocoa. The Orient uses its opium and haschich, Northern Europe introduces into the South its beer and whisky, while the South sends north its spoiled maize; each one of these products being responsible for numerous deadly brain poisonings. Deadly also are the ether, the morphine, and the codein, which under the guise of medicine, given at the hospitals, proceed to disturb the peaceful home of the citizen and lay snares for his mind in the same way as has been done for centuries by wine....

Regarding crime, he is more optimistic, predicting a dramatic decrease through the 'lifelong confinement of incorrigibles', and the 'seclusion of insane criminals in an insane asylum'.[306] He predicts:[307]

> The coming century will provide on a large scale agricultural colonies for abandoned and neglected children, shelters for the unemployed and vagrants, decent shows at a reasonable price for the frequenters of saloons, and will introduce fines, warnings by the judge, work in the open air, shower baths, confinement in the home in place of the degrading prisons, which tend to increase crime instead of making it rarer.

Through today's eyes, Lombroso's predictions are both naive on some points and uncannily astute on others. Lombroso points toward the emerging Progressive reforms in considering the penology of the future:[308]

> And it will be shown to the criminaloid, and to the criminal moved by passion, that, nothing is done to curb him, but everything is done for his good. When they feel that their own personality is no longer crushed, and see that they are directed to some useful occupation, treated like human beings, and not like slaves under a convict number, the prison discipline will not only improve, but the case of backsliders will very much decrease.

5.8.5 Disorders of the will

While scholars as diverse as the historian of psychiatry German Berrios (1996) to the philosopher Sarah Stroud (writing in the *Stanford Encyclopedia of Philosophy*) are consistent in their describing the marginal status of 'the will' in conceptions in psychiatry and moral psychology,[309] a quick review here will, I hope, convince readers that this dismissal is less strong than suggested by Berrios. True, the 'will' is a feebly represented term in contemporary neuroscience or psychiatry; but its family of *concepts* lives on, providing the same stumbling blocks to understanding the relationship between thought and action that have been present from its beginnings. The centuries, in the meantime, have introduced many related terms of uncertain metaphysical status: desire, appetite, volition, conation, motivation, drive, impulse, and goal-directedness, to name a few.

What anyone means by 'the will' is very much still a focus of the debate. Thomas Pink, writing in *The Routledge Encyclopedia of Philosophy* defines it as:[310]

> As traditionally conceived, the will is the faculty of choice or decision, by which we determine which actions we shall perform. As a faculty of decision, the will is naturally seen as the point at which we exercise our freedom of action—our control of how we act.

In ordinary discourse, the will is very much alive, in our concern for the 'will of the people', considering the ramifications of 'free will', or appealing to 'God's will', to name a few examples. Berrios does identify a psychopathology-specific problem, however:[311]

> At the end of the nineteenth century, it [the will] came under attack. 'the domain of the voluntary, *reified under the name of will* in popular language was adopted by the primitive psychology of faculties' [italics mine]. Experimentalism, psychoanalysis, and behaviourism accelerated its fall, and by the end of the First World War, the will was no longer a fashionable concept. This created a conceptual vacuum in the 'domain of the voluntary' which has since been unsatisfactorily filled by notions such as 'instinct', 'drive', 'motivation', 'decision-making', and 'frontal lobe executive'.

As a consequence, the will was sectioned, partitioned, redefined, blended, and swallowed up by new sciences, theories, and philosophies, and disorders of will faded in psychiatric discourse after the nineteenth century, and the family of related concepts like drive, instinct, volition, motivation, and conation occupied empirical and philosophical psychology.

In the philosophical traditions, the Greeks addressed the will, albeit in indirect ways through concepts like *akrasia*, or 'weakness of will', which described the problem of a person choosing an alternative action over the best possible action, with all things considered.[312] Such seemingly irrational action demanded understanding, and the debate continues into the present. St. Augustine identified the will as an executive faculty oriented toward the carrying out of sin or virtue, and St. Thomas Aquinas identified the will as a distinct faculty.[313]

By the end of the eighteenth century the notion of the will as a psychological faculty, with diverse variations, consolidated it alongside the faculties of intellect/cognition and affection/emotion, promulgated by modern-philosophical luminaries like Locke, Condillac, and Kant. The eighteenth-century 'common-sense' philosopher Thomas Reid sketched out the component features of the will:[314]

> Reid advised that the defining features of the will should be obtained from introspective analysis: (*a*) every act of will must have an object, (*b*) this must be some action of our own, (*c*) it must be believed to be within our power, (*d*) 'volition is accompanied with an effort to execute that which we willed', and (*e*) there must be something 'in the preceding state of the mind that disposes or inclines us to the determination'.

Reid's work allows us to detect many of the sources of philosophical objection and revision to the will concept: feelings or emotions for (e), intentionality for (a), with concepts like motivation, drive, and volition, scattered among (b) through (e), depending upon the theorist.

The congealing of the will as a faculty of the mind and part of ordinary explanations of human conduct naturally led to its assimilation into nineteenth-century psychopathology, as did the notion of weakness of will find its way into discussions of criminal/moral responsibility. Berrios[315]notes that psychopathological symptoms like abulia, impulsive dyscontrol, and compulsions were attributed to disorders of the will. As might be expected, Esquirol assimilated a disturbance of the will into various of his monomanias; with lypemania or depression associated with diminished will, while in instinctive monomania the perversion of the will was the core disturbance.[316] Berrios attributes a strong influence to Théodule-Armand Ribot (1839–1916) on the emerging psychology of will. Ribot framed psychopathologies of will as of excess or deficiency; impulsive action or instinctive monomania being examples of the former, and agoraphobia and abulia for the latter. Deviant preoccupations like pyromania or kleptomania were attributed to failures of select intellectual functions in addition to excessive will.[317]

The emerging sciences of physics, chemistry, and to a lesser extent physiology, contributed to the core metaphors associated with the actions of the will, recalling the hydraulics of the id, superego, and ego of Freud, the relation of the neural impulse to the impulsive action, and the notion of desire for Krafft-Ebing's sexual deviations. Patients succumbing to these disorders are cast as failing to resist pressures to act in maladaptive ways. While the attribution of disorders of the will largely disappeared by the twentieth century, the conceptual residuum of will concepts can be found in disorders such as intermittent explosive disorder and the other impulse control disorders, the paraphilias, and perhaps even tic, obsessive-compulsive, and eating disorders. Moreover, the notion of the will still haunts courtroom dramas around the insanity defense, reduced capacity, and irresistible impulse claims.

Berrios laments the passing of the will as a psychological faculty through the substitution of more contemporary, but no less ill-defined, concepts:[318]

The decline of the will left psychiatry without a model to account for the pathology of action. Some of the disorders once associated with the will have been reconceptualized away (e.g., obsessions), others (e.g., impulse) remain unexplained, yet others (e.g., aboulia) have been quietly dropped out of circulation. Categories such as lack of 'motivation' or disorders of 'drive' and 'desire' are not more illuminating than the old term disorder of the will. The fashionable neuropsychological notion of 'frontal lobe executive' is not free from the very same conceptual objection (regression *ad infinitum*) that once was considered as fatal to the concept of the will.

5.8.6 Homicidal insanity and the confounding of psychological faculties

... The frame of reference of the human monster is, of course, law. The notion of the monster is essentially a legal notion, in a broad sense, of course, since what defines the monster is the fact that its existence and form is not only a violation of the laws of society but also a violation of the laws of nature. Its very existence is a breach of the law at both levels. . . . However the monster emerges within this space as both an extreme and an extremely rare phenomenon. The monster is the limit, both the point at which law is overturned and the exception that is found only in extreme cases. The monster combines the impossible and the forbidden.[319]

Foucault's 'monster' has been, perhaps less poetically, described in professional and popular culture as the homicidal maniac, the serial murderer, and the psychopathic killer. While a derivative concept of 'homicidal insanity' does not exist today in official psychiatric taxonomies, for the purposes of this book the notion warrants its own section and treatment for Foucault's reasons as well as several others. As Foucault suggests, the homicidal lunatic as monster poses a challenge to law and psychiatry as well as to public comprehension and apprehension.[320] For law, the homicidal maniac poses a question of distinction from the more-ordinary criminal murderer. For psychiatry, the challenge is to understand and explain human behavior that embodies 'evil' and begs to be understood outside the bounds of naturalistic science. As a murderer without discernable motivation or passion, homicidally insane people raise our darkest doubts about ourselves as we wonder if we too are subject to such dark forces and bloodlust. As (often) neither deliberate nor passionate killers, the homicidal insane pose an enigma for the clinics and the courts because they seem to fit neither the praxis of the court nor the science of psychiatry. As will be shown, homicidal insanity is an excellent center point for discussion of faculty psychology, which emerged in the seventeenth and eighteenth centuries and was consolidated in the nineteenth century up to the present day.[321] As an exemplar category, homicidal insanity poses the metaphysical, scientific, and legal constraints of faculty psychology-based psychopathology. Finally, we'll see that a Foucauldian monster is only part of homicidal mental illness, as a variety of other psychopathologies associated with murder pose a confusing array of phenomena within the VMDR.

The concept of homicidal insanity has not been extensively studied in the history literature, and for this section I am heavily dependent upon Janet Colaizzi's groundbreaking history of American homicidal insanity,[322] as well as Isaac Ray's aforementioned *Treatise* of 1844, which goes into some detail on the problem of homicidal insanity. Providing a succinct summary of the spectrum of terms and phenomenologies of homicidal insanity is quite challenging; the historian Colaizzi resorts to organizing her discussion around a chart presented early in her book, which I have redrawn and updated as Figure 5.1, 'Psychiatric Categories Associated with Homicidal Insanity, 1800–2000'.[323] Colaizzi herself was writing in the mid- to late-1980s and only includes studies through 1985. Curiously, she also ignores the DSMs, which by 1980 were in three editions, with DSM-I appearing decades earlier in 1952. My adaptation and expansion of her graphic and analysis includes considerations up to DSM-IV in 2000 and provides cross-references to faculty psychology metaphysics outside of her three original 'pigeonholes' of Intellectual Insanity, Emotional Insanity, and Volitional Insanity. By the DSM-III era, the intellectual/emotional/volitional vocabularies were still present, though the taxonomic picture was becoming increasingly complex, as DSM diagnostic categories and criteria differentiated, spanning all three of the nineteenth-century faculties. (See Figure 5.1.) Throughout this discussion, the figure will be referred to and elaborated upon.

The notion of homicidal insanity arose in the context of the nineteenth-century discourses on the partial insanities and monomanias which have been discussed above, as well as the historical nomenclature of intellectual disability, most notably moral imbecility, also discussed earlier. As can be seen from Figure 5.1, the problem of mad homicide arose in a variety of clinical contexts and phenomenologies by 1800. For instance, consider the setting of what today would be postpartum psychosis ('puerperal mania'); in the context of Esquirol's instinctive monomanias, with delusions as the primary symptom; in the context of Pinel's *manie sans délire* and what today are still called crimes of passion; as well as through the complications of the more familiar melancholias and manias of the time. By midcentury, American psychiatry was increasingly open to European psychopathology, and in particular the influence of Esquirol in France and Kraepelin in Germany. Kraepelin's textbooks increasingly found their way into translation and influence on American soil, promoted by Adolf Meyer[324] and ultimately well-recognized in US psychiatry by the early twentieth century.[325]

The pre-eminent theorist of homicidal insanity in America, Isaac Ray, summarizes the homicidal insanity nomenclature this way, exhibiting his enthusiasm for Esquirol:[326]

It [homicidal insanity] has received the various appellations of *monomanie-homicide, monomanie-meurtriere, melancholie-homicide, homicidal insanity, instinctive monomanie*. Esquirol, in his valuable memoir published in the shape of a note in the French translation

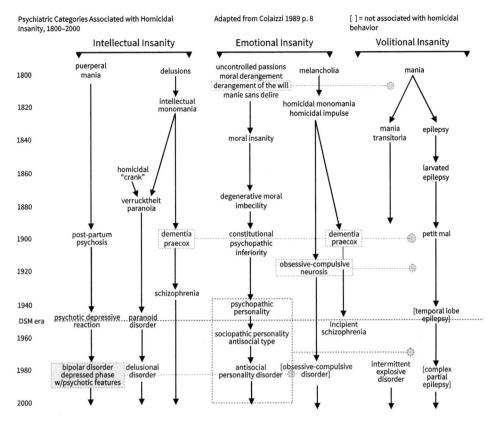

Figure 5.1 'Homicidal Insanity'

of Hoffbauer's work, observers [sic] that homicidal insanity, or *monomanie-homicide*, as he terms it, presents two distinct forms, in the former of which the monomaniac is always influenced by avowed motives more or less irrational, and is generally regarded as mad; in the latter, there are no motives acknowledged, nor to be discerned, the individual being impelled by a blind, irresistible impulse. It is with the latter only that we are concerned, for the other is clearly a form of partial intellectual mania; but as this division has not been strictly made by nature, cases often occurring that do not clearly come under either category, the subject will be better elucidated by noticing all the forms of this affection, and seeing how intimately they are connected together.

Ray distinguishes one kind of homicidal insanity which springs from, for instance, persecutory delusions which provoke the patient to retaliate against his imagined persecutor. The other kind, which Ray advocates as the core homicidal insanity concept, involves the motiveless, impulsive, unpredictable killer who even acknowledges his offense, his wits otherwise fully intact, and exhibits varying degrees of remorse for the lethal actions, from none to substantive remorse. In other words, this second type is a Foucauldian monster. As his cases that follow demonstrate, the cleavage between instinctive-impulsive homicidal insanity and deliberate-delusional cases is not sharp. His case 136 briefly describes the former:[327]

A young lady who had been placed in a *maison de sante*, experience homicidal desires, for which she could assign no motive. She was rational on every subject and whenever she felt the approach of this dreadful propensity, she shed tears, entreated to have the straight-waistcoat put on and to be carefully guarded, till the paroxysm, which sometimes lasted several days, had passed.

Case 143, a Jacques Mounin, had been restrained by his family on account of his numerous acts of 'violence and fury:'[328] but escaped partially clad and took to the fields to escape, leading to a killing spree of victims of chance encounter:[329]

. . . His flight having excited considerable alarm, as after some epileptic attacks he had formerly given many signs of a blind fury . . . On arriving at a field where many laborers were at work at a distance from one another, Mounin first threatened a man who was driving a cart, and immediately after pursued Joseph Faucher and pelted him with stones. The latter having escaped, he then made up to an old man almost blind, named Mayet, whom he knocked down and killed by beating him on the head with a large stone. He next attacked a man who as digging at a little distance, and killed him with a spade. A few minutes afterwards he met Propheti on horseback, whom he struck down with stones, but was obliged to leave him in consequence of the cries of his victim. He then chased some children, who saved themselves by hard running, but he overtook a man at work and slew him. On being questioned during his confinement, Mounin said he well recollected having killed the three men, and especially one, a relative his own, whom he greatly regretted; he added that in his paroxysms of phrensy he saw nothing but flames, and that blood was then most delightful to his sight. At the end of a few days' imprisonment, he seemed to have entirely recovered his reason, but subsequently he relapsed.

Ray recounts Georget's case of Henriette Cornier,[330] the sensational French case previously mentioned by Foucault as a 'monster' exemplar, which further complicates the phenomenology of 'homicidal insanity':[331]

In the month of June, 1825, a singular change was observed in her character; she became silent, melancholy, absorbed in reverie, and finally sank into a kind of stupor. She was dismissed from her place, but her friends could obtain from her no account of the causes of her mental dejection. . . . In the month of September she made an attempt to commit suicide, but was prevented. . . . In the following October she entered into the service of Madame Fournier [who] endeavored in vain to ascertain its [her melancholic disposition's] cause; the girl would talk only of her misfortunes in losing her parents at an early age, and of the bad treatment she received from her guardian . . . [days later] her mistress went out for a walk, having told Cornier to prepare dinner at the usual hours, and to go to a neighboring shop kept by dame Belon, to buy some cheese. She had frequently gone to this shop and had always manifested great fondness for Belon's little girl, a beautiful child nineteen months old. On this day she displayed her usual fondness for it, and persuaded its mother, who at first was rather unwilling, to let her take it out for a walk. Cornier then hastened back to her mistress's house with the child, and laying it across her own bed, severed its head from its body with a large kitchen knife. She subsequently declared that while exacting this horrid deed, she felt no particular emotion—neither of pleasure, nor of pain.

Cornier, when confronted later, tossed the child's head out the window into the street, confessing later the premeditation of persuading dame Belon to 'entrust her with the child'. She provided no reason for the act, that the idea had 'taken possession of her mind' and that she 'was destined to do it'.[332] The first trial was deferred because testimony could neither determine Cornier's sanity or insanity; the second trial found her guilty of 'committing homicide voluntarily but not with premeditation', and she was sentenced to life at hard labor.[333]

Ray's series of homicidal insanity cases concludes with a discussion of the core clinical features. The premier feature is 'the *irresistible, motiveless impulse to destroy life*'.[334] He goes on to describe seven other common features, though these shouldn't be construed to describe all cases, and certainly not contemporized into 'diagnostic criteria': (1) the murderous acts are preceded by various mental changes of a melancholic or manic character; (2) the impulse to destroy is triggered by weapons, favorable circumstances, or some feature of the victim that elicits negative feelings in the offender; (3) the victims are either unknown to the patient or cherished friends or family; (4) most regret their actions, but some express no grief or regret; (5) most confess readily and cooperate with their arrest, but a few flee and deny their act; (6) outside the window of pre- and post-murderous actions, the subjects are rational; and (7) some plead insanity or ignorance of their actions; others claim no mental disturbance; and most acknowledge 'a perturbation of mind'.[335]

To twenty-first-century eyes these descriptions do little to ascertain either diagnosis or criminal responsibility and are so variable to raise the legitimate question of whether 'homicidal insanity' could ever qualify as a taxon of disorder under contemporary diagnostic practice. In foreshadowing Foucault's opening quotation about the challenge of the monster, Ray, however, believed that the homicidal maniac should be acquitted by reason of insanity, and concludes:[336]

When, therefore, as in the case of jurors generally, the mind is not fitted by any of this preparation so necessary to a successful investigation of difficult cases, it seizes only on some of the most obvious though perhaps least important points which they present, and of course the verdict will often be deplorably at variance with the dictates of true science.

The disconnect between criminal responsibility and the utility of diagnosis in this regard will arise in my later deliberations about the VMDR.

A major motif of Colaizzi's work is that the variations of homicidal insanity were driven by the epistemic frames of three mental faculties of: reason/cognition, emotion/affect, and volition/conation. These three faculties served as conceptual frames to organize observations as well as theorizing, an epistemic motif that will be become even more important in the next section which considers the birth of 'sexuality' and sexual perversions.[337] I refer interested readers to Colaizzi's book for her detailed historical discussion. A brief summary of the development of psychopathological concepts associated with murder will suffice for present purposes. As a general comment, over the 200-year period it can be noted that the entire concept of a homicidal monomania was increasingly marginalized as a category unto itself, and the problem of murder by a mentally disordered individual receded from formal classification, along with most all of the other monomanias. The mad killer transitioned from a taxon to a complication of other conditions.

Influenced by Esquirol and like-minded European theorists of partial insanities, two core varieties of intellectual insanity are presented by Colaizzi. The first, no doubt provoked by high-profile murders by young women like Henriette Cornier, was puerperal mania though this variety was of course limited to the postnatal context. Kraepelin had identified a postpartum psychosis in his turn-of-the-century texts, this entity being split later into 'psychotic depressive reaction' in the Adolf Meyer-influenced DSM-I and II, and still later with DSM-III into 'Major Depression with Psychotic Features' and the more contemporary 'Bipolar Disorder, Depressed Phase with Psychotic Features'. The latter was to address contemporary 'homicidal insanity' cases like Texas' Andrea Yates, who drowned her five children in 2001 in a postpartum delusional state.[338] In 1980 the framing of Bipolar Disorder as an 'affective' (and later 'mood') disorder shifted the emphasis of postpartum disorders into the faculty realm of emotion/affection.[339]

The other variety of intellectual insanity emerged from Esquirol's elaboration of delusions. A so-called 'intellectual monomania', was characterized by a relatively systematized delusional system and the absence of disturbances of reason in thought-content domains outside of the particular delusion. By 1880 and the fading of the monomania concept, Kraepelinian influence promulgated the bifurcation of paranoia and dementia praecox, the former resembling the earlier intellectual monomania, delusions with the preservation of reason, and the latter of course being Kraepelin's favored term for the condition(s) we call schizophrenia today. Following Eugen Bleuler's coining of the schizophrenia concept, the latter has gone through revision in the DSM systems, with today's concept largely defined as a chronic, deteriorating condition characterized by a disturbance of thought process, hallucinations, delusions, and 'negative' symptoms like hygienic neglect and lack of motivation. For dementia praecox and the various iterations of 'schizophrenia', homicidality was a peripheral feature or complication of the condition. Regarding paranoia, the condition was considered rare by the turn of the twentieth century and, therefore, infrequently implicated in murder cases. Nevertheless the concept has persisted, with minor variations, into the present, in DSM-I and II as 'Paranoid Disorder' and 'Paranoid State Disorder',[340] and even as a nondelusional 'Paranoid Personality Disorder' in DSM-III forward.[341]

Regarding the development of 'emotional insanity' from the past 2 centuries, murderous behavior within the domain of this faculty was also bifurcated into two sets of rather encompassing and vague threads; one leading to 'moral insanity' later in the nineteenth century, the other encompassed by 1800 as 'melancholia', which at the time was too much of a catch-all term for partial insanities of various phenomenologies.

The development of the concept of moral insanity was characterized by a group of conditions, not all of which constituted a disorder. For instance, the alienists recognized the idea of crimes of passion, and courts then and now contended with this condition as an excusing or mitigating condition in the context of murder.[342] Pinel's concept of *manie sans délire* was coined in reference to criminal offenders, and the idea that some murderous offenders were led by urgent and uncontrollable impulses was recognized. The popularization of the concept of moral insanity by Prichard and others, including Benjamin Rush and Isaac Ray in the United States, made it an influential concept in early American forensic psychiatry, though one which was always controversial, and interwoven with metaphysical and religious issues. The latter is exemplified by the rejection of the concept by John Gray, then-editor of the *American Journal of Insanity* and one of America's most influential nineteenth-century psychiatrists. Gray believed that the concept was poorly sketched and described. Gray's biggest reservation about moral insanity concerned the contradiction the concept posed to his deeply held Christian beliefs in an immortal soul, a soul which could not be polluted by disease, especially a disease that affected the capacity to serve right and wrong. Only the brain could be diseased, and Gray's implicit disjunctive folk metaphysics of soul/mind made a disease of the mind a nonsensical concept, a category error. The ramifications required the rejection of the general notion of a psychological disorder by like-minded Christian alienists.[343] Apparently concepts like moral insanity also combined 'the impossible and the forbidden'!

The notion of moral imbecility was a contemporaneous concept, influenced by Morel's degeneracy theory and Lombroso's notions of born criminals,[344] contributing to public fear of the intellectually impaired. Adolf Meyer, among others, popularized a general notion of 'psychopathic disorders' by the turn of the twentieth century; these conditions referred to a general nonpsychotic disturbance of emotion and conduct. However, not until midcentury with Hervey Cleckley's[345] detailed description of 'psychopathy', as a disorder crystallized in public and professional circles. Cleckley's psychopathy was characterized by shameless criminal offenses; lack of empathy; inability to follow through with responsibilities; a general ease with lying, cheating, and manipulating others; and in some cases, murder and multiple murder. Cleckley's version of the murderous psychopath is exemplified today by figures like Ted Bundy, the young, smart, and handsome law student who killed approximately 30 women in the 1970s[346] with tepid motivations.

By the latter twentieth century and into the twenty-first, the psychopathic concept was refined through the defining research of psychologist Robert D. Hare, who developed a nuanced and psychometrically robust instrument (the Psychopathy Checklist—Revised[347]) that discerned four statistically derived factors in his construct of Psychopathy, not all of which were associated with criminal violence, much less motiveless carnage. Despite widespread use of an instrument that dominated the field of clinical research on psychopathy, Hare's work failed to make a substantive influence on the DSM-III forward. The APA manuals favored a version of psychopathy that emphasized the social/interpersonal aspects of the condition; explicitly emphasizing antisocial and criminal misconduct in its diagnostic criteria.[348] The resulting construct, Antisocial Personality Disorder, remains a more vice-laden construct than the Hare construct of psychopathy, which could admit more-or-less law-abiding citizens within its rubric. Both the DSM constructs of Antisocial Personality Disorder and Hare's psychopathy raises questions not just about normative function of the emotion faculty, they also raise questions about a disturbance of will or volition faculty, through emphasizing various sorts of impaired behavioral controls and impulsivity.

In regard to the latter, conditions dominated by impulsive antisocial behavior led to the splitting off of psychopathy, developing the contemporary category of 'Intermittent Explosive Disorder'[349]—the expression of episodes of rage and violent behavior out of proportion to environmental provocation. 'Rage attacks' in the nineteenth century became associated also with epilepsy, with interest in the relationship between epilepsy and episodic, explosive violence persisting into the present through concepts such as 'episodic dyscontrol syndrome'.[350] In the mid-to-late-twentieth-century, the concept of 'minimal brain dysfunction'[351] linked the precursors of contemporary Attention-Deficit Hyperactivity Disorder to episodic dyscontrol and rage attacks as well.[352]

The journey of late-eighteenth-century melancholia as an emotional disorder associated with homicidal insanity (as in the 'differential diagnosis' of Henriette Cornier) into homicidal impulse, and, almost 100 years later, dementia praecox, and obsessive-compulsive disorders is explained by Colaizzi as the confluence of Karl Menninger, Kraepelinian, and Freudian influences. According to Colaizzi, citing Menninger's *The Vital Balance* (1964), the idea of a homicidal impulse shifted from not a monomaniacal disease in itself, but a symptom of other diseases. Prominent forensic cases of the time associated dementia praecox psychosis with homicidal impulses. Degenerationism could also manifest with homicidal impulse, springing from older concepts like moral imbecility and constitutional psychopathic inferiority, which in turn led into our more contemporary family of psychopathic/sociopathic disorders (absent the degeneracy etiological baggage). By the turn of the twentieth century, Kraepelin's notions of dementia praecox were increasingly influential, and the dynamic psychiatry of Freud and his followers, and the growth of outpatient psychiatry, contributed to the identification of cases of homicidal impulse governed by 'neurotic' disorders like obsessive-compulsive neurosis. Colaizzi summarizes:[353]

> As a symptom instead of a disease, the homicidal impulse became identified with two distinct mental conditions. In constitutional psychopathic states, a name given to the conditions brought about by a degenerating nervous system, the homicidal impulse, and impulses in general, were believed to be stigmata of degeneracy. In dementia praecox, alienists saw the homicidal impulse as evidence of the emotional indifference,

deterioration of the will, and the impulsive as well as purposeless behaviors that were often destructive and dangerous.

Dementia praecox, nee schizophrenia, came to be increasingly conceived as a disorder which affected all three faculties—cognition, affection, and conation, all conspiring to generate the potential for homicidal impulse. Clinical lore and public fears increasingly led to beliefs in the dangerousness of the condition, beliefs which were not seriously challenged until systematic studies by H. J. Steadman and others were conducted in the second half of the twentieth century, addressing the empirical evidence about the dangerousness of severe mental illness.[354]

The connection between obsessive-compulsive neurosis and impulsive homicide had to do with the common presence of violent obsessions in persons with obsessive-compulsive neurosis. Whether or not the patient acted upon the violent obsession was a matter of prominent debate between Freud and his colleague Pierre Janet. Freud insisted that obsessionality contributed to impulsive action; Janet claimed the opposite: 'In more than 200 cases, in which criminal impulses were present, he did not observe a single real occurrence, he did not observe a single crime committed nor a single suicide.'[355] At least according to today's viewpoints, Janet was right, the person with Obsessive-Compulsive Disorder is not likely to act on the violent obsession.[356]

In terms of volitional insanity and homicidal insanity, the eighteenth century considered mania as a perturbation of the will, and because manias (e.g., lunacy or total insanity) were often found to be associated with homicidal actions (see discussion of the insanity defense earlier), the eighteenth-century concept has been associated with mad homicide. By the early nineteenth century, however, early concepts of epilepsy generated a persistent link between seizures and homicidal insanity; the link to volition was the stereotypy, automatisms, and unresponsiveness of the patient with fits. Nineteenth-century epilepsy was viewed as a dangerously unpredictable condition—the EEG had not yet been invented, and dynamic psychiatrists and psychologists were eager to formulate the etiology of epilepsy in psychological terms. As might be expected from such formulations, the epileptic individual was subject to stigma, as well as imputations into defects of character (fueled likely by degeneracy concerns), here summarized by Noyes in 1934:[357]

> As maturity is approached the earlier characteristics are accentuated and the patient is frequently an irritable, selfish, egotistic, impulsive, asocial, rigid personality with a considerable mixture of cruelty and sadism.

While challenged by some alienists and neurologists, the belief in the dangerousness of the epileptic was perpetuated until the proliferation of the use of the electroencephalogram in the 1930s, and the discovery of abnormal brain waves in epileptic subjects. The use of phenytoin, phenobarbital, and other drugs for treatment was a further advance in reducing stigma and claims to dangerousness, though this belief faded slowly as revelations of psychotic complications of epilepsy were described, rekindling concerns about dangerous epileptics in midcentury.[358] By the end of the century, even these concerns faded as seizure characterization technologies proliferated and epileptology as a subspecialty of neurology generated reams of clinical research on the condition.

Of note under 'volitional insanity' is the relatively short-lived phenomenon of mania transitoria, an early version of the idea of psychosis related to epilepsy. Advocated by Henry Maudsley in the UK, and Isaac Ray in the United States, mania transitoria was a short-lived violent psychosis, lasting only a few hours to a few days, then resolving. However, many American psychiatrists rejected the condition of scientific grounds, seeing it as a relapse into monomanias and moral insanities, and criticizing it as a diagnosis of convenience for attorneys serving defendants accused of just about any crime.[359]

The lessons of 'homicidal insanity' are many. We can see over the nineteenth into the twentieth century the difficulties provoked by diagnosis on the basis of single- or single-groupings of symptoms, what I call 'monosymptomatic' disorders. From Esquirol to Ray into the present, diagnostic categories like 'homicidal insanity' were glued together by a single common, and often infrequent, symptom, resulting in widespread diagnostic confusion. In the 1800s, psychiatric diagnostic science had not yet developed even the modest advances that characterize our current era: psychology as science was exemplified by narrative theorists like Freud and introspectionist psychological philosophers like William James, whose research consisted largely of systematic observation, insightfully performed but methodologically impoverished as science. Syndrome description a la Sydenham was informal and variable from observer to observer. Mathematical statistics, the science that permitted the empirical grouping of related diagnostic descriptors, had not yet been invented; probability concepts, not yet arrived; the Gaussian distribution, newly discovered.[360] Diagnostic constructs were as often promulgated through the charismatic bravado of figures like Esquirol as well as by systematic observers like Kraepelin. Monosymptomatic disorders were confounded by few standards for clinical examination, so that some observers found additional clinical features while others did not. Like our own monosymptomatic disorders today, the single symptom admits an enormous amount of diverse causes of mental disturbance, called 'etiological heterogeneity', and like the diagnosis of 'headache', confuses profound disease with everyday foibles.

In the legal setting monosymptomatic disorders are especially problematic. In the absence of etiological defining features, or more detailed independent diagnostic features, folk understandings of behavior ('crimes of passion') seem as adequate to juries as highfalutin' concepts proffered by psychiatrists; the latter's variability in diagnosis and formulation only undermined their credibility in addressing important legal matters like criminal responsibility. The antagonistic polarities of the criminal trial fostered the use of the insanity defense on feeble diagnostic constructs—fostering varying public reaction from sympathy for, to outrage about, offenders.

Psychiatric disagreement about fundamental clinical features like diagnosis only fueled public skepticism about the field.

By the end of the twentieth century, American psychiatry turned away from the 'science of psychopathology'[361]—the study of abnormal mental states, and while the discourse in DSM classifications maintained its presupposed faculty psychology apparatus, the latter became increasingly remote and occult in its influence, becoming a set of sedimented metaphysical assumptions rather than metaphysical commitments that were open to direct debate. Kraepelinian nosology became the blueprint for most of the major mental disorders in the DSM-III,[362] making the classification 'neo-Kraepelinian' and, thereby, based upon a nineteenth-century psychopathology.[363] Instead, late-modern psychiatry favored formulations based upon a proliferation of therapeutic theories, whether pharmacological/neurobiological/genetic or psychoanalytic, cognitive/behavioral, or family systems (or others). Diagnostic constructs in the broad sense of providing holistic as well as focal appraisals of 'what is going on' with the patient[364] became relative to what 'orientation' one had toward caring for patients—despite the formal influence of the DSMs, which favored biomedical approaches.[365] Diagnosis and nosology increasingly became relative to one's preferred etiological theory and/or therapeutic modality.[366] McHugh and Slavney, responding to this lack of scientific unity, invoked a 'perspectivism' of psychopathological parallels—description varied under one of four perspectives.[367] Other theorists tried to assimilate diverse etiological theories of psychopathology into general systems theory, as George Engel did with the 'biopsychosocial model'.[368] Into the twenty-first century, contemporary theorists like Paul McHugh and Philip Slavney, David Brendel,[369] Kenneth Kendler and Peter Zachar,[370] Bradley Lewis,[371] and Nassir Ghaemi[372] provide their own synthetic visions of 'models' for psychiatry. What remained of the science of psychopathology persisted in Continental Europe, tied to philosophical traditions like Husserlian and Jaspersian phenomenology.[373] Even these traditions of philosophical psychopathology faded in Europe by mid-twentieth century, only to resurface in Europe and the United States with a 'renaissance' of the philosophy of psychiatry in the late-twentieth century,[374] permitting the writing and promulgation of works like this one. The impact the new psychopathologists and phenomenological psychiatrists will have in the twenty-first century is too early to tell.

The significance of the science of psychopathology for the VMDR concerns the focus on the experience of mental illness, and the engagement in understanding patient's experiences, and the fleshing out of capabilities and incapacities without presupposed theoretical structures or reified categories (e.g., abstract descriptions of 'disorders' which are presumed to be real, as too often is the case with the DSM use[375]). As will be discussed in later chapters, an elucidation of capabilities and incapacities may be more important to an accurate assessment of criminal responsibility than the assignment of a particular diagnosis.

As a final focus of brief discussion, we can see how the nineteenth-century faculty psychology as exemplified in the 'homicidal insanity' concept relates to the issue of criminal responsibility and excuse discussed in Section 5.7.2. Legal standards for excuse were found there to favor 'total insanity', where at minimum 'intellectual insanity' and the later 'psychosis' conditions elicited the most sympathy from juries considering excuse. The backlash against monomanias, moral insanity, and partial insanities after their initial reception in the United States is relevant today when we consider the inapplicability of the insanity defense to monosymptomatic contemporary conditions like Kleptomania, Pyromania, Antisocial Personality Disorder, and the Paraphilias. While explored as a vehicle for criminal excuse and the moderation of sentences, even legal standards involving analogues to 'volitional insanity'—such as 'irresistible impulse'—are at best variably successful in mitigating guilt and/or punishment.

5.8.7 Victorian sexual deviance and the birth of sexual identities and paraphilias

In this final discussion of core concepts in the history of the VMDR, I turn to the area of sex-related disorders and 'sexuality' in the nineteenth and twentieth centuries. In the discussion of the history of morality, I showed that the social regulation of sexual morality through religion, government/rulers, and the state was quite, and even perhaps, the most variable over the ages. Theft and murder have been perennially wrong, though pederasty, adultery, and even sexual hedonism have much more complex and ambivalent moral histories, as discussed in the prior chapter.

What is philosophically and morally fascinating about the history of sexual disorders, sex offenses, and the concept of 'sexuality' is that all of these ideas were birthed in parallel with larger social changes and related changes in folk psychologies and folk metaphysics. The moral and metaphysical status of (for instance) pederasty and sodomy changed in the early nineteenth century. Before this epoch, these concepts referred primarily to behaviors, that, depending on the era, were abominations (as described in the Holy Bible's Leviticus book), or rites of passage (as in ancient Greece) or sinful temptations (as in Augustine and Aquinas). These behaviors were part of human nature; all humans were 'eligible' to indulge in them, as with any other sin or temptation. In the late eighteenth and early nineteenth centuries, behaviors such as pederasty and sodomy were slowly recast within Anglo-European culture and became part of a bigger picture. What was this bigger cultural picture?

To summarize briefly, sexuality, sexual 'perversions', and sexual disorders arose at a time corresponding to the development of the modern self, accompanied by related ideas such as personal identity, the psychological concept of 'personality', and a metaphysical distinction, particularly in the West, of the individual from the family, culture, and collective.[376] In early America, the nineteenth century marked the cultural movement away from the family as culturally central, and more toward the individual as the core unit. As described by earlier sections, this was an era marked by a number of social changes that contributed to a transformation in how we conceive ourselves: (1) The development of market-based economics, industrialization, the economic theory of capitalism, and bourgeois business, shifting the social equilibrium away from cooperation and toward competition and individual 'initiative'; (2) the rise of modern science and the diminishing of religious authority, and the subsequent redefining of social deviance as illness, impairment, or ignorance rather than sin or possession; (3) the promulgation and wide acceptance of Enlightenment ideas about individual liberty, the worth of the individual, and the right of freedom from intrusion by others; (4) the development of cities and the creation of urban loneliness and disengagement from extended family; and (5) equally important, but perhaps less appreciated, development of a cheap and available written communication system—the postal mail system, which in combination with the new phenomenon of personal advertisements ('lonely hearts') in newspapers and magazines, enabled the now-isolated and lonely moderns to discover and communicate with each other privately and over long distances.[377]

With this social/cultural transformation of self and selfhood, sexual behavior came to be assimilated into a concept of the I, the self, or 'myself', thus giving birth to not just sexual behavior but sexual experience incorporated into social and personal identities—'lifestyles'—with their own independent sense of community and belonging. Instead of the Biblical antinomies of sexual sin and reproductive sex, sexual practice as play, as personal identity, as individual mode of expression, as social membership, was added to the mix. In a word, 'sexuality' was born.[378] These cultural changes posed the opportunity for people to find each other who had been historically constrained by religious or other traditional attitudes about sex. People of differing sexualities could create communities of fellows who shared sexual predilections. These communities, during these modern transitions, united through a bond-generating sense of social ostracism and even oppression by others. In the nineteenth century, Western culture transitioned from the idea of sexual behavior— moral, criminal, or virtuous—to the idea of 'sexuality'—the idea that one's sexual desires, consciousness, practices, values, and narrative self-talk represented a portion of one's own personal identity or sense of selfhood. While I consider the nineteenth-century birth of sexualities here, the implications and carryover of many of these processes continue in 2022 and beyond with, for example, transgender communities focusing on rights and noninterference, and the cultural appearance of the gender-nonbinary in ordinary discourse.

The development of communities, secret or otherwise, based around sexuality and sexual practices was seized upon by the new psychiatrists, neurologists, psychologists, and 'sexologists' resulting in publications centered around sexual themes, sexual cultures, sexual disorders, and 'perversions' from European authors like Sigmund Freud, Havelock Ellis, Richard Krafft-Ebing, and lesser-known pioneers like Valentin Magnan (the coiner of the term 'sexual perversion'), Károly Mária Benkert, Albert Moll, Magnus Hirschfeld, Karl Ulrichs, Karl Maria Kertbeny, and others.[379] By the turn of the twentieth century, sexuality not only had a name but also a rapidly expanding scientific and popular literature.

From the standpoint of iconic ideas, the era's most significant figure for the VMDR might be Richard von Krafft-Ebing, a Viennese psychiatrist, textbook author, and nosologist of sexual perversions. Harry Oosterhuis, Krafft-Ebing's biographer,[380] makes the important point that for some twentieth- and twenty-first-century advocates for sexual freedom and acceptance of diversity, Krafft-Ebing may be viewed as a cruel oppressor of Viennese-Victorian sexual minorities. However, Oosterhuis provides, as does Krafft-Ebing himself in *Psychopathia Sexualis*, abundant historical evidence that Krafft-Ebing was, in the globally repressive context of the time, a great liberator of individuals with sexual deviance from heteronormative moral standards. Before Krafft-Ebing, individuals who violated sexual norms were outcasts, criminals, and sinners, worthy of ruthless ostracism, persecution, and punishment. Krafft-Ebing improved their (still stigmatized) social status to that of sick people in need of compassion and treatment. Krafft-Ebing's publications pioneered the autobiographical clinical case narrative.[381] The circulation of these case narratives led to a lessening of the then-perverts' shame, isolation, and alienation. In reference to this liberatory cultural transformation, consider this brief text from an 'urning' (homosexual person) of the era:[382]

> It was as if the scales had fallen from my eyes, and I bless the day this enlightenment came to me. From that day I saw the world with different eyes; I saw that many others were cursed with the same fate, and I began to learn, as well as I could, to be content with my lot.

While far short of today's LGBTQ+ liberatory zeal, Krafft-Ebing pioneered what historian Thomas Laqueur calls the 'humanitarian narrative', the story that elicits empathy in the reader, and the resolve to address such matters of human pain through social action.[383] Of course, Krafft-Ebing's contribution to a greater acceptance of sexual diversity is transitional in the arc of history, as the movement to further destigmatize sexual difference was yet to arise in the form of feminism, gay liberation, transgender recognition, and related movements in the latter half of the twentieth century and on into the twenty-first century.

To be sure, Krafft-Ebing (K-E), however, in *Psychopathia Sexualis*,[384] wrote about many conditions and practices that even today's most tolerant and generous people might find objectionable—although perhaps no longer shocking. Indeed, his text, which underwent many editions, originally featured the case material written in Latin as to avoid prurient readings by the laity, and was not fully translated into English until 1965, English-language case details intact.

Such meticulous detail in K-E's text cannot be adequately summarized here, nor needn't be for the purposes of this book.[385] A degenerationist, Krafft-Ebing distinguished perversion—a degenerative constitutional disorder fully integrated into the personality—from perversity, the indulgence in ordinary immoral sexual conduct, and historically labeled as sin or temptation. Like many of his religious predecessors, K-E defined normal sexual behavior as (heterosexual) coitus with the intent of reproduction. Subsequently, he considered reproductively unnecessary sex play or pleasuring as abnormal, but not perverse.[386] K-E considered a wide range of sexual deviance, but focused on four main perversions: sadism, masochism, fetishism, and 'contrary sexual feeling'. The latter term, coined by Moll, was also referred to as 'urning' and 'sexual inversion' by others, and referred to the persistent desire for same-sex couplings. The 'homosexuality/heterosexuality' distinction, introduced by Austro-Hungarian journalist Karl Maria Kertbeny in 1869, however, is a great illustration of how the 'discovery' of the homosexuality–heterosexuality distinction was interdependent.[387] In order to have a crystallized concept of heterosexuality, a contrast-concept like homosexuality was needed. In this sense, 'heterosexuality' in its contemporary sense didn't exist prior to the nineteenth century either! Prior to these Western conceptual revolutions, all that could be thought and articulated was normative reproductive sexual practice and sin/deviation/transgression.

K-E liked these newer terms and incorporated the term 'homosexuality' in his later editions. K-E himself coined the terms 'sadism' inspired by de Sade's work, and 'masochism' from Leopold van Sacher-Masoch's scandalous novel of 1870, *Venus in Furs*. K-E also coined the term 'pedophilia'. Despite the popular image of Victorian Europe as sexually repressive, it was the era of the birth of modern (e.g., printed, massively reproduced) pornography, and an explosion of new scientific-sexual terminology for sexual phenomena, some of which persisted into the present (and much that didn't): exhibitionism, bestiality, pedophilia, incest, necrophilia, urolagnia, coprolagnia, androgyny, paranoia sexualis, and notably, a variety of French terms referring to pinching, rubbing, flogging, and spanking—to name only a few. The Germans, however, own the term, *Zopfaschneider*, for men who indulge lusts for cutting off and stealing women's hair buns![388] One might speculate such linguistic prolixity was a carryover from the monomanias and the nineteenth-century predilection for monosymptomatic disorders.

These trends arose in the context of nineteenth-century European psychiatry and culture. Matters were different in the young United States. In the eighteenth and nineteenth centuries, American culture was dominated by an often religious and a self-abnegating 'puritanical' mindset. Norman Dain explains:[389]

> American psychiatrists shared the old Jeffersonian prejudice that rural life was healthier than urban life. This conviction was associated with the idea that everything man-made, complicated, and not of nature was corrupt. . . . This approach, though predating Puritanism, conformed to the Puritan suspicion of easy living. Psychiatrists thought practically everything that enhanced life was injurious to mental stability. Drinking, sex, smoking, snuff, novels, poetry, drama, imaginative thoughts, study, financial speculation, and luxurious living in general were either positively harmful or became so if indulged beyond 'moderation'.

No wonder that masturbation was identified as a common cause of insanity and even warranted its own category, 'masturbatory insanity'. Such prudery made the lurid perversities of K-E's and Freud's cases unthinkable, much less clinically useful.

Both had to wait until the post–World War II era to have widespread influence on American psychiatry.

While European psychiatrists and psychologists were exploring sexuality and perversions at the turn of the twentieth century, American psychiatrists' reactions to the literature of sexology and sexual psychopathology were conservative and traditional. Vern Bullough, the distinguished historian of sex and sexuality, summarizes American attitudes toward the new sexology:[390]

> American sex research differed from that in England or on the continent in its concentration on basic heterosexual problems. Richard von Krafft-Ebing, Magnus Hirschfeld, and Havelock Ellis all originally had major concerns with variant sexuality. So did Sigmund Freud. . . . Generally, the American medical establishment itself was reluctant to deal with sexual issues, and when an English version of Havelock Ellis's work on sexual inversion first appeared, an American reviewer stated that Ellis was too inclined to fill his book with the 'pornographic imaginings of perverted minds rather than cold facts . . .'.

Such American discomfort with the unveiling of diverse sexual culture persisted well into the mid-twentieth century and beyond. One need only consider the controversy that was to surround Alfred Kinsey's pioneering sex research decades later.

The late-nineteenth-century was a time that Americans were dealing with their own social issues as never before. The nation was recovering from the shattering aftermath of the Civil War and contending with the end of slavery and struggling with the integration of the new African American freedmen and women. However, racism was hardly eradicated. For instance, Whites claimed that Blacks were too primitive to be mentally ill and were largely excluded from asylums. Institutions for lunatics, imbeciles, and the poor were overcrowded, underfunded, stressed to the breaking point, and the beginnings of humanitarian activism and twentieth-century Progressive era reform were spreading.[391] The aforementioned problems of urban crowding and industrialization were associated with expanding public concerns of moral turpitude, such as prostitution, drug and alcohol addiction, the recognition of syphilis and 'venereal' diseases, and the inbreeding of degenerates, as discussed in earlier sections. The nation was posed to reassess its moral standards on many fronts.

Over the ensuing 30 years, from roughly 1880–1910, public concern about moral conduct and moral activism sprang up all over the country. Perhaps the 'purity movement'[392] could be understood as spearheaded by Anthony Comstock, a Yankee postal worker and politician who founded the New York Society for the Suppression of Vice, one of the many organizations intended to clean up American society. With Congress' passing of the Comstock Law, transportation of pornographic material was made illegal, as well as information on birth control. As welcomed by churches as he was spurned by artists and writers, Comstock cut a controversial figure in early twentieth-century life. George Bernard Shaw coined the term 'comstockery' to refer to censorship owing to the perception of obscenity or lewdness; Shaw's plays being a prominent recipient of comstockery scorn.[393] Comstock, however, was only a prominent example; morality/purity movements proliferated nationwide.

Sexual vice was not the only target; gambling, liquor and drugs of abuse were also on the moral reformer's checklists, culminating in 1906's Pure Food and Drug Act, regulating abusable substances like alcohol, cocaine, cannabis, and (opioid) narcotics, and 1919's Volstead Act, and the US Eighteenth Amendment to the Constitution—Prohibition—banning the manufacture, sale, or transportation of beverage alcohol (to be repealed in 1933 through the twenty-first amendment).[394] America's 'Cowboy Philosopher', Will Rogers, appraised the Prohibition movement's success, famously stating 'Prohibition is better than no liquor at all.'[395] The purity movement can be considered as still another manifestation of the push for humane social reform that characterized the post–Civil War period, and persisting well into the early twentieth-century Progressive era. Needless to say this reform, like any social reform, reflected the prevailing values of the community of the time.

Formal classification by the Americans in the twentieth century began with the Committee on Statistics of the American Medico-Psychological Association in 1916; producing a proto-DSM involving 22 general categories of psychopathology, intended mostly for institutional record-keeping and not as a diagnostic guide. The manual resulting from this committee work, the Statistical Manual for the Use of Institutions for the Insane,[396] in keeping with the marginalizing of sexual disorders, did not have its own categories for perversions or paraphilias; instead, sexual deviations were listed under the category 'Psychoses with Constitutional Psychopathic Inferiority',[397] mentioned earlier in reference to homicidal insanity. This listing underwent multiple editions until the movement that resulted in DSM-I in 1952, though as Grob[398] notes, the scientific classification of psychopathology was not a compelling interest of early twentieth-century psychiatrists.

With the development of Nazism in Germany in the 1930s, and the resulting second World War, Freudian expatriates emigrated to England and especially America. Younger psychiatrists during the war period utilized Freudian psychoanalytic and Meyerian psychobiological thinking to show substantial successes during WW II in returning the GI's to the battle lines, returning 'psychoneurotic' casualties to the front in 2–5 days.[399] The influx of these new psychiatrists into the new GAP contributed to the promulgation of the psychodynamic model in training programs in midcentury, and the building of a golden era of psychodynamic outpatient psychiatry in the United States. Grob argues that these changes within American psychiatry, and the renewed interest in medical education, combined to provoke the development of DSM-I and kindle greater interest in diagnosis and classification of mental disorders.[400]

By the time of DSM-I, the breaking of the silence of sexual culture in the United States had only begun. In the post–WWII era, influential research led by Alfred Kinsey and others, as well as an increased recognition of Havelock Ellis's sexology, began to take cultural hold.[401] Kinsey's initial book-length report, *Sexual Behavior in the Human Male* (1948), was a popular sensation in terms of book sales and cultural influence. Given its stolid recitation of behavior counts and relative narrative poverty, a book whose sales were extraordinary in midcentury turned out to be a crashing bore to contemporary readers. Kinsey's difficult road in his achievements have been well-documented in the above references and elsewhere; his initiative paved the way for sex research of all kinds and opened the door for investigators of normal and abnormal sexuality from John Money to Masters & Johnson. Perhaps more importantly, it opened new avenues of cultural discussion about sexuality for the nation as a whole.

These changes in the field in midcentury, however, had not yet raised the profile of sexual deviations in DSM-I. The latter's entry for its lone category, Sexual Deviation, reads in complete below:[402]

> This diagnosis is reserved for deviant sexuality which is not symptomatic of more extensive syndromes, such as schizophrenic and obsessional reactions. The term includes most of the cases formerly classed as 'psychopathic personality with pathological sexuality'. The diagnosis will specify the type of the pathological behavior, such as homosexuality, transvestism, pedophilia, fetishism, and sexual sadism (including rape, sexual assault, mutilation).

Notably, Krafft-Ebing's concepts had now found their way into the DSM, although as subtypes. Interestingly, rape, sexual assault, and (presumably sexual) mutilation were listed as diagnosable subtypes along with the more familiar categories to contemporary eyes. This latter is resonant with the aforementioned discussion of a new openness to psychiatry to treating criminal conduct as psychopathology.

In 1968, DSM-II was published, which again specified 'Sexual Deviations' as its superordinate category, and listing Homosexuality, Fetishism, Pedophilia, Transvestitism, Exhibitionism, Voyeurism, Sadism, Masochism, and others/unspecified sexual deviations as its subtypes. With the publication of the seventh printing in 1974, 'Homosexuality' had been removed from the manual as a category of mental disorder; reflected the 1973 vote by the APA membership to remove it. The issue was a *cause célèbre* within APA as well as the public, inspiring news and scholarship about what it means to create or undo a category of psychopathology.[403] The story of the removal of the disorder needn't be recounted here, as it has been told many times, other than to note that organized gay and lesbian activism was influential in moving this issue forward professionally and publicly.

What was substituted in the seventh edition of DSM-II was a new category, 'Sexual Orientation Disturbance [Homosexuality]'.[404] This was described as 'individuals whose sexual interests are directed primarily toward people of the same sex and who are either disturbed by, in conflict, with or wish to change their sexual orientation'.[405] This condition was modified to 'Ego-dystonic Homosexuality' in DSM-III.[406] By DSM-IV in 1994 it had been relegated to the catch-all category 'Sexual Disorder Not Elsewhere Classified'[407] and noted to concern 'Persistent and marked distress about sexual orientation'.

The DSM-III, however, introduced new techniques of diagnosis, using the 'operationalized' criteria under a new term, 'Psychosexual Disorders'. In addition to the new categories of 'Transsexualism', 'Gender Identity Disorder of Childhood', and 'Atypical Gender Identity Disorder', DSM-II renamed the set of disorders previously identified as sexual deviations as 'Paraphilias', which has now persisted into the DSM-5 present, albeit in a form distinguishing sexual diversity (Paraphilias), from disordered conditions (Paraphilic Disorders). These latter developments are discussed in later chapters. The DSM-III also introduced, in addition the detailed diagnostic criteria sets, a substantial amount of discussion about the classified conditions, including essential features, associated features, and considerations of impairment, complications, predisposing factors, prevalence, sex ratios, familial patterns, and the like.

DSM-III marked a new subtlety in psychiatric diagnosis and the description of psychopathology. In addition to offering a general definition of mental disorder, each section, including the Paraphilias section, discussed the qualifiers, disqualifiers, and cultural nuances involved. I have remarked elsewhere[408] that despite the DSM-III's intention to be user-friendly and minimize obfuscating jargon, the manual, when used properly, encourages subtle cultural judgments before making a diagnosis. Unfortunately, the nuanced approach of the DSM-III and its followers has too often been overlooked by its critics. Such is the case with the Paraphilias section.

The introductory discussion of the Paraphilias note that 'the essential feature of disorders in this subclass is that unusual or bizarre imagery or acts are necessary for sexual excitement'.[409] Through this the DSM-III authors presumably intended to exclude the many cultural variations of sexuality and sexual pleasure that are practiced between 'consenting adults' behind (mostly) closed doors. The 'obligatory' aspect of variant arousal may have been helpful in isolating disorders from fun-loving sexual diversity but was to prove problematic later as research found many people who engaged in ongoing paraphilic practices could also function quite well with more conventional sexual partners and practices. DSM-III specified a distinction between consenting and nonconsenting partners. This was well-intended but also problematic when considering the contemporary diversity practices of the bedroom, involving varying degrees of deviant intent—from simple play-acting to more serious injury and intent to harm the partner (as well as callous disregard for the impact on nonconsenting others). However, while DSM-III notes the importance of consent in sexual practices, this concern does not find its way into diagnostic criteria for the disorders 'at risk' for nonconsenting partners: Sexual Masochism, Sexual Sadism, Pedophilia, Exhibitionism, and Voyeurism.

For my purposes of the analysis of the VMDR, I've made the stipulation that some paraphilic practices may involve nonconsenting partners that are harm-inducing; my term has been to call these 'victimizing' paraphilias to specify that harm is done to the partner by definition. I acknowledge that some sexual behaviors that might perceived as harmful but are not, as practiced (as in some mutually consenting, culturally self-regulating sadomasochistic communities),[410] but to address that some

paraphilic behavior does in fact result in nonconsenting harm to others—victims—
and in those cases represents a criminal transgression. Nevertheless, what constitutes
victimizing in any particular sexual engagement may be, and has been, problematic.

By DSM-IV in 1994, the obligatory/exclusive nature of paraphilic arousal was
modified to permit any particular individual to have periods of more normative
function interspersed with paraphilic arousal:[411]

> For some individuals, paraphilic fantasies or stimuli are obligatory for erotic arousal and
> are always included in sexual activity. In other cases, the paraphiliac preferences occur
> only episodically (e.g., perhaps during periods of stress), whereas at other times the
> person is able to function sexually without paraphiliac fantasies or stimuli.

DSM-IV also added the 'clinical significance criterion' to the Paraphilias, specifying that
the diagnosis must be associated by the patient's distress or functional impairment:[412]

> The behavior, sexual urges, or fantasies cause clinically significant distress or impairment
> in social, occupational, or other important areas of functioning (Criterion B).

In contrast to DSM-III's diagnostic criteria sets, all of the Paraphilias in DSM-IV had
specific 'Criterion B' criteria added, making distress and impairment a requirement
for diagnosis. This of course was to become a later cause of discussion in the DSM-
IV-TR and DSM-5 era, as the importance of the clinical significance criterion was
debated—see Chapter 3.

5.9   Conclusions

In concluding this long chapter, I will focus primarily upon the changes that characterize the past two centuries of psychiatry, madness, and morality; as before, organizing them around a series of iconic summary points to consider for the remainder
of this book.

1. *Colonialism & practical community solutions.* The early American colonies, in
   eking out an existence in the face of harsh physical conditions and limited resources, did not concern themselves with social deviance (madness, crime, delinquency, poverty) per se but rather offered practical community solutions to
   the difficulties offered by their mad, criminal, widowed, and orphaned peers.
2. *Colonial religious charity.* A prevailing Christian-religious and charitable orientation toward the needy framed the moral ethic of the Colonists' preface to
   'social care'.
3. *Three psychological faculties.* By the end of the eighteenth century, philosophy
   and the emerging psychology had consolidated around three faculties: reason/
   cognition, emotion/affection, and will/conation, providing the metaphysical

vocabulary for describing psychopathologies. Notably, discussion of morality as a faculty was marginal, yet found its way into a few of the developing psychiatric categories, nonetheless.

4. *Ambivalence about secular/medical madness.* While the eighteenth century exhibited the proliferation of modern science in Western Europe, this Enlightenment trend was still novel to colonial America; witchcraft, pagan religion, and madness were still linked together in many American colonial minds. Culturally, madness was still often viewed as a consequence of sin, a viewpoint that continued well into the nineteenth century and up to the twentieth century, where it dispersed into various subcultures.

5. *Limitations of descriptive diagnosis.* Early American psychiatrists like Pliny Earle recognized the limitations of diagnosis based solely upon clinical presentation and symptomatology.

6. *Modernism breeds suspicion of deviancy.* In the transition from the colonies to the early United States, the growth of major cities, urbanization, bourgeois business, and the appearance of factories disrupted the previously close-knit family and community fabric, creating new numbers of widows, orphans, transients, rogue opportunists, and madpersons, while provoking more suspicion and intolerance of them among established community members.

7. *Mens rea and actus reus.* Considerations of *mens rea* (criminal intent) and *actus reus* (criminal acts) permeate Western considerations of criminal responsibility/excuse going back as far as Greek and Roman law.

8. *Establishing the need for psychiatric expertise in the courtroom.* Pinel's late eighteenth-century description of *manie sans délire* set the stage for the formulation of 'partial insanities', the differentiation of milder forms of psychopathology, and the need for forensic psychiatric experts to detect subtle forms of psychopathology in the courtroom setting.

9. *Particular mental states as a consideration for criminal responsibility.* British jurists like Hale and Coke however, described 'partial insanities' as early as the late 1600s under considerations of criminal responsibility. Coke sorted out four kinds of mental disturbances relevant to criminal responsibility: global static impairments like idiocy, temporary impairments related to medical illness or personal catastrophe, willful impairments like drunkenness, and periodic impairments with lucid intervals, like manic-depressive insanity.

10. *Idiocy and madness.* Intellectually impaired children and adults (who managed to survive) were lumped together with the mad in the American colonial response to the socially marginal. With population growth and urbanization these populations transitioned to the first almshouses, workhouses, and ultimately the asylums and schools for idiocy.

11. *Modernism moves the (moral) education of children.* The above changes in American society moved the center of gravity in moral and general education away from the Church/family and into the newly established schools by the mid-eighteenth century.

12. *A rejection of harsh English punishments.* Colonial criminal offenders were humiliated through mechanisms like the stocks; repeat offenders were extruded from the community or (infrequently) hung; but the religious colonists tended to reject the harsh treatments of native England and embraced the new penal theories of humanists like Beccaria and Bentham.

13. *Beginning child welfare programs.* The failure of early American almshouses to protect needy children provokes the adaptation of English poor laws to establish legal means for the state to protect child welfare. The legal precedents then persist, in large degree, today: concepts like *parens patriae*, institutions like orphanages, and principles like local care, family involvement, and distinguishing between deserving and undeserving dependency.

14. *Conflict between early juvenile justice reform & families.* Early American law and culture tends to protect the sanctity of American family life; emerging efforts to develop juvenile courts provoke pushback from families who view them as intruding into private affairs.

15. *Moral responsibility, will, and reason frame the concept of criminal excuse.* Beginning in the 1700s and continuing into the present, various tests and procedures for considering criminal excuse were developed, all based in large part upon a moral model of criminal responsibility and resting upon the fundament of human reason and the freedom of will.

16. *Early debate on the insanity defense.* Nineteenth- and twentieth-century debates about the 'insanity defense' revolved around the rationality of the defendant, the ability of the defendant to regulate his/her own actions, and the question of a causal relationship between the mental condition and the criminal action.

17. *The persistence of 'the will'.* While often disparaged by psychology and neuroscience today, the eighteenth-century concept of the will persisted in both psychiatry and criminal justice, through such variant concepts of weakness of will (*akrasia*), impulse control, abulia, behavioral compulsion, and 'irresistible impulse'.

18. *The establishment of reform-oriented prisons.* The rejection of harsh punishments and the death penalty stimulated the early Americans to establish prisons with the goal of both incarcerating and reforming criminals by the early nineteenth century, which facilitated more guilty verdicts for defendants, as juries no longer needed to acquit in order to avoid the extreme punishment of execution for guilty criminals.

19. *Commingling of reason and morality.* The commingling of Enlightenment moral psychologies of the will with older, Aquinian Christian morality lead to the formulation of moral disorders of the will, which married a failure to resist sin/temptation with the failure to act rationally.

20. *Orphan children exploited.* At the turn of the nineteenth century, orphaned children were increasingly compelled into indentured service with unrelated families, for economic benefit to the family, not the child.

21. *Idiocy education.* Civic leaders such as Howe, Wilbur, and Séguin, in the early nineteenth century, persuade the US public that the intellectually impaired are educable and need schools, not asylums or prisons. Early attempts at classifying intellectual impairment set the stage for professional rivalries over education/treatment versus custodialism for this population.

22. *Immigrants contribute to the demand for social institutions.* In the early eighteenth century, the aforementioned changes of urbanization and industry were complicated by the new immigrants, whose lack of community roots and tenuous economic status contributed to the need for social institutions, such as almshouses and workhouses, that collectively addressed the needy.

23. *Enlightenment science & secularism rise in the United States.* The American churches were unprepared to address the social challenges of the new United States; and secular influences of the European Enlightenment imported optimism about the power of science and reason to address the problems of society.

24. *American individualism and social deviance.* Industrialization, American democratic theory, and secularism, among other factors, fomented the cultural beliefs in American individualism and personal responsibility, contributing to the differentiation of institutions for the socially deviant.

25. *Hospitals and asylums.* The new scientific medicine and alienism imported from Europe contributed to the early eighteenth-century enthusiasm among the Americans for hospitals, in general, and asylums for care of the mentally ill, in particular.

26. *Emergence of debate around therapeutics versus custodianship.* The moral therapy and other humanistic approaches of the early US asylums were rapidly challenged and ultimately undermined by the unremitting influx of immigrant, aged, and chronic patients, contributing to an algebra of chronicity, overcrowding, and custodianship, overwhelming therapy efforts.

27. *State-supported asylums.* Crowding and abuse in private asylums provoke social reformers' political success in establishing state-supported asylums in the early eighteenth century.

28. *Moral imbecility and moral insanity.* The open sexuality of the feebleminded, their perceived association with violent crime, and degeneracy theory provoke the category of the 'moral imbecile' in American psychiatry. Lombroso's theory of atavism contributes to a related concept of 'moral insanity' that catches hold in the new United States under the influence of Isaac Ray and Benjamin Rush.

29. *From moral insanity to Antisocial Personality Disorder.* Benjamin Rush's vice-specific version of moral insanity provides an American historical root for later concepts like constitutional psychopathic inferiority, psychopathy, and Antisocial Personality Disorder.

30. *Monomanias.* Esquirol's mid-nineteenth-century notion of monomania ushers in the requirement for psychiatric expertise in the courtroom through

American intermediaries like Isaac Ray. Monomanias provide a vehicle for medicalizing vice and initiate the validity problems of monosymptomatic categories of mental disorder that persist into the present.

31. *Homicidal insanity and faculty psychopathology.* The ill-fated nineteenth-century concept of homicidal insanity was emblematic of the psychiatric transition from psychopathologies primarily affecting a single faculty or mental function, to psychopathologies affecting multiple faculties and functions.

32. *Controversy around the soul and psychopathology.* Nineteenth-century American psychiatry is divided metaphysically into psychiatrists disapproving of the notion of a psychological or moral 'disorder', based upon the Christian belief in the immortal soul (mind), and psychiatrists who are more secular in their casting of psychopathology, recognizing the insights of the new psychology and Enlightenment philosophy.

33. *The homicidal lunatic as 'monster'.* A popular conception of the (Foucauldian) 'monster', an individual whose crimes defy rational explanation or understanding, emerges from nineteenth-century descriptions of homicidal insanity.

34. *The dissipation of 'homicidal insanity'.* Sharing a fate with most of the monomanias, homicidal insanity dissolved into other potentially violent disorder categories by the turn of the twentieth century, some of which have sustained concern in their risk for violence (e.g., postpartum psychosis, psychopathy), with others subsequently debunked as posing violence risk (e.g., epilepsy).

35. *Europeans turn sour on American prison innovations.* In the post–Civil War era, the reform ideals of the American prison were progressively diluted by underfunding and overcrowding, leading the initial European praise for the American prison approach to transform into bitter criticism based on humane grounds.

36. *Degeneracy and atavism.* Degeneracy theory and Lombroso's atavism theory augment the suspicion and fear of idiots, insanity, and criminality, and set the stage for American eugenics.

37. *The feebleminded and eugenics.* Degeneracy theory and moral panic about the sexuality of the feebleminded contribute to the development of a eugenics movement and compulsory sterilization laws around the turn of the twentieth century.

38. *Backlash against eugenics.* By the first decade of the twentieth century, criticism and rejection of eugenics and sterilization laws also spread; rejection of eugenics in America became essentially complete by the time of Hitler's Nazi eugenics and the Holocaust in the 1930s.

39. *The birth of the self and of sexuality.* A transformation in Western culture in the eighteenth century, characterized by new cultural ideas about the individual, self, personality, and personal identity, contributed to changing ideas about sexual behavior. Once simply moral, criminal, or virtuous, sexual behavior now became integrated into the psychological self through the concept of

'sexuality'—the idea that one's sexual desires, behavior, consciousness, practices, values, and narrative self-talk represented a portion of one's own personal identity or sense of unique selfhood.

40. *New communications enable subcultures.* The eighteenth-century development of more rapid communications like the postal system and 'personals' in newspapers enables 'sexual deviants' to find each other, develop subcultures, and be described by the new psychiatrists, psychologists, and sexologists, founding new categories of psychopathology as well new ramifications of the stigma of mental illness and the mad-bad debate.

41. *American politicization and moralization of psychopathology.* The development of sexualities in Victorian Europe were late in influencing the more prudish and religious American psychiatrists, who were still under the influence of monomanias, often characterizing social noncompliance as psychopathology, such as 'masturbatory insanity' and 'draepetomania'.

42. *Psychiatrists contribute to purity and temperance movements.* Many late-nineteenth and early twentieth-century psychiatrists were suspicious of urbanization and modernization, seeing this trend as contributing to moral turpitude, madness, and degeneracy, provoking psychiatric involvement in the purity and temperance movements of the era.

43. *Reform brings indeterminate sentencing and parole.* By the latter quarter of the nineteenth century, prison reform movements led to new innovations in bolstering reform and improving prison conditions, including the use of 'indeterminate sentencing' and parole as a way of encouraging convicts to exhibit good behavior in order to earn hospital privileges and ultimately shorten their sentences.

44. *Indeterminate sentencing expands the role of psychiatrists & psychologists.* Indeterminate sentencing was associated with other prison reforms such as extensive use of psychologists and psychiatrists, and in some cases educators, in both prognosticating who was ready for parole and release, as well as to build educational programs to develop convicts' skills and readiness for the 'outside' world.

45. *Federal prisons raise the bar.* The establishment of the Federal prison system in 1897 raised the bar for prison conditions and programs: establishing a classification system for convicts based on the severity of their crimes as well as their potential for reform, as well as establishing minimum standards for prison conditions.

46. *New institutions for child welfare.* Social reforms concerning child welfare at the end of the nineteenth and the turn of the twentieth century were exemplified by the founding of the Society for the Prevention of Cruelty to Children, the Children's Aid Society in New York, and the federal Children's Bureau, all concerned with child welfare, abuse, neglect, and delinquency.

47. *The appearance of universal compulsory education.* The development of compulsory education for children during the latter half of the nineteenth century

contributed the social regulation of street delinquency and child labor, as well as created a new social problem of 'truancy'.

48. *From mothers' pensions to welfare mothers.* The creation of 'mother's pensions' to help single and widowed mothers was intended to enable women to be home and raise their children; thereby diminishing delinquency. Debate ensued about whether such programs provided relief or simply bred dependency upon government resources. Mother's pensions grew into the federal AFDC programs in the mid-twentieth century, generating public ambivalence about 'welfare mothers' that persists into the present.

49. *Turn-of-the-century prison rioting.* An irony emerging from the development of federal prisons was their role in inspiring outbreaks of prison rioting over the poor conditions of state prisons.

50. *Reciprocal growth.* The new alienist/psychiatrists reciprocally benefit from the growth of American asylums, as well as the American prison, and to a lesser extent, the development of services for the intellectually impaired.

51. *American scientific/organized medicine.* Alienists take the lead in American organized and scientific medicine, through establishing early medical journals and the first American medical specialty organization.

52. *The 'soul' and psychopathology.* Some early American alienists' ties to the Christian soul imposed metaphysical limits on understanding and classifying of psychopathology, contributing to a debate on secular versus 'Christian' psychopathology. The mind/soul could not be diseased for many clinicians, because of the immortal nature of the eternal soul.

53. *A critical American neurology arises.* The turn of the twentieth century brings the demand for reform from within American psychiatry, as well as from the new neurologists, who voice stern criticism about the alienists' science and humanism.

54. *The Child Welfare Movement.* The child welfare movement of the early twentieth century stimulated the development of public/private charitable organizations and their regulation by the states.

55. *The Mental Hygiene Movement.* Clifford Beers, Adolf Meyer, and Thomas Salmon founded the Mental Hygiene Movement in the early twentieth century, and struggled over its objectives: humane reform of asylums for Beers, versus the development of outpatient care and psychopathic hospitals for the doctors.

56. *Education versus custodianship for the mentally retarded.* The early twentieth century brings debate around the proper care of the intellectually impaired; splitting into factions oriented toward education and accommodation by society (led by the new American Association for the Study of the Feeble-Minded), and a custodianship-oriented faction led by the asylum psychiatrists.

57. *IQ testing and psychologists.* The development of the IQ test by Binet contributes to the classification of the intellectually impaired, as well as contributes

to the special role of the new psychologists in assessing and classifying this population.

58. *Problems with classifying mentally retarded people.* Both asylum doctors and the educators of the intellectually impaired struggled with the proper methods to classify their populations. Turf battles, as well as difficulties in assimilating the nosological significance of dimensional psychological properties, contributed to a flux in classification schemes among both groups.

59. *Debates about juvenile justice.* The development of the juvenile justice system at the turn of the twentieth century stimulated new debates and resentments about government intrusions into family affairs, this time manifested by the probation system and the use of probation officers to assist and provide oversight to juvenile offenders.

60. *DSMs are developed.* The development of the first DSM in 1952 addressed both the classification of mental illnesses, as well as MR, though the early editions were intended more for institutional and administrative use, and not so much for the scientific classification of disease. The release of DSM-III in 1980 changed that orientation and intended to aid in the development of a scientific psychiatry.

61. *Disparities in early child welfare.* The early child welfare efforts were marked by gender, class, and racial disparities. Fathers were de facto excused from childrearing responsibilities; the poor were disproportionately represented in abuse/neglect and delinquency settings; and the new African Americans, struggling to find a place in a postslavery United States, were overrepresented in all these systems. Even delinquents themselves were 'gendered': boys were expected to be thieves, and girls, promiscuous.

62. *Recidivism and the birth of the Child Guidance Movement.* Progressives' concern about persistent delinquency recidivism prompted the child guidance movement and the birth of child and adolescent psychiatry as a subspeciality.

63. *Social science supports child welfare reforms.* Coupled with the momentum of the mental hygiene movement, child guidance Progressives generated the first sets of social scientific data to explore the causes of delinquency and child abuse, providing empirical support for child welfare reforms.

64. *Splintering of child and adolescent psychiatry.* The splitting of child psychiatry is manifested by the development of the American Academy of Child and Adolescent Psychiatry in 1952; with the American Orthopsychiatric Association retaining its social, multidisciplinary focus and membership, and the newer AACAP catering to private and academic, biomedically oriented psychiatric practitioners.

65. *Cycles of mental health care reform.* A series of reform cycles over the first 2 centuries of psychiatry characterizes a sociopolitical flux between the pursuit of expensive but humanistic care ideals, the decline of the quality of care, and the withdrawal of public, political, and financial support for mental health

care because of the failure to meet these ideals. Patients are caught in the middle of these cycles.

66. *Cycles of overcrowding & underfunding.* An algebra of overcrowding and underfunding for asylums, as well as prisons, invokes institutional reform movements in the latter half of the nineteenth century (and again and again in the twentieth), invoking debates over therapeutics/reform versus custodianship in the mental health sector.

67. *Reform and mid-twentieth-century new media.* Mid-twentieth-century public awareness of crime, feeblemindedness, mental illness, and poverty exploded in large part by the development of new media, especially the development of popular magazines, photojournalism, radio, and television. This new public awareness was often channeled into humanistic reforms in the institutions addressing these forms of social deviance.

68. *The rise of outpatient, psychodynamic psychiatry.* By the mid-twentieth century, an influx of new psychodynamically oriented, politically astute psychiatrists come to dominate academic medicine and psychiatric leadership. They develop an outpatient-oriented, neurosis-centered, prevention-aware mode of psychiatric practice, and in effect marginalize institutional, asylum psychiatry, while establishing new resources such as the National Institute of Mental Health.

69. *DSM-I and Paraphilias.* The new outpatient psychiatrists contribute to greater interest in classification, culminating in DSM-I, and a new American sexology brings paraphilias into American psychiatry by the mid-twentieth century, though not fully until 1980s DSM-III.

70. *A new crime/delinquency agenda.* The aforementioned twentieth-century psychodynamic psychiatrists develop a social psychiatry agenda, intending to address the problems of crime and delinquency through preventive, social intervention, and therapy.

71. *From reprobate to victim.* Many of the postwar psychiatrists, together with social workers and the new criminologists, recast the criminal offender from moral reprobate to a traumatized, neglected, and diseased victim, offering new therapeutics for crime and criminals.

72. *Return of some civil liberties to prisoners.* Mid-twentieth-century reforms return a number of civil liberties to prisoners, including the *writ of habeus corpus*, freedom of religion, and new constraints on warden's powers.

73. *The birth of 'effective parenting'.* The Child Guidance and Child Welfare movements stimulate public awareness and concern about delinquency prevention, developing and promulgating education efforts about effective parenting, and inculcating an ethos of parenting skills and conscientiousness though the new popular media of the mid-twentieth century.

74. *Deinstitutionalization.* A cluster of factors shape the development of 'deinstitutionalization' in the mid-twentieth century, including the development of Medicare and Medicaid, the public influence of 'anti-psychiatry' critical

concerns about psychiatric/hospital abuses, the vision of a community mental health movement to treat the ill in their communities, and the rise of a promising new psychopharmacology, providing opportunities for stabilizing even chronic, severely mentally ill patients.

75. *From classifying pathology to classifying social care.* The American Association on Mental Retardation (AAMR, now the American Association on Intellectual and Developmental Disabilities (AAIDD)) departed from the individual psychopathology model of the DSMs in their late-twentieth-century classifications. In carrying out the spirit of 'normalization' from midcentury, the new AAMR/AAIDD classifications focus on a social demand model, and the kinds of social care posed by their population.

76. The 1973 by-member-vote decision by the American Psychiatric Association to 'declassify' homosexuality as a mental disorder is a major victory for the gay liberation movement, provoking an ongoing discussion of the issue of moral judgments in psychiatric diagnosis, as well as a providing a challenge to the scientific status of psychiatric classification.

77. *Increases in homeless and incarcerated mentally ill.* By the end of the twentieth century, deinstitutionalization, cost restrictions on community psychiatry, a failure to parse out criminal offenders from mentally ill offenders, public policy and attitudes to be 'tough on crime', and the failure to effect cures for mental illness all contribute to a large problem of the homeless mentally ill, as well as the overpopulation of the mentally ill in jails and prisons in many US states.

78. *US leads in per capita incarceration rates.* In the second half of the twentieth century, American prisons experienced explosive growth to make the United States the leader in incarceration rates per capita in the free world. Factors that contributed to this complex phenomenon included tough-on-crime politics, extraordinary numbers of drug-related convictions and sentencing to prison, an economic structure that favored harsh punishments over reform and drug treatment, as well as the shifting of offender-management costs from local communities to the state and Federal systems.

79. *Psychiatry responds to growing stigma of mental illness.* In the latter twentieth century, American psychiatry increasingly distances itself from its historic criminal-reform commitments because of anticrime public sentiment, as well as a felt need for psychiatry to address the stigmatizing of mental illness as manifested by burgeoning homelessness, addiction, overcrowding of facilities, and the faltering of outpatient public sector care.

80. *New penal settings and sentencing reforms address prison crowding.* In response to prison overrun, but with varying success, states and the federal government institute greater dependence on parole and probation, increasing the use of psychiatry and clinical psychology; develop new levels of security based on the degree of dangerousness of criminals, and implement alternatives to prisons such as house arrest, work-release, electronic monitoring (ankle bracelets),

and sentencing reforms such as community service and compulsory outpatient mental health treatment.

81. *A psychiatric medical-industrial complex.* In the latter half of the twentieth century, the explosive growth of psychopharmacological approaches fed into a 'MIC' which converged financial causal vectors from business, the NIMH, insurance companies, commercial advertising, and wanton big-business lobbying of Congress, culminating in a powerful economic domination of American psychiatry and the transformation of psychiatrists' clinical role from the holistic captains of mental health care to (too often) the mere dispensers of pills.

82. *Ineffective treatments for vice-laden disorders.* Despite unparalleled expenditures for psychiatric research in the past 50 years, the group of disorders identified in this book as 'vice-laden' identify a group of psychiatric conditions with the worst research base, treatment opportunities, and outcomes in the field.

83. *Clinical significance criterion in sexual disorders.* In the DSM-IV era of the late-twentieth century, the issue of the clinical significance criterion (a requirement for a disorder to be associated with distress and/or impairment) becomes a significant source of discussion for sexual disorders and the paraphilias.

84. *Psychiatry dominated by 'theoretical orientations'.* By the end of the twentieth century, the eighteenth-century faculty-oriented psychopathology had been in large part confounded and replaced by a psychiatry dominated by 'theoretical orientations', both articulated and railed against by influential theorists such as Leston Havens, George Engel, Paul McHugh and Philip Slavney, David Brendel, Bradley Lewis, Kenneth Kendler and Peter Zachar, and Nassir Ghaemi.

As I hope is evident from these 84 summary points, many, perhaps most, of these iconic ideas are still alive today in various forms, through different populations, constituencies, and cultures. They still play out in our contemporary discourse, whether that be the popular media, the courtroom, the consultation room, or the legislation room. With this detailed cultural background, I will now turn to our VMDR contemporary scene through several perspectives.

Notes

1. Rothman (2002a, p. 3).
2. Grob (1994; Rothman 2002a).
3. Nielsen (2012).
4. Hunter & MacAlpine (1963, pp. 66–67).
5. Pliny Earle, quoted in Grob (1983, p. 35).
6. Rothman (2002a).

7. ibid, p. 101.
8. As we'll see in Chapter 6, English and American l debate the boundary between immoral and illegal conduct up to the present.
9. Rothman (1995, 2002b).
10. Rothman (1995, 2002a). This severity of punishment in the earlier colonial era was to change with mounting resentment of the British and their 'ways' later in the eighteenth century, as American revolutionary fervor mounted, and a Zeitgeist of humanistic and democratic reform coalesced.
11. Hacsi (1995, p. 162).
12. Kendi (2016).
13. Jarvis (1842, p. 119); see also Deutsch (1949).
14. Cartwright (1851).
15. Gonaver, W. (2018).
16. Summers (2010); see also Simon (1978).
17. Grob (1983, 1994).
18. McConville (1995).
19. Rothman (1995, 2002a, p. 6).
20. Rothman (2002a, p. 29).
21. Grob (1994).
22. See McConville (1995); Nielsen (2012); Rafter (1997a, b); Rothman (2002a).
23. Grob (1994, p. 24).
24. ibid, p. 25.
25. Wallace (1994, p. 47); see also Sigerist (1951, 1961); Simon (2008).
26. Grob (2008a); Rothman (2002a).
27. Grob (2008a).
28. Grob (1994, 2008a); Rothman (2002a, 2002b).
29. Deutsch (1949, Grob (2008a, 2008b); Rothman (2002a).
30. Grob (2008b, p. 533).
31. Barton (1987).
32. Deutsch (1949); Grob (1994); Rafter (2007a, b); Rothman (2002a, 2002b).
33. Grob (2008b, p. 536); see also the original source: Worchester State Lunatic Hospital, *Annual Report*, 61 (1893) p. 70.
34. This 'algebra of chronicity' will be a recurrent theme for this history and this book.
35. Deutsch (1949); Grob (1983, 1994, 2008a 2008b); Rothman (2002a, 2002b). An interesting historical question is: Where did the acute patients go when the asylums were full? We'll see later that the founding of outpatient psychiatry provides one part of the answer but in the transition the question remains.
36. Grob (2008b, pp. 538–539).
37. Grob (1983, 1994, 2008a).
38. Grob (2008).
39. The medical specialty that 'owns' the demented elderly is ambiguous today, often played out in the domains of psychiatry, neurology, and internal medicine. The old saw from the mid-twentieth century that held that as somatic causes are discovered, the patient population moves out of psychiatry, seems to be breaking down.
40. Grob (1983).
41. Grob (1983, p. 62).
42. Shorter & Fink (2010, p 23).
43. Grob (1983).
44. Rothman (2002b).
45. Winter (2004).

46. Grob (2008b).
47. Grob (1983).
48. Grob (1983, 2008a).
49. Grob (2008b, p. 547).
50. These APA Task Force reports have been a valuable resource from which this book has drawn and referred.
51. Goldman & Morrissey (1984, 1985).
52. Talbott (2004).
53. The 'antipsychiatry' label was often, perhaps usually, resisted by its 'members', justifiably so in that their views were diverse and unified only in the view that psychiatry was in need of reform, revision, or in some cases, rejection. In some ways, the legacy of the antipsychiatrists lives on within psychiatry today through the 'critical psychiatry' network: http://www.criticalpsychiatry.net/. Outside of psychiatry, another 'legacy' organization of antipsychiatry might well be Mind Freedom International http://www.mindfreedom.org/.
54. Grob (2008a, b).
55. Grob (1994).
56. Morrissey & Goldman (1984, 1985).
57. Goldman & Morrissey (1985, p. 728).
58. Grob (1994).
59. Stevens (2008).
60. At least in the United States, concerns about abuse of human subjects in clinical research settings did not arise in a profound way until the 1960s, several well-publicized cases came to professional/scientific and public attention generating congressional intervention. See Emanuel et al. (2008); Rothman & Rothman (1984).
61. Healy (1997, 2002).
62. Goodman et al. (2003); Greene (2007); Healy (2003).
63. Kovel (1980).
64. Healy (2003); see also Eisenberg (1986); Relman (1980).
65. Potter (2010); Potter & Penniman (2017). Wendell Potter's 2010 book on how corporate pharmaceutical companies manipulate messaging to sell pharmaceuticals is a persuasive analysis from an industry insider. He went on to crusade against the corrupting influence of 'big money' on democracy in general in his 2017 collaboration with Nick Penniman.
66. See Sadler (2013) for a detailed discussion of the contemporary mental health MIC, and its links to the DSM. See also Rothman 2012.
67. Stevens (2004).
68. See Healy (2002, 2004); Relman (2007).
69. Sadler (2009).
70. See Larry Davidson (2013) for a comparison of the 'cure' model of mental disorder and the 'recovery' model of mental disorder, and Kirk & Kutchins (1992).
71. Sackett et al. (2000).
72. Gupta M. (2009).
73. See Insel & Wang (2010); National Advisory Mental Health Council's Workgroup (2010).
74. See for instance Leichter (2003); Minkler (1999); Resnik (2007); Wikler (2002).
75. Minkler (1999).
76. Parens & Johnston (2011).
77. This claim can be verified simply through the examination of current psychiatric textbooks.
78. Harris & Rice (2006); Millon et al. (1998).
79. Laws & O'Donohue (2008). Zonana et al. (1999).
80. Hill & Maughan (2001).
81. Cited in Rothman (2002a, p. 76).

82. Rothman (1995, 2002a).
83. Rothman (1995).
84. ibid.
85. Rothman (1995, p. 106).
86. Rothman (1995).
87. Dickens, quoted in Rothman (1995, p. 111).
88. Morris (1995); Tonry (2004).
89. Rothman (1995, 2002b); Rotman (1995).
90. Rotman (1995).
91. ibid.
92. Report quoted in Rotman (1995, p. 155).
93. See the American Correctional Association's website: www.aca.org.
94. Meskell (1999); Rotman (1995).
95. Rotman (1995).
96. Goffman (1961); Rotman (1995).
97. Morris (1995).
98. ibid.
99. Liptak (2008).
100. The Pew Center on the States, The Pew Charitable Trusts (2009).
101. ibid; Liptak (2008).
102. Tonry (2004, p. 21).
103. Liptak (2008).
104. Tonry (2004).
105. ibid.
106. ibid.
107. Beckett (1997).
108. Tonry (2004, p. 41).
109. Morris (1995).
110. Morris (1995, p. 228).
111. Noll & Trent (2004); Trent (1994).
112. Rothman (2002a).
113. Trent (1994, p. 11).
114. Noll & Trent (2004).
115. Jean Etienne Dominique Esquirol (1772–1840) a French alienist will become an influential theorist of 'monomania' and can be considered one of the founders of Forensic Psychiatry.
116. Séguin quoted in Trent (1994, pp. 45–46).
117. Trent (1994, pp. 51–52).
118. ibid, p. 53.
119. Brigham quoted in Rafter (1997a, b p. 24).
120. 'Report of Committee on Classification of Feeble-Minded', reproduced in Noll and Trent (2004, p. 87), from the 1910 publication in the *Journal of Psycho-Asthenics*.
121. Rafter (1997a, b).
122. Deutsch (1949); Rafter (1997a, b).
123. Rafter (1997a, b).
124. Trent (1994).
125. Rafter (1997a, b), quotes mine.
126. ibid, p. 68.
127. Rafter (1997a, b, 2008).
128. Rafter (1997a, b).
129. Noll & Trent (2004); Rafter (1997a, b).

130. Ray (1838, p. 123).

131. ibid, p. 124.

132. Rafter (1997a, b).

133. Rush (1786, pp. 1–2). Dr. Rush's distinction here is prescient to contemporary cognitive neuroscience's distinction between 'fast' moral intuition and the slower moral reflection.

134. Metzel quoted in Noll & Trent (2004, pp. 420–444); Rafter (1997a, b).

135. Noll & Trent (2004); Rafter (1997, 2008); Trent (1994).

136. Dwyer (2004) Rafter (1997a, b); Trent (1994).

137. Trent (1994, p. 160).

138. ibid, p. 164.

139. Goddard quoted in Trent (1994).

140. Deutsch (1949); Trent (1994).

141. Trent (1994, p. 193.

142. ibid, pp. 197–198.

143. Trent (1994).

144. ibid.

145. Trent (1994, p. 231).

146. Trent (1994).

147. ibid, p. 243.

148. Nielsen (2012).

149. Noll & Trent (2004); Scheerenberger (1987); Trent (1994).

150. See Danforth (2011); Danforth, Slocum, & Dunkle (2010); Goodey (2005); Mather & Morris (2011) McClimens (2007).

151. Trent (1994).

152. Grinnell (2011).

153. APA (1952, p. 100).

154. Scheerenberger (1987, p. 12).

155. APA (1968, p. 14).

156. Scheerenberger (1987, pp. 12–13).

157. ibid.

158. Scheerenberger (1987, p. 13).

159. APA (1980, p. 36).

160. ibid, p. 8.

161. APA (1987, p. 32).

162. APA (1994).

163. APA (2000).

164. AAMR, (2002, pp. xi–xii).

165. American Psychiatric Association (2013); Nielsen (2012).

166. I thank, and give credit to E. Jane Costello, Ph.D., for her presenting the Office Krupke song from *West Side Story* as an introduction to her lecture on the epidemiology of conduct disorder. Dr. Costello also gave valuable input into this section. I should also note the appearance of cross-dressing and gender ambiguity in *Officer Krupke*, identifying gender ambiguity with delinquency. A half a century later gay/lesbian/bisexual/transgender/queer advocacy had moved gender ambiguity from delinquency/deviance to an expression of human diversity. As this book was completed in 2022, social debate about LGBTQ+ rights, healthcare, and civil liberties persists.

167. Grossberg (2002, p. 6).

168. Grossberg (2002); see also Friedman (2005); Jones (1999); Rothman (2002a).

169. Kymlicka (1990).

170. Grossberg (2002, p. 6).

171. Friedman (2005); Kelly (1992).

172. Pleck (1987); also quoted by Grossberg (2002, p. 8).

173. Grossberg (2002); Jones (1999).

174. ibid.

175. Grossberg (2002).

176. Jones (1999).

177. https://unos.org/transplant/history/. Last accessed 12/29/21.

178. Tanenhaus (2002); see also Jones (1999).

179. Tanenhaus (2002, p. 59).

180. Baker (1910).

181. See http://www.law.cornell.edu/uscode/42/666.html. Last accessed 11-1-21.

182. Jones (1999, p. 8).

183. Jones (1999); Tanenhaus (2002).

184. Deutsch (1949).

185. ibid, p. 323.

186. Deutsch (1949); Horn (1989).

187. George Stevenson MD, quoted in Deutsch (1949, p. 325).

188. Deutsch (1949).

189. Jones (1999).

190. Dillaway & Paré (2008).

191. Paolucci & Violato (2004).

192. Healy, quoted in Jones (1999, p. 45).

193. Adapted from Healy (1915). Breckinridge & Abbott (1912).

195. ibid, p. 10.

196. Jones (1999).

197. From the American Orthopsychiatric Association website, www.aoatoday.com/ortho.php last accessed 10/23/11, which is now defunct, having been superceded by their renamed organization, Global Alliance for Behavioral Health and Social Justice https://www.bhjustice.org/. Last accessed 12/29/21.

198. See their website: https://www.bhjustice.org/. Last accessed 12/15/21.

199. Jones (1999, p. 33), quoted from statute.

200. Horn (1989); Jones (1999).

201. Jones (1999).

202. Maier (2003).

203. Parent-Teacher Association, founded 1897 as the National Congress of Parents and Teachers: https://www.pta.org/home/About-National-Parent-Teacher-Association/Mission-Values/National-PTA-History; http://www.pta.org/1164.asp. Last accessed 12/29/21.

204. Pinel, quoted by Goldstein (2001, p. 172).

205. Prosono (2003, p. 18).

206. Hale, Emly, and Wilson 1736. Available online https://archive.org/details/historiaplacitor01hale/page/n3/mode/2up. Last accessed 12/29/21).

207. Coke (1791). Coke's book is available online as a Google E-book: https://www.google.com/books/edition/The_First_Part_of_the_Institutes_of_the/_x00AQAAMAAJ?hl=en&gbpv=1&dq=Sir+Edward+Coke%E2%80%99s+The+First+Part+of+the+Institutes+of+the+Laws+of+England+or,+a+Commentary+upon+Littleton+&pg=IA1&printsec=frontcover. Last accessed 12/29/21.

208. Friedman (2005); Plucknett (1956); Robinson (1996).

209. Coke (1628) quoted in Robinson (1996, p. 118); bracketed translations from the Latin are mine.

210. Garner (2004, p. 39).

211. Erickson & Erickson (2008) have emphasized the ideological frame of morality lent by the *mens rea/actus reus* language in English common law, coupled with the concept of free will, then create a religious metaphysics undergirding Law, which they then contrast with the blameless,

deterministic metaphysics of behavioral science and medical explanations of misconduct. These considerations will receive more attention in the concluding chapters.

212. Prosono (2003); Robinson (1996).
213. Porter (2002).
214. Jackson (1983); Radden (2000).
215. Goldstein (1998, 2001).
216. Simon & Shuman (2002).
217. Robinson (1996). Professor Robinson's book is an excellent general reference for the history of the insanity plea.
218. See Prosono (2003); Robinson (1996).
219. See "State Insanity Defense Laws, (U.S.) Public Broadcasting Service (PBS), http://www.pbs.org/wgbh/pages/frontline/shows/crime/trial/states.html, last accessed 11/14/21. See also FindLaw.com, "The Insanity Defense Among the States," https://www.findlaw.com/criminal/criminal-procedure/the-insanity-defense-among-the-states.html. Last accessed 11/14/21.
220. Ray (1838).
221. ibid, p. 169.
222. ibid, pp. 172–173.
223. The relevance of this description to contemporary Hypomania and/or Narcissistic Personality Disorder are striking to twenty-first-century readers.
224. Ray (1838, p. 186–187).
225. In Foucault's later *Abnormal* (1999) collection of lectures, he describes three domains of abnormality in nineteenth-century France. Of most interest here he calls the 'human monster', the seemingly rational author of inconceivable crimes, an individual who defies the law, as well as the laws of nature: 'The field in which the monster appears can thus be called a "juridico-biological" domain. . . . The monster is the limit, both the point at which law is overturned and the exception that is found only in extreme cases. The monster combines the impossible and the forbidden' (p. 56).
226. Prosono (2003); see also Robinson (1996).
227. Gariepy (1994).
228. I.F.R., 1872.
230. Rogers (2008).
231. Slovenko (2002).
232. American Law Institute. http://www.ali.org/index.cfm?fuseaction=about.overview. Last accessed 11/27/11.
233. ALI, quoted in Gutheil and Appelbaum (2000, p. 276).
234. Slovenko (2002).
235. See Sadler (2002) for a detailed discussion.
236. Slovenko (2002).
237. ibid.
238. ibid.
239. Sadler (2002); see also Morse (1998).
240. Wallace (1994).
241. ibid.
242. Hunter & MacAlpine (1963).
243. ibid.
244. Benjamin Rush, *An Inquiry into the Influence of Physical Causes Upon the Moral Faculty*, 1839, p. 1, available online through NIH Digital Collections: https://collections.nlm.nih.gov/catalog/nlm:nlmuid-57020900R-bk. Last accessed 12/29/21.
245. Rush (1839, pp. 6–7).
246. ibid.

247. Hunter & MacAlpine (1963, p. 715).
248. Hunter & MacAlpine (1963).
249. Prichard (1835), from Hunter & MacAlpine (1963, p. 839).
250. ibid, pp. 839–840.
251. ibid, p. 840.
252. Millon, Simonsen, & Birket-Smith (1998).
253. Hunter & MacAlpine (1963, p. 838).
254. Dain (1964).
255. Millon, Simonsen, & Birket-Smith (1998).
256. ibid, p. 10. See also Kraepelin (1904).
257. Blashfield (1982, 1984).
258. Healy & Bronner (1926).
259. Partridge (1930).
260. Millon, Simonsen, & Birket-Smith (1998, p. 16).
261. Patrick (2006).
262. Cleckley (1988, pp. 337–338).
263. Widiger (2006).
264. Esquirol (1845, p. 320).
265. ibid.
266. ibid.
267. ibid.
268. Esquirol (1845, p. 335).
269. ibid, p. 351.
270. ibid.
271. Singy (2009), and personal communication (2011).
272. Foucault (1999).
273. Esquirol (1845, p. 362).
274. Goldstein (1987, 1998).
275. Hunter & MacAlpine (1963).
276. Ray (1838, pp. 162–163).
277. ibid, pp. 164–165.
278. ibid.
279. ibid, p. 167.
280. Gamwell & Tomes (1995, p. 80).
281. ibid, p. 81.
282. Cartwright (1851); see also Haller (1972).
283. Goldstein (2001).
284. Goldstein (1998, 2001).
285. Goldstein (2001).
286. Kraepelin (1904). For a more extended discussion of monomania in contemporary Psychiatry, see Sadler (2015).
287. Bynum (2003).
288. Glueck (1916).
289. Abelson (1989).
290. O'Brien (1983).
291. Anonymous (1897).
292. Abelson (1989), quotation the author's, in original article.
293. Geller, Erlen, & Pinkus (1986).
294. Hunter & MacAlpine (1963).
295. Stekel (1911).

296. Geller, Erlen, & Pinkus (1986).

297. ibid, p. 223.

298. Liégeois (1991).

299. Rafter (1997a, b).

300. See Rafter (1997a, b, 2008) for detailed discussions of the spread of degeneracy theory in the United States. Foucault (1999) provides a discussion for France, and Shorter (1997) and Zilboorg (1941) for general discussions.

301. Rafter (1997a, b).

302. Ferri (1917).

303. See Rafter (1997a, b) for details.

304. Lombroso (1912); Rafter (1997a, b).

305. Lombroso (1912, pp. 57–58).

306. Lombroso (1912, p. 60).

307. ibid.

308. ibid.

309. German Berrios (1996); Stroud & Zvirsky (2021).

310. Pink (2000, p. 929).

311. Berrios (1996, p. 351), original citations omitted.

312. Stroud & Tappolet (2013).

313. Irwin (1992).

314. Reid, quoted in Berrios (1996, p. 353).

315. Berrios (1996).

316. Esquirol (1845).

317. Berrios (1996).

318. Berrios (1996, p. 364).

319. Foucault (2003, p. 56).

320. Adshead (2008). See also her book-length study with Horne (2021).

321. Berrios (1996).

322. Colaizzi (1989).

323. Original in Colaizzi (1989, p. 8).

324. Deutsch (1949).

325. Blashfield (1984); Colaizzi (1989).

326. Ray (1838, pp. 199–200).

327. ibid.

328. Ray (1839, p. 204).

329. ibid, p. 205.

330. Foucault discusses Cornier as a 'monster' at some length in *Abnormal* (1999).

331. Ray (1838, pp. 218–219).

332. ibid, p. 221.

333. ibid, p. 223.

334. ibid, p. 229, italics in original.

335. ibid, p. 231.

336. ibid, pp. 233–234.

337. Davidson (2001).

338. Resnick (2007).

339. American Psychiatric Association (1980).

340. American Psychiatric Association (1952, 1968).

341. American Psychiatric Association (1980, 1987, 1994, 2000).

342. Kelly (1992).

343. See Dain, (1964).

344. Rafter (1997a, 2008).
345. Cleckley (1941).
346. Michaud & Aynesworth (1999).
347. Hare & Neumann (2006).
348. American Psychiatric Association (1980, 1987, 1994, 2000).
349. American Psychiatric Association (1980, 1987, 1994, 2000).
350. Gordon (1999).
351. Wender (1971).
352. Elliott (1982, 1992).
353. Colaizzi (1989, p. 84).
354. See for instance Steadman & Cocozza (1978); Steadman & Felson (1984); Steadman, Mulvey, Monahan et al. (1998); Steadman, Robbins, Silver et al. (1999).
355. Colaizzi (1989, p. 117); quoting Dercum, (1917) p. 195.
356. American Psychiatric Association (2000).
357. Noyes, quoted in Colaizzi (1989, p. 117).
358. Paine (1923); Slater & Beard (1963).
359. Colaizzi (1989).
360. Hall (1970).
361. Andreasen (2007).
362. Blashfield (1984).
363. Not until contemporary philosophy of psychopathology did conceptual refinement of phenomenological concepts reappear. See for instance Lysaker & Lysaker (2008); Parnas, Sass, & Kendler (2008); Ratcliffe (2008); Stanghellini & Fuchs (2013); Stanghellini (2004).
364. Sadler (2005).
365. Sadler (1997).
366. Havens (1973).
367. McHugh & Slavney (1998).
368. Engel (1977, 1980).
369. Brendel (2006).
370. Kendler (2008); Zachar (2000); Zachar & Kendler (2007).
371. Lewis (2011).
372. Ghaemi (2003, 2010).
373. Jaspers (1997).
374. Fulford, Stanghellini, Sadler, & Morris (2003).
375. Frances (1994).
376. Davidson (2001); Garton (2004); Irvine (2005); Laqueur (1990); Martin & Barresi (2006); Oosterhuis (2000); Porter & Hall (1995).
377. Of course, the potential for communication with highly selective social groups was to experience another quantum leap in the late-twentieth century with the explosion of the Internet, digital communication, and most recently 'social media'.
378. Garton (2004); Laqueur (1990); Nye (1999); Porter & Teich (1994).
379. See Bullough (1994a, 1994b); Irvine (2005); Oosterhuis (2000). Even the term in early Sexual Psychiatry, 'perversion', reveals through its negative connotation the residuum of moralizing about deviating from sexual conventions. It was a transitional concept—less awful than 'abomination', but not as comparatively accepting as 'sexual diversity' and other terms we might use in the early twenty-first century.
380. Oosterhuis (2000).
381. ibid.
382. ibid, p. 227.
383. Laqueur (1989).

384. Krafft-Ebing (K-E) (1965).

385. Sorry to disappoint some of you.

386. K-E (1965); Oosterhuis (2000); Porter & Teich (1994).

387. Oosterhuis (2000).

388. Oosterhuis (2000, p. 45).

389. Dain (1964, p. 91).

390. Bullough (1994b, p. 303), original citations omitted.

391. Deutsch (1949); Rothman (2002b).

392. Bullough (1994b).

393. LaMay (1997).

394. Friedman (2005).

395. Behr (2011).

396. American Medico-Psychological Association (1918).

397. ibid, p. 27.

398. Grob (1991).

399. ibid, p. 427.

400. Grob (1991).

401. Allyn (1996) Bancroft (2004); Bullough (1990, 1998, 2004, 2006); Granzig (2006); Irvine (2005); Pryce (2006).

402. American Psychiatric Association (1952, pp. 38–39).

403. See especially Bayer (1981, 1987); also Sadler (2005).

404. American Psychiatric Association (1974, p. 44).

405. ibid.

406. American Psychiatric Association (1980, pp. 281–283).

407. American Psychiatric Association (1994, p. 538).

408. Sadler (2005).

409. American Psychiatric Association (1980, p. 266).

410. Seidman, Fischer, & Meeks (2006).

411. American Psychiatric Association (1994, p. 523).

412. ibid.

6

The legal and criminal justice context of the VMDR

With this chapter I move into the contemporary realm and sketch the conceptual background necessary to understanding the vice/mental disorder relationship (VMDR) from the legal/court and criminal justice/penal system perspectives. In the first section I compare critically the aims, methods, and some of the metaphysical assumptions of law and medicine/psychiatry. In places, I consider medicine and psychiatry separately. While many of the aims, methods, and metaphysical assumptions of medicine in general and psychiatry-in-particular are shared, particular aspects of psychiatry differentiate it from general medicine, as will be seen. As I have argued elsewhere[1] psychiatry poses a special case of medical practice in some domains—domains I will show are critical for the VMDR.

One domain of consideration here calls attention to the social problem of the widespread incarceration of the mentally ill in the US penal system—a heartbreaking and growing problem, though one, I will argue, that is closely related to inadequate treatment opportunities in the mental health system, combined with inadequate diversion by the criminal justice system (CJS) into mental health care and other factors. These failures fall particularly on the poor, and therefore often, perhaps typically,

Vice and Psychiatric Diagnosis. John Z. Sadler, Oxford University Press. © Oxford University Press 2024.
DOI: 10.1093/oso/9780198876830.003.0006

are racialized, contributing to systemic racism in the mental health and CJSs. From these standpoints, the incarceration of the mentally ill has less to do with psychiatric diagnosis and the VMDR than it has to do with the disarray of our mental health, criminal justice, and other social welfare systems. These in turn are embedded in larger social, political, and economic structures, leading to failures in the humane management of patients, offenders, and prisoners and too often failing the public at large. The concluding two sections ask two simple questions: (1) What do the law, and the courts, want from psychiatric diagnosis? (2) What does the criminal justice and penal system want from psychiatric diagnosis? As might be expected, the questions are easy to ask but more difficult to answer, given the aforementioned metaphysical differences in the two fields, as well as the problem of jurisdictional diversity in the United States.

6.1 The law and the criminal justice system—background

Some preliminary and cautionary notes are in order for this section. In the following analyses of US law and medicine, my intent is not to formulate an original or revisionist account of these disciplines—rather, the intent is to capture a plausible and relatively noncontroversial account of their goals, methods, and procedures. Stated differently, my reader needs a straightforward understanding of the goals, content, and relationships of these systems. With this understanding, the presentation of the following goals of law, medicine, and psychiatry are not intended to be philosophically critical, but instead, conventional; normative in the 'standard' sense of the term, and not the 'prescriptive' sense of the term. If I and my readers are to understand the law/medicine context of the VMDR, then a descriptive account of these fields is needed. A critical and prescriptive account will be addressed in later stages of this book.

6.1.1 Comparing law and medicine

Considering the history provided in Chapters 4 and 5, it would appear that lawyers and doctors have always had an uneasy relationship. They differ in aims, in methods, and most importantly, in many of the metaphysical assumptions about the nature of being human and how knowledge or the 'truth' is ascertained. Mental disorders that are associated with wrongful or criminal conduct confound both disciplines in at least two directions. For the vice-laden mental disorders that are the primary consideration in this book, they commingle concepts of disease with concepts of morality, the latter traditionally being a core background for the law.[2] The other direction, that of patients with non-vice-laden disorders who criminally offend, the legal notions of culpability, intent, and excuse commingle with clinical notions of (ir)rationality and cause-effect relationships. Law and medicine, I'll show, come at 'truth' in these contexts from quite different directions, an understanding that will help clarify some of the confusion about the VMDR.

6.1.1.1 The aims of law, medicine, and psychiatry

In this section I will compare and contrast the aims, or goals, of law and medicine, beginning with the former; and concluding about the special case of medical psychiatry. A few introductory comments are required. American law, for my purposes, has several varieties pertinent to the VMDR. The baldest distinction is between common, statutory, and civil law. Common law is the body of law developed over time based upon judicial decisions and precedents and handed down for judicial interpretation and application to new cases.[3] In the United States, common law addresses many facets of the VMDR, and is derived partly from English common law 'brought over' by the British colonists, as well as a huge body of judicial decisions scattered among the 50 states as colonial America developed and grew into an independent country. The local nature of common law in the United States makes for a dizzying array of variations for the nation at large. Statutory law is made up of laws that are passed through political action—legislation—by governing bodies, like Congress or state legislatures.

Civil law, in contrast, is a system of laws that address particular kinds of cases— typically, private disputes or binding agreements between individuals or groups of individuals. These include contract law, tort law, family law, and property law. Tort law, typically derived from common law, addresses disputes between people involving compensation for damages (and excluding violations of contracts). Tort law is familiar to clinicians in cases of malpractice and personal injury lawsuits. Criminal law, of significant interest to the VMDR theorist, is made up of both common law and statutory law elements, where common law fills in the gaps that are not explicitly addressed by the statutory instructions of legislation. Of course, criminal law is focused upon the issue of crime, which is conceptualized as offenses against the community or polity. Torts address disputes between individuals; criminal law addresses disputes between an individual and society.[4]

Goals of Law. Before we can understand the aim of the law, a discussion of the meaning of 'law' and 'crime' provides a useful background. Perhaps an obvious place to start is to examine what a contemporary textbook of criminal law has to say about the aims and goals of criminal law. Here I use Matthew Lippman's text from 2009.[5] Lippman presents this discussion as fundamental introductory material to his text. He describes the nature of crime as:

> . . . an act that is officially condemned by the community and carries a sense of shame and humiliation. Professor Henry M. Hart, Jr. defines crime as "conduct which, if . . . shown to have taken place will result in the 'formal and solemn pronouncement of moral condemnation of the community' ". (p.2, editing in original text)

In this description, the relationship of community morality to law is explicit, posing a philosophical and normative question to be examined in more detail later, namely, Should the law be governed by a community morality?

In his discussion of the purpose of criminal law, Lippman appeals to a few statements from various state legislatures. I have selected his extract from New York State as an example here because of its multifaceted description of the reach of criminal law:[6]

> The primary purpose or function of criminal law is to help maintain social order and stability. . . . The New York criminal code sets out the basic purposes of criminal law as follows:
>
> - *Harm*. To prohibit conduct that unjustifiably or inexcusably causes or threatens substantial harm to individuals as well as to society
> - *Warning*. To warn people both of conduct that is subject to criminal punishment and of the severity of the punishment
> - *Definition*. To define the act and intent that is required for each offense
> - *Seriousness*. To distinguish between serious and minor offenses and to assign the appropriate punishments
> - *Punishment*. To impose punishments that satisfy the demands for revenge, rehabilitation, and deterrence of future crimes
> - *Victims*. To insure that the victim, the victim's family, and the community interests are represented at trial and in imposing punishments

In reading between the lines, the reader can recognize motifs that were introduced in Chapter 5 concerning the historical development of law: preservation of the public order (Harm), deterrence from offending (Warning), framing responsibility and culpability (Definition), Punishment, and involvement of the victim(s). As we come to understand more about the CJS, we'll see that several of these elements of law will be challenged, as well as some of the metaphysical assumptions that underlie them.

Even from Lippman's brief discussion of the nature and purposes of law one can see that criminal law has a potential for many meanings, purposes, and social roles. Criminal law should be understood within the context of law broadly conceived, which at this point I will mark with a capital 'L', with 'Law' meaning the law in the broadest historical sense. The distinguished American legal scholar, Roscoe Pound, in his *An Introduction to the Philosophy of Law*,[7] identified 12 senses, or meanings, of Western Law. These conceptions of Law are summarized in Table 6.1 below. As we'll see, only a handful of these are of contemporary significance for a discussion of the VMDR. However, all of them are of significance in the potential for confounding scholarly, professional, and lay discussions of Law as one definition or sense may blend into another, confounding analysis and understanding. Pound provides only limited historical connections to these senses of the law, and I will remark on these when given. Otherwise, I will interpret them and cross-reference them to material from Chapters 4 and 5. I should note that these twelve senses do not represent a

Table 6.1 Roscoe Pound's Twelve Conceptions of Law

1. Law as divinely ordained rule(s) for human action

2. Law as divinely tolerated traditions and customs for human action

3. Law as the received wisdom of the aged and the ages

4. Law as a philosophically derived system of principles expressing the nature of things, to which humans should conform [natural law$_1$]

5. Law as an eternal and immutable moral code discoverable through reason [natural law$_2$]

6. Law as a system of agreements governing interpersonal relations within a political society

7. Law as a reflection of divine reason: one arm of 'oughts' or moral laws apropos to humanity, and the other arm of 'musts' suitable to the rest of creation [Aquinas' Natural Law, natural law$_3$]

8. Law as a 'body of commands of the sovereign authority' (Pound 1959, p. 27)

9. Law as a system of 'precepts' (p. 28) which, once discovered by humanity, maximize freedom of will for all

10. Law as a body of philosophical and juridical discourse intended to harmonize the collective will of humanity

11. Law as a system of rules imposed by the empowered to advance their own interests

12. Law as the expression of social rules derived from social science with the aim of regulating social conduct and assuring justice

linear development of Law, but more like an historical family of concepts, culture-bound and differentiated in various directions.[8]

The first sense identified by Pound is linked to the idea of a divine ruler or authority who issues one or more proclamations for worldly human beings to respect. Pound cites the Code of Hammurabi[9] as an example.

The second sense of Law for Pound is one bound up with tradition—Law as a set of customs or mores established by humans and presumably tolerated or authorized by the gods. I interpret this sense as reflected in Sophocles' ancient Greek conflict between Antigone and Creon.[10] In this account, Antigone, in defiance of King Creon's earthly command to leave the conquered dead to rot, instead seeks to respect the gods by providing the traditional burial of her dead brother. Antigone's rejection of earthly law in favor of divinely approved tradition exemplifies Pound's second sense of Law.

Pound presents the third sense as the received cultural wisdom from the sages and elders of the society. He cites Demosthenes and the ancient law of Athens, and I would add Confucius's sense of custom as a prevailing governing power in societies.[11] One can recognize a preliminary relationship of this sense to centuries-later concepts of common law discussed earlier.

The fourth sense of Law introduces human reflection and reason, and to my reading introduces an early concept of 'natural law' into these senses of Law—listed in Table 6.1 as 'natural law$_1$'. Pound describes this sense as reflected in early Roman law, acknowledging both the divine roots, but also the reconciliation with the prevailing political ideas of the time, all articulated though philosophical reason. Derivative from this fourth sense of Law is Pound's fifth sense, in which the natural law is given, through philosophical reflection, greater metaphysical weight through, to use Pound's terms, 'a body of ascertainments and declarations of an eternal and immutable moral code'.[12] While Pound provides no explicit example here, this sense of law seems to me to be reflected in the relationships between the Stoics' metaphysical natural order and a subsequent, derivative moral order, briefly described in Chapter 4, Section 4.2.4.2. In Table 6.1 I identify this idea as 'natural law$_2$'.

The sixth sense of Law introduces what contemporary eyes might recognize as a more secular, modern sense of law, where law is explicitly political: where a people put together a 'body of agreements'[13] to govern human relations. Pound refers to the Minos dialogue of Plato as an example, and to my reading introduces a preliminary notion of a social contract.

Thomas Aquinas' Roman Catholic notion of natural law (identified in Table 6.1 as 'natural law$_3$') is linked to Pound's seventh sense of Law, where law is a reflection of divine reason governing the cosmos, split into (1) moral law governing people and (2) causal law which governs the rest of God's creations.[14]

The eighth sense introduces the idea of Law as directives from a sovereign political authority, and Pound provides multiple examples, ranging from Justinian law[15] to French and English notions of royal authority in the sixteenth and seventeenth centuries, and on down to parliamentary/democratic notions of political authority emerging from the American Revolution and Enlightenment philosophers. I would identify Hobbes[16] as an exemplar resource here, in his emphasis on combining both the social-contractual elements of law along with the prevailing authority of the sovereign.

The ninth sense of Law reflects the burgeoning diversification of human culture and philosophies. Pound describes it as an interaction between sovereign authority, human biopolitical potential, and juridical activity, which, writ large as a societal endeavor, will generate an emergent, perhaps inevitable, result: a maximizing of human freedoms. I read this as propounding a kind of progressive arc to Law, analogous to that of scientific progress, where the methodological activities of Law (science) progressively approximate justice (for Law) and knowledge (for science).[17]

The tenth sense of Law, again more contemporary, secular, and philosophical, where political theorizing and juridical decision combine to harmonize the 'individual in action' with the community.[18] I interpret this sense as exemplified by the nineteenth and twentieth century efforts to provide systematic philosophical accounts of justice, such as those by John Rawls,[19] Ronald Dworkin,[20] Martha Nussbaum,[21] and Robert Nozick[22]; accounts which are both deeply philosophical as well as engaged with ongoing developments and decisions in Law.

Pound casts his eleventh sense as an 'economic' one, though to my twenty-first-century reading it resonates with theories of social power articulated by Karl Marx or Michel Foucault.[23] Pound acknowledges that this sense of law has many varia-tions. He describes it as 'a body or system of rules imposed on men in society by the dominant class for the time being in furtherance, conscious or unconscious, of its own interest'.[24] Pound's discussion of this sense of Law as a 'class struggle'[25] evokes Karl Marx without explicitly citing him. Moreover, he notes that this sense of Law explicitly brings in the social sciences in understanding the meaning of Law. Indeed, the concept of 'normalizing' in Foucault and his interpreters[26] expands the reach of social theories of law to include not just economics, but psychiatry as part of the power relations which shape social conduct into increasingly homogenized norms.

The twelfth sense of Law according to Pound is described as a social product sub-ject to the analysis and interpretation by the sciences, whether they be biology or the social sciences. Earlier[27] Pound relates this sense of Law to legal positivism, the idea that law emerges from its sociohistorical sources, not from its value as a system of ideas. Here the law loses much of its autonomy and instead becomes a manifestation of larger social forces which the biological, psychological, and social sciences can explicate.

In reflecting upon Pound's senses of Law, and with a twenty-first-century, post-modern, post–critical theory, post-Foucauldian mind set, we can recognize that many of Pound's senses apply to criminal law today, but in combinations, in a dy-namic simultaneity. For example, we can recognize, in the altogether, the contem-porary need for protection of the polity from the dangerous mentally ill (sense 6), legislation that protects the civil liberties of the mentally ill (senses 9 or 10), the po-litical marginalizing of the mental health system and the overrepresentation of the mentally ill in jails and prisons as an expression of economic interests of the priv-ileged (sense 11), and the recognition that mental health law both empowers and dis-empowers particular individuals at different points in time, in different contexts, and in different ways (sense 12).

However, Pound's discussion of the senses of Law is more definitional, and less prescriptive or normative, as a discussion of the conventional goals of Law would be. Moreover, and as a matter of focus for this book, a discussion of goals, functions, or ends of the law should address the *criminal* law specifically; this is the domain of Law most relevant to the VMDR.

The history of 'independent' disciplines often makes for both ironies and corres-pondences. Such is the case for this phase in considering the goals or functions of *criminal* law, the British 'Wolfenden Report' of 1957.[28] In the sense of timing and in surrounding controversy, the Report anticipates the decriminalization of homosex-uality by the American Psychiatric Association (APA) in 1968 and indeed expresses overlapping concerns and controversies.[29] The Wolfenden Report was prompted by a series of publicized and embarrassing vice convictions of some prominent British citizens. In response, the British government appointed a committee, named after its chair, to address the current status of British law concerning the matters of ho-mosexuality and prostitution. The Committee's deliberations and report turned out to be a (controversial) benchmark in British, and ultimately American law[30] around the issue of what relationship the law should have to community morality. That is, should criminal law enforce morality? If so, which aspects of morality and determined by whom? If not, why not?

A thorough discussion of the Wolfenden Report and its aftermath warrants its own review and book, which of course cannot be done here. However, the deliberations and controversy around the Report aid in understanding the contemporary issue of morality and criminal law; the ramifications of which resonate throughout the United States (and UK) today through such considerations of laws concerning elective abortion, hate crimes, sodomy, gay and transgender rights, polygamy, and sex offenders.

Kelly[31] notes that in the considerations of the criminal status of homosexuality and prostitution, the Wolfenden Committee declared a philosophical position about the function of criminal law, a viewpoint that commentators have likened to John Stuart Mill's earlier position:[32]

> [The function of the criminal law in these areas] is to preserve public order and decency, to protect the citizen from what is offensive or injurious, and to provide sufficient safeguards against exploitation and corruption of others, particularly those who are specially vulnerable because they are young, weak in body or mind, inexperienced, or in a state of special physical, official or economic dependence.
>
> It is not, in our view, the function of the law to intervene in the private lives of citizens, or to seek to enforce any particular pattern of behavior, further than is necessary to carry out the purposes we have outlined . . . [We think to be decisive] the importance which society and the law ought to give to individual freedom of choice and action in matters of private morality. Unless a deliberate attempt is to be made by society, acting through the agency of the law, to equate the sphere of crime with that of sin, there must remain a realm of private morality and immorality which is, in brief and crude terms, not the law's business.[33]

In my review of the philosophy of (criminal) law, this is one of the earliest theoretical descriptions of its goals or functions outside of case decisions proper. The Wolfenden Report supported the decriminalization of homosexuality and supported the ongoing criminal status of prostitution.[34] It since has generated a substantial body of literature in English and American Law, and found its way into hundreds of legal opinions.[35]

My use here of the report is not to take sides in its analysis and critique, but to highlight the pragmatically clear statement of a common point of view about the function of criminal law. A few points of clarification and emphasis help us understand the associated controversy. First, the opening statement notes that criminal law is oriented toward both 'public order' and 'decency'. The former, 'public order' suggests a potential for a morality-neutral formulation of criminality—an example being stop-sign traffic legislation which prevents car accidents but does not meet my earlier discussed notion of a 'moral' value. Stop signs are a practical intervention which indeed preserves public order. However, the latter expression, 'decency' to my interpretation brings in the moral world; 'decency' and 'indecency' lose their meaning as word-concepts if we attempt to remove the moral evaluation from their meaning.[36] To be decent is a moral good, to be indecent is immoral. 'Decency' is moral-value-laden in a way that stop signs are not.

So the Wolfenden Committee recognizes that at least some component of morality contributes to criminal law. Similarly, in the reference to 'offensive' and 'injurious' related to criminal law, 'injurious' situations suggest a practical harm to the public order, while 'offensive' situations suggest negative values in the arena of the aesthetic (e.g., making highway billboards a criminal offense because they are ugly) or moral (the aforementioned prostitution because it is exploitative or demeaning). The reference to vulnerable individuals is of less interest to us here, other than as potential crime victims (see below) and is likely directed to the cases of homosexuality and prostitution as particular criminal offenses under consideration.

In the second Wolfenden paragraph reproduced above, an important distinction is introduced concerning the content of morality in law. The authors note that the [criminal] law is not to intervene in the citizen's private life, nor to enforce any particular 'pattern of behaviour' at least insofar the criminal law serves the functions of the first paragraph. The authors distinguish crime from sin, though they don't close the door on society electing to make that equivalency. Rather, the authors emphasize this as an important competing value is the preservation of 'individual freedom of choice and action in matters of private morality'. They conclude by acknowledging a 'realm of private morality and immorality' which is outside the function of criminal law.

What remained, and remains, to be debated is the extent that morality and immorality should be regulated by criminal law, and how such intrusion by the State into the moral lives of its citizens could be justified and delimited.[37] The debate revolves around the interest of the State to preserve order, as against the unreasonable intrusions by the State in the private lives and moralities of its citizens. To make this more concrete in terms of contemporary life, some examples of currently criminal activities that (arguably) cross into the realm of private life and personal morality include elective abortion, use of pornography, polygamy, sodomy, and euthanasia. We can immediately see the analogous ambiguities in the arena of psychiatric diagnosis—psychiatry has categories that are 'pathological' or 'sick' yet cross into the area of personal morality—the immoral and criminal conduct associated with Conduct Disorder, and the realm of private 'morally deviant' sexual practices such as paraphilic transvestism or fetishism being only a few examples.

The details of the debate needn't be reviewed here and have been considered elsewhere.[38] Judge Patrick Devlin, in his 1959 response to the Wolfenden Report, noted that indeed, current law was shot through with moral pronouncements. The presence of consenting partners, for instance, had not been sufficient to decriminalize suicide pacts, euthanasia, or sibling incest. For Devlin, English law reflected a public, largely Christian morality, and had done so for hundreds of years. For this reason, he was opposed to the theory that public morality could be expunged from the law—on practical grounds. Later, he clarified his position by stating that there was no theo-retical limit to law reflecting public morality; however, there were 'elastic principles' that as a practical matter could remove moral content from law, even consistent with the Wolfenden recommendations.[39] Kelly summarized neatly this later position:

> These principles, briefly, were 'toleration of the maximum individual freedom that is con-sistent with the integrity of society'; a recognition that 'the limits of tolerance shift'; a re-spect, as far as possible, for the privacy of individuals; and an acceptance that 'the law is concerned with the minimum and not with the maximum'—as he put it, 'there is much in the Sermon on the Mount that would be out of place in the Ten Commandments'.[40]

H. L. A. Hart, in his responses to Devlin, noted that some shared morality reflected in law is acceptable, even crucial, but that is quite different from maintaining that mo-rality is an identity with law. Moreover, from an empirical standpoint, a social toler-ance for degrees of immorality does not necessarily precipitate a total breakdown of society.[41]

We are left in current law with an acknowledgment that public morality penetrates into the law in a limited and variable fashion, and that in controversial cases the dis-tinction between protecting the functioning of society and imposing moral orders on private citizens can, should be, and are disputed. In the United States, we can recognize that laws governing sexual conduct have moral content as well as substantial political content, leading to the wide variations nationwide in different states' treatments of the aforementioned elective abortion, sodomy laws, and hate crime legislation.

While this debate was going on across the Atlantic, a Stanford Law professor, Herbert L. Packer, was approaching the function of criminal law from a different direc-tion, that of 'models' of criminal procedure.[42] Packer's approach for framing the 'crim-inal sanction' described a kind of social dialectic between two idealized models: one being the 'crime-control' model, with the other being the 'due process' model. These models described, and perhaps prescribed, the operation of criminal law and the CJS in terms of dueling polarities. (Over the years these dueling polarities have become more an interactive complex of competing value systems operating within criminal law[43]). The crime control model was driven by the values of efficiency and efficacy in bringing criminal offenders to punishment (and protecting society), while the due process model was oriented to protecting civil liberties and governmental abuse of the accused (and preserving civil stability). The two models in some ways address them-selves to different categories of crime—the crime control model being more suited to violent and property crimes like murder, rape, burglary, and larceny, while the due process model addresses (allegedly) victimless crimes like obscenity, illicit drug use, and prostitution. In his critical review of models of criminal process, Kent Roach de-scribes Packer's theoretical innovation as well as the two models:[44]

> Models serve multiple purposes. They provide a guide to judge the actual or positive op-eration of the criminal justice system. Packer's crime-control model suggested that most

cases end in guilty pleas or prosecutorial withdrawals whereas his due process model suggested that the cases that go to trial and are appealed were the most influential. Models can also provide a normative guide to what values ought to influence the criminal law. Packer was somewhat reticent in this regard, but it is clear that his crime-control model was based on societal interests in security and order while his due process model was based on the primacy of the rights of the individual in relation to the state. Models of the criminal process can also describe the ideologies and discourses which surround criminal justice. The most successful models have become terms of art so that people in public discourse now debate and advocate the crime control and due process values that Packer identified. At a discursive level, Packer's models have become self-fulfilling prophecies.

The latter function of the models, concerning their description of the public discourse, can be exemplified today by the political media's dichotomization of 'conservative' 'tough-on-crime' concerns about capturing, controlling, and punishing offenders, and the 'liberal' concern about protecting civil liberties and the avoidance of convicting innocent citizens. Packer's influence extends into later considerations when new models of criminal justice are considered, such as the restorative justice model.

Roach, in his 1999 review[45] and critique of Packer's influential work, reviews the limitations of this two-model polarity in the ensuing 35 years following its original publication. Perhaps most importantly Roach notes that applicability of the crime-control model is significantly compromised by a series of victimization studies in the 1980s and 1990s that indicate that only a small number of crimes are actually reported by victims. These data undermine Packer's assumption that criminal prosecution and punishment are the primary means of regulating criminal deviance because the crime-control path (e.g., policing) to justice contributes only a small portion of crime regulation. Roach also notes research examining the impact of punishment and the frequent occasions of its actually increasing criminal activity (hence contemporary anxiety about prison terms 'hardening' criminals through traumatizing them and inculcating them with more effective skills in community offending and evading police detection). In considering the actual practice of the due process model, Roach cites studies that indicate defense attorneys infrequently invoke due process rights in criminal procedure, undercutting the relevance of the due process model to contemporary law practice. For minor offenses, the effort involved in seeking due process protections are more arduous and expensive than simply pleading guilty. Practical limitations, then, limit the use of due process constraints. Finally, Roach notes that contemporary criminal law utilizes other models of criminal sanction or procedure that do not share either set of values embodied in the crime-control and due process models. These alternative models include restorative justice, community justice, diversion and therapeutic jurisprudence, and Aboriginal justice. However, delving into these models of law and criminal justice brings us away from the focus on criminal law proper, and will be considered later. At this juncture I turn to the goals of medicine.

Goals of medicine. While the considerations of the ends of medicine go back to the Hippocratic, contemporary reflections by philosophers of medicine address more contemporary challenges. Pellegrino,[46] in a critical essay on the goals and ends of medicine, cites the following from Hippocrates, *The Art*:

> First I will define what I conceive medicine to be. In general terms, it is to do away with the sufferings of the sick, to lessen the violence of their diseases, and to refuse to treat those who are overmastered by their diseases realizing that in such cases medicine is powerless.[47]

Like the early and simplistic injunction for law to 'keep the peace', the ensuing centuries have proven that doing away with the sufferings of the sick is complicated. In earlier chapters I emphasized a fundamental difference in the disciplines of law and medicine; that being that law in its core is a social practice, constituted and delivered by groups of people, inspired by social needs and developing social ends. Medicine, on the other hand, has a more primordial nature—a response to illness, inspiring both self-care and care by others. Ancient medicine is dyadic in a way that the beginnings of law were not; even today, many philosophers of medicine cast 'the clinical encounter' as a fundamentally dyadic interaction between doctor and patient, with the role of others being complementary and supplementary.[48] Moreover, if we think of the foundational disciplines of Law as philosophy and rhetoric, the founding disciplines of medicine might include those two as well, though with the emphasis on natural philosophy, which in the seventeenth century evolved into the 'science' we know today (and as considered in Chapter 4).

The relation of science to medicine has been a subject of much discussion, some of it my own. Developed at some length in the introduction to *Values and Psychiatric Diagnosis*,[49] where I drew upon Ronald Munson's paper on 'Why Medicine Cannot Be a Science',[50] which argues—persuasively in my immodest assessment—that medicine, while crucially dependent upon the truth-seeking and knowledge base of the sciences, is much more than just 'applied science' but rather driven by explicitly moral, ethical, and practical goals in caring for patients. Scientific knowledge, in this assessment, is a tool of medicine but not the end of medicine.

This view is confirmed by philosophers of medicine such as Pellegrino,[51] who is distrustful both of efforts to mechanize medicine into value-empty natural processes and technical procedures, as well as 'social construction' accounts of medicine, which strip away the invariant and permanent moral essences of the practice, relativizing the field. For Pellegrino, what makes medicine universal to human beings is the experience of illness or injury, prompting the 'need of sick persons for care, cure, help, and healing'.[52] The corruption of the ends of medicine by 'goals' or 'functions', like assisting in torture or executions, is what worries Pellegrino about social constructionist accounts of the field. Pellegrino explicitly identifies himself as an essentialist regarding the ends of medicine and as such is suspicious about what he calls social constructionist revisions of the ends of medicine. These core tasks—caring, curing, helping, and healing—are practical interventions, which in their practicality share key elements with Law. Pellegrino also emphasizes two more ramifications of these simple ends of medicine: (1) the 'covenant of trust' with the patient, where patient needs prevail over personal, economic, or political needs,[53] and (2) the 'moral community'[54] of medicine, which supports and protects these ends of medicine.

Perhaps as in law, medicine does not have a rich literature of foundational questions about their respective goals or ends. In the mid-1990s the premier US independent and nonpartisan bioethics think tank, the Hastings Center, organized an international panel to consider the 'Goals of Medicine'.[55] Representing more of an international consensus statement rather than a detailed philosophical analysis or theory, the collected articles making up this Special Supplement to the *Hastings Center Report* converged upon four goals (Table 6.2):[56]

While recognizing the added complexity of biomedical technologies, economically driven delivery systems, medicalization and enhancement, complex healthcare delivery systems, and the differential and unbalanced emphases of these four goals as practiced in contemporary healthcare today, this Report reads, like Pellegrino, with the physician at the center of the goals of medicine with ethical and practical essences intact.

More recent authors addressing the goals of medicine in a more philosophical mode, Bengt Brülde[57] and Lennart Nordenfelt[58] take issue with the ideals of an essential goals or ends of medicine, not from a social constructionist viewpoint (which Pellegrino criticizes) but more from a conceptual-analytic approach examining how medicine is actually practiced and functions socially. A common and crucial point from Brülde and Nordenfelt is that 'medicine' as a discipline today blends seamlessly into 'health care systems' which collect and utilize a wide variety of disciplines of study and practice—nursing, pastoral care, social work, various specialized therapists, and administrators). The health care system, in turn, tends to overlap or transition into general social welfare concerns when observed from an even broader perspective.

Nordenfelt in particular contrasts medicine with social welfare.[59] By 'social welfare' Nordenfelt means much the same as the social welfare efforts described here in Chapter 5, namely, the provision of aid and economic support for the poor and needy, assistance with housing and employment, and protection from social adversities like crime and child abuse. For Nordenfelt, medicine and social welfare share the

Table 6.2 The Hastings Center's Four Goals of Medicine

The prevention of disease and injury and promotion of the maintenance of health

The relief of pain and suffering caused by maladies

The care and cure of those with a malady, and the care of those who cannot be cured

The avoidance of premature death and the pursuit of a peaceful death common feature of improving 'the ability of a person'. [60] That is to say, medical efforts and social welfare efforts aim to maintain, restore, or increase the individual's capabilities to act or function in the world. As was illustrated in Chapter 5, the demarcations between medicine and social welfare today are often very difficult to draw—the VMDR being only one vivid example. Treating vice-laden conditions may be a way of diminishing criminal offending and enhancing the public welfare. Providing clean air and water surely fits into the social welfare equation, though the health-promoting benefits are obvious. Addressing poverty with clean, safe housing diminishes animal-vector-related and other infectious diseases. Nordenfelt notes that fundamental social welfare efforts, such as safe housing, public exercise and sports facilities, and crime prevention, have health-promotion and preservation benefits as well. Public health interventions perhaps best exemplify the blurring of medicine and social welfare functions. Finally, Nordenfelt emphasizes that medicine is an enterprise made up of collectives or teams; not only do physicians contribute to the accomplishment of the goals of medicine, but other health care workers do as well (e.g., nurses, social workers, respiratory therapists, and dieticians), as mentioned earlier.

From these analyses an important set of perspectives can be recognized. First, physicians experience a primordial moral complexity in that their traditional ethic is directed to the patient—Pellegrino's doctor-patient dyad—while at the same time physicians work in the context of a larger health care system which in large part controls or constrains human resources, practices, facilities, and the physician's payment. The business interests of the healthcare system may or may not support the physician's dyadic 'moral mission'. In the context of the United States' nonuniversal, commercially dominated health care system, where profit motives by healthcare organizations compete with the moral content of these fourfold goals of medicine, and approximately 15% of people in 2019 have no health insurance or guaranteed healthcare at all,[61] physicians can, and often are, caught between the financial interests of the corporation and payer and the interests of the patient. Efforts to control costs (and protect profits) through limiting care provide a common example.

Second, in recognizing the broader context of medicine as a specific kind of social welfare effort, the physician's role as moral agent is dissipated through complex healthcare delivery systems where molar interventions (e.g., physical examination, administration of medicines, administration of other therapies, and preventive efforts) are spread among a wide range of people, diluting the centrality of the doctor-patient relationship. As we saw in Chapter 5, little of the social welfare effort with medical ramifications is delivered by organizations that are *not* business- or government-related. The physician is a team member working within a larger system with not just traditional medical goals described above, but also with other goals imposed by others (e.g., government interest in community hospital employment, 'stewardship', and cost controls, not to overlook profit-making for shareholders).

The third and final ramification is that the boundaries between medicine-as-moral-practice and medicine-as-social welfare are fuzzy, contributing to a highly politicized public discourse about the goals of medicine.[62]

Goals of psychiatry. Perhaps nowhere is the issue of physician identity diffusion, and the politicizing of the goals of medicine, more acute than in psychiatry or mental health care taken broadly. While psychiatrists might well endorse the Hastings Center's and Pellegrino's goals or ends of medicine, actual scholarly writing and research on the 'goals of psychiatry', the 'ends of psychiatry', 'the role of psychiatry', or 'the purpose of psychiatry' generates only a few, mostly peripheral, papers on the subject on Google Scholar or Ovid search engines. Even within the emerging philosophy of psychiatry field the topic is absent.[63] While not attempting such a philosophical treatment for the goals of psychiatry, I offer a few comments about what is distinctive about the goals of psychiatry as a medical specialty.

Four goals for psychiatry, but it's complicated. Making sweeping claims about (even) one's own field without some definitive survey data is always risky business, but I'll hazard one here: most psychiatrists would likely have few strong complaints about the four goals of medicine from the Hastings Center, listed in Table 6.2. American psychiatrists today have a strong physician identity.[64] Given these assumptions, I can start about the 'distinctive' goals of psychiatry from these benchmarks. As can be seen from the following discussion, despite my endorsement on behalf of American psychiatrists for the Hastings Center's (HC's) mostly noncontroversial goals of medicine, application of these goals to psychiatry is complicated.

Treating maladies. The first complication is recognized by the Hastings authors. In one of the Report papers, they specify the language of the goals of medicine in not treating diseases, disorders, illnesses, and sicknesses, but instead as 'maladies':[65]

> The term 'malady' is meant to cover a variety of conditions, in addition to disease, that threaten health. They include impairment, injury, and defect. With this range of conditions in mind it is possible to define 'malady' as that circumstance in which a person is suffering, or at an increased risk of suffering an evil (untimely death, pain, disability, loss of freedom or opportunity, or loss of pleasure) in the absence of a distinct external cause. The phrase 'in the absence of a distinct external cause' is meant to distinguish the internal sources of malady from a continuing dependence upon causes clearly distinct from oneself (e.g., the pain caused by torture or civil violence). The harm, in short, comes from within the person, not from the outside.

Not only reminiscent of post-*Diagnostic and Statistical Manual of Mental Disorders* (DSM)-III definitions of mental disorder ('increased risk of suffering an evil'; harm 'comes from within a person'),[66] I would suggest that 'malady' is intended to be inclusive of mental or psychological disorders and to have as few metaphysical or causal commitments as possible (e.g., malady as biological, psychological, social, and environmental).[67] In specifying malady, the authors are recognizing that the kinds of things that psychiatrists treat may not necessarily emerge from biological defects of various sorts, but by pathological (harmful) results of higher order processes which may, or may not, be functioning typically (e.g., psychological, social, and cultural).

Psychiatry's catholic approach to explaining and understanding mental distress generates ambiguities for the goals of psychiatry: 'Just what is 'it' that we treat?'. Psychiatry's pluralism also generates reams of philosophical questions for the field, from how to precisely define 'mental disorder' to what counts as 'evidence' in the determination and management of mental disorder (Phenotypes? Biomarkers? Structure and content of patient narratives? Patterns of communication and behavior? Quantitative scoring on psychological tests?). Moreover, the fluidity of even more precisely defined mental disorders, as in conditions that meet carefully applied DSM criteria, commonly bleed into other conditions that are more dubiously 'medical', reminding us of Nordenfelt's points about close relationships with social welfare concerns. For instance, clinicians familiar with working with depressed patients in impoverished domestic settings commonly observe worsening (and improvement) in DSM depressive symptoms in tandem with the fluctuation of social stressors like money problems, acting out children, abusive spouses, or threatening neighbors. (Hence the inclusion of ratings for stressors in the post-DSM-III multiaxial system, at least until DSM-5.)

Being and having. In a paper describing the significance of the 'personal self' in psychiatry[68] I considered the common linguistic practice of referring to people with mental disorders as '*being*'. That is, patients say 'I *am*' schizophrenic, depressed, or alcoholic, for example. Compare these expressions to the common practice in general medicine to refer to one's illness as *having*, as in *having* a heart attack, AIDS, a cold, or a broken leg. For some, this metonymic usage collapses the affected person's identity into a disease or disorder and is, therefore, offensive to many psychiatric service users as well as clinicians.[69] Granting this piece of identity politics, however, I believe this usage also conveys important information about the nature of mental illness.

However stigmatizing or politically incorrect these references to *being* rather than *having* may be, the commonality of this language use betrays an important feature of mental disorders, or (otherwise) the conditions that psychiatrists treat. I called this feature the 'self-illness ambiguity'—the difficulty that patients, psychiatrists, and others have in separating out the features of oneself from features of one's mental disorder.[70] Our cultural formulation of mental distress seems powerfully linked to one's cultural sense of self or personal identity in a way that having a heart attack, AIDS, a cold, or a broken leg does not. The absurdity of saying a patient 'is' a broken leg or a myocardial infarction contrasts with the familiarity of saying a patient 'is' a schizophrenic. Psychiatric conditions can be a part of the person's 'being' in a way that other disease states are just things people 'have': relatively external, even foreign to the embodied self.[71]

If people who 'are bipolar' are among psychiatry's patients, then psychiatrists are not just in the business of treating a depersonalized, anonymous, and meaningless disease state, but rather compelled into the business of positively transforming the selves of their patients. This was exemplified by me earlier through the common query clinicians hear from their patients: 'Is this my illness talking?' Psychiatrists, then, if they are to be effective in their practice of caring for and curing maladies, may well enter into the caring for and curing of selves, identities, and problematic turns in people's life trajectories. Psychiatry's dialogues with the selves of its patients may not be a primary goal, but certainly constitutes a distinctive mode of reaching conventional medical goals, and perhaps more importantly, adds a unique perspective to 'that which psychiatrists treat'.

Existential distress. One needn't be an existential philosopher or anthropologist to recognize that human nature possesses some universal features: pain, anxiety, sadness, joy, love, loneliness, and dread, to name a few. Orthopedic surgeons, pediatricians, and radiologists deal with only a few of these in the context of their professional duties, and not typically as an everyday occurrence nor as a primary clinical focus. For psychiatrists, however, the varieties of existential distress (as well as the absence of existential positives) encountered by all people constitute a confusing albeit central feature of everyday practice.

Existential distress in psychiatry is confusing for several reasons: (1) These existential features of human nature bleed—often seamlessly—into subtle and even frank psychiatric disorder.[72] One of the core debates concerning DSM-5 at the time of its development was the status of 'grief' as a normal human experience or as a potential mental disorder.[73] Any psychiatrically sophisticated married couple who has suffered a heated, angry argument can recognize how quickly interpersonal perceptions can degrade into the psychotic range, only to 'remit' once the dust has settled, conflicts have resolved, bad feelings have ebbed, apologies made, and making-up has occurred. Patients and psychiatrists alike wonder how much and what kind of anxiety is normal and adaptive or not. (2) Even people with 'everyday' existential distress feel the need to share, discuss, and gain perspective on these problems in living, and seek psychiatric and other kinds of assistance to address them. No 'disorder' is necessary to seek help here.[74] Who else to ask but a psychiatrist (or other mental health professional) about whether my anxiety is extreme? (3) Existential distress follows straightforward mental illness, in the impact the disorder has on the patient's life, on loved ones, and on prized personal activities and work. Psychiatric management also provides existential damage control after the onslaught of mental illness does its dirty work.

The significance of existential distress as a core consideration in psychiatric practice is that its status as a malady is dubious. Psychiatrists' care of patients often extends beyond the caring and curing of maladies and into the care of existential distress. This is in contrast to general medicine where a firm gap exists between a disease and the human existential response. Is addressing the pains of existence a legitimate goal for psychiatry? I would argue yes, if for no more reason than the practical difficulty in expunging it from good clinical practice, for all the reasons mentioned above.

Distress dimensional and categorical. Already mentioned is the tension in psychiatry between categories (either/or conditions with tight definitional boundaries: in medicine, pregnancy is an example) and dimensions (continuously variable features between two or more extremes: in psychiatry and psychology, intelligence is the paradigm example).[75] Coupled with the private and subjective nature of our most important psychological features (like the existential features of being human mentioned earlier), dimensional concepts in our field pose questions about what features of the patient warrant clinical attention as well as treatment. Given that many psychiatric treatments pose significant risks of their own, unjustified treatment is a core ethical concern for the field. Psychiatrists have to decide whether to remove the excesses of pain, anxiety, and sadness or instead to help the patient tolerate existential pain more effectively. For example, treatment of Borderline Personality Disorder often focuses on helping the patient with affect tolerance[76] and grief care consists of helping, even simply accompanying, and witnessing, the person through the process.[77]

Goals of treatment for each patient not presupposed. Conventional medical treatments often are governed by standards particular to the disease or injury process, not the person as a whole. Textbooks recommend treatments for diagnostic groups of individuals that share common features. Treatment by diagnostic group is established by the use of the randomized clinical trial (RCT) in evaluating drug treatment in a group of patients selected not for their individuality, but because of their commonality in sharing a similar disease or disorder condition. Psychiatry also depends upon the controlled RCT in developing its scientific 'evidence base'. However, as I argued in my 2007 paper,[78] the close relationship between mental disorders and the patient's sense of selfhood often requires the clinician to not simply apply standard population-directed treatments, but rather tailor treatment to the individual. Instead, the goals of treatment often require negotiation with the patient, as the patient stands to lose something in the treatment process that may be, at minimum, currently valued or important to them: think about the pride of narcissism, the fascination of hallucinations, the increased energy of mania as examples.[79] Thus the negotiation of goals for treatment in psychiatry goes beyond that negotiated in general medicine, as the element of the transformation or alteration of the self is largely absent in general medical therapy.

Philosophical content of practice. The abovementioned characteristics of psychiatric practice impose philosophical demands on the clinician. Only a couple of the philosophical aspects of psychiatric practice can be mentioned here, even with setting aside the issue of ethical judgments in the field. Psychiatry requires complex clinical judgments which are often, perhaps usually, only partly guided by empirical science. Many of our patients' most significant or crippling symptoms are private experiences which the clinician may only access indirectly. Determining whether the severity of anxiety is a normal part of being human or an extreme of normal anxiety requires observation, application of relevant science, and reasoned judgment. The demand is one of philosophical hermeneutics—the principles and practice of interpretation.[80] The application of diagnostic criteria in the DSM requires layers of judgment about matching criterion to patient experience, the accuracy of the criterion in describing the patient's experience, and inference into patient and clinician bias in applying criteria, as well as the potential for social factors to provoke various kinds of 'spin' and clinical masquerades.[81] For an example of the latter, consider the needy patient whose symptoms do not fit into the approved diagnosis for acceptance into a particular treatment program, and who manipulates the reporting of symptoms in order to gain the assistance needed. More pertinently for the VMDR, consider the criminal defendant whose clinical presentation is filtered by a desire to be acquitted.[82] A philosophical practice also enters into the treatment dialogue, as practical, ethical, religious, and existential value preferences are elicited, negotiated, and staged with the patient before, during, and even during the termination of treatment. The development of insight into one's unconscious scripts or limiting cognitive schemata, to the processing of the restored or new self in response to psychopharmaceutical response[83] complicate the goals of psychiatry by implying that psychiatry's goals involve the pursuit of a deliberate perspective about one's experience of being ill and one's response to treatment. How that fits into the care/cure goals of medicine is complex.

Unique goals of forensic psychiatry. When we consider the unique goals of forensic psychiatry, the subspecialty of psychiatry that interfaces with the law and CJS, the application of the HC's and Pellegrino sets of goals for medicine become even more problematic. While little in the way of philosophical analysis about the goals of forensic psychiatry has been written, a window into the goals of the field can be provided by the discussion of the ethics for the field. The role, purpose, and interests served by forensic psychiatry are the basis for building an ethics, albeit these considerations of role, purpose, and interest may be assumed rather than argued.

Writing from a British perspective, Gwen Adshead and Sameer Sarkar describe forensic psychiatry as operating under two 'ethical paradigms',[84] though they distinguish the ethical framework in the UK from the ethical framework in the United States. One paradigm, that of welfare, frames forensic psychiatry in a familiar ethical role: a 'beneficent ideal that has been central to the ethical identity of doctors since Hippocratic times'.[85] The authors are careful to note even in traditional medicine, circumstances may demand that physicians act 'paternalistically' and act in the best interests of the patient when the latter lacks autonomy, resulting in practices like involuntary seclusion and treatment.[86] In the case of forensic psychiatry, however, Adshead and Sarkar note that '... it is not just *patient* welfare that justifies detention and coerced treatment in psychiatry. The welfare of *others* is also considered a justification for overriding the autonomy of psychiatric patients'.[87] The authors note that in the UK, the practice of forensic psychiatry emerged from the need for care of the mentally ill in prisons, only later to develop the role as expert witness familiar to Americans. From this standpoint the British forensic psychiatrist, (which would be called the correctional psychiatrist in the United States) tends to patients under the traditional goals of care and cure, just in the prison setting. In this setting, the question of confinement and punishment has already been settled, and the forensic psychiatrist is a prison doctor.

In Adshead and Sarkar's counterpoint, the 'American way' of forensic psychiatry pits the welfare paradigm against the second paradigm, that of a justice paradigm. In contrast to the origins of forensic psychiatry in British prisons, in the United States the role of forensic psychiatry grew out of expert testimony in the prosecution and trial phase within the CJS[88] as in Chapter 5's discussion of Isaac Ray's pioneering of US forensic psychiatry. Here the psychiatrist's expertise is utilized in the service of the administration of justice, through mechanisms like determinations of competency to stand trial, the 'insanity defense', or the state of mind of the defendant at the time of the offense. The primary goal of the formative American forensic psychiatrist is not the welfare of the patient or the provision of patient benefits, but rather service to society in assisting in the pursuit of criminal guilt or innocence and the overall administration of justice.[89] Adshead and Sarkar acknowledge the dual roles today in both the UK and United States; posing ambiguities about forensic psychiatry's purpose. Moreover, non-forensic psychiatric practice has its own coercive elements of involuntary seclusion and treatment: general psychiatrists appear to have a duty, albeit not a primary goal, to the public welfare too.

These tensions have been debated in US forensic psychiatry, and are explicitly addressed in the American Academy of Psychiatry and the Law (AAPL) ethics guidelines of 2005.[90] Several points of these guidelines are relevant to our considerations here:

1. The AAPL notes that their ethics guidelines apply also to 'psychiatrists practicing in a forensic role'.[91] They identify forensic roles as 'civil, criminal, correctional, regulatory, or legislative matters, or in specialized clinical consultations such as risk assessment or employment'. General psychiatrists are recommended to use these guidelines.
2. The AAPL recognizes the conflicts of duty and goals characterizing the field. 'Psychiatrists in a forensic role are called upon to practice in a manner that balances competing duties to the individual and to society'.[92]
3. The AAPL specifies that when treatment relationships exist, as in correctional settings, the 'usual physician-patient duties apply'.[93]
4. In the setting of forensic evaluations, special attention is called to clarifying the limits or absence of confidentiality with the evaluee, and psychiatrists should explain to the evaluee who is requesting the evaluation and 'what they [psychiatrists] will do with the information'.[94] The AAPL calls special attention to 'explicitly inform the evaluee that the psychiatrist is not the evaluee's "doctor"'.[95]
5. Regarding consent, AAPL specifies that the 'nature of purpose of the evaluation and the limits of confidentiality' be disclosed to the evaluee.[96] For compulsory court-ordered evaluations, the psychiatrist should explain that the evaluee's refusal becomes part of the report.
6. Attention to due process of the law, and an explicit prohibition against participating in torture are part of the guidelines.

7. Significant for the discussion of medical and psychiatric methods and legal methods to follow, the AAPL ethics guidelines emphasize that bias provoked by the adversary system should be avoided as much as possible and honesty and objectivity remain a goal of psychiatric participation in the legal process.
8. The AAPL explicitly advises against psychiatrists providing treatment serving as an expert witness for the patient in the court setting.

The AAPL ethical guidelines were preceded by a heated debate in the forensic psychiatry literature triggered by a former APA President, Alan A. Stone. While not a forensic psychiatrist himself, Stone had distinguished himself as a scholar at the interface of law, ethics, and psychiatry. When his paper 'The ethical boundaries of forensic psychiatry: A view from the ivory tower'[97] was published, it provoked brisk responses from the forensic psychiatry community and ongoing discussion about forensic psychiatry ethics into the present.

Stone's concerns about the ethics of forensic psychiatry were fivefold:[98]

First, there is the basic boundary question. Does psychiatry have anything true to say that the courts should listen to?

Second, there is the risk that one will go too far and twist the rules of justice and fairness to help the patient.

Third, there is the opposite risk that one will deceive the patient in order to serve justice and fairness.

Fourth, there is the danger that one will prostitute the profession, as one is alternately seduced by the power of the adversarial system and assaulted by it.

Finally, as one struggles with these four issues—Does one have something true to say? Is one twisting justice? Is one deceiving the patient? Is one prostituting the profession?— There is the additional problem: forensic psychiatrists are without any clear guidelines as to what is proper and ethical, at least as far as I can see.

In addition to raising, in his own way, the tension between the welfare and the justice aims later articulated by Adshead and Sarkar, Stone also raises the issue of the state of psychiatric science and practice and worries about the potential for unfulfilled, or perhaps unfulfillable, promises that could be made by forensic psychiatry. Further, Stone emphasizes through his rhetorical emphasis and choice of metaphors ('prostituting', 'seduced', and 'assaulted') the serious difficulty of even the most sincere and conscientious forensic clinician in avoiding bias or frank manipulation of the proceedings. As a latter instance, he identifies the notorious Texas forensic psychiatrist James Grigson, 'Dr. Death', whose confidently gloomy predictions for reoffending by convicted murderers sent some to Death Row, justified by, at best, feeble science.

In a 1997 response, Paul Appelbaum, a *bona fide* forensic psychiatrist and an APA president, responded in detail to Stone's challenge in the setting of his Presidential Address for the 1996 AAPL annual meeting.[99] Appelbaum responded with a theory of ethics presented to the literature. Appelbaum took Stone's concern for a moral and ethical foundation very seriously, and was equally concerned about a field that could have wanton practitioners carrying out an anything-goes practice.

The details of Appelbaum's theory are of limited utility for my purposes and needn't be recounted here. However, there are several points of Appelbaum's which are relevant to the VMDR and the goal(s) of forensic psychiatry that warrant discussion. However, in my reading, Appelbaum's theory is in prevailing agreement with the AAPL ethics guidelines presented above, and very likely influenced their development and specifics.

(1) *The ethics of 'settings'*. Appelbaum wants to justify the psychiatrist's potential acting against the patient's interests (e.g., contributing to a conviction, prison sentence, death sentence, or other censure) not just from an ethic of justice and truth but also in comparison against other, perhaps less controversial, physician practices. In the latter regard, Appelbaum compares the dual loyalties of forensic psychiatry to the dual loyalties of the physician-scientist: the clinical investigator. In these settings, the goals of the practice change and other, morally desirable, values may limit or even trump the care/cure goals of medicine at large. In the case of forensic psychiatry, the welfare of the patient may be limited or trumped by the need to protect the citizenry, as discussed earlier. In clinical research, the therapeutic care or cure goal may be trumped by the need to develop scientifically credible facts from a formal research protocol that prohibits the tailoring of 'treatment' to the needs of the individual.[100]

(2) *A grounding in social values*. Appelbaum, to my reading, appears to support the idea that the core identity of a physician remains unchanged while the goals of the physician's role can be different in different contexts. However, this context-relativism of the Appelbaumian goals raises an important question, which is only elliptically addressed by him: What limits are there where context demands moral action incompatible with physician identity and goals? In other words, are there social contexts or demands for physician practice which *in spite of* competing values, however worthwhile, the physician should not tread? In his theory Appelbaum doesn't directly raise this issue, but addresses it in this passage:[101]

> To determine which moral rules and ideals a group of professionals ought to observe with particular zealousness, we look to the values that society desires that profession to promote.

So, the 'grounding' of physician goals comes from the larger society in which the physician is operating. In my interpretation, the determination of the bounds of appropriate physician roles and goals, we should look to the values embraced by the larger society.

The grounding of physician goals in social values is where the panic of Appelbaum's critics sets in. In an editorial for the *American Journal of Psychiatry* entitled 'Ethics in Evolution: The Incompatibility of Clinical and Forensic Functions',[102] Appelbaum notes 'Forensic psychiatrists, however, work in an entirely different ethical framework, one built around the legitimate needs of the justice system. Their duties are to seek and reveal the truth, as best they can, whether or not that advances the interests of the evaluee.'[103] In a reply to this editorial as well as Appelbaum's (1997) *Theory* paper, Halpern, Freedman, and Schoenholtz raise the issue of 'limits to the overriding goal of the forensic psychiatrist's professional activity to advance the interests of justice'.[104] These authors had a specific physician role in mind as offensive: the participation of psychiatrists in capital punishment or the death penalty. Later, they raised the issue of Soviet psychiatrists 'treatment' of dissidents who were in conflict with the prevailing social values of that time and place.

Appelbaum's response to the issue of psychiatric involvement in the death penalty followed:[105]

> . . . Now, to what I suspect is the actual motivation for this letter, Dr. Halpern and colleagues—opponents of the death penalty—have been vociferous advocates of the position that psychiatrists should neither evaluate the competence of prisoners to be executed nor treat those found incompetent. Although I am in agreement with them on the latter, I differ on the former, because I believe that their position reflects a fundamental misconception of the psychiatrist's role. As in other forensic settings, psychiatrists are providing information regarding subjects' mental state, with judicial decision makers passing judgment on the implications of those data for the issue at hand. Indeed, one might expect opponents of the death penalty to favor psychiatric involvement, since one of the consequences of psychiatric evaluation may be the postponement, perhaps indefinite, of the sentence of death.

Perhaps ironically, Appelbaum invokes Edmund Pellegrino as an authority in the latter's acknowledgment of '[t]he subject-physician relationship [i.e., in the forensic evaluation context] does not carry the implication or promise of the primacy for the patient's welfare that [is] intrinsic to a true medical relationship'.[106]

Appelbaum specifies the treatment relationship as the domain in which considerations of forensic matters should not intrude; indeed, he raises concerns about treating clinicians having any business participating in courtroom proceedings. The irony that I referred to has to do with Pellegrino's explicit stance against relativistic positions about the ends of medicine that were raised earlier: that the ends of medicine shouldn't be subject to the whims of social change or political allegiances; the physician cares, cures, helps, and heals the ill regardless of politics, era, and culture. To my reading of each man's positions, Appelbaum's grounding of the forensic role in society's values and Pellegrino's essentialist view of the ends of medicine are incompatible. From the Pellegrino perspective, once the physician steps out of the cure/care/help/heal role relative to the patient, as in a forensic evaluation, the physician has stepped away from the moral identity of the profession into a new moral identity framed by encompassing societal values that are nonmedical. For Pellegrino, the goals or ends of medicine cannot be simply changed like a suit of clothes when social values shift.

From Appelbaum's perspective, the sociomoral legitimacy of the need for social justice and crime control provides an ethical basis for forensic psychiatry. But Appelbaum and Halpern et al. fail to identify explicitly the underlying larger problem, of which capital punishment and Soviet-era psychiatric abuse are only examples: What if the societal values are corrupt, evil, or wrongful? Are they still legitimate grounds for forensic psychiatrists' participation? Grounding the forensic psychiatrist's role through societal values makes the forensic psychiatrist a political actor in a way that the Pellegrino medically moral physician would never tolerate.

I do think there is a potential to provide a stronger foundation for forensic psychiatry goals and ethics; albeit one that does not refute or resolve the conflict with Pellegrino's essentialist conception of physicianhood. What I would suggest, but don't have space to elaborate here, is rejecting the idea that societal values writ large provide a basis for forensic psychiatry. The problem, in my view, is not with having a political forensic psychiatry but having just *any kind* of politics or social values 'underwriting' forensic psychiatry. Forensic psychiatry, by its nature as contributing to the goals of civil order, public protection, and goals of the State can't help but be bound up by State politics.

What is needed is an explicitly political-philosophical account of forensic psychiatry, justified within democratic theory and practice, and subject to censure and regulation by a democratic polity. Soviet or North Korean Communist totalitarianism would not qualify as a legitimate political basis for forensic psychiatry; a specific set of morally justifiable political processes and practices would be required, likely embracing not just civil liberties for all, but also supporting the potential for conscientious civil disobedience for a forensic psychiatrist. Such a democratic-political theory of forensic psychiatry's identity, goals, and ethics would tightly rein in the power and responsibility of forensic psychiatrists and indeed, could decide that perhaps physicians are not the apropos experts to serve criminal law in the role currently occupied by forensic psychiatry.[107] Indeed, such a political-theory account may end up defending a Pellegrinian physician essentialism and prefer criminological psychologists (nonclinical) to perform the functions of forensic psychiatrists today. Such nonclinical experts could draw upon the knowledge base of psychiatry, psychology, criminology, biology, and other relevant sciences to address the needs of courtroom justice, with 'treatment' not part of their expertise or practice. But I digress.

In summary, both general psychiatry and forensic psychiatry can find themselves in controversial situations where the care/cure/help/heal identity of the physician is questionable and questioned. For general psychiatrists, the involvement in involuntary seclusion and treatment along with courtroom testimony are good examples. For forensic psychiatrists, participation in any component of torture or executions provides central examples. These ambiguities contribute to the problematic nature of the VMDR and will be considered in more detail later.

6.1.1.2 Truth, justice, the American way: Methods of law, medicine, and psychiatry

> In my view the law is not a static order built on certitude, but a dynamic order built on process.
>
> —Judge David Bazelon (1978, p. 144)

From the goals of law, medicine, and psychiatry I turn to the methods of these fields. While some commonalities exist between law methods and medicine and psychiatry methods, the prevailing point of this section is to illustrate not just procedural differences but more profound metaphysical differences in how the two fields conceive and approach their goals.[108] The discussion of metaphysical differences will be elaborated in the next section and reappear in the next chapter, when public perceptions of the VMDR are considered.

As with the prior section, I shall consider the methods of law first, followed by considerations of medicine and psychiatry.

Methods of criminal law and criminal procedure. As in the earlier section, consideration of the disposition of the convicted offender (e.g., punishment, rehabilitation) will be left to the later section on the CJS, while this section focuses on criminal procedure leading up to sentencing.

As suggested in the development of morality and law discussed in Chapter 5, the determination of criminal guilt in Western law changed shortly before and during the Enlightenment era. Prior to the Enlightenment, determining the truth of criminal charges emerged from divine proclamation or intervention, examples being medieval trial procedures such as trial by battle, or by ordeal (e.g., burnings at the stake, near-drownings). The basic idea was that God, or the gods would determine the fate of a defendant; the innocent would prevail and the guilty would have their judgment and sentence rolled into the same process.[109] Our contemporary recognition of the foregone doom of those charged with witchery and tried at the stake brings with it our presumption in favor of a rational procedure that has the possibility of two or more outcomes (guilt/innocence). This assumption that a trial should depend upon rational process is in contrast with medieval European folk metaphysics, where no threat to the innocent would prevent them from divine protection, if indeed they were innocent.

Sward[110] describes this metaphysical viewpoint of the medieval and prior eras as the failure to distinguish law from fact. The struggle of the law to establish facts through law has occupied the field since. Today we might view the defendant's death in a trial by battle as the outcome of the defendant's inferior fighting skills, but in the medieval period such outcomes indicated God's will and were unchallenged. With the Enlightenment and the rise of reason over faith, methods for the determination of the truth of criminal acts were needed, methods that were grounded in reason. The concept of evidence codeveloped in law and in science, often by the same philosophers such as Locke, Bacon, Hume, Descartes, Spinoza, and others.[111] Reasoning from observable, demonstrable evidence became the core of rational law and science, with truth emerging from such rational methods.

Philosophers of law recognize the epistemological challenge posed by criminal procedure. Recently, Pardo described this challenge:[112]

> The trial is fundamentally an epistemological event. We want jurors and judges to know. And we want to know what they know. And we also want to know the conditions when they know, and when, if at all, these conditions obtain.

At the same time, a second value competes with truth in criminal-legal method, and that value is justice. In my reading of the methods of criminal law, a kind of dialectic appears where the values of truth and justice are jointly pursued, yet often get into each other's methodological way. We will see how this tension unfolds.

Two interrelated methods serve both truth and justice in contemporary American criminal law. One is delivered through judicial authority and interpretation of common and civil criminal law. The other is the 'adversary process' in criminal procedure. In the discussion following, first I'll describe the adversarial ideal, its problems, and some of the amendments to the adversary process that attempt to deal with these problems. Later in this chapter I will describe alternatives to the adversarial model that are practiced in other Western countries. A discussion of the role of the judiciary in criminal law follows.

In her comprehensive review of the adversary system in American adjudication, Ellen Sward describes the importance of the adversary system:[113]

> The hallmark of American adjudication is the adversary system. The virtues of the adversary system are so deeply engrained in the American legal psyche that most lawyers do not question it.

The American Bar Association *Model Code of Professional Responsibility*[114] describes the duty of attorneys to the adversarial system:

> Our legal system provides for the adjudication of disputes governed by the rules of substantive, evidentiary, and procedural law. An adversary presentation counters the natural human tendency to judge too swiftly in terms of the familiar that which is not yet fully known, the advocate, by his zealous preparation and presentation of fact and law, enables the tribunal to come to the hearing with an open and neutral mind and to render impartial judgments. The duty of a lawyer to his client and his duty to the legal system are the same; to represent his client zealously within the bounds of the law.

The adversarial ideal is that truth, and derivatively, justice, can be secured by two sides, the criminal defense and prosecution, which (in the United States) mostly control the investigation and presentation of evidence to a judge and jury, the former serving as a moderator of criminal procedure, with the jury deciding about innocence or guilt. This generalization is most accurate for severe or felony crimes; misdemeanors or lesser crimes may not involve a jury and expand the judge's role to adjudicate guilt and sentencing. My discussion here focuses on severe crimes. Regardless, in the adversary system, the two attorneys, or adversaries, provide the best case from their point of view, and through the deliberation of the jury (or judge in 'bench' (nonjury) decisions), the truth, and justice, is determined. 'Criminal procedure' is a method to decide the defendant's guilt or innocence, and as we'll see, the practice of criminal procedure has been amended over the centuries to address 'offenses' to truth and justice that emerge from a wanton adversarial process.

Davis and Elliston, in their 1986 *Ethics and the Legal Profession*, identify three senses of the 'adversary system'[115] in their introduction to the section on this topic. The first sense is the more commonsense concept, that of a method of trial that recognizes two or more opposing parties. They acknowledge that even American law, with its commitment to the adversarial model, has elements of law practice that are not adversarial (e.g., legal procedures like adoption or name-changing). However, some elements of American law are adversarial compared to Western European practices; they mention impartial contract negotiations in Europe as an example, in contrast to the standard opposing counsel in American contract law.

Davis and Elliston's second sense of 'adversarial system' has to do with legal procedure, at trial and immediately preceding the trial. Attorneys are primarily responsible for presenting the best case for their client at trial. With the adversarial method, the judge is largely not involved in trial preparations, not involved in collecting and interpreting evidence, and has comparatively little involvement in which witnesses are called, or what questions will be posed to them. The judge in American criminal procedure may even depend, in significant part, on the opposing attorneys to cite the relevant law.[116] This at-trial sense of an adversarial system is in contrast to the method of criminal law in most of Western Europe, which is labeled the inquisitorial model.[117]

The third sense of the adversary system identified by Davis and Elliston they call a 'style of lawyering'.[118] They describe this style as:[119]

> Lawyers act as if all persons but their client were potential (or actual) adverse litigants and all questions of law or justice should be left to be decided by trial.

To my interpretation this describes the pugnacious professional demeanor practiced by many criminal attorneys, and as the authors note, is not dependent upon the first two senses of adversary. One can be a pugnacious lawyer in the inquisitorial setting just as easily as a deliberate and patient one. The adversarial lawyer depends upon the other structures of the criminal trial to buffer his wanton advocacy, with the truth presumably winning out.

However, Sward, addressing primarily civil disputes, notes that truth is difficult to determine, and the court depends upon a congruence between truth and the persuasiveness of one or the other side:[120]

> Our procedural system must resolve conflicts in such a way as to achieve a true characterization of the events out of which the conflict arose. Because truth is elusive, however, it is not always possible to be sure of the past. Witnesses may differ in what they think they saw; or there may be no witnesses on a significant issue so that the past must be reconstructed from circumstantial evidence; or, in some cases, witnesses may deliberately lie. Once the evidence is presented, it must be interpreted, leaving room for further indeterminacy. These problems with reconstructing the past are a primary reason for the existence of burdens of proof. Each party to a dispute must try to persuade the trier of fact that his version of the facts corresponds to truth, and someone must bear the risk of nonpersuasion. Failure to persuade the trier of fact does not necessarily mean that one's position is untrue; it means simply that the party has failed to convince the court of its truth. A procedural system ideally should resolve conflicts in such a way *that truth (to the extent it can be known) and persuasiveness correspond more often than not* [emphasis added].

So criminal procedure can be framed similarly, with one of the aims of criminal procedure to maximize the correspondence between truth and persuasiveness as promulgated by the adversaries. The criminal trial is the stage in which the drama of justice is played out:[121]

> First, the parties [opposing attorneys] themselves are responsible for gathering and presenting evidence and arguments on behalf of their positions. Second, the decisionmaker [judge/jury] knows nothing of the litigation until the trial, when the parties present their neatly packaged cases to him.

Philosophers of law have recognized the inherent flaws in accomplishing the ideal; that is, coherence of truth and persuasiveness[122] under even a revised, supplemented, and regulated adversarial system. Why? Some attorneys have more rhetorical skills than others or are better at selecting sympathetic jurors. Some witnesses are more credible than others. Some attorneys are better at coaching dubious witnesses into credible ones. One side may be more competent in the search for and assimilation of evidence than the other. Juries may find out about the case from media accounts and develop attitudes about the defendant in advance of the trial. Witnesses may lie. Experts may be mistaken, incompetent, or bought. Attorneys may hide unfavorable evidence or gain new witnesses during the trial. The list goes on.

The value of justice manifests in criminal procedure in various ways. One is determining guilt and the administration of a sentence (punishment) as a consequence for wrongdoing. A second is the assurance that the criminal procedure is fair (see the earlier discussion of Herbert Packer on the 'due process' arm of criminal justice) for the defendant as well as parties involved in the crime. This latter concern, about fair procedure, has led to modifications to a pure adversarial process that addresses many of the sources of unfair advantage mentioned in the previous paragraph.

The regulatory procedures in American criminal law are multiplex and cannot be adequately reviewed here, nor can the intellectual debate about them be captured adequately. Moreover, for the purposes of this chapter I seek to neither condemn nor praise the adversarial method, just sketch it out for criminal law for reference in considerations of the VMDR. However, some of the more general facets should be mentioned to deepen the understanding of how modifications to an unfettered adversary model can increase the coherence between truth and persuasion.

One of the most significant of these are the rules about discovery, that is, the reciprocal disclosure of relevant evidence by both sides. For example, if through either accident or skill, one prosecutor in the courtroom may have better evidence; such an imbalance of evidence may tip the scale in favor of the prosecution, but having better or more evidence could easily obscure the truth and convict an innocent defendant, or in converse circumstances, acquit a guilty defendant. Discovery rules, then, address timely requirements for sharing of evidence with the other side.[123]

The judge and the judiciary are crucial actors in criminal procedure because of another epistemic problem: the law is not determinative; meaning criminal legislation and common law do not interact in formulaic ways so that a simple calculus can be invoked to determine the right selection and interpretation of law and precedents. Both common law and civil law require interpretation, often by precedent, and by precedent that is jurisdictional, meaning a judicial interpretation here in Dallas doesn't determine a judicial interpretation there in New York. Hence the concept of criminal appeals; where higher level courts are involved to address arguments about allegedly wrongheaded judicial interpretation and conclusion at the original trial.

Other examples of regulation of criminal procedure include perjury, the crime of false testimony by a sworn witness. The crime of perjury reflects an effort to secure accurate testimony from witnesses and minimize the telling of falsehoods. The courts use various techniques to address bias from the supposedly neutral decisionmakers, judge and jury.[124] One well-known technique is jury selection, when the lawyer-adversaries are allowed to reject a potential juror out of concern for bias; each lawyer deselects (strikes) their own set of would-be jurors; the remainder are presumably nonpartisan, or at least minimally damaging to one side's case. Still another bias-controlling practice is the criterion of selection of jurors who are ignorant about the case, and the later protection of the jury from media or other sources of potentially biasing information about the case. Only the attorney-adversaries are able to proffer case information. The sequestration of the judge from pretrial information about the case is another measure to prevent judicial bias before the case has started. Suggested earlier about the development of the concept of evidence in science and law, the requirement that legal procedure be *rational*—reasonable—represented a departure from earlier trial processes based upon faith and accidents of circumstance.

Methods of medicine and psychiatry. As with law, medicine has had a relatively limited number of philosophical reflections upon its methods. Medicine has had its share of articulators of methods for portions of the field; but a holistic account of the methods of medicine (and psychiatry) remains yet to be done. One of the defining volumes of the then-developing philosophy of medicine, Pellegrino and Thomasma's *A Philosophical Basis of Medical Practice* gives methodology a mere mention,[125] nor will I provide a holistic account of the methods of medicine and psychiatry here; just enough to get a sense of the deep differences between these fields and criminal law.

Earlier in this chapter and in *Values and Psychiatric Diagnosis* I described medicine, echoing Ronald Munson, as a moral practice dependent upon, but not the same as, science. I'll simply refer to those prior claims and let interested readers pursue them in more detail.[126]

I should mention the concept of the 'professional stage' that I'll be using later in comparing law and medicine. The professional stage—where the practical action of criminal law takes place—is (primarily) the courtroom, as might be inferred from the foregoing pages. The professional stage, however, for the physician is the clinic or the hospital; the doctor's defining practical actions take place in those two kinds of (closely) related places. A professional stage, then, is the tangible center of practical action for a profession. Because of the centrality of psychiatric diagnosis to the professional stages of the courtroom and the clinic, these locations are the settings where the substance of the VMDR play out. (Another professional stage, the penal or CJS, is more diffuse in spatial location and will get its own VMDR due in later sections.)

The reader might be wondering, the methods for what aspects of medicine? The foregoing discussion of the professional stage of medicine, the clinic, helps to answer this question and sharpen the focus of this section. A brief reflection upon the methods of medicine broadly conceived allows us to recognize that methods are relative to particular tasks. medicine, as suggested earlier, is dependent upon the sciences in developing factual knowledge that is relevant to the healing task. The field of philosophy of science is rich in the analysis of the methods of biology and the social sciences like psychology, anthropology, and sociology.[127] While a very basic analysis of the scientific basis of medical practice will be provided here, the philosophical details are not so pertinent in understanding the methodological differences between law and medicine, to be highlighted in subsequent sections. Indeed, the focus of these sections is not to provide cutting-edge insights, but a descriptive account of medical methods that any practitioner could recognize easily and without controversy.

In reference to Munson's insights, while the methods of science are crucially important to the methods of medicine, epistemically successful scientific methods in isolation do little to cure, care, help, and heal. The latter tasks involve selecting scientific knowledge that is *relevant*, as well as practical and moral activities with their own methods—medicine applies science in pursuit of health-related goods. Regarding the latter, the moral methods of medicine, the methods of medical ethics and ethical decision-making, will also not be focused on here, again because they are not central to understanding the key methodological differences between law and medicine. Indeed, the methods of moral reasoning and ethics in law and medicine are unlikely to differ dramatically; what makes medical and legal ethics distinct are the different goals and methods for each field, in addition to their substantially different social contexts; not ethical theory or modes of ethical analysis of their professional practices.

So the key focus of medicine's methods here is on the *practical activity* framed by medicine's professional stage, the clinic, and perhaps the main vehicle for medical methods, the clinical encounter.[128] By the 'clinical encounter' I mean the meeting of the physician and patient in the 'professional stage' setting, where the task of medical care plays out. Just as the adversarial approach to finding truth and justice frames the practical activity of the criminal court, the clinical encounter demands its own methodological account of medicine's practical activity.

What methods does the physician draw upon in the clinical encounter that advance the tasks of caring, curing, helping, and healing? As I did for law, perhaps the first step is to turn to what a textbook of medicine has to say about the methods of the clinical encounter. In this case I draw from the first chapter of *Harrison's Textbook of Internal Medicine*:[129]

> Deductive reasoning and applied technology form the foundation for the solution to many clinical problems. . . . When a patient poses challenging clinical problems, an effective physician must be able to identify the crucial elements in a complex history and physician examination; order the appropriate laboratory, imaging, and diagnostic tests; and extract the key results from the crowded computer printouts to determine whether to 'treat' or to 'watch'. . . . This combination of medical knowledge, experience, intuition, and judgment defines the art of medicine, which is as necessary to the practice of medicine as is a sound scientific base.

While the 'art of medicine' may be as necessary to practice as science is, according to this passage, the latter is given far more elaboration than the former in this text, in medical education, and in medicine in general. Indeed, articulating the 'art of medicine', the methods of the clinical encounter, has proven to be elusive and difficult for the field, and has been left to medical theorists and philosophers. While I stick to my claim that holistic accounts of methods for the clinical encounter are few; nevertheless, a rich literature exists that addresses facets or components of this broader question. Let's consider some examples:

Evidence-based Medicine (EBM). In a sentence, Sackett et al. describe the thrust of this methodological movement in medicine:[130]

> It's about integrating individual clinical expertise with the best external evidence.

The 'best external evidence' referred to in this short description of EBM is scientific evidence in the form (preferentially) of controlled clinical trials of treatments, and the use of meta-analyses (statistical analysis of collected studies to find the major data trends) in guiding treatment decisions. EBM is methodologically built upon a hierarchy of evidence, with clinical trials at the top (meaning the best evidence) descriptive or observational studies[131] in the middle, and clinician expertise and reasoning at the bottom. The patient's values and preferences are to be given credence once the evidential assessment is made. The EBM movement is focused on providing a formal method for making treatment decisions in patient care, based upon the best current science. EBM has generated its own share of controversy, though its major tenets have become assimilated into clinical parlance and formally assimilated into medical education.[132] Because of its focus on clinical decision-making around the scientific evidence for various treatments, EBM is incomplete as a method for navigating the clinical encounter. The practical features of diagnosis and clinical intervening, the doctor-patient relationship, interactions with the healthcare system, as well as an account of 'patient values' remain for others to figure out. As a potential outgrowth of this limitation, more recent scholars outside of psychiatry have focused on developing 'shared decision-making' (SDM) as a practice model.[133] Beginning with standard discussions of informed consent in treatment, the authors of SDM elaborate on the practical implications of treatment negotiations and provide some structural elements and techniques to facilitate these. In this regard, SDM completes a sketch of negotiating treatment with the patient that is mostly overlooked by EBM.

'Models' for integrating the sciences of medicine. Two popular accounts, so popular, in fact, that they are part of everyday clinical parlance today, are the 'biomedical'[134] and the 'biopsychosocial'[135] model. The former model refers to a process of developing medical knowledge based upon the methods of the biological sciences in explaining the causes of disease, the scientific development and administration of disease treatments, and the scientific prediction of disease behavior. The biomedical model per se has little to say about clinical decision-making and other practical methods for medicine, and so again is of limited value in navigating the clinical encounter. In 1977 George Engel articulated a critique of the biomedical model and presented an alternative, the biopsychosocial model. Based in part on the organization of the sciences in von Bertalanffy's General Systems Theory,[136] the biopsychosocial model advocated that not only were the biological sciences relevant to the understanding, prediction, and treatment of human disease, but other system levels as well, each with their own relevant sciences (e.g., chemistry, psychology, and anthropology). Engel intended the biopsychosocial model to be more humanistic as well as more holistic and comprehensive in its scientific approach to patients. In his 1980 elaboration of the clinical application of the model, Engel presented a case study and analysis that incorporated some elements of a hermeneutic method to the clinical encounter (more on hermeneutic methods later).[137] Engel showed that considering the interactions of the differing system levels (biological, psychological, and social) could enable a physician to anticipate novel aspects of disease presentation and behavior that would facilitate care.

Both the biomedical and biopsychosocial models place the metaphysical weight of medical methods on the sciences and undertheorize the practical aspects of the clinical encounter[138] as well as the issue of navigating healthcare systems.

Medical hermeneutics. As I've noted, much of clinical methodology is assumed, tacit, and not explicit. In the 1980s and 1990s a small group of physicians and philosophers sought to elaborate the methods of the clinical encounter through focusing on the hermeneutical philosophy of interpretation.[139] Generated by medieval theologians as a method toward understanding the meaning of scripture, 'hermeneutics' as a concept and method was appropriated over the following centuries by philosophy and other scholarly disciplines in Western culture. Cooper,[140] drawing from Palmer,[141] listed six definitions of hermeneutics which have evolved beyond the original theological sense:[142]

1. A theory of biblical exegesis.
2. A theory of general philological methodology.
3. The science of all linguistic understanding.
4. The methodological foundation of *Geistewissenschaften* (a German term for the human sciences; including philosophy, history, philology, social sciences, and arguably, law and theology).
5. The phenomenology of existence and human understanding.
6. The systems of interpretation, both recollective and iconoclastic, used to reach the meaning behind myths and symbols.

Leder,[143] accurately, I believe, described the then-contemporary interest in medical hermeneutics as a reaction against the:

> . . . .lens of a positivist philosophy of science. The doctor is portrayed as an impartial investigator who builds diagnoses like scientific theories via a process of induction and experimental verification.[144]

In medical hermeneutics a key task of the clinical encounter—to interpret the various sources of relevant information and human expression—is the cornerstone of medical methods.

In medical hermeneutics the patient's presentation is *analogized to a text* which requires interpretation. While a complete explication of this literature is not feasible here, presentation of two of the 'fourfolds' of clinical hermeneutics may give a sense of how the methods of philosophical hermeneutics may be brought to bear upon interpreting the clinical encounter. A common thread within hermeneutics, whether philosophical or clinical, is the 'hermeneutic round' or 'hermeneutic circle'.[145] This simply means that understanding is not given fully, that as our relationship with the text (or the patient) deepens, we find that our initial impressions of meaning are modified by subsequent experiences, in a recursive fashion. The part informs the whole, and the whole informs the part. While a brief summary here cannot do justice to this tradition in the philosophy of medicine, a few brief comments can indicate the distinctive approach to interpreting the clinical encounter and acting on the medical 'professional stage'. The evolutionary, process-orientation of clinical practice, clarified by medical hermeneutics, provides a crisp contrast to the either/or culpability determinations of criminal law, as we'll discuss later.

Stephen Daniel's version of a medical hermeneutics is literally derived from the medieval fourfold used in the interpretation of scripture.[146] For scripture or the clinical encounter, there are four senses of meaning: the literal, the allegorical, the moral, and the anagogical or mystical. Daniel explains them in application to the concept of Jerusalem:

> The classical illustration of the method is the interpretation of the scriptural word 'Jerusalem', which is literally the historical city in Palestine, allegorically the Church, morally the individual Christian soul, and anagogically the heavenly city of God.[147]

Daniel then analogizes this to the clinical encounter:[148]

> ... four aspects or steps in the interpretive process, as suggested by the medieval fourfold sense: (1) the object of interpretation (corresponding to the literal), (2) the mode of interpretation or interpreter's way of coming to know the object (corresponding to the allegorical), (3) the praxis or life-affecting activity following from interpretation (corresponding to the moral), and (4) the change of life-world brought about through interpretation (corresponding to the anagogical).

Applied to the clinical encounter literally, Daniel's fourfold applies to the patient as object of interpretation, the diagnosis as mode of understanding, the therapy as the practical or moral, and the healing as the revelatory change.

In contrast, Drew Leder's fourfold account of medical hermeneutics includes the experiential, the narrative, the physical, and the instrumental.[149] The experiential account is delivered by the patient to the physician, having had its own revisions and amendments done by the patient's own self-interpretation. The patient may deliver her own (experiential) account in the frame of cultural convention or idiom of distress: for example, a 'common cold', a 'heart attack', or *ataques de nervios*. The narrative account, according to Leder, is a complex, unfolding story 'composed' by three authors: one is the diseased body of the patient, the second, the patient's account of his bodily experiences (including, of course, the psychological) with the third being the doctor, who presumably provides new and illuminating turns to the story based upon her education, expertise, and experience. The third account, the physician's, involves not just the observation of the patient's appearance, comportment, behavior, and the physical examination, but also assisted by technologies that directly extend the physician's perceptions such as the stethoscope or magnetic-resonance imaging. The last account, the instrumental, refers to the use of remote technologies that further elaborate the presentation of disease: laboratory studies, physiological tracings like the electrocardiogram, and imaging studies of various kinds. In psychiatry this might well including the use of psychological testing.

For the integration of these accounts, what Leder calls the 'hermeneutic telos',[150] he offers three criteria: coherence, collaboration, and clinical effectiveness. Coherence emerges from fitting the patient's 'text' into the context of clinical diagnosis and the prevailing scientific and practical knowledge of the disease or condition(s). *Coherence* emerges throughout the clinical encounter, as the clinician's foreknowledge structures her unfolding framings of the clinical encounter.[151] The coherent interpretation of the clinician, however, is insufficient in itself, if the patient does not accept or is not engaged with the clinical process, little effective action is likely to occur. The element of *collaboration* is then the engagement of the clinician with the patient as they co-constitute new accounts of the clinical problem(s). Finally, the test of the adequacy of interpretation is *clinical effectiveness*, which introduces a pragmatic criterion—the provision of caring/curing/helping/healing.

Phenomenological methods. The phenomenological approach to psychiatry, using the methods of Edmund Husserl, among others, has been influential in the contemporary philosophy of psychiatry movement.[152] The primary focus of the contemporary phenomenological psychiatry literature, developed vigorously in the Oxford International Perspectives in Philosophy and Psychiatry series over the past 20 years, has been on illness experience, and more recently on broadly conceived clinical methods.[153] However, two American collaborators, a psychiatrist and a philosopher, working in the phenomenological tradition, have written a series of papers that address clinical methods directly;[154] which I can only briefly sketch here.

The inspiration of Michael Schwartz and Osborne Wiggins (S&W) on clinical methods was in part a response to George Engel's objective to merge humanism with science in medicine.[155] In their 1986 and 1988 responses to Engel, they frame the mistake of modern-medical accounts of clinical methods through a critique of the starting point of these methods. That starting point for clinical method is the abstract, theoretical sciences. Instead, S&W recommend beginning from the concrete experiences of patient and clinician and adapting scientific methods to these primordial experiences. They situate clinical method in 'communicative interaction'[156] with the patient where a critical phenomenological attitude is cultivated; considering not just the evidence of the empirical sciences but also the experiential evidence as presented to the clinician through the patient's communications, behavior, comportment, and the clinician's own reactions to the patient. Drawing from the interpretive methods of Karl Jaspers,[157] S&W present 'six laws'[158] that aid in interpreting the meanings in the clinical encounter, drawing inspiration from Jaspers. In this focus on interpretation and understanding, the S&W account is in the spirit of the earlier medical hermeneutics approaches:[159]

1. Empirical understanding is an interpretation.
2. Understanding opens up unlimited interpretations.
3. Understanding moves in a deepening spiral.
4. Opposites are equally meaningful.
5. Understanding is inconclusive.
6. To understand is to illuminate and expose.

Explicating these laws in detail would be a paper, even a book, in itself.[160] They suggest that the understanding of the patient and clinical encounter is provisional, evidence is not monolithically determinative, understanding the patient is a developmental process, and true understanding opens up possibilities rather than closes them off. Like Jaspers in the German tradition, S&W distinguish between 'understanding' (*Verstehen*) and explanation (*Erklären*), the latter being more characteristic of causal science, while the former, understanding, is more characteristic of the unique understanding of singular events, as in historical and literary interpretation. Both are necessary to the clinical encounter, and both are directed toward the pragmatic and moral interests of healing. Of significance later is the distinction that in medicine, clinical understanding doesn't close, but remains open to revision, but in the criminal courtroom, closure in the form of a verdict is a requirement, practical as well as epistemic.

While S&W provide a sketch of methods for the clinical encounter, their focus, like that of the biomedical and biopsychosocial models, emphasizes the comprehension and interpretation of the clinical encounter. However, there is little attention paid to practical intervening at this point in their work. The 'art of medicine' remains in development by a new generation of scholars, with coherent accounts of understanding and intervening taken up later by twenty-first-century phenomenological psychopathologists like Stanghellini, cited in endnote 158.

Decision analysis. Beginning in the late 1970s a group of scholars led by Arthur Elstein[161] and Jerome Kassirer[162] began a research program that had several components. The first was to understand and model normative clinical reasoning and clinical problem-solving. The second, to compare clinician reasoning against Bayesian and other probabilistic computerized models for diagnosis and later models for use of diagnostic tests, treatments, screening techniques, and prevention techniques. The third component promoted these probabilistic models for clinical use. Like other models of clinical methods discussed here, the decision-analytic approach contributed to the EBM movement, yet its methodological scope once again as limited to primarily diagnostic considerations and marginalized the transactions of the doctor-patient relationship, with their values, preferences, social-community interests and limitations, and other difficult-to-quantify contextual features.

Contemporary pluralism and integrationism for psychiatry. Psychiatry, as the branch of medicine that arguably draws more, and depends more, upon the social sciences and humanities than other medical specialties, has long struggled with the diversity of theoretical approaches to its scientific basis as well as the craft and moral aspects of its practice. In recent years many theorists of psychiatry have sought pluralism—the (hopefully wise and informed) use of multiple theories and methods, and integrationism—a metamethod for organizing multiple theories and methods into a synthetic whole. In this selective and whirlwind review of some of these thinkers, I cannot do justice to all aspects of their work but have selectively drawn key points about clinical method from them.

Recent synthetic work by Kenneth Kendler and Peter Zachar, separately and collaboratively, have made substantial theoretical contributions to a 'comprehensive etiological understanding of psychiatric disorders'.[163] Similar to the biomedical and biopsychosocial models that preceded this work, the focus for these authors is on the integrating or coordinating of scientific explanations for mental disorders. The methods described by Kendler and Zachar however, are focused on synthesizing the sciences of psychiatry, and again are marginal in the moral-practical considerations of the clinical encounter. However, three other contemporary accounts addressing practical intervening raise some important points about the methods of psychiatry for the purposes of this book.

The first of these is Nassir Ghaemi's 'pluralistic approach to the mind and mental illness', presented formally in his 2003 book[164] Ghaemi draws from his mentors McHugh and Slavney's perspectivism[165] Leston Havens,[166] and the philosophy of psychiatry articulated by Karl Jaspers in the previously mentioned *General Psychopathology*.[167] Ghaemi's book addresses a broad number of conceptual and philosophical issues in psychiatry, but prominent is the advocacy of his brand of pluralism:[168]

> Finding the right method for the right problem: This is the imperative of pluralism.

Ghaemi's major methodological worry for psychiatry is eclecticism: the idea that in its manifold theories and methods, all are created and exercised equally and thoughtlessly. The treatment trope of 'medication and psychotherapy' for most all of the major mental disorders he finds a particularly offensive example of eclecticism run amok. Such a motto and practice inappropriately presume that these combined approaches are effective, both overgeneralizing from particular scientific studies as well as ignoring the particular circumstances that generate this instruction in the scientific literature.

Instead, Ghaemi puts forward a version of Jasper's methods of *Verstehen* and *Erklären*, the sorting of the clinical problems by whether they demand causal explanation, *Erklären*, or whether they demand holistic understanding in narrative or interpretive terms, *Verstehen*. In the midst of this work, Ghaemi offers much in clinical wisdom pertinent to practice, themes that will be echoed by his colleagues discussed below. However, the actual instruction in the use of his pluralistic approach to the clinical encounter is limited to a few pages in his last chapter. There he advocates for a clinical practice that is informed by multiple empirical sciences and facts and suggesting that clinical expertise govern the formation of treatment plans, rejecting the common assumption that a single 'treater' is better than multiple ones. Finally, he concludes with an instruction to humility:[169]

> For [the pluralist] there are no finished systems. There are no ideologies to which he can cling. He sees the mind as complex, yet he still seeks to be clear in his attempts to explain and understand it. He cannot claim to know anything for certain. Yet he must reject all

relativism. He is the eternal skeptic, yet he is also always open to belief. Belief for him is not an ideology, though; it is faith in James' definition: the need to make choices because the decisions are momentous, even in the absence of sufficient evidence.

Ghaemi's approach to pluralism, however, does not have much to say about the role of the patient and doctor-patient relationship in formulating decisions in the clinical encounter. For this we turn to two of his contemporaries.

In the title to his *Healing Psychiatry: Bridging the Science/Humanism Divide*, psychiatrist and philosopher David Brendel[170] appeals directly to George Engel's mission from 30 years back. However, at this point the resemblance to the biopsychosocial model ends; Brendel seeks a different set of philosophical resources than his predecessors: that of American pragmatism, the philosophy of (chiefly) William James, Charles S. Peirce, and John Dewey. In summarizing these philosophers' work, Brendel offers the 'fundamental principles' of the 'four p's':[171]

> They include (1) the *practical* dimensions of all scientific inquiry; (2) the *pluralistic* nature of the phenomena studied by science and the tools that are used to study those phenomena; (3) the *participatory* role of many individuals with different perspectives in the necessarily interpersonal process of scientific inquiry; and (4) the *provisional* and flexible character of scientific explanation.

Of particular note here is the emphasis the third p, of participation, which in the setting of psychiatric practice, emphasizes the role of (especially) the patient, as well as others involved: for example, other members of the healthcare team or the family. Often, the patient is the determinant in what can, should be, and is, done.

In synthesizing the four p's around the issue of clinical judgment, Brendel neatly summarizes the challenges of the clinical stage:[172]

> Drawing on James' notion of a pluralistic universe, they must have multiple explanatory tools available at all times. Meanwhile, drawing on the strengths of the explanatory sciences, they must choose their diagnostic and therapeutic models carefully, with serious consideration of any available scientific evidence and expert consensus. To ensure good patient care, clinicians need to have many explanatory concepts at their disposal, but they should then use sound clinical judgment to refine their diagnoses and treatments in a practical direction. Clinical judgment, of course, is very difficult to define, but its core elements would include evidence-based hypothesis formation, consideration of a wide range of diagnostic possibilities, careful observation of a broad spectrum of clinical phenomena, flexibility to revise a clinical formulation on the basis of new evidence, and open-mindedness to consultation with other colleagues in situations that are characterized by complexity, confusion, and uncertainty.

Brendel enlightens through his emphasis of the practical ends of the clinical encounter, and his portrayal of psychiatric practice as not just a theorizing clinician-expert but also as a component of a rich interpersonal array of actors, all of whom contribute to clinical action.

My last contemporary theorist of psychiatric pluralism is psychiatrist-philosopher Bradley Lewis,[173] whose 'Narrative Psychiatry' approach is perhaps the most vigorous in emphasizing the role of the patient in clinical judgment. Like his colleagues and predecessors, Lewis rejects simple-minded reductions of complex phenomena and complex clinical decision-making. He frames the metaphysical aspects of the clinical encounter as the presentation of different 'stories'. The task of treatment in his account is the (metaphorical) rewriting of these stories that patients tell themselves. The new stories offer new perspectives, directions, and outcomes that are healing or liberating. For Lewis, stories can come not just in the form of spoken or literary narratives, as in a patient's 'history', but even bioscientific causal explanation can be a kind of 'story'. Thus Lewis's account is pluralistic like his predecessors. Perhaps more than his predecessors, Lewis focuses on the clinician's path to selecting a clinical account, or story, that is effective in achieving treatment goals. Like McHugh and Slavney and their students, Lewis frames his pluralistic account as the potential for multiple modes of storytelling—multiple 'perspectives'—but what is distinctive in Lewis's account is the fundamentally interpersonal aspects of his clinical method. Rather than clinical method being centered around a clinician's thought process and reasoning, Lewis's narrative method assimilates the patient as an equal actor on the clinical stage. The process of clinical problem-solving becomes an ongoing dialogue with the patient in defining clinical problems as well as exchanging perspectives about how the clinical problem can be understood and addressed. Reminiscent of formal informed consent procedures, the process of clinical method becomes an ongoing, exploratory, and elaborate consent process with the patient. The clinician offers alternative perspectives or 'storying' of the patient's problems, and the patient considers their appeal, coherence, applicability, and potential for therapeutic change. In these features, Lewis's account bears resemblances to the work of Stanghellini mentioned earlier.

In his book, Lewis uses a published fictional source, Chitra Divakaruni's *Mrs. Dutta Writes a Letter*,[174] as his demonstration narrative; an example which then is reinterpreted through multiple substories, from the explanations of biological psychiatry to multiple psychotherapeutic, cultural, and spiritual perspectives. To bring this narrative labor to more life, Lewis speculates about how a 'true-life' Mrs. Dutta might respond to this or that narrative perspective; finding that she is more receptive to some perspectives than others. Through this collaborative negotiation of narrative perspectives, clinical decisions are made, and clinical actions taken. Like Brendel, the benchmark for the 'correct' story is pragmatic: effective treatment is the meeting of the goals of treatment. If one narrative perspective is rejected, fails, or stalls, this is an occasion for the dyad of doctor and patient to reinterpret the clinical process. In this explicit account of a method for clinical decision and action, Lewis's account is among the most novel of the literature on psychiatric method.[175]

In concluding this section, a few comments are indicated to summarize these very brief sketches of medical and psychiatric clinical methods. (1) Medicine and psychiatry are based upon a moral and practical imperative to care, cure, heal, and help their clients: patients. (2) The methods of the sciences, primarily the biological and social sciences, provide an essential component to clinical method. This contribution is complementary to the moral and practical aspects of medicine. The contribution of the sciences is the contribution of approaches to ascertaining truth about disease identity, cause, and behavior, and matching disease concepts to patient presentation (diagnosis), not to overlook the contribution of the sciences to evaluating and predicting the patient response to treatments. (3) A dilemma in clinical practice is how to apply the manifold findings of the sciences (to paraphrase Ghaemi, finding the 'right method') to the singular, unique patient (paraphrasing Ghaemi again, finding the 'right problem'). (4) The sciences provide general knowledge about populations of people, and so are always questionable in how they apply to the unique individual facing the unique clinician. For this, clinical methods require components that address interpretation and practical action. (5) These latter challenges move the core of the clinical method beyond the clinician alone, but to the interpersonal field involving (most elementally) the doctor and patient. The patient is the key epistemic as well as practical partner in treatment planning. However, the interpersonal field more comprehensively includes other caregivers, significant others of the patient, and by extension, larger systems and communities. (6) The interpersonal field implies competing interests, priorities, and values, which extend the moral-ethical content of clinical method beyond that of the provision of narrowly construed care/cure/help/heal, but into the moral and ethical interests outside of medicine. A key example of this extension of the moral beyond the core-clinical interpersonal field is the VMDR. Most directly, the interface of clinical method with the demands of the law and CJS pose multiple new moral ambiguities which were discussed in Chapters 1 and 2. With this understanding, I turn now to comparing and contrasting the methods of criminal law and medicine, and through that, showing the hazards and challenges lurking in the interdisciplinary space overlapping the two professional contexts.

Contrasting the methodological elements of American criminal law & medicine. With this discussion of the methods of law and medicine as background, a direct comparison of the methods around common themes in law and medicine will help crystallize the important differences between the fields. Leading into the next section on the metaphysical assumptions of law and medicine, I present several common epistemological and practical themes in their methods. While these themes or elements of law and medicine practice present an appearance of similarity, each section describes the substantial differences in which these superficial resemblances bring into focus. These elements are presented in alphabetical order for simplicity and reference' sake. Except when noted, the comparisons address the place of the defendant for criminal law, and the patient for medicine and psychiatry, as the respective 'clients'.

Advocacy. The role of advocate is a central one to the method of the criminal lawyer, as presented earlier, especially in light of the adversarial model. In the United States, the role of advocate not only addresses the lawyer's moral obligation to the client but constitutes a major epistemological role in the determination of the 'truth', and relatedly, justice, as discussed in the methods section for criminal law. Moreover, the prevailing value of criminal law is service to social justice, and in the US the adversarial system, however flawed and amended, is considered a core component in securing truth, but also (and perhaps more importantly) justice. Recall that this dual aspect of advocacy in criminal law sets up an ethical tension in the field, where client advocacy and advocacy toward truth and/or justice may conflict. This dual modality of advocacy is moderated and buffered by the judge's regulatory guidance and enforcement of criminal procedure. The dual modality of advocacy is also reflected in legal ethics and regulatory policies as well as debates about the bounds of advocacy.

In medicine and psychiatry, the role of advocate is also central to the moral duties of the physician to his 'client'—the patient. However, the enactment of those duties is different for medicine and psychiatry. First, the advocacy to the patient or client means that the physician is the patient's chief agent in furthering caring/curing/helping/healing. The goals of physician advocacy then are circumscribed to a narrow range of the patient's interests. The physician-as-advocate is not concerned with the patient's guilt or innocence regarding criminal acts; is not concerned with the patient's tax status or political attitudes, at least not until these infringe on the patient's health. Medical advocacy is circumscribed by the patient's health interests, but also distinct from criminal law's goals of truth and justice. Moreover, medical advocacy is anchored to the moral goals of medicine; as Pellegrino specified earlier, a goal of medicine is promoting health in the patient. Deviating from that role as a healer compromises one's very status as a physician. Thus, the conflicts between medical advocacy and the advocacy in criminal law set up deep tensions in forensic psychiatry, which were described earlier concerning Paul Appelbaum's framing of forensic psychiatry ethics.

Cause. Cause or causation is an important concept in criminal law but is entangled with two related terms that are of equal interest but also equal potential to confuse. Those terms are culpability and responsibility. Like cause, these terms are used in ordinary (lay) language, but in the criminal law setting each has a technical meaning. To complicate things further, the relationships between these concepts and even their meaning are contested by legal theorists and philosophers of law. Thus, in their actual use on the courtroom stage, different meanings may prevail resulting in jurisdictional and judicial variation in application of these concepts, with resulting confusion in courtroom discourses.[176] To narrow a considerable range of discussion, and for my purposes here, a noncontroversial, everyday-legal sense of each term is needed, hence the following references to *Black's Law Dictionary*.[177] The defining causes of interest in criminal law are *human* causes, not natural or mechanical ones. Otherwise, criminal law deals causally in defining coincidences: these are of interest for not-guilty decisions. Cause, in criminal law, is typically broken into two related concepts, 'cause-in-fact' and 'proximate (or legal) cause'. *Black's* defines 'cause-in-fact' as 'The cause without which the event could not have occurred.'[178] 'Proximate or legal cause' requires a wordier definition:[179]

1. A cause that is legally sufficient to result in liability; an act or omission that is considered in law to result in a consequence, so that liability can be imposed on the actor.
2. A cause that directly produces an event and without which the event would not have occurred.

Already, definition (2) looks a lot like cause-in-fact, so for our purposes; definition (1) should be the focus.

In contrast, the concept of 'culpability' in criminal law has to do with whether the defendant is blameworthy for the criminal act:[180]

> Blameworthiness; the quality of being culpable. Except in cases of absolute liability, criminal culpability requires a showing that the person acted purposely, knowingly, recklessly, or negligently with respect to each material element of the offense.

Moore[181] notes that a fundamental interest of criminal law regarding causation is to assess the degree or amount of moral blameworthiness of the offender's action. This determination aids in prescribing proportionate punishment. An offender who had a small role to play in a crime should, proportionately, suffer a lighter sentence than an offender who played a major role in the crime. For example, the driver of a getaway car in a bank robbery should suffer a lighter sentence than the robber who shot one of the tellers in the bank.

The last related concept, responsibility, or criminal responsibility, also has a technical meaning:[182]

1. Liability.
2. Criminal law. A person's mental fitness to answer in court for his or her actions. See Competency. . . .

In the discussion section of this *Black's* entry, the authors note that responsibility has two common meanings in criminal law: One being accountability or being subject to censure or paying consequences. The other has to do with the ability of people to 'control their actions and conform to law'.[183] The gist of the insanity defense controversy then, has to do with whether a mentally ill offender is culpable—blameworthy for the crime—which of course is intertwined with the offender's responsibility: whether the defendant should be held accountable and/or was capable of conforming his/her/their actions to the requirements of law. Only responsible, culpable defendants can be a cause of the crime, because then only the 'sufficient' conditions for liability are met. These stipulations are nestled into the concept of *mens rea*, or criminal intent, which was introduced in Chapter 5.

Criminal law, at base, addresses two kinds of acts: it requires people to not do something (as in not stealing or murdering), or it requires people to do something (as in paying your taxes or stopping your car at the red-light traffic signal). To decide if a criminal offense has occurred, an assessment of cause is involved. In the case of bank robbery, the bank lost money *because* John Dillinger took cash from the safe at gunpoint. In the case of nonpayment of income taxes, Al Capone was found guilty of tax evasion *because* of his accountant's evidence of income not reported to the Internal Revenue Service, and, therefore, taxes were not paid. However, making these determinations of cause in practice can be quite difficult. Moore[184] gives the vivid example of a woman stabbed in the chest by a man. The woman, bleeding out, refuses medical care which is immediately available. She dies quickly. What was the cause of her death, her stabbing or her treatment refusal? The ambiguity introduced by this case is just the tip of an iceberg of case variations which makes the philosophy of criminal causation very complex indeed.[185]

Remember conventional criminal law practice in the US depends upon two requirements regarding causation: (1) cause-in-fact and (2) legal or proximate cause.[186] According to Moore[187] cause-in-fact is sometimes referred to as 'scientific' causation because it often depends upon scientific explanation: the woman died *because* of blood loss from the knife wound. In this frame, the woman died from the consequences of her stabbing, looking at the aftermath of the stabbing. However, proximate cause is typically the cause immediately preceding the criminal event. Did the woman's refusal of medical care cause her death? From this latter example of proximate cause, Moore suggests that cause-in-fact is often more 'objective' or easier to determine, while legal or proximate cause requires a judgment or evaluation based upon the facts and situational details of the case. However, he later develops the case that both concepts, cause-in-fact and proximate cause, pose deep philosophical difficulties as well as practical difficulties in the courts.

In American law, the prevailing test of cause-in-fact is the *sine qua non* of the American Law Institute Model Penal Code: the 'but-for' test.[188] This test asks a counterfactual question: 'but for the defendant's action, would the victim have been harmed?'[189] In Moore's stabbed-woman example, the 'but-for' test is helpful, because the woman would not have died without the stabbing, even if she refused medical treatment. So the stabbing would be the cause-in-fact. So far so good. However, numerous problems have been identified in theory and practice with cause-in-fact assessments. These problems are too many to discuss here. Many of them stem from the steep demands of criminal prosecutors, who carry the burden of proof, to establish evidence 'beyond a shadow of a doubt'. They also emerge from the ambiguities of counterfactual reasoning, which depends upon speculations about how things would be different if the facts of the case changed. Moore explains:[190]

> Counterfactuals by their nature are difficult to prove with any degree of certainty, for they require the fact finder to speculate what would have happened if the defendant had not done what she did.

Crudely, playing 'let's pretend' in the courtroom poses deep challenges to juries who are trying to find a judgment beyond a reasonable doubt. I recommend Moore's review for more in-depth discussion and critique of legal-cause reasoning and the American Law Institute (ALI) handling of cause in their *Model Penal Code*. Ironically, Moore notes that juries don't seem to have nearly as much difficulty in recognizing causes in an intuitive way as do legal theorists in dissecting these judgments into their conceptual elements!

In summary, causal judgments in law, however ambiguous, are important because they implicate guilt or innocence for a criminal event, as well as provide a proportional estimate of blameworthiness for the punishment phase of court judgments. Causes in legal settings are framed typically by but-for counterfactual reasoning, along with proximate cause, which is a practical judgment made by juries in assessing the most salient human contributions to the criminal event.

For medicine, the notion of cause has scientific roots, particularly for the cause of diseases, and moral-practical roots, in that medicine's interest in causes is driven by the ethic of therapeutics. Interest in causes in medicine range from the diagnostic (what caused this person's affliction) to the prescriptive (how can I, the physician, cause improvement in the patient's condition). Importantly, medicine's therapeutic interest in causes is overwhelmingly *prospective*: As a physician I am interested in manipulating causal factors in my patient's future—that is, providing effective therapy. I want to provide an intervention that is causally sufficient for the patient to improve in the future. This is a sharp contrast to the law's interest in causes: in criminal law as well as torts, the law wants to know the causes of *past* events: the law's interest in causes is retrospective.[191]

However, the future-orientation of therapeutics does not imply that medicine has no interest in understanding the causes of past events. Earlier I discussed Munson's idea that medicine is dependent upon the sciences for providing much of the factual knowledge base for intervening in the clinical encounter. So while in the clinical encounter the physician's causal interest is prospective, the sciences from which the physician draws often derive their utility from retrospective analyses of causes of diseases. Epidemiology studies the causes of diseases in (past) affected populations, and the biological and social sciences study the causes of diseases (etiology), often in the past through mechanisms like descriptive studies or 'retrospective chart reviews', in addition to present- and future-oriented causal studies: that is, experiments. However, the generation of this knowledge from the sciences bears fruit through its informing the physician in the clinical encounter. For this use of knowledge in effecting change in the future, 'writing a prescription' in medicine gains both literal and metaphorical meaning.

The discussion of cause in clinical-encounter reasoning has taken many forms in physician's discourses. Doctors talk about diseases being 'multifactorial', that is, having multiples causes or 'factors'. Which of the multiple factors becomes important in the clinical encounter depends upon the practical potential or practical utility of intervening with therapy. The doctor may recognize that poverty is a causal factor in clinical depression, but for most contexts the doctor's ability to amend a patient's impoverished environment is limited to none. Such a practical limitation means the doctor turns her attention to other factors, such as intervening with cognitive-behavioral therapy to undo the negative cognitions that are another causal factor in depression or intervening by prescribing an antidepressant which address neuro-chemical factors in depression.

So a part of practical clinical skills for physicians is identifying causal factors which may provide practical opportunities for clinical intervening with therapeutic intent. Because of these practical interests, physicians are typically open to considering all kinds of causal factors. Removing one factor from a chain or network of pathogenic events may be therapeutically definitive. For example, lead poisoning in children in toxic lead–containing environments would warrant removal of lead from the environment, or removal of people from said environment, but the practical physician will treat the poisoned child with chelating agents to remove the lead from the patient's body.

Earlier in this section we considered a variety of theories of clinical reasoning. Much of the challenge in clinical reasoning has to do with identifying manipulable causes of disease and then planning the proper sequence of clinical intervention. The practical reasoning of the clinician often provokes a rejection of intervening with some causes. This rejection of some causes and not others emerges from practical reasoning: utility judgments. For example, a patient may not want to take a medication, and prefer psychotherapy; an intervention which requires frequent visits may be rejected because the patient may have transportation difficulties. Helping the patient with transportation permits the patient to obtain the treatment she needs. Transportation difficulties may not cause her depression, but it might pose a cause of treatment failing in this circumstance.

Philosophers of science and medicine have offered much more nuanced and sophisticated analyses of 'cause' in medicine, though for my purposes here (pointing out fundamental differences in causal understanding in law and medicine) reviewing these is not necessary. Interested readers should consider Nordenfelt and Lindahl[192] and Kendler and Parnas.[193] For my purposes here, a few implications and conclusions can be drawn about 'cause' in law and medicine:

1. *Prospective versus retrospective.* The practical interests in cause in criminal procedure involve a looking back in time (are retrospective) regarding the events surrounding the crime. In medicine, cause in the clinical encounter involves looking forward in time (is prospective) in aiming toward effective treatment.
2. *Culpability versus therapy.* Criminal law's interest in cause is driven by the demand to find culpability, or blameworthiness for the criminal event. The link of the event to the defendant is provided by causal accounts. In contrast, medicine's interests in causes are driven by the demand of providing therapeutics to the patient.

3. *Punishment versus cure or care.* Related to (2) criminal law's interest in causes is framed by the moral ends of punishing wrongdoers, restoring victims, and protecting the public. Medicine's interest in causes is framed by its moral ends of care/cure/helping/healing.

4. *Singularity versus multiplicity.* In criminal procedures culpability is derived through courtroom debate about the causal role of a single or few crucial factor(s), typically the defendant's actions. In medicine, causal relevance is determined by the utility of multiple factors in informing practical therapeutic interventions with patients.

5. *Role of responsibility.* In law, criminal responsibility has to do with the defendant's accountability for the crime, and his/her/their mental capability to conform to the rule of law. In medicine, concepts of responsibility are implicated with the patient's causal contributions to their illness and their duty of participation in therapy.

These differences are morally profound. Criminal law, to the degree that its ends are defined by punishment, restoration to victims, and incapacitation of offenders, is effectively pointed toward causing harm to the criminal offender toward a 'greater good' of providing protections against public harms. Medicine's ends are quite the opposite—indeed one of its prevailing moral maxims is 'First do no harm.' Law's focus on culpability means that it dwells upon the defendant's contributions to the event-of-interest to the relative exclusion of all other causal factors, making for a practical environment that is foreign to a clinician's typical reasoning around multiple causal factors converging to explain an event.

Division of labor. Criminal law and medicine and psychiatry share some commonalities concerning the division of labor in executing each profession's duties. Both depend upon an extended infrastructure that supports their respective missions. For criminal law, this includes policing, a legal staff to assist in investigation and collection of case information, the administrative trappings of the courts, the jail system for holding offenders prior to trial, the jail and prison system for short- and long-term sentences respectively, the probation and parole systems, to name a few. Medicine and psychiatry are disciplines embedded in different set of large systems, each involving piecemeal contributions to medicine's mission. Among others, these systems include the healthcare system of hospitals, clinics, and private practices; the public health system; administrative and funding systems, including the insurance and managed care companies; the Veteran's Administration healthcare system; and in psychiatry, the public sector mental health system. Healthcare itself is a team effort involving not just physicians but nurses, various therapy specialists (e.g., occupational, respiratory, rehabilitative, and psychotherapists) and clerical staff and administrators. Medical systems were considered earlier when I discussed Nordenfelt on medicine and social welfare.

For both professions' relationships with clients, the lawyer and the doctor serve in most capacities in 'center stage' being in large part responsible for the success of each endeavor and also being at the center of the professional stage—the courtroom and the examination room, respectively. To be sure, both the criminal attorney and the clinician are subject to regulatory input, censure, and even removal from each of their professional stages: for the criminal attorney, the judge may alter the courtroom proceedings, just as a hospital administrator may transform, redefine, even exclude a physician's participation in the hospital stage. However, in terms of the professional-client relationship, the attorney, and the physician both have clients to whom they are primarily and selectively responsible in ways the judge and the hospital administrator are not.

The important difference between the two professions has to do with the culmination of their collective activities: for criminal law, the collection of evidence and the enactment of a persuasive performance in convicting or acquitting the defendant, and for medicine, the provision of assessment, counseling, and therapeutics. For the project of criminal law, the courtroom trial has a dramaturgical character—theater in playing out the narrative conflict of the adversarial model. In cases of severe or violent crime, the theater of criminal law even has an extended audience—the jury and courtroom visitors. The moral center of this drama is the potential for punishing wrongdoing, protecting the public, and perhaps, providing revenge for the victimized. This theatrical character shapes the participants of the pretrial stage of criminal law into contributors to a production. The trial itself constitutes a performance aimed at persuading the judge and jury. For medicine, the supportive participants are continuously engaged in another kind of ritual which is to battle certain existential facts of human existence: death, disability, and suffering. I argue that the character of the typical clinical encounter lacks most of the features of theatricality. Indeed, the clinical encounter is a series of private and often very personal interactions between two people, doctor and patient, augmented by other caregivers in hospital settings. This difference between criminal law and medicine is most vividly played out on the 'professional stage' discussed further below.

Evidence. The concept of evidence is perhaps the most pliable and confusing element in describing the differences between legal reasoning and medical reasoning. In these two professional practice domains, the uses, formulation, practical interests, and treatment of bias about evidence are notably different. For this reason, and to keep the differences as crisp as possible, I will break out the discussion of evidence for both professions into four categories: (a) practical interests in evidence, (b) evidential judgments (evaluating evidence), (c) constraints on evidence, and (d) the handling of evidential bias. From these four perspectives, I intend that quite different meanings of evidence will emerge for each of the two fields. A summary of the considerations of evidence in law and psychiatry is provided in Table 6.3.

(a) Practical interests in evidence: law. Criminal Law's interest in evidence emerges from the context of the criminal trial, where preparations for the trial involve collecting evidence by the prosecution and defense, which is then presented at trial in an effort to bring the accused to justice and truth. Because the

372 Vice and Psychiatric Diagnosis

Table 6.3 Contrasting Evidence in Criminal Law and Psychiatry

Aspect of Evidence	Criminal Law	Psychiatry
Practical interest in evidence	*Retrospective*—the crime largely concerns events in the past *Unbalanced interpretation of evidence*—judge and jury are primary interpreters *Case-particular narratives*—must be material and probative *Lay-oriented*—evidence must be comprehensible to the public	*Past, present, & future oriented*—evidence from all time frames are typically relevant *Dialogical*—evidence gather in collaboration (active or passive) with patient *More balanced interpretation of evidence*—patient and doctor interpret together *Narrative & scientific evidence together*—unique narrative as well as scientific generalizations are always considered together *Mutuality of evidence*- given and taken between doctor & patient
Evaluating evidence	*Multiple evaluators*—from arrest through trial *Complex procedural rules of evidence* *Final arbiters of evidence*—are the judge and jury	*Science & the doctor-patient dyad*—evidence is evaluated from the vantage of scientific process and the doctor-patient dialogue *Diagnosis linked to summaries of evidence*—Science provides stylized, clinically relevant evidence, based upon diagnosis *Use of evidence is negotiated*—in the doctor-patient relationship
Constraints on evidence	*Time*—high demand for efficient gathering and processing of evidence *Endpoint*—evidence converges upon a conviction or acquittal *Standard criterion*—'beyond a reasonable doubt'	*Time*—patient need may constraint time for 'adequate' evidence *Death as endpoint*—clinical deliberations about evidence typically end at the patient's death *Multiple criteria*—clinical evidential judgments depend upon scientific as well as narrative criteria
Handling of evidential bias	*Adversary system*—an ongoing critique of evidence *Criminal procedure*—regulatory norms and oversight to diminish bias *Rules of evidence*—particular guidance on use of evidence	*Social elements of scientific process* *Peer review and consultation* *Professional regulatory structures*—professional associations and conflict-of-interest rules

development of a criminal case is in large part prepared through looking into the past—developing evidence in retrospect—the securing and use of legal evidence lacks the empirical immediacy of medical evidence within the clinical encounter. The important exception to the retrospective quality of criminal law evidence is the uncommon situation where a witness presents an unanticipated revelation in the here-and-now of the witness stand. Here the evidence presented (as a most blatant example, where a witness confesses to the crime thus exonerating the defendant) may, in the here-and-now, transform the proceedings. Judges may consider factors around the use of evidence, such as the admissibility of evidence, or evidence as future precedent. However, these judicial actions do not characterize the attorney-client relationship and are important but noncentral to the role of evidence in criminal procedure. However, for the most part, the use of evidence in criminal law consists of *reconstructing* events of the past, be it through, for example, eyewitness memories, analysis of the crime scene, murder weapons, and incriminating circumstances.

A second important practical interest of the criminal court revolves around the requirement that evidence be *material* (relevant and significant to the case at hand) and *probative* (contributing to the proof of something, e.g., the guilt or innocence of the defendant). The latter means that the evidence should not address a general state of affairs, but the particular charges that have been raised against the defendant. Legal evidence is directed toward unique circumstances, unique events, and unique persons. In its orientation around a crime narrative in the past, legal evidence more closely resembles the evidence of history than the evidence of scientific experiment and research. Model- or rule-governed scientific generalizations are by and large not material or probative in law, because as generalizations they may, or may not, apply to the unique and particular trial case at hand.[194]

The last practical interest by criminal law concerning evidence is perhaps the most important: Criminal trials for severe crimes like murder and larceny are decided by juries consisting of laypersons; therefore, all evidence that is presented must be comprehensible by the lay jury. This means technical evidence requiring extensive education or specialized background knowledge or experience is not admissible unless delivered by an expert witness whose role is to assist the Court and jury in understanding such technical aspects of the relevant evidence.

(b) Evaluating evidence: Law. The criminal law has multiple structural elements and procedural elements that serve to evaluate the relevance, quality, and utility of evidence. These structural and procedural elements pose a complex and often ambiguous set of demands as well as conclusions. One source of evidence evaluation may precede the trial completely. If the evidence collected by police is too weak or flawed, the judge or prosecutor may elect to not prosecute the case altogether and dismiss the charges. Alternatively, a grand jury may consider, on a preliminary basis, evidence of a crime before deciding whether a criminal charge is warranted—if so, an indictment is issued, thus demanding a criminal trial. These procedures both impose standards for quality evidence as well as control the volume of criminal cases for formal trials. In medical terms, the grand jury provides a 'triage' function about whether further prosecution is warranted by the current evidence.

One of the most important skills of the criminal attorney is the ability to anticipate and address the ramifications of evidential procedure. A criminal attorney must anticipate how her opponent as well as the judge will respond to her collection, delivery, and use of evidence. One of the evaluative elements of evidence in criminal law emerges from the aforementioned adversarial model. The opposing sides are looking for ways to challenge, disqualify, or otherwise criticize each other's evidence. This is played out most obviously in the cross-examination of witnesses presenting various pieces of evidence (e.g., testimony about the events related to the crime, the salience of various sources of evidence).

In 1975 the US developed the Federal Rules of Evidence (FRE),[195] which were originally developed for the US Federal Court system, but since then, and under no obligation, many individual states have assimilated or adapted them to their state court systems. The FRE offer rules about admissibility of evidence, use of expert witnesses, what counts as 'hearsay' evidence, and guidance about what kinds of evidence are stronger, and weaker, in the criminal court setting. With 67 rules under 11 articles, the FRE are a concrete example of the complexities about what counts as evidence and what doesn't. The third element that evaluates evidence in the criminal setting could be inferred from the earlier comment about not all states (or jurisdictions) having to use the FRE. States develop their own precedents and laws about proper use of evidence in criminal courts through the vehicle of judicial decisions.

Many of these rules of evidence in the FRE and other jurisdictions are discretionary, and so the fourth element of evidential evaluation comes from courtroom judges, who choose to apply such guidelines, and generally make judgements about admissibility of evidence when the latter is challenged by attorneys through objections or other mechanisms. Much discussion in the literature has been made of the use of the *Daubert* guidance on admissibility of expert witness evidence, which depends upon a judge's discretion.[196] Recognizing these regulatory structures and procedures gives only a clue about the complex thinking that goes into criminal trial procedure vis-a-vis evidence.

(c) Constraints on evidence: law. Perhaps the most obvious constraint on the presentation of evidence in both law and medicine is time. Both the attorney and doctor have to be aware of time constraints in assembling evidence. Often, the judge is the arbiter about the appropriate timeframe for the presentation of evidence, and precedents develop in local jurisdictions about the use of evidence that is too time-consuming or complex for a jury proceeding. More importantly, a significant difference with law as opposed to medicine is that criminal law has a concrete, definitive endpoint—a conviction or an acquittal. In this setting, the demand made of the evidence of the case is high; hence, the concrete instruction to the jury regarding evidence: that a conviction should be based upon evidence that leads the jury to be 'beyond a reasonable doubt'. As we'll see shortly, no such time-limited demand for decisive evidence characterizes medicine, at least outside of life-or-death emergency care decisions.

(d) Handling of evidential bias: law. Both law and medicine have the potential for evidence, or its interpretation, to be biased. However, each has different procedures for handling or preventing such biased evidence. I've already noted the screening for the adequacy of evidence by judges, prosecutors, and grand juries. However, once the case comes to trial, the stylized rituals of the criminal courtroom are the primary mechanisms where criminal law deals with bias. These mechanisms have already been introduced. The adversary system serves to expose and nullify bias in the opposing side's arguments and evidence. The judge administers the trial process and regulates bias through application and enforcement of jurisdictional and FRE—adjudicating whether a piece of evidence or testimony is admissible, material, and has probative value. The jury sits in final judgment of the defense and prosecution's evidence, and approaches the evidence presented with their own common-sensical approaches to discovering bias.[197]

From these four perspectives in law—practical interests in evidence, evaluating evidence, constraints on evidence, and handling of evidential bias, I turn to the comparable processes in medicine and psychiatry.

(a) Practical interests in evidence: medicine. Law and medicine share an imperative to translate their technical concepts and procedures into communications that the lay public can comprehend and take meaningful action upon. In the case of law, the jury must make a judgment about guilt or innocence of the criminal defendant. In the case of medicine the physician presents a diagnosis to, and negotiates a treatment plan with the patient, which requires varying degrees of action by the patient, ranging from passive acceptance in the extreme (as in a comatose patient) to an active, egalitarian, shared-decision-making mission that involves engagement and labor from both parties—physician and patient (as in a diet, medication and exercise program for a patient with diabetes). Both law and medicine are dependent upon evidence of various kinds to persuade both the jury and the patient respectively. Moreover, for both criminal law and medicine evidence is collected and assimilated outside of the setting of the professional stage. However, the similarities around evidence between law and medicine largely end here.

The physician applies scientific evidence collected in research settings which describe the behavior of disease processes and their responses to treatments; recall the earlier discussion of EBM. The scientific generalizations about disease behavior and response to treatments become part of the physician's expertise that is shared with the patient. Moreover, the physician is also responsive to clinical evidence gathered with the participation of the patient and other informants (e.g., family, parent, relative, friend, and medical record) sometimes called 'collateral' evidence. In medicine this evidence is collected and especially interpreted with the patient—recall the earlier discussion of the hermeneutics of medicine—and these clinical interpretations, in concert with the patient's consent and participation, shape the clinical actions of diagnosis and treatment. The physician, as medical expert, carries the greater burden of interpretation, because the patient has come to the physician expecting one or more alternative interpretations of the patient's illness experiences, placing the patient's experience within the context of medical theory, science, and practice.[198]

In criminal law the hermeneutics of action are posed to the jury by rival attorneys (the prosecution and defense), and each side tries to convince the jury of the inferiority of his/her/their rival's interpretive account. In this sense, the jury carries *a greater burden of interpretation than the medical patient*, in that the jury is left with rival interpretive accounts that only the jury can reconcile on their own, with minimal assistance from the judge. Even with more minor cases, the judge still suffers a burden of interpretation in receiving the rival accounts from the prosecution and defense.

In contrast, the medical patient appeals to the physician for assistance in understanding and acting on the new interpretive account (a re-interpretation of the medical evidence), which involves a dialogue characterized by a mutuality of mission and purpose.[199] This mutuality of the medical interpretive mission is not comparable to the interpretive demands made by the dueling advocates of the legal/adversarial model. With these quite dichotomous epistemic procedures, it should not be surprising that physicians experience the criminal law setting as distorting of the truth, and attorneys find physician testimony often gratuitously complex, nonmaterial, and nonprobative. Both professions are founded upon fundamentally different methods and interests in evidence.

A second substantive difference in the pragmatics of evidence involves the direction of interpretation. Criminal procedure is (mostly) retrospective in focus in respect to the defendant. The criminal court procedure tries to determine what happened in the past, at the time of the crime.[200] The dueling accounts of the past criminal event are presented to the jury for their consideration. Medicine, on the contrary, focuses on three temporal directions of evidential interpretation past, present and future, that interplay into medical decision-making. One consideration is diagnostic, which tries to account for what is happening to the patient *now*, in which evidence from the *past* (the patient's history) is crucial, but also evidence in the *present* which is also crucial (e.g., the clinical examination and current laboratory studies). Another interpretive clinical task—that of therapy—is *future* directed, where the physician uses collected evidence to predict the patient's response to treatment. The task of the clinical encounter then, is triply temporal for the physician: evidence informs interpretations of the past, present, and future.

A final difference between the practical interests in evidence concerns the earlier-mentioned distinction between narrative interpretation in law, and the synthetic interpretation of the sciences in medicine. In law, the professional stage is dominated by adversarial attorneys who elicit evidence from witnesses, aiming for the kind of holistic, particular understanding characterizing historical interpretation and generalization. While expert witnesses from the technical and scientific disciplines may contribute insights from the sciences for the Court, these are intended to be facts that serve the purposes of building a historical-narrative account. (Remember that expert testimony must be material and probative—that is, experts must be able to speak to THIS case, and not just general populations or clinical situations. A requirement for material and probative evidence means that the evidence must fit into a unique narrative account.) In contrast, a physician's interpretations in the clinical encounter perform a dance involving narrative (first-person patient history) and scientific generalizations and models (generated from third-person research in relevant populations) as partners in building a diagnosis and therapy.

(b)   Evaluating evidence: medicine. Earlier I noted that criminal law has three sources of evidential evaluation that interact in complex ways across various jurisdictions: the adversarial criminal procedure (including the respective strategies of the prosecution and defense attorneys), the interpretations and directions from the judge, state and other jurisdictional rules and conventions around evidence, and the FRE.

In medicine, the evaluation of evidence moves through the procedures of medical science, and this corpus of knowledge is brought to the clinic by the physician and then critically evaluated again through the hermeneutic lens of the clinical encounter and the patient's unique characteristics. The scientific contributions to medical-evidential judgment are processed by a large corpus of systems, procedures, and processes: the peer-review system for scientific research grants and research publications, the continuing medical education system for disseminating new knowledge, the synthetic efforts of services like Cochrane reviews and diagnosis and treatment guidelines from medical professional organizations, to name a few. Physicians as 'life-long learners' are expected to keep up with new scientific developments in their field, though today the interpretive and memory tasks are supplemented by hand-held and electronic medical record assistance and surveillance of emerging scientific data.

So, the evaluation of scientific evidence for physicians is highly stylized and often delivered in concise summary format to facilitate assimilation. Moreover, the massive critical evaluation of these complex bits of evidence is done outside of the clinical stage of delivery (e.g., bedside or consulting room), making for a notable difference between law and medicine. For law, the evaluation of evidence is shifted more into the here-and-now procedures of the trial. In medicine, the preprocessed scientific information is then brought by the physician to the clinical encounter in a stylized set of 'standards of care'. At this point the diagnosis and treatment dialogues then serve as a final round of evaluation, as patient and physician dialogue about the applicability, differential value, of the scientific as well as personal information and values provided by the patient. What is novel to medicine here is the prevailing evaluative power of the doctor-patient relationship, where clinical judgments are made largely in terms of education, negotiation, and agreement within the doctor-patient dyad. Contrast with the courtroom setting where a much more open field of evidence evaluation operates.

(c)　Constraints on evidence—medicine. In the comparable law subsection above, I discussed the time considerations with the two professions, that evidence is constrained by time considerations for both fields. Importantly, the requirement for criminal law to arrive at a definitive conclusion provides a concrete stopping point in the consideration of evidence. Medicine's use of evidence, however, is more provisional and practical, and may develop over time as the patient course and treatments develop over time.[201] Important exceptions exist for this generalization, however—as with urgent or emergent medical care where prompt action is required.

(d)　Handling of evidential bias: medicine. In the law section, I mentioned the contributions of criminal procedure and the adversary system in addressing evidential bias. For medicine, evidential bias is addressed in the scientific domain through the mechanisms of scientific methods (e.g., use of control groups, experimental design), and perhaps more importantly the social elements of science (e.g., peer review, openness to criticism, equality of opportunity to participate, and epistemic freedom to study what one desires).[202] As implied earlier, evidence is not just evaluated by the scientific process, but bias is regulated through the process as well. More recently, research regulatory procedures governing 'responsible conduct of research'[203] and the rise of a more explicitly articulated clinical research ethics also contribute to the minimizing of scientific bias—consider the recent discussions and regulations concerning conflict-of-interest in basic, clinical, and translational research.[204]

In regard to the evidence considered in the clinical encounter, the potential for evidential bias is not as closely regulated, theorized, or considered. The patient herself provides a service to the physician by evaluating the aptness of the physician's formulations, often bringing up amendments to her history in response to diagnostic wrong turns ('I should have told you that there was blood in my urine.'). The avoidance of bias in the clinical encounter is governed by the clinical skills (both examination and interpretive) of the physician, the physician's integrity in adhering to the evidence, and the quality of the doctor-patient relationship.

(e)　Special considerations about psychiatric evidence. The distinctiveness of the medical perspectives on evidence are preserved in psychiatry. However, psychiatric practice poses some differences in emphasis regarding the balance between narrative and scientific interpretation. As Mona Gupta has pointed out in a series of publications[205] the exclusively empirical-based EBM approach is less suited to psychiatric practice. When one turns to psychiatric practice, while population-based, empirical evidence offered by the sciences are crucially important, important limitations in applicability and generalizability prevail. In psychiatry the interpretive, narrative facets of clinical reasoning and inference, as well as contextual determinants, are much more prominent, for the reasons discussed earlier—such as the relationship of psychopathology to human existential limitations. In this latter case the clinician doesn't simply interpret the applicability of scientific data but must place the scientific data into a human existential and practical context and appraise the normative status of the patient's experience and behavior.[206]

The weight of the interpretive challenge is even more pronounced in the forensic/criminal justice setting. Here the interpretive challenges are deepened by the psychiatrist's requirement to remain skeptical about the veracity of the evaluee's account. The general presumption of truth-telling and honesty in the therapeutic doctor-patient relationship may be lost in the forensic setting, where incentives to avoid punishment (or in some cases, to re-enter prison) are powerful. Moreover, in the forensic setting, the clinician's focus may more often be retrospective, and therefore heavily historical and narrative in structure, as apropos to a forensic examination focusing on a defendant's state of mind at the time of the criminal event. Similarly, in the psychotherapeutic setting, clinical reasoning may tip toward the use of narrative interpretations of clinical data.

Interpretation. In criminal law, the tasks of interpretation of the evidence vary by the role of the key participants: the opposing prosecution and defense attorneys, the judge, and the jury. Moreover, in criminal law the Court's interpretation is definitive in that the aim of criminal procedure is a verdict—to determine guilt or innocence—a categorical distinction not permitting intermediate determinations. One is either guilty or not guilty—no in-betweens, even after a chain of appeals. The judge and/ or jury are the final interpreters of the evidence, although just for the single trial. If the case is 'appealed' then it moves to appellate courts where determinations are typically made by a panel of judges. Ultimately the appeal process comes to a final determination, and in the case of the United States, that final stopping point is the US Supreme Court.

In the context of a first-time criminal trial, the adversary-attorneys prepare and process their evidence and present a stylized, persuasive, and coherent story from either the prosecutorial or defense perspective, intended to sway the jury toward each side's largely predetermined interpretation. What the (US) judge does, among other things, is interpret the rules of evidence and criminal procedure so that the excesses of the adversarial system do not inappropriately sway the jury away from truth and justice.[207] In the case of criminal law, the interpretation is always directed to the culpability of the defendant—determining what the defendant's role was, if any, in the past criminal event.

In summary, in criminal law interpretation is definitive (a final verdict must be made): emergent (the definitive interpretation emerges from the combined efforts of judge, attorneys, witnesses, jury, and even perhaps the courtroom audience),[208] and

Table 6.4 Interpretation in Criminal Law and Psychiatry

Criminal Law	Psychiatry
Emergent—jury interprets from courtroom process	*Ongoing*—health and disease as continuous process
Definitive—verdict determines interpretation	*Pluralistic*—valid interpretations are > one
Singular—only one interpretation prevails	*Evolutionary*—interpretation changes over time

singular (a verdict determines the 'winning' interpretation). Table 6.4 briefly summarizes these distinctions between criminal law and medicine.

In the case of medicine, I have already discussed at some length the various models of clinical interpretation. Suffice to say the (psychiatric) clinician, in aiming toward a future effective therapy, must interpret the case-relevant science, collect the patient's narrative account of her illness and interpret it in light of the clinician's knowledge of psychopathology and a normative understanding of being human, consider contextual and practical factors, and then interpret how to bridge the patient's view from the clinician's 'expert' view(s),[209] all aiming toward selecting an effective therapeutic strategy that the patient will engage with and support. The patient's involvement doesn't appear at the end as suggested here: the patient is involved, ideally, at nearly every stage of thinking. The clinician negotiates clinical interpretations in doctor-patient relationships, and a hermeneutic 'check and balance' process occurs where a mutuality of interpretation between doctor and patient is the ideal. This does not occur in criminal law—the attorneys and judge do not negotiate the verdict with the jury; the opposing views are presented and the jury (or with minor cases and appeals, the judge[s]) make a unilateral determination.

In summary, in medicine and psychiatry, interpretation is ongoing (new interpretations of disease processes and treatment options are ever-present), pluralistic (more than one interpretation of the patient's malady is permissible, and even desired), and evolutionary (illness process and identity can change over time).[210]

Objectivity. The notion of objectivity, the ideal of minimizing bias or prejudice in interpretation, is discussed (indirectly) above in the context of evidential handling of bias. I mention objectivity as a separate issue here just for completeness' sake.

Professional stage. Earlier I introduced the concept of the professional stage. The professional stage is the practical location where each profession executes its activities, services, and responsibilities. In the most obvious sense, the professional stage for criminal law is the courtroom, while for medicine the professional stage is the hospital or clinic (office). Of course, I should acknowledge that these professional stages extend into other spaces (e.g., the jail, the health fair, and public health efforts), but for the purposes of this contrasting of the professions these two locales place the discussion for the two professions—pardon the pun—stage-center.

In the criminal courtroom I mentioned that a theatrical or dramaturgical character is ever-present. A criminal trial, because of the opposing attorney's rhetorical
intent to persuade the jury one way or other, has performance characteristics distinctive from the medical professional stage. First, the criminal trial is defined as
a moral drama by the charges at question. While the charge of tax evasion may not
command as much moral indignation as a murder charge, the criminal court offers a
morality play where wrongdoing is considered and suitably addressed (or not). Each
attorney's personal view about the guilt or innocence of the defendant is not particularly relevant to the performance characteristics of the trial process. Each attorney
attempts to serve her client's interests regardless. The circumstances of the evidence
may shape one side's strategy, but again the attorney's view of the 'truth of guilt' is not
particularly important. For example, a defense attorney may decide to plea-bargain
on behalf of her client, not (just) because she may think the client is guilty, but because the defendant has an unfavorable case, having, for example, much convincing
evidence against him. In presenting the client's case, each attorney presents him/
herself in a sympathetic light, marshaling the best rhetorical techniques to persuade
the jury or judge of his/her/their point of view. In this sense, the criminal attorneys
must always present an advocacy performance regardless of their personal moral
viewpoints, lending another dimension of pathos in the potential for a criminal attorney to act inauthentically—in opposition to one's own moral perspective. Indeed,
as an adversarial advocate, the criminal attorney's ethic is to resist or set aside such
inner turmoil and advocate for the client. The slang language about the determination of guilt reveals the frame of mind that allows for such a tolerance of personal
inauthenticity—an attorney 'wins' her case. As in a game, where there are winners
and losers, and where the players are rivals and if not enemies, are at least competitors, criminal attorneys win or lose. The professional stage of the courtroom then
sets up a particular kind of drama where the primary participants are competitors in
which the jury—the 'audience'—makes the determination who 'wins' and the judge
serves as a kind of referee. All protagonists serve justice, and in that sense the aim of
justice ennobles the methods to get there.

Milner Ball[211] provides a detailed analysis of the criminal courtroom as theater.
Formal elements of the criminal court are theatrical. First, he views the courtroom
itself as a 'theatrical space'[212] where actors perform in costume and in ceremony.
Second, the courtroom has seats for an audience. The jury is always an audience,
but the courtroom may have spectators in the audience as well. Indeed, a courtroom open to the public is a constitutionally protected procedure.[213] Moreover,
in other sorts of proceedings, the judge may be the only member of the audience.
Third, courtroom procedure provides the format of drama. 'Protagonist and an-
tagonist confront each other, present conflicting versions of the past and establish a problem to be solved.'[214] Fourth, and citing John Dewey, Ball notes that the
advocate-attorney's logic is one directed to particular consequences, not of complete syllogistic antecedents and conclusions. Rather, the attorney builds arguments
based upon selected facts that support her predetermined conclusions, coupled

with a presentation that presents such a consequential logic in the most plausible and compelling manner. Fifth, the performance of the advocate-attorney has similar metaphorical content as does the play:[215]

> The passage from fact to metaphor is what the advocate seeks. It is the passage from the materials of fact and law (the text) by means of courtroom presentation (the performance) to a persuasive statement of what ought to be done in a given situation (the metaphor).

Medicine and psychiatry possess their own performance, persuasive (rhetorical) habits and technique.[216] Indeed, a core aspect of medical, and particularly psychiatric, training is the building of a therapeutic alliance as a core feature of the doctor-patient relationship.[217] At its core, the therapeutic alliance has to do with the cooperative, collaborative relationship between the patient and doctor, though the literature is replete with variations on the concept depending upon therapeutic modality, clinical theory, and treatment.[218]

While much of the therapeutic alliance may consist of true reciprocal, egalitarian, and cooperative interactions, psychiatric practice, Jonathan Bolton argues, is characterized by the Aristotelian rhetorical triad of *ethos*, *pathos*, and *logos*.[219] 'Logos' refers to the reason the clinician uses to persuade the patient; 'ethos' refers to the qualities of the speaker's (clinician's) character in persuading the patient; and 'pathos' addresses the emotional state provoked by the speaker which favors the persuasive intent. Moreover, the performance aspects of the clinical professional stage are augmented by its own 'sets' (the trappings of health care) the attire of the clinician, most dramatically the white coat as 'costume'. A patient enters the professional stage with countless signals that healing is expected.[220]

However, the features of the legal professional stage are nonetheless quite different from the medical professional stage. In the medical setting, the doctor and patient, the primary and typically collaborative protagonists, enter into a relationship in which the outcome is the patient's improvement in health. The aim to health, a positive value, compares in law with the aims of justice (also a positive value) and punishment for wrongdoing (a debatably positive value at best, depending on personal opinion[221]). The public outcomes, and occasionally the public process, of the criminal courtroom contrast with medicine's stage which is aimed at privacy and confidentiality. One does not find out about one's health in the newspaper but might find out about one's verdict there. Doctors don't win cases, they succeed in healing or helping a case: the patient. While doctors may find themselves occasionally acting against their own values and beliefs on behalf of a patient (e.g., healing a criminal offender, performing an elective abortion), the option for a clinician to refer the patient elsewhere is always open. This option is not so easily done by an attorney in the context of a criminal proceeding. In this sense, the potential for inner conflict or turmoil around authenticity or moral integrity is lessened in medicine compared to the criminal law setting. Finally, while doctors no doubt use their powers of persuasion to influence their patients to engage in health-promoting behaviors, a dramaturgical character for the clinic is largely absent. There is no audience, costuming is relatively scant, the logic is deductive and inductive, and the decisions about treatment are bilateral and collaborative.

Perhaps most importantly, the performance rules for each professional stage are markedly different.[222] While the white coat of the clinician and the gown of the patient provide for some costuming, these features are not required and not an essential component of the doctor-patient relationship, especially in psychiatry, where preferably clinical management is conducted while fully and conventionally clothed! While the attorney-client relationship shares some aspects with medicine (i.e., confidentiality, advocacy), the doctor-patient relationship in medicine is primary in a way that the attorney-client relationship isn't—the attorney's social roles as attorney are multiple—persuader of client, judge, jury, and even courtroom audience.[223]

The rules for each professional stage also differ markedly. The criminal court has an extensive and stylized routine with involves presentation of the accused, the preparation and rules of evidence, the jousting of objection, the subtext of precedent in interpreting common and civil law, and the sequencing of trial events, as well as other facets of criminal procedure. Moreover, the 'cast'—the relevant parties in the criminal decision-making process, are large, often diverse, and complex. For medicine, constraints and rules are posed by professional ethics, scientific evidence, local practice standards, and the relationship with the patient. A much smaller cast for the case of medicine and particularly psychiatry, and much of the burden of role performance loads onto the doctor. In summary, the professional stages of criminal law and medicine differ in regard to authenticity, integrity, role complexity, rules of 'engagement', privacy, strategy, and performance characteristics.

Relation to the sciences and technical knowledge. Both criminal law and medicine and psychiatry depend upon the sciences to advance their aims. In terms of procedures, however, they differ. Science plays a role in legal strategy (e.g., what persuades juries, use of expert witnesses, prediction of juror behavior, and scientific facts salient to the criminal events) but because of the requirement that legal evidence be material and probative, as well as narrative in structure in interpreting the past, no scientific data addressing general trends, or the behavior of populations, are admissible in the criminal courtroom.[224] Science, however, plays a role in the forecasting (prediction) of illness behavior and treatment outcome. Third-person knowledge collected by medical science contributes to clinical estimates of probabilistic trends in populations of diagnostically similar individuals. As such, this third-person knowledge is completely relevant and even crucial to the practice of medicine and psychiatry.

In summary, criminal-legal epistemology is largely historical in character, accounting for a particular and unique event that occurred in the past. The question of legal knowledge, while always commingled with an aim to justice, is ultimately settled by the jury or judge(s). Medical epistemology is both model-driven (drawing from the generalizations of the biological and human sciences) and narrative-driven (in application to the unique patient) in its forward-looking approach to prognosis and therapy. Medical knowledge, like scientific knowledge, is rarely settled.

Typically, medical knowledge is in process or evolving as new information and new disease or patient behavior raise the potential for new understandings.[225]

Truth. As discussed earlier, criminal law harbors an uneasy tension between truth and justice. Which value should prevail, and the possibility of conflicts between the two, are major sources of debate for philosophers of law and criminal procedure. However, medicine also has an uneasy relationship with truth, though for different reasons. Medicine's discomfort with truth resides in its evanescent quality. In contrast to law, where definitive case action is required, and some practical kind of 'truth' is determined (or at least settled), in medicine the truth of disease is often never determined. The development of a medical case evolves over time. Some formulations may be more helpful or effective than others. The disease may change over time; the patient may develop new problems independently or in response to treatments (e.g., side effects, partial responses to treatment, and toxicities). Often, physicians don't know for sure that their approach and case understanding is true until the patient responds favorably to treatment, and even in that case, the truth is determined by a strictly pragmatic criterion. In this sense criminal law's and medicine's truths are instrumentally true—affirmed by their practical outcomes and not by some epistemic benchmark or universal 'God's eye view' of truth.

The context of criminal law and the context of medicine/psychiatry provide for significant distinctions in their methods, and ones which pose potential for misunderstanding and conflict. I now turn to the difference in their worldviews, or metaphysical assumptions about the nature of being human.

6.1.1.3 Metaphysical assumptions of law, medicine, and psychiatry

Metaphysical assumptions are fundamental beliefs, often presupposed, about the nature of reality and of human existence—what it means to be human. Many of the metaphysical assumptions of law and medicine have been revealed in the analysis of the preceding sections of this chapter. This section summarizes the core lessons. These summary comments are most relevantly addressed to the institutional cultures of law, medicine, and psychiatry, and do not represent the cultural diversity of metaphysical assumptions held by particular individuals or subcultural groups among both professionals and their clients. These latter 'folk-metaphysical assumptions' will be important in later chapters.

Legal historian Theodore Plucknett, in his *A Concise History of the Common Law*, explains the significance of Judeo-Christian morality on medieval English law:[226]

> ... And finally, the Church brought with it moral ideas which were to revolutionise English law. Christianity had inherited from Judaism an outlook upon moral questions which was strictly individualistic. The salvation of each separate soul was dependent upon the actions of the individual. This contrasted strongly with the custom of the English tribes which looked less to the individual than to the family group of which the individual formed a part. ... With the spread of Christianity all this slowly changed. First, responsibility for actions gradually shifted from the whole group to the particular individual who did the act;

and then the Church (and later the law) will judge that act, if necessary, from the point of view of the intention of the party who committed it.

This brief account introduces what I believe is a crucial difference between the metaphysical assumptions of law and medicine: the roots of Anglo-American law in Judeo-Christian-Islamic (Abrahamic) morality and the roots of contemporary medicine in secular philosophy and science. This distinction was introduced and described in more detail in Chapter 4 (Section 4.2.6) when Abrahamic, (primarily Christian in Europe) folk beliefs based on Church dogma split from Enlightenment assumptions and values in the seventeenth century.[227] Plucknett adds the important point that the tribal wars that characterized medieval Europe likely fostered folk beliefs in a shared responsibility for evil; with the burgeoning spread of the Christian Church, Christian metaphysics provoked not just a conversion to monotheism but also a cultural conversion from a moral metaphysics of collectivism to one of individual responsibility, free will, and desert.[228] This particular moral metaphysics was advanced in Jewish and Islamic traditions as well. This cultural-metaphysical transition not only changed viewpoints about the nature of wrongdoing, but also imported into English (not to overlook continental European and later, American) law a Judeo-Christian set of moral tenets which are very much present today and exemplified by landmarks such as (1) the Wolfenden Report mentioned in Section 6.1.1.1 earlier in this chapter, (2) the ongoing debate in the philosophy of criminal law regarding the proper relationship between law and morality,[229] and (3) manifesting in both professional and lay debates about the meaning, specifics, and application of so-called natural law (see various discussions of natural law in Chapter 4) and more.

Jumping to late in the twentieth century, psychologist-attorney (and philosopher by practice) Stephen Morse illuminates this schism between the account of human nature in law and the account of human nature in scientific medicine, psychology, and psychiatry, through the practical challenges encountered in court:[230]

> When one asks about the human action, 'Why did she do that?' two distinct types of answers may therefore be given. The reason-giving explanation accounts for human behavior as a product of intentions that arise from the desires and beliefs of the agent. The second type of explanation treats human behavior as simply one more bit of the phenomena of the universe, subject to the same natural, physical laws that explain all phenomena.

Morse calls, in keeping with contemporary philosophy and psychology, the reason-giving account 'folk psychology', depending as it does upon the interactions of human desires and beliefs—the folkish stuff of common sense. He goes on to characterize psychology and psychiatry explicitly:[231]

> The social sciences, including psychology and psychiatry, are uncomfortably wedged between the reason-giving and the mechanistic accounts of human behavior. Sometimes they treat behavior 'objectively', treating it as primarily mechanistic or physical; other

times, social science treats behavior 'subjectively', as a text to be interpreted. Yet other times, social science engages in an uneasy amalgam of the two.

One example of this 'uneasy amalgam' might be the explicitly pragmatic approach of psychiatry in adapting understandings of patient phenomena in terms that support effective therapeutic intervening, as exemplified by the discussion of clinical hermeneutics, and the crosstalk between scientific psychiatry and the narrative aspects of the clinical encounter, considered earlier in this chapter. That is, psychiatrists may use medications situated in the mechanistic explanation of human behavior simultaneously with psychotherapies which emerge from narrative, nondeterministic, albeit theoretical models of behavior like psychoanalytic or cognitive-behavioral theory. The pluralistic theoretical approaches to human behavior that characterize psychiatry (e.g., biological psychiatry, psychoanalytic psychiatry, cognitive-behavioral psychiatry, and family systems psychiatry) consider and reconsider Morse's tension between mechanistic explanation and hermeneutic, narrative-driven understanding in many ways and varieties. However, the tension persists, differing mainly in a diversity of theoretical terms and postulates[232] and empirical rules and generalizations.[233]
    In contrast, Morse characterizes law:[234]

Law, unlike mechanistic explanation or the conflicted stance of the social sciences, views human action as almost entirely reason governed. The law's concept of a person is as a practical reasoning, rule-following being, most of whose legally relevant movements must be understood in terms of beliefs, desires, and intentions. . . . the law presupposes that people use legal rules as premises in the practical syllogisms that guide much human action.

These differing sets of metaphysical assumptions are crucial to understanding how we got to the confusion of the VMDR. Law depends upon a human nature involving free will, personal rather than collective or multisystem responsibility, goal-directed behavior based upon beliefs and desires, and the moral concept of desert. Psychiatry, on the other hand, depends upon its multiplex theoretical orientations and unsettled and pluralistic accounts of human nature each with varying admixtures of determinism, cashed out in terms of multiple causal vectors and, more recently, recursive, multilevel systems and 'models'. These dueling sets of metaphysical assumptions underlie different formats and contexts throughout this book.

6.1.2 The contemporary displacement of the mentally ill into the criminal justice system

Before I depart from a comparison of criminal law and medical psychiatry, I should acknowledge the massive public health and social service problem of the disproportionate population of the mentally ill in jails and prisons. By way of background, in

Table 6.5 Prevalence of Mental Health Problems among US Prison and Jail Inmates[230]

	Percent of Inmates			
	In State Prison $n = 14,499$		In Local Jail $n = 6982$	
	% With Mental Problem	% Without Mental Problem	%With Mental Problem	% Without Mental Problem
Selected Characteristics and Criminal Record				
Current or past offense	61%	56%	44%	36%
3 or more prior incarcerations	25	19	26	20
Substance dependence or abuse	74	56	76	53
Drug use in month before arrest	63	49	62	42
Family background				
Homelessness in year before arrest	13	6	17	9
Past physical or sexual abuse	27	10	24	8
Parents abused alcohol or drugs	39	25	37	19
Charged with violating facility rules*	58	43	19	9
Physical or verbal assault	24	14	8	2
Injured in a fight since admission	20	10	9	3

*Includes items not shown.

Adapted from James DJ, Glaze LE (2006). Bureau of Justice Statistics Special Report: Mental Health Problems of Prison and Jail Inmates. US Department of Justice, Office of Justice Programs.

2007, 26.2% of American adults aged 18 years and older had suffered some form of mental illness over their lifetime. A smaller portion of the US population, 6% suffered 'serious' mental illness in that year.[235] According to the US Bureau of Justice Statistics, in midyear 2007, more than half of all prison and jail inmates had a mental health problem: 56% in state prisons, 45% in federal prisoners, and 64% in jails.[236] Table 6.5 summarizes data from an influential US Bureau of Justice Statistics report. The data were based upon a definition of 'mental health problem' as involving a history of mental health care (diagnosis or treatment) and/or DSM-IV defined symptoms over the preceding 12-month period. By 2012 matters had improved some; about 50% of prisoners and 36% of jail inmates reported no indication of a mental health problem.[237]

In a 2010 comprehensive review from the National Center for Addiction and Substance Abuse at Columbia University, prison and jail inmates are seven times more likely to meet medical criteria for a substance abuse disorder. Almost two-thirds (64.5%) of the inmate population in the United States have a substance abuse disorder. One-third (32.9%) of prison and jail inmates have a diagnosis of a mental disorder. Prisoners that carry both diagnoses, substance abuse and mental disorder, constitute one-quarter of the prison population (24.4%). Considering women as an 8.4% subpopulation of this group, they are more likely to have a substance abuse disorder compared to male inmates (66.1% compared to 64.3%) and much more likely to have a mental disorder than male inmates (40.5% versus 22.9%). Only 11.2% of the overall population had received any treatment for their conditions, and inmates using substances in prison is outgrowing the overall US population by a factor of 3.5 over the period from 1996 to 2006.[238]

By way of comparison, the prevalence of serious mental illness among US adults in 2020 is approximately 5.6%,[239] and the 12-month prevalence for any mental disorder is 21.0%, compare with the Kessler et al. study.[240] A review by Merikangas and McClair indicates the 12-month prevalence of alcohol dependence as 12% and for other drugs of abuse 2%–3%.[241] The National Institute for Drug Abuse notes the prevalence of substance abuse disorder complicated by mental illness is 37.9%, and the reverse, mental illness complicated by substance abuse was 18.2% in 2017.[242]

This extraordinary overrepresentation of mental illness in the incarcerated population has many causes which cannot be discussed here, though a number of resources appear in this endnote.[243] The problem is relevant to the VMDR: by definition, vice-laden mental disorder categories assure overlap of populations in the mental health system and the CJS. Moreover, as we have seen, the gap between the multicausal, multidetermined, naturalistic metaphysics of medicine and psychiatry and the morality-laden, free will metaphysics of criminal law sets up a polarity that makes for a problematic overlap between the two systems, including their institutional structures that predetermine and maintain such an overlap.

6.2 What do the courts want from psychiatric diagnosis?

As I head into a summing up of this chapter and the perspectives of the criminal law and the CJS, a couple of practical questions deserve attention: for this section, the question is: What do the courts want from psychiatric diagnosis? As the following discussion demonstrates, what the courts want from psychiatric diagnosis is a messy endeavor indeed because the wants are relative to person and perspective. These persons and perspectives range from the philosophical ideals of criminal justice to the various parties involved in the criminal procedure (e.g., judge, prosecution, defense, and victim). Nevertheless, I shall keep the answers short, building upon the detailed discussion in the earlier portions of this chapter.

6.2.1 Lawyers and criminal courts want a persuasive performance

Criminal court dockets are overloaded, and the efficient movement of cases through is crucial.[244] Psychiatric diagnostic categories are one of the means through which psychiatric expert witnesses contribute to the trial phase of criminal procedure. Those expert witnesses should be decisive, transparent in the applicability of their expertise to the criminal questions at hand, and perhaps most of all during the trial, be able to present a rhetorically persuasive performance for the judge and jury.

6.2.2 Courts want clarity about mental disease/defect

Psychiatric diagnostic categories are relevant to criminal procedure in the investigatory, evidence-gathering, pretrial, trial, and sentencing phases. In investigations, the courts want consistent and reliable diagnosis of the defendant, not a jumble of migrating diagnoses over time and across examiners. The court wants clear relationships between the particulars of a mental disorder and questions about responsibility, rationality, 'hard choice', and the defendant's ability to participate in his/her own defense. That is, psychiatric diagnosis should map onto these mental functions in an empirically rigorous and reliable way. Indeed, these mental functions have been argued as more fundamental to criminal procedure than diagnosis proper.[245] However, one should not discount prematurely the cultural resonance of DSM diagnostic categories in providing the rhetorical persuasion needed for moving the jury to one or another conclusion. For instance, claiming a defendant has a severe mental illness, or suffers from Schizophrenia or Bipolar Disorder, are cultural tropes which resonate not just in mental health settings but carry meanings, often highly stigmatized ones, from everyday media and popular culture settings. The label of Antisocial Personality Disorder can mark a defendant as an unremitting threat to the community, as the earlier mention of James 'Dr. Death' Grigson illustrated.[246] What might be important for the criminal court as a whole may only be a relative advantage for one or another side, however. When the features of psychiatric participation in criminal courts are played out through the dueling rhetoric at-trial characteristic of the adversarial approach to criminal law, the utility of diagnostic formulations may contradict or cancel each other.

6.2.3 Courts want sharp boundaries of impairment

The appeal of DSM-style diagnostic categories in part resides in their either/or status, however misleading the DSM categorical approach to diagnosis may be. Making a DSM diagnosis means that either the patient/defendant meets the criteria or doesn't. While this certitude in diagnosis is more promissory than reality,[247] and this certitude mutates over history and DSM revision,[248] courts want the diagnosis to do the work of distinguishing the areas, severity, and boundaries of impairment that questions about responsibility, culpability, mitigation, and hard choice require. Unfortunately, and usually,[249] the diagnosis does not provide much help in this regard. As Morse has argued, careful assessment of the defendant's rationality and burden of hard choice at the time of the criminal event is much more important than clarification of what diagnostic category the defendant falls into.

6.2.4 Courts require an assessment of intent and blameworthiness

Often, psychiatric expert witnesses can illuminate and clarify the issue of criminal intent and culpability, though diagnostic categories are probably not an effective tool to do this. However, the fog of dueling rhetoric between the defense and prosecution is often delivered by a prosecutorial focus on diagnostic categories, which can distract attention away from the more crucial questions about rationality and hard choice, issues which may 'favor' the defense, if explicitly addressed. The prosecution may benefit from quizzing the expert about diagnosis as a smoke-and-mirrors technique to distract jury attention away from the questions of intent, hard choice, and rationality that are more key to the determination of guilt and appropriate sentencing. Moreover, grilling the expert on diagnostic fine points serves to cast doubt on the expert's competence for the jury.

6.2.5 Courts want crisp determination of causes

The courts, in order to convict the defendant, require the determination of a component of the causes of the crime to be attributed to the defendant. This establishes culpability (remember the 'but-for' test). However, as with the earlier 'wants', the reality is more complex, as the adversarial model shapes the issues. For example, in the trial setting, a causal nexus (network of causal action) as explained by a clinical expert witness, using the concepts of multiple causation and naturalistic forces, can be obfuscating to the culpability-finding mission. As such, multicausal clinical explanation may be of value for the defense, as a defendant who is the pawn of complex-causal circumstances is one more likely to be acquitted.

6.3 What does the criminal justice system want from psychiatric diagnosis?

The second practical question addresses quite different needs. If we consider the CJS as involving the police, crime detection, and prevention as an early phase in the criminal justice cycle, with jail being a second phase; with criminal procedure, trial and sentencing a third (covered in the preceding sections), and punishment, deterrence, rehabilitation, and/or incapacitation as a complex fourth phase, what the CJS wants from psychiatric diagnosis proves to be at least as complicated as what criminal law wants from psychiatric diagnosis.

6.3.1 Background for the criminal justice system

Much has been written here about the perspective of criminal law, but criminal law is set in the context of a more encompassing CJS. In recent reviews, Tonry and

Cavadino and Dignan[250] note that CJSs in the Western world share many common features: legislated criminal codes, police systems, criminal trial and judicial procedures, and various pretrial, incarceration, and custodial systems.

However, the United States is distinctive from many Western industrialized countries in its CJS. One of these differences is the United States' embrace of the 'expediency principle',[251] where prosecutors are not obligated to prosecute all credible criminal cases (called the 'equality principle'[252]), but rather select cases for prosecution based upon practical and policy considerations. A second significant difference between the United States and other Western industrialized countries (other than Switzerland) is the political status of most judges. In the United States, judges are elected or appointed with strong political considerations and obligations, whereas in other countries judges are nonpartisan civil servants whose everyday work has little political significance. As discussed earlier, US criminal law is dominated by the adversarial system, as opposed to the inquisitorial system of continental Europe. Another significant difference is that US states and territories have complex state and federal jurisdictional rules and policies. As a concrete example, the 50 US states have a variety of approaches to the insanity defense, ranging from relatively permissive attitudes toward its use, to excluding the insanity defense from criminal proceedings entirely in some states.[253]

Tonry[254] identifies three crucial features that distinguish the US CJS from the rest of the developed world. The first is the aforementioned politicization of the US CJS. Politicization of the CJS means that public discourse places crime, policing, and criminal punishment as major political considerations in government elections and policymaking. For many decades and into the present, one of the most damaging public perceptions for a US political candidate is to be 'soft on crime'.[255] The ongoing threat of public perceptions of being soft-on-crime drives criminal justice politicians (e.g., judges, prosecutors, and police commissioners) to increase the harshness of punishments and to apply existing criminal justice policy in severe ways. The ironic corollary here is this pressure persists despite actual crime rates and evaluations of the crime-suppressing efficacy of tough-on-crime policies. That is, crime rates have declined in the United States over the past 30 years despite the waxing and waning of tough-on-crime policies. Being 'tough on crime' doesn't make a heck of a lot of difference in crime rates.

The second major difference, according to Tonry, is consequent to the above. American state legislatures pass laws of unparalleled severity concerning crime, compared to all other developed countries. Four good examples can be mentioned briefly here. 'Three-strikes laws' require a minimum sentence of 25 years to life after a third felony conviction. These felonies may be major—like murder—or may be minor, such as selling marijuana. Three-strikes laws are a significant contributor to the United States' overcrowding of prisons and its status of having the highest incarceration rate in the world, particularly of young African American men. A second example is 'sexual predator' laws that address sex offenders, which typically require lifetime public registration of the offender, may prolong the offender's incarceration, and/or forbid establishing a residence within a specified distance from residential areas or schools.[256] A third example, life-without-the-possibility-of-parole (LWOP) laws have been enacted in most US states. Tonry notes,[257] 'In 2008, 41,000 people were serving LWOPs, 7,000 of them for offenses committed by people who were minors at the time.' Finally, at the time of his writing, 48 of 50 states do not allow prisoners to vote (Maine and Vermont the exceptions),[258] and many convicts lose their right to vote even after their sentence is served. Only in recent years have the swelling rolls of prisons and prisoners inspired discussion of criminal justice and penal reform.

The third major difference for Tonry is the harshness and severity of American punishments such as the death sentence, LWOPs, or long mandatory sentences. The consequence of these policies is that the United States has a year 2019 incarceration rate of 629 people per 100,000 (down from 730 in 2000). Table 6.6 lists selected 2019 incarceration rates per 100,000 by rank and nation.[259]

One might infer from these data that the United States has a greater crime burden than other countries. The conclusion may appear obvious given the American inundation of media coverage of violent crime and the vigorous and on-going popularity of violent crime stories in our cultural entertainments. The thesis of a greater crime burden in the United States, however, is false. For example, according to the 2004–2005 International Crime Victims Survey,[260] the crime rate for all offenses, from 1989 to 2005, remained remarkably similar across Western European countries, Canada, Australia, and the United States, ranging from a low in Switzerland in 1989 at 13.0, and a high in Estonia in 1996 at 28.3. Over the same period, the US rates decreased from 25.0 in 1989 down to 17.5 in 2004–2005.[261] As a second example, according to the US Bureau of Justice Statistics,[262] both violent and property crimes have steadily diminished in the US from a high in 1993 to across-the-board lows in 2020, a finding that holds for Western industrialized countries in general[263] into the present, despite politicians' claims to the contrary. In 2020 the downward trends for both violent and property crime continued.[264] This decrease in crime has not been accompanied by proportionate decreases in the incarceration rate, however.[265] I shall be discussing the reasons for these findings in the next chapter, which concerns public attitudes and beliefs about crime and mental illness.

US criminal justice jurisdictions have local, state, and federal components. Given that each of these are largely self-supporting through regional taxation, local prosecutors are often incentivized financially to seek higher level charges and sentences in order to shift the financial burden to the state and federal levels. This practice is also politically appealing to voters because the prosecutor is tough on crime AND is (seemingly) diminishing the taxpayer burden. Unfortunately, however, this practice often does not provide adequate service and relapse-prevention to mentally ill offenders, who are often dependent upon probation-related support programs, mental health courts, and other diversion alternatives that are provided at the local level. The mental health baby gets thrown out with the criminal bath water. These

Table 6.6 Selected Prison Population Rates
According to the World Prison Brief ICPS, 2019

Rank, Highest to Lowest	Country	Rate per 100,000
1	Burundi	90
4	UK: Scotland	138
5	UK: Northern Ireland	83
6	UK: England & Wales	132
11	Russian Federation	321
19	France	102
39	New Zealand	150
50	India	35
52	Australia	165
113	China	119
120	United States	629
125	Finland	50
151	Switzerland	73
157	Saudi Arabia	207
177	Iran	228
181	Canada	104
186	Israel	234
190	Ghana	42
217	Syria	60
223	Cuba	510

https://www.prisonstudies.org/highest-to-lowest/prison-populat ion-total?field_region_taxonomy_tid=All.

For information on interpreting these data: https://www.prison studies.org/about-us.

trends not only contribute to recidivism of crime (and illness-related morbidity and mortality) but also the disproportionate representation of the mentally ill in jail and prison populations. The public pays for this service failure in other ways (e.g., property loss, indigent-population health care costs, and revolving-door mental health readmissions).

The arc of an offender's stay in the CJS could end in recovery and reintegration into society. Unfortunately, a prison stay too often simply provides an abusive and harsh context in which the offender is both traumatized psychologically while learning more effective skills in violating and dodging social norms. This so-called 'hardening' of criminals then leads to the commission of one or more additional crimes and re-entering the system.[266] The handling of US sentencing and postpunishment services for the convict varies considerably from state to state and jurisdiction to jurisdiction. The postincarceration phase for the convicted offender is framed by the approaches to criminal justice discussed earlier (e.g., the model of criminal justice discussed briefly in Section 6.111 earlier in this chapter). At this point I briefly review these alternative models of criminal justice disposition as they can shed new light on the VMDR.

6.3.1.1 Retributive justice

Black's Law Dictionary[267] defines 'retributivism' as:

> The legal theory by which criminal punishment is justified, as long as the offender is morally accountable, regardless whether deterrence or other good consequences would result. According to retributivism, a criminal is thought to have a debt to pay to society, which is paid by punishment. The punishment is also sometimes said to be society's act of paying back the criminal for the wrong done.

Retributive justice (also known as the 'just deserts' model) is the prevailing mode of administering criminal justice in the United States and UK today.[268] Packer's crime-control theory of criminal procedure, discussed earlier, builds upon the assumptions of a retributive justice model. The idea of justice as retribution is ancient, going back to the Code of Hammurabi (Chapter 4, Section 4.2.2.1) and the rule of *lex talionis* 'an eye for an eye' (Exod 21:24). Built upon a psychology of vengeance, in more recent times retributivism has found adherents couching the concept in the context of utilitarian ethics.[269] The basic utilitarian argument is: Offenders deserve punishment; civil society should not increase human suffering; but punishment prevents crime such that its net effects are less suffering for all.[270] Today, among the lay English-speaking public, retributive justice is equated with criminal justice: an individual commits a crime; that person is captured and convicted in a court of law; and a punishment is delivered.

Emerging from the criminal justice theories of Beccaria and Bentham (Chapter 4, Section 4.2.6.2) retributivism is built upon criminological 'choice theory',[271] the idea that criminal acts are deliberative choices based upon the criminal's appraisal of the risks of apprehension and the potential benefits of offending. Choice theory resonates with the Judeo-Christian roots (e.g., personal responsibility and desert) of Western criminal law: wrongful choices that harm others are particularly subject to sanction in order to preserve the stability of society. The preventive arms of the CJS, like policing, derive concepts of *deterrence* from retribution: if the punishments are sufficiently severe, or the chances of apprehension are so high, then the potential offender will choose not to offend.[272]

Multiple elements of retributive justice, however, are a cause for controversy: Centuries ago, Beccaria[273] believed that if punishments were too severe (meaning out of proportion to the offense), then such policy would paradoxically increase more serious crimes because the rewards for 'larger' crimes would override the deterrence potential of super-harsh punishments. Therefore, the concept of *proportionality* has been often utilized in modern society to determine the severity of punishment (e.g., determine sentencing policies)—more severe crimes implicate more severe punishments. A third function of retribution is *incapacitation*—the idea that removing the criminal from society (as in placing the offender in jail or prison), constitutes both punishment through the deprivation of freedom and prevention of ongoing crime. The ultimate incapacitation of an offender is, of course, execution or the 'death penalty', which is justified by advocates, because of reports of re-offending of violent crimes like murder after release from prison[274] as well as the often-overwhelming persistence of *lex talionis* sentiments by criminal justice officials and the public alike.

Pettit[275] discusses the current sociopolitical context that reinforces and stabilizes the retributive justice model in the United States. Pettit reminds us that the assumption that harsh punishments reduce crime has turned out to be prevailingly false not just in the United States but internationally, if scientific evidence is considered.[276] Pettit explains the contemporary genesis and persistence of the retributive justice approach to an 'outrage dynamic'[277] first described by Oliver MacDonagh in 1958. The outrage dynamic consists of three elements:[278]

> In each area there is an evil to be dealt with by policy, usually an evil associated with the industrial revolution and the results of that revolution for the organization of social life. And then three elements come into play in sequence. First, this evil is exposed, usually in the more or less sensational manner of the developing nineteenth century newspapers; the exposure of the evil may be triggered by some catastrophe or perhaps by the work of a private philanthropist or fortuitous observer. Second, the exposure of the evil leads to popular outrage; this outrage connects with the increasing humanitarian sentiments of people in nineteenth century Britain, sentiments in the light of which the evil appears as intolerable. And third, the popular outrage forces government to react by introducing legislative or administrative initiatives designed to cope with the evil; this reactiveness of government is due, no doubt, to the increasingly democratic character of nineteenth century British government.

One can readily identify contemporary social phenomena through this social process. The aforementioned three-strikes laws, the development of sexual predator laws, and LWOP laws all arose as a response to repeat offenders and heinous but rare crimes against children, and horrific crimes in general (respectively). More recently, then Vice President Joe Biden had been directed by then President Obama to formulate a policy response to the December 2012 shooting at Sandy Hook Elementary School, where 26 people, including 20 first-grade students, were murdered by a single gunman wielding a semiautomatic rifle.[279] Biden's task was to formulate an expedient and feasible response regarding gun violence, mental illness, and other factors that contribute to this and similar tragedies. (Unfortunately, this political response has still not yet appeared.)

A quote from Biden from the above news story is 'Even if . . . we can only save one life, we have to take action . . .', indicating that the government must react to cope with the evil of mass shootings. In the setting of the outrage dynamic, considerations of cost benefit and efficacy get lost in the fever to 'do something'. Doing a political 'something', likely a very costly 'something', that saves one life is, correspondingly, not a good use of social resources. The rhetoric implies that no cost is too high to deal with horrific events—even though phenomena like mass school shootings, while rising, are still rare in the much larger setting of gun violence, where school shootings account for less than 2% of the annual homicides of youth aged 5 to 18 years.[280] Unfortunately, in the ensuing years into the 2020s, school and mass shootings unfortunately have grown, with gun-violence reform crippled by a parallel outrage dynamic by 'gun rights' and the gun lobby, opposing gun-violence reform. Thus, outrage dynamics can interact with each other in complex ways.

How do outrage dynamics contribute to greater government controls and bureaucratic regulations? Pettit, again interpreting MacDonagh, describes how the outrage dynamic evolves within a democratic society to increase government duty and bureaucratic responses to social problems. The developmental steps toward a bureaucratic response to social wrongs[281] can be summarized:[282]

Phase 1a: An intolerable social wrong is identified and comes to wide public attention.

Phase 1b: A legislative response is generated through popular demand: laws are passed to address the intolerable social wrong.

—[usually] years pass—

Phase 2a: Further examples of the social wrong come to light; provoking a new public scandal and concern that the prior legislative interventions have failed to curtail the intolerable social wrong.

Phase 2b: An administrative response follows: individuals and groups are appointed to study the social wrong and recommend how it can be reduced or eliminated.

Phase 3a: The administrative response concludes that the prior legislation is inadequate.

Phase 3b: Amendments or new laws are recommended, usually more centralized and including a systematic collecting of data on the social wrong, and the appointment of centralized (e.g., federal) program officers to monitor the information, inform, and advise regarding control of the social wrong.

—more time passes—

Phase 4a: New examples of the social wrong come to public attention and horror. The polity is newly concerned about the inadequacy of prior responses. A recognition develops that the social wrong cannot be eliminated by a definitive legislative-administrative agenda.

Phase 4b: Ongoing intervention requires a 'regulative bureaucracy' which monitors, reviews, and intervenes in the manifestations of the social wrong. Professional expertise emerges in the context of the regulative bureaucracy, and a new domain of governmental function has fully matured, and a surrounding social network of professionals, guilds, training, regulatory agencies, and academics blooms.

Space does not permit detailed examples of the outrage dynamic in contemporary life. However, a few brief examples can be mentioned, and sources cited, for interested readers to do their own applications of the outrage-dynamic model. In 2012, the Obama administration was entertaining policy for national mandatory screening for individuals purchasing guns, suggesting a Phase 4 of the United States' periodic engagement with gun control legislation. This consideration is still being debated into the 2020s, illustrating the often-slow growth of bureaucratic regulation.

A second, more historical, example that vividly illustrates the outrage dynamic is the development of human research ethics regulation in the United States in the period from the mid-1960s to the early 1980s. Early recognition of clinical research abuses such as the Tuskegee experiments by the US Public Health Service,[283] the 'Willowbrook Wars' involving dangerous nonconsented hepatitis research with intellectually disabled people,[284] and the expose of unethical mainstream clinical research studies by Henry K. Beecher in 1966[285] among other examples, led Congress to pass the National Research Act in 1974. This trend led to the establishment of federal offices overseeing human subjects protections, leading to a nationwide regulatory bureaucracy for human subjects research in 1981.[286] The resulting Institutional Review Boards and Human Subjects Protection Programs evident everywhere in clinical research today continue to be subject to periodic review and reform, through NGO agencies like the Association for the Accreditation of Human Research Protection Programs, Inc. (AAHRPP). Another example of the additional layers of clinical research regulation is the need for clinical trial registries, such as ClinicalTrials.gov to police the withholding of negative studies by pharmaceutical sponsors, among other scientific publication abuses.[287]

The foregoing sketch very briefly summarizes the prevailing model of criminal justice today. Before ending this section, I will briefly consider alternative models for criminal justice.

6.3.1.2 Alternative models of criminal justice

Over several decades, international scholars, human rights advocates, social scientists, and others have provided substantial critiques of retributive justice. Reviewing these for this book would not be feasible, and references appear in endnote 276. However, I can give an overview of the international critique of retributive justice and sketch some of the common features of the many alternatives offered.

As the foregoing discussion suggests, academic, professional, and public discussion has generated much criticism of the retributive justice model. A search for credible alternatives has been inspired by these critiques. Earlier in this chapter I outlined Kent Roach's critique of the crime-control (retributive) model, and those points included (1) punishment has not proven uniformly effective in deterrence, and indeed, may increase reoffending through the hardening process; (2) victim- ization studies show that many, perhaps most, victim crimes go unreported and, hence, an effective retributivist response is undermined; (3) the due process of crim- inal procedure is too often not invoked by the defense because of pressures to close minor offense cases and the delay and expense in invoking due process objections; (4) the relative exclusion of victims of crime in the justice process, denying them perspective, compensation, and healing; and (5) the marginalizing of attention to the actual losses (material, emotional, and economic) suffered by victims, and the absence of a response to compensate victims for such losses.

However, much of the criticism of retributivism is centered on ethical con- siderations. The claim that retribution—just deserts—is justified as a good in its own right has been repeatedly challenged, along with utilitarian arguments sup- porting punishment.[288] This debate around retributivism and its alternatives is complex and ongoing and cannot be reviewed here, much less settled. The re- sponse of restorative justice and its many variations and iterations implies its own collective and emergent critique. The vigorous popular interest in alternatives to retributivism has contributed to a proliferation of terms, practices, and concepts. What are some examples?

Restorative justice. The concept 'restorative justice' is complex, regional, and evolving. Often treated as an umbrella term for various alternative approaches to criminal justice, it is invoked in different countries, jurisdictions, criminal and do- mestic settings, cultures, and applied in different ways and with different particu- lars. Most discussions using the 'restorative justice' language, however, have some common threads and certainly some common values. Daly and Proietti-Scifoni or- ganize, in a recent review, these common values under a 'master term' rubric.[289] They describe the master term as the 'starting point' for alternative accounts; in my reading, they could easily be labeled the prevailing or guiding value(s) for alterna- tive justice accounts. Daly and Proietti-Scifoni identify three master terms, which can be elevated or combined depending upon the particular author, context of ap- plication (e.g., domestic offenses, international crime, political crime, and violent crime), and community or jurisdiction. As will be shown, the three master terms are all overlapping in meaning, differing mainly in emphasis of component elem- ents or values.

The first master term is 'reparation'. Reparation may be material, such as paying money or giving material goods to the victim (called restitution) or repairing or re- turning property. Reparation may be symbolic, such as the offender providing an apology to the victims and/or community (adding a shame psychology to the mix) or performing a compensatory action such as entering a drug treatment program or providing community service.

The second master term is 'restoration'. Daly and Proietti-Scifoni note that this concept is more diffuse and diverse in its use and application. My take is that restoration has to do with making the victim whole or returning the victim to a prior state of integrity. Restoring wholeness to victims is a more abstract concept that reparation, the latter implying a particular transaction between parties. Restoration transcends efforts such as apology, restitution, and literal replacement of property. It implies a renewal of trust and redefining the relationships of the offender relative to the victim(s) as well as the larger community. A concept of restoration that would include only financial compensation, as in the Western tort/civil law system, would be inadequate to account for the aim of restoring emotional and psychological wholeness to the victim and community at large, under the 'restoration' rubric. In this sense, restoration poses a more complex social practice than simply paying money to victims. The restoration is a process involving interpersonal, meaningful engagements among stakeholders.

'Making amends' is the third master term, according to Daly and Proietti-Scifoni. This concept emphasizes a substantive process of apology. Making amends is not just saying you're sorry, but a negotiation between the involved parties (victim, offender, and community). This negotiation involves assuring that the offender's acknowledgment of harm is sincere, and the offender participates in planning, action, and evaluation in restitution, punishment, or other elements that emerge in the collective discussion. Making amends involves taking personal action that expresses regret not just in words, but in deeds. Making amends introduces the potential for a punishment element in the process; making amends often has an element of penitence and may manifest in self-sacrifices of the offender's property, time, and/or labor.

The restorative justice concept and ideal plays out, as noted earlier, in multiple settings. In international law, truth commissions to address political wrongs to particular members of the population are well-known, as in the South African Truth & Reconciliation Commission.[290] Community tribunals reflecting local community restorative practices were inspired by traditional tribal practices (in, e.g., Australian and New Zealand Aboriginal and US Native American settings).[291] These can be applied widely, from domestic violence situations to community property crimes.

Other examples of restorative practices include victim-offender mediation, which are post-plea discussions among offender and victim(s), usually hosted by a trained facilitator.[292] Restorative practices are prominently and diversely explored in youth justice and criminal court settings.

From this very brief sketch of the US CJS, I return to the question of what these systems want from psychiatrists and/or Behavioral Science. As before with the Criminal Law section, using the foregoing discussion as background, I mention these points as summaries.

6.3.2 Mechanisms for behavior control

The CJS wants tools from psychiatry and behavioral science to identify offenders (e.g., criminal profiling). The CJS wants techniques and technologies to manage behavior in prison settings, and to retain parolees and maintain their good behavior.

6.3.3 Prediction of future offending

The CJS wants to know if past offenders will offend in the future, and if so, where, where, how, and whom. While the CJS may recognize psychiatry's limitations in this regard,[293] these predictive goals remain an ideal, if a far-from-realized one.

6.3.4 Opportunities for rehabilitation, therapeutics, and recovery

The law, CJS, the mental health system, and the public remain ambivalent about the proper handling of criminal deviance. This ambivalence is reflected by the huge diversity of approaches to rehabilitation and therapeutics, only touched upon earlier in this chapter. Moreover, these systems as human collectives are variable as to who exactly is in charge of rehabilitation and therapeutics. Smith, Gendreau, and Swartz and Weisburd, Farrington, and Gill,[294] recently reviewed 'what works' in criminal rehabilitation, acknowledging the often-lacking political will to implement these evidence-based procedures. These and other considerations in rehabilitation will be considered again in the concluding chapters of this book.

6.4 Concluding comments

Several lessons emerge from exploring Criminal Law and criminal justice from the vantage point of the VMDR. Perhaps most important is the fundamental, and truly radical, differences in conceiving human nature in these systems and practices. Springing from the medieval metaphysics of individualism, personal responsibility, and just desert, the Western Criminal Law and justice systems are centered on culpability rather than complex understanding, punishment rather than rehabilitation, and marginalization/exclusion rather than integration and social inclusion. The retributive model of justice is a process aimed at harming criminal offenders, a bold contradistinction between the clinical objectives of helping, healing, caring, and curing—leading to the banal reality of clinicians' moral distress in participating in the CJS.[295] The social handling of criminal offending has not always been this way; the threads of restoration have a history going back to the ancients.

Notes

1. Radden & Sadler (2010); Sadler (2005, 2007); Sadler & Fulford (2004).
2. Dworkin (1966, 1986); Hart et al. (2012); Hayes & Carpenter (2012); Husak (2010); Kelly (1992); Pound (1959).
3. Plucknett ([1956] 2010).
4. Lippman (2009, 2012).
5. Lippman (2009).
6. ibid, pp. 3–4 (editing is mine).
7. Pound (1959).
8. Adapted from Pound (1959); bracketed notes mine. See internal page references in the Table. I should note that the implications of Pound's work in the international setting is beyond the scope of this project.
9. See my Chapter 4, Section 4.2.2.1.
10. Discussed in Section 4.2.4.2 of Chapter 4.
11. Again, see Section 4.2.4.2 in Chapter 4.
12. Pound (1959, p. 27).
13. ibid.
14. See Chapter 4, Section 4.2.5.1, subsection c. 1000–1500 for more on Aquinas.
15. ibid, subsection c. 500–1000 AD.
16. Chapter 4, Section 4.2.6.1.
17. See my discussion of Bentham (Chapter 4, Section 4.2.6.2, under 'Enlightenment').
18. Pound (1959, pp. 28–29).
19. Rawls (2005).
20. Dworkin (1986).
21. Nussbaum (1999; 2006, p.130; 2013; 2019).
22. Nozick (1974).
23. Foucault (1980); see also Gutting (1994).
24. Pound (1959, p. 29).
25. ibid.
26. Arrigo & Milanovic (2008); Connolly (1987, 1993); Gutting (1994); Foucault (1980); Sadler (2002, 2005).
27. Pound (1959, pp. 22–23).
28. Report of the Committee on Homosexual Offences and Prostitution, § 13 (1957).
29. See Bayer (1987) for a history of the declassification of homosexuality as a mental disorder.
30. Dworkin (1966, 1977).
31. Kelly (1992).
32. Dworkin (1977); Kelly (1992).
33. Kelly (1992, p. 444), quoting the original report, editing and bracketed material Kelly's.
34. The former is the interesting happenstance mentioned earlier, given its close temporary proximity to the removal of homosexuality as a mental disorder from the DSM in 1968 (Bayer 1987).
35. See Dworkin (1966, 1977) and Hart (1963) for a framing of the issues.
36. See Sadler (1997, 2005) for detailed philosophical discussions about the analysis of value-laden concepts.
37. Cohen (1940); Dworkin (1977).
38. See Devlin (1965); Dworkin (1966, 1977); Hart (1963).
39. Kelly (1992, p. 447).
40. ibid, p. 445, quoting from Devlin (1965).
41. Hart (1963); see also Kelly (1992).
42. Packer (1964, 1968).

43. Luna (1999).
44. Roach (1999, p. 672), internal citations omitted.
45. ibid.
46. Pellegrino (1999).
47. Hippocrates cited in Pellegrino (1999 p. 61). See also Hippocrates, *The Art* (1923).
48. See Shelp (1983) for multiple perspectives on the clinical encounter.
49. Sadler (2005).
50. Munson (1981).
51. Engelhardt & Jotterand (2008); Pellegrino (1999); Pellegrino and Thomasma (1981).
52. Pellegrino (1999, p. 60–61).
53. ibid, p. 65.
54. Pellegrino (1999, p.65).
55. Callahan 1996; Hastings Center (1996).
56. ibid, Executive Summary, p. 2.
57. Brülde (2001).
58. Nordenfelt (2000, 2001).
59. Nordenfelt (2001).
60. ibid, p. 23.
61. Kaiser Family Foundation (2020). With the ongoing roll-out of the Obama Administration's Affordable Care Act, this proportion of the uninsured was shrinking, only to be, at least, partially undone years later by the Trump Administration policies.
62. Hanson & Callahan (2000).
63. While discussions about the goals of psychiatry may be impoverished in its professional literature, a plethora of studies discuss the presupposed purposes of psychiatry—e.g., 'models' of psychiatry. Many of these will be discussed in the later sections.
64. See for instance Reynolds et al. (2009).
65. Hastings Center (1996, p. S9).
66. See the definitions of 'mental disorder' offered in the DSMs: APA (1980, 1987, 1994, 2000).
67. See Culver & Gert (1982).
68. Sadler (2007).
69. See Radden & Sadler (2010); Sadler (2007).
70. Sadler (2007 p. 115).
71. See Sadler (2007) for a more complete discussion and defense of this account.
72. ibid.
73. See Clark (2002) for a discussion of phenomenological extremes as a marker of psychopathology.
74. At the time of this writing, the DSM-5 committees and the community were debating the status of the relationship between Major Depression and grief. See Shear, Simon, Wall et al. (2011).
75. See Millon & Klerman (1986) and Sadler (2005) for detailed discussions of categorical versus dimensional diagnostic approaches.
76. Whelton (2004).
77. Worden (2009).
78. Sadler (2007); see also Gupta (2014, 2007, 2009, 2011); Radden & Sadler (2010).
79. Sadler (2007.
80. A more-detailed discussion of medical and psychiatric hermeneutics follows in this chapter.
81. Sadler (2005.
82. Calcedo-Barba (2010).
83. See Kramer (1993).
84. Adshead & Sarkar (2005).
85. ibid, p. 1011.
86. ibid, p. 1012.

87. Adshead & Sarkar (2005, p.1012)
88. See Chapter 4, Section 4.8.
89. A later discussion will address the problematic nature of truth and justice when the methods of the criminal law and psychiatry are contrasted.
90. AAPL (2005).
91. ibid, p. 1.
92. AAPL (2005).
93. ibid.
94. ibid.
95. AAPL (2005, p. 2).
96. ibid.
97. Stone ([1984], 2008).
98. ibid, pp. (167–168).
99. Appelbaum (1997a).
100. In the research ethics arena, Appelbaum has been a pioneer in clarifying 'the therapeutic misconception' where a research subject often misconstrues participation in a clinical research protocol as standard-of-care practice. See Appelbaum, Lidz, & Trisso (2004); Appelbaum, Roth, & Lidz (1982); Appelbaum, Roth, Lidz et al. (1987). The goal of US human subjects research regulation is to minimize risk to human subjects, including assuring adequate informed consent. These two distinctions don't apply to the goals of the State for forensic psychiatry, consent for a forensic evaluation does not apply, and an assurance of avoiding harm to the evaluee does not exist, indeed, the evaluation as discussed early may well contribute to harm, through a punitive sentence, for the evaluee. My conclusion here is that the comparison to clinical research is a false analogy.
101. Appelbaum (1997a, p. 238).
102. Appelbaum (1997b).
103. ibid, p. 445.
104. Halpern, Freedman, & Schoenholtz (1998, p. 575).
105. Appelbaum (1998, p. 576).
106. Pellegrino cited in Appelbaum (1997a, p. 243).
107. Advocacy for this position is unlikely to win me any friends in the forensic psychiatry field! However, this points to the potential for self-interest to interfere with physicianly beneficence ethics. Forensic psychiatrists have practical and financial interests in maintaining their professional role as expert witnesses in the prosecution phase of criminal law.
108. 'Metaphysical' here means the nature and constitution of reality. In the sphere of interest in this section, it would include concepts about human nature.
109. Sward (1989) and Chapter 4.
110. Sward (1989, p. 325).
111. See Sward (1989) and Chapter 4.
112. Pardo (2005 p. 321).
113. Sward (1989, p. 301).
114. American Bar Association (1980, p. 51), internal citations omitted.
115. Davis & Elliston (1986 p. 185).
116. ibid, p. 186.
117. Judges in the inquisitorial method are much more active. They alone or as part of a panel will organize at least a preliminary investigation, oversee the collection of evidence and witnesses, and structure the questioning of witnesses. The role of attorneys in the inquisitorial method is mostly to be the interpreters of evidence and law for the benefits of their clients (defendant and state's prosecution).
118. Davis & Elliston (1986, p. 186).

119. ibid.

120. Sward (1989, pp. 304–305), internal citations omitted, bold added by me for emphasis.

121. ibid, p. 312.

122. See Dubber (1999); Roach (1999); Stuntz (1997); Sward (1989).

123. Lind et al. (1973); Stacy (1991); Stuntz (1997, 2006). I'm grateful to Tom Mayo, J.D., for the important point that discovery rules are complex on the one hand, and in some jurisdictions, one side may suffer a greater discovery burden. For example, federal law requires an asymmetric requirement for the prosecution to provide the defense any exculpatory evidence obtained.

124. See Sward (1989).

125. Pellegrino & Thomasma (1981, p.13).

126. Sadler (2005, Chapter 3); Munson (1981).

127. Most any philosophy of science textbook addresses many elements of the methods of science.

128. Shelp (1983).

129. Longo et al. (2012).

130. Sackett et al. (1996, p. 312); see also Sackett, Richardson, Rosenberg, & Haynes (1997).

131. Descriptive and observational studies are forms of clinical research where observations are systematically made and recorded, in order to characterize a phenomenon through shared features. Consider a series of 200 patients with a particular disease—an observational study might document the various clinical features exhibited by the patients, and their response to particular treatments. No experimental manipulation is made; only the naturalistic behavior of the phenomena is recorded.

132. Coomasaramy & Khan (2004); Khan & Coomasaramy (2006); Phillips & Sadler (2021); Straus et al. (2018); van Dijk et al. (2010). For a comprehensive critical discussion of EBM in psychiatry, see Gupta (2014).

133. See for instance Elwyn et al. (2012).

134. Seldin (1977).

135. Engel (1977, 1980).

136. von Bertalanffy (1969).

137. Engel (1980).

138. See Sadler & Hulgus (1989, 1992) for the arguments in this regard.

139. See for instance Baron (1990); Daniel (1986, 1994); Leder (1990); Lock (1990); Svenaeus (2000); Thomasma (1994, 2001).

140. Cooper (1994).

141. Palmer (1969).

142. Cooper (1994, p. 152); the description of *Geistewissenschaften* is mine.

143. Leder (1990).

144. ibid, p. 9.

145. See Phillips (1996) for a concise review of hermeneutics in psychiatry, while Jaspers (1963, 1997a, 1997b) provide an influential treatment from the last century.

146. Daniel (1986).

147. ibid, p. 200.

148. ibid, p. (200–201).

149. Leder (1990).

150. ibid, p. 19.

151. Sadler and Hulgus (1989), drawing upon some earlier work with Frederick Grinnell, proposed a 'hermeneutic spiral' as a three-dimensional metaphor for the manner clinical understanding evolves and changes over time.

152. The Oxford University Press's International Perspectives of Philosophy and Psychiatry book series has published an excellent range of new books in phenomenological philosophy of

psychiatry. See Matthews (2007); Ratcliffe (2008); Stanghellini (2004); Stanghellini & Rosfort (2013); Stanghellini & Fuchs (2013).

153. Stanghellini & Fuchs (2013.
154. See Schwartz & Wiggins (1986, 1987a, 1987b, 1988a, 1988b, 1997, 2005).
155. Engel (1977, 1980, 1997).
156. Schwartz & Wiggins (1988, p. 162).
157. Jaspers (1963, 1997a, 1997b).
158. Schwartz & Wiggins (1988, pp. 153–154).
159. ibid, pp. 153–155; see also Jaspers (1963/1997a, 1997b).
160. See Sadler & Hulgus (1991) for an explication of only #3. 'Understanding moves in a deepening spiral.' Work on phenomenological psychiatry and psychopathology has exploded in the past 10 years, too much literature to review here. See Stanghellini et al. (2019) and Stanghellini & Fuchs (2013) for extensive related discussions; the latter book is explicitly dedicated to re-appraising Jaspers's work. For an 'applied' phenomenological approach in the context of psycho-therapy, see Stanghellini (2016); Stanghellini & Mancini (2017).
161. See Elstein & Schwartz (2002) for a review.
162. See Kassirer (1989); Kassirer et al. (1987).
163. Kendler (2008); Kendler & Parnas (2008); Zachar (2000); Zachar & Kendler (2007).
164. Ghaemi (2003).
165. McHugh & Slavney (1998); see also Chisolm, Lyketsos (2012).
166. Havens (1973, Havens and Ghaemi 2004).
167. Jaspers (1963, 1997a, 1997b).
168. Ghaemi (2003, p. xviii).
169. ibid, p. 308.
170. Brendel (2006).
171. ibid, p. 29.
172. ibid, p. 40.
173. Lewis (2011).
174. Divakaruni (1999).
175. More recently, Douglas Heinrichs has articulated a clinical method for interacting and negotiating treatment with the patient based upon scientific model-building. See Heinrichs (2015).
176. Morse (1998).
177. *Black's Law Dictionary*, 8th edition, Garner (2004). See also Alexander (2002); American Law Institute (1962); Schaffner (1985); Hart & Honoré (1985); Moore (2011).
178. Garner (2004, p. 234).
179. ibid, cross-references and discussion omitted.
180. Garner (2004, p. 406), discussion and cross-references omitted.
181. Moore (2011).
182. Garner (2004, p. 1338).
183. ibid.
184. Moore (2011, p. 170).
185. See Moore (2011) for a review.
186. American Law Institute (1962); Averbach (1957); Brennan (1987); Danner & Segall (1977); Moore (2011).
187. Moore (2011, pp. 170–171).
188. American Law Institute (1962); Moore (2011, p. 170).
189. Moore (2011, pp. 170–171).
190. ibid, p. 171.

191. In criminal and tort law, this is not always true, a prominent exception being the judge's interest in precedent-setting for the future of similar cases. However, even in this example, the prospective causal interest is relatively independent of the focus on determining guilt or innocence of the defendant.

192. Nordenfelt & Lindahl (2012).

193. Kendler & Parnas (2008).

194. Eisenberg (2001); Gutheil et al. (2003); Mosteller (1996); Shuman (2001); Slobogin (1998).

195. The text of the FRE is available online: http://www.law.cornell.edu/rules/fre/.

196. For reviews, see Gianelli (1993); Mosteller (1996); Shuman (2001); Slobogin (2003).

197. Lippman (2012).

198. Sadler & Hulgus (1992).

199. Zaner (1990).

200. While the aim of criminal law is retrospective, this is not to say that attorneys don't think about the future course of the trial as a strategic consideration in developing their cases. A counselor must anticipate arguments made by opposing counsel in the future and consider practical strategies to block or counter these opposing arguments. Also, the judge considers the implications for the future regarding past precedents around use of a particular piece of evidence.

201. Sadler & Hulgus (1989); Sadler (1992).

202. Sadler (2005).

203. See http://ori.hhs.gov/, the US Office of Research Integrity, for discussion and materials about the 'responsible conduct of research'.

204. See Rothman (2012) for a recent review.

205. Gupta (2007, 2009, 2011, 2014).

206. Sadler (2005).

207. Ball (1975); Bradley & Hoffman (1996).

208. Sadler & Hulgus (1989).

209. Sadler (2007).

210. Sadler & Hulgus (1992).

211. Ball (1975).

212. ibid, p. 83.

213. ibid, p. 86.

214. ibid p. 88.

215. ibid, p. 91.

216. Bolton (2011a, 2011b).

217. Catty (2004).

218. Catty (2004); McGuire, McCabe, & Priebe (2001); Elwyn et al. (2012).

219. Bolton (2011a).

220. Biddle (1986).

221. The debate is about the ethical appropriateness of retributive punishment as a consequence of criminal wrongdoing; relevant are the alternatives models of justice introduced later in this chapter.

222. I'm grateful to Jonathan Bolton for this point in our personal conversations on rhetoric in medicine.

223. Ball (1975).

224. I admit that scientific discourse, and the use of science in the clinic, has a narrative structure too, but that doesn't mean the narrative structure of (say) EBM claims is the same as the retrospective storying of a criminal case.

225. Sadler (1992).

226. Plucknett (([1956] 2010), pp. 8–9). See also Seidentop (2014) for a detailed study of the historical role of Christianity in founding fundamental legal concepts like the individual, personal responsibility, and just desert.

227. See Sadler (2013) for a brief summary account of these historical roots of contemporary criminal law and contemporary medicine.

228. Plucknett ([1956] 2010).

229. Dworkin (1977).

230. Morse (1998 p. 338).

231. ibid.

232. Jaspers (1963); Sadler (2005).

233. As yet psychiatry doesn't have something resembling a comprehensive field theory of psychopathology, so the field is dominated by a series of competing theoretical models and empirical research programs, mostly nonintegrated and representing various kinds and degrees of reductive determinisms.

234. Morse (1998 p. 339).

235. Bronson and Berzofsky (2017); Kessler, Chiu, & Demler (2005); Sundararaman (2009).

236. US Department of Justice (2006).

237. Adapted from James & Glaze (2006).

238. CASA (2010).

239. See https://www.nimh.nih.gov/health/statistics/mental-illness.

240. Kessler et al. (2005).

241. Merikangas & McClair (2012).

242. See https://nida.nih.gov/publications/research-reports/common-comorbidities-substance-use-disorders/introduction

243. Erickson & Erickson (2008); Lamb & Weinberger (1998); NAMI: https://www.nami.org/Advocacy/Policy-Priorities/Stopping-Harmful-Practices/Criminalization-of-People-with-Mental-Illness; Slate & Johnson (2008).

244. I'm grateful to Bill Bridge, Professor of Law at Southern Methodist University School of Law, for this provocative and ultimately, fecund formulation.

245. See Meynen (2009, 2010a, 2010b, 2012); Morse (1998, 1999, 2002).

246. Ewing (1983).

247. DSM disorders vary in severity, often possessing dimensional, continuously variable properties; see Sadler (2005).

248. Margolis (1994).

249. See Shuman (1989, 2002).

250. Cavadino & Dignan (2006); Tonry (2011a, b).

251. Tonry (2011a, p. 3).

252. ibid.

253. ibid. See also Findlaw (2019).

254. Tonry (2011a).

255. See Cavadino & Dignan (2006) and Tonry (2011a) for reviews.

256. See Laws & Ward (2011); Winick & La Fond (2003); Wright (2014); and Zonana et al. (1999) for detailed studies of so-called sexual predator laws.

257. Tonry (2011a, p. 5), internal citation omitted.

258. See https://www.sentencingproject.org/publications/felony-disenfranchisement-a-primer/.

259. https://www.prisonstudies.org/country/united-states-america. While the World Prison Brief by the Institute for Crime & Justice Policy Research may represent the best data on incarceration rates, the raw rate per 100,000 population in the right column of Table 6.6 can be misleading, as the top-ranked countries are don't have the highest population rates. The rankings

represent a complex calculation of estimates based on available data, and other forms of imprisonment such as pretrial/remand imprisonment. Keep in mind that these estimates are also dependent upon reporting by country, which in themselves can be variable by dates and data accuracy in reporting.

260. Van Dijk et al. (2010).

261. See also Tonry (2011b).

262. See https://bjs.ojp.gov/content/pub/pdf/cv01.pdf. By 2019 the violent crime victimization rate had declined to 21.0/1000 persons aged 12 years or older, and to 16.4/100 in 2020. https://bjs.ojp.gov/library/publications/criminal-victimization-2020.

263. See also Tonry (2011a, 2004). For very recent crime rate data, see the Pew Research Center article online: https://www.pewresearch.org/fact-tank/2020/11/20/facts-about-crime-in-the-u-s/.

264. See Bureau of Justice Statistics, Criminal Victimization 2020 summary: https://bjs.ojp.gov/sites/g/files/xyckuh236/files/media/document/cv20_sum.pdf.

265. Cavadino & Dignan (2006); Tonry (2006, 2011a). See also Table 6.6.

266. See Kupers (1996); Parsons (1918); Pizarro, Stenius, & Pratt (2006).

267. Garner (2004, p. 1343).

268. Boonin (2008); Caruso (2021); Garland (2002); Haney (1980); Kurki (2000); Minow (1998); Roach (1999).

269. Boonin (2008); Tadros (2011).

270. Samuel-Siegel (2019).

271. Fisher (2014).

272. The calculus of crime, with the criminal as rational actor, flies in the face of so much contemporary psychological and psychiatric theory and empirical evidence one does not know where to start in terms of citations.

273. Beccaria ([1766] 1986).

274. Siegel (2006).

275. Pettit (2002).

276. The scientific literature shows substantially the failure of retributive punishment policy in reducing criminal recidivism. See also Baumer (2011); Caruso (2021); Gordon (2001); Raynor (2007) Tonry (2006, 2011b); Weisburd, Farrington, & Gill (2017).

277. Pettit (2002 p. 430); see also Timasheff (1937).

278. Pettit (2002 p. 430).

279. See Jackson (2012), and https://www.cnn.com/interactive/2012/12/us/sandy-hook-timeline/. https://www.usatoday.com/story/news/politics/2012/12/20/obama-biden-gun-control-effort-newtown/1782257/.

280. Flannery et al. (2013). Unfortunately, in the 8 short years following this study, the phenomenon of mass shootings, including school shootings, has increased. Sanders & Lei (2018), using a novel advanced statistical technique, estimate that the annualized increase in public mass shootings in the United States since 1982 have at least doubled, and possibly, quadrupled.

281. I substitute 'social wrongs' here to extract the drama of terms like 'evil', and provide a more neutral, less rhetorically persuasive example.

282. Pettit (2002).

283. Reverby (2009).

284. Rothman & Rothman (2003).

285. Beecher (1966).

286. See Bulger, Heitman, & Reiser (2002); Porter & Koski (2008).

287. See Califf et al. (2012) for a description of the implementation and success (or not) of ClinicalTrials.gov.

288. Berman (2013); Boonin (2008); Duff (2013); Grisso (1996); Haque (2013); Husak (2010); Kurki (2000); Murphy (2007); Tadros (2011); Tanguay-Renaud (2013); Zaibert (2013).

289. Daly & Proietti-Scifoni (2011, pp. 230–231).
290. Potter (2006).
291. Braithwaite (1999); Kurki (2000).
292. Daly & Proietti-Scifoni (2011).
293. Bazelon (1978).
294. Smith, Gendreau, & Swartz (2009); Weisburd, Farrington, & Gill (2017).
295. See for instance Greenberg & Shuman (1997); Peternelj-Taylor (2004); Ward & Brown (2004).

7

The public interest context of the VMDR

7.1 Public attitudes toward mental illness, crime, and their relationships

For this chapter, I survey the literature and appraise US public attitudes and beliefs about crime and mental illness and their relationships. Understanding these public attitudes are important in addressing the vice/mental disorder relationship (VMDR) described in previous chapters. They provide a set of background attitudes that contribute to responses to vice-laden mental illness categories. The first section is largely a descriptive review of social science studies which describe public attitudes and beliefs toward crime, criminals, and mental illness. I explain and use social science concepts like 'cultural literacy' and 'stigma' in understanding these relationships. This first section (7.1) describes the 'what' regarding public views on the VMDR. The second section (7.2) addresses the 'whys' for the phenomena that are described in the earlier section. A subgroup of these latter studies, concerning the influence of media accounts of crime and mental illness, gets its own section because of the considerable amount of literature in this regard, and its importance in understanding the current status of the VMDR. The concluding section draws upon these insights to consider the epistemic and practical power these findings have in shaping public policy in multiple domains: public policy and legislation proper, research funding allocations, funding for criminal justice and mental health programs, and—of course—the *Diagnostic and Statistical Manual of Mental Disorders* (DSM).

Vice and Psychiatric Diagnosis. John Z. Sadler, Oxford University Press. © Oxford University Press 2024.
DOI: 10.1093/oso/9780198876830.003.0007

7.1.1 The concept of cultural literacy

In the early 1980s, an English professor at the University of Virginia, E. D. Hirsch, Jr., articulated his concept of 'cultural literacy', a concept which was to become a call to action as well as a focus of great controversy in American higher education—a controversy that persists into the present day. Perhaps his most seminal paper is 'Cultural Literacy'.[1] Lamenting the decline of literacy in American schools, he recounted several of his own empirical studies examining the relationship between what philosophers call 'background knowledge' and the understanding of a particular standardized text. Background knowledge is the prior knowledge one brings to new learning situations. Background knowledge was to be crucial in understanding cultural literacy. Moreover, it constitutes a big part of what citizens bring to public affairs.

Hirsch was interested in the question of whether the amount and quality of background knowledge had an effect on what readers understood and retained of standardized texts. He conducted several empirical studies to address this question. He compared the same text against high- and low-background knowledge in otherwise-similar samples of people. He had, for instance, American and (South Asian) Indian populations exchange readings of otherwise-similar accounts of American and Indian weddings. What he uniformly found was that greater the (relevant) background knowledge for each group, the greater the speed, comprehension, and retention of the novel narrative material. His *Cultural Literacy: What Every American Needs to Know, with an Appendix: What Literate Americans Know*[2] explored the ramifications of his findings in reference to then-current American educational practices, which emphasized the stylistic, formal elements of reading and writing, and not specific 'contents' of literature. Hirsch argued that educational practices of the time, which de-emphasized traditional background knowledge (the academic 'canon'), were the cause of declining US literacy. Instead of expanding their knowledge base of great literature, students were learning about the relatively few formal elements of good writing, eschewing any particular set of iconic, 'core', or canonical literature. Under the then-current circumstances, the books read in English classes could be anything deemed worthy by teachers, school administrators, or for that matter, politicians. Indeed, the diversification of English course work to include a pluralistic, multicultural perspective, an educational trend contemporary with Hirsch' concerns, represented a shift away from what was depicted as a 'dead white male' canon of content for English curricula. The depth of Hirsch's insight into learning, combined with a relatively traditional prescription for what English curricula should include as canon, sowed the seeds for the controversy to follow.

Hirsch's 1983 paper summarized his insight about the importance of background knowledge in understanding new readings:

> Briefly, good style contributes little to our reading of unfamiliar material because we must continually backtrack to test out different hypotheses about what is being meant or

412   Vice and Psychiatric Diagnosis

referred to. Thus, a reader of a text about Grant and Lee who is unsure just who Grant and Lee are would have to get clues from later parts of the text, and then go back to re-read earlier parts in the light of surer conjectures. This trial-and-error backtracking with unfamiliar material is so much more time-consuming than the delays caused by a bad style alone that style begins to lose its importance as a factor in reading unfamiliar material. The contribution of style in such cases can no longer be measured with statistical confidence.[3]

This research hardly constitutes what I would consider a counterintuitive result—any philosophy professor teaching (for instance) Jean-Paul Sartre to undergraduates has the same kind of problem that the psychiatric geneticist has in teaching behavioral genetics to psychiatry residents. Learning new material requires suitable background knowledge. Applied to the general education context, Hirsch's idea of cultural literacy was this: in educating competent students, a substantial amount of cultural knowledge of a more-or-less factual nature is necessary for efficient and effective new learning to take place.

So far so good. What was, and is, controversial about Hirsch's work is following out the implications, especially in a multicultural, pluralistic society. The key questions in response to Hirsch's proposals have been: Who gets to decide what knowledge-content is required for 'cultural literacy', and what might that knowledge-content be? While the discourse about cultural literacy in American education is vigorous and very interesting for any educator, for my purposes the stripped-down idea of cultural literacy as crucial background knowledge is the core idea that I want to utilize in discussing public understandings of crime and mental illness.[4]

Hirsch's influential idea of cultural literacy launched a new direction in educational research and scholarship. One consequence was the diversification of 'literacies', which now included, among others, health, mental health, and crime literacy, which are my primary interest here. What my review will show is that the public's mental health and crime literacy is low, at least as defined by contemporary social scientists.

7.1.2 Mental health and crime literacy

One can instantly recognize that Hirsch's concept of cultural literacy is dimensional (what people need to know may be more, or less) and context-specific (what you need to know to understand Sartre's philosophy is different than what you need to know to understand behavioral genetics). As I mentioned earlier, one of the legacies of Hirsch's concept of cultural literacy has been the appearance in the academic literature of all kinds of 'literacies': 'health literacy' being perhaps most prominent for medical audiences.[5] For our interest here, I'll review the modest literatures on mental health literacy, and the even more modest literature in crime/criminology literacy. The question of what the public needs to know to be informed and competent participants in public policy debates on the VMDR is one of the key ones for this

chapter. Moreover, the notion of mental health and crime literacy will prove important in understanding the 'whys' of public attitudes toward crime and mental illness
to follow later in the chapter. I consider, at the end of the chapter, the contribution to
crime and mental health literacy to the VMDR.

7.1.2.1 Mental health literacy—what the public does and doesn't know

Studies of mental health literacy are relatively recent and quite limited, particularly in the United States and the UK. Moreover, the literature is primarily descriptive (what the public does and does not know) with even fewer studies addressing
why the public does/doesn't know. The dean of mental health literacy studies in the
English-speaking world is unquestionably Anthony F. Jorm, a social scientist at the
University of Melbourne. Jorm defines 'mental health literacy' as 'knowledge and
beliefs about mental disorders which aid their recognition, management or prevention'.[6] Jorm's research is primarily motivated by the clinical goal of increasing use
of mental health services by those who need, or will need, them. I have organized
the discussion of mental health literacy around related themes or questions, starting
with treatment-seeking.

Treatment-seeking for mental disorders. For my purposes, what is most striking,
and disturbing, about mental health literacy research is the uniform finding of poor
participation in mental health services.[7] Perhaps the definitive work in this area is
the World Health Organization (WHO)'s World Mental Health survey component,[8]
which addressed delays in treatment-seeking, as well as failure to seek treatment,
after the onset of anxiety, depressive, and substance use disorders. Table 7.1 lists
some sample results out of 15 countries and over 76,000 participants in the surveys.
The authors used trained laypersons in diagnosing episodes of any DSM-IV anxiety disorder, any mood disorder, and any substance abuse disorder, then queried
treatment-seeking within 1 year and extrapolated for a 50-year span.

Table 7.1 WHO Delay/Failure in Treatment-Seeking Sample Data—2007—Excerpt

Country	% Treated in 1 y			% Treated w/in 50 y			Median Delay in y		
	ANX	DEP	SUBS	ANX	DEP	SUBS	ANX	DEP	SUBS
France[a]	16.1	42.7	15.7	93.3	98.6	66.5	18.0	3.0	13.0
Germany[a]	13.7	40.4	13.2	95.0	89.1	86.1	23.0	2.0	9.0
Israel	36.4	31.9	2.0	90.7	92.7	48.0	3.0	6.0	12.0
Japan	11.2	29.6	9.2	63.1	56.8	31.0	20.0	1.0	8.0
Mexico	3.6	16.0	0.9	53.2	69.9	22.1	30.0	14.0	10.0
Netherlands[a]	28.0	52.1	15.5	91.1	96.9	66.6	10.0	1.0	9.0
New Zealand	12.5	41.4	6.3	84.2	97.5	84.8	21.0	3.0	17.0
Spain[a]	23.2	48.4	18.6	86.6	96.4	40.1	17.0	1.0	6.0
USA	11.3	35.4	10.0	87.0	94.8	75.5	23.0	4.0	13.0

Note: a = screened for major depression rather than 'any mood disorder'.

The participant samples by country ranged from a low of 2,372 for the Netherlands to a high of 12,992 for New Zealand. The authors used the statistical technique of survival analysis[9] to calculate the probabilities of the 1- and 50-year treatment-seeking. What is striking is the uniformly poor utilization of treatment across all countries, the low percentages of those accessing care within one year of illness, and the median delay in accessing care for all three groups of disorders. In the United States, the rates of treatment-seeking within 1 year were 11.3% for any anxiety disorder, 35.4% for mood disorder, and 10.0% for any substance use disorder. At best, only a little over a third (in the case of mood disorder) of ill people sought help from the mental health system within a year. The median delays (in weeks) were equally disturbing, being 23.0, 4.0, and 13.0 respectively for each disorder group. Jorm reviews additional studies showing poor treatment-seeking on the part of the public.[10]

Recognition of mental illness in self and others. The WHO data raise many 'why' questions. For Jorm, chief among them is the question of whether laypersons can (or are willing to) recognize mental illness in themselves or others. In a 2010 review,[11] Gulliver et al. summarize 15 qualitative and quantitative studies of young people's attitudes toward mental health, including the subjects' self-reported barriers and facilitators of care. The authors identified 'barrier' themes (what gets in the way of help-seeking) and 'facilitator' themes (what aids in help-seeking). Of note for the issue of recognition of mental illness, the third-most prominent barrier theme for Gulliver et al. was 'identifying the symptoms of mental illness',[12] which appeared in five out of the thirteen studies reviewed. In a 2008 study by Thompson et al.,[13] their sample subjects took an average of 6.9 years to recognize that subjects had experienced an anxiety disorder. In Jorm's 2012 review, he notes common patterns of poor recognition of mental disorders by the surveyed public in countries including the United States, Canada, Australia, India, Japan, Sweden, and the UK.[14] Individuals in these surveys referred to their problems as 'stress' or 'life problem', in effect de-medicalizing the condition.[15] Jorm notes that the early onset in life for many mental disorders provides a context for young people to believe that their suffering is a norm, a fact of life, or the 'human condition', rather than a personally impairing illness.

Preferred helpers for mental distress. The inability to recognize the symptoms of mental illness, as well as the experience of their mental distress as existential norms leads many, perhaps most members of the public to seek assistance 'on their own' or with family, friends, and neighbors.[16] Moreover, in the studies in Jorm's 2012 review, the subjects of surveys had high regard for family, friends, and neighbors as sources of assistance for mental distress, compared to mental health professionals.

Understanding of mental health services and therapies. The prevailing preference for friends and family as helpers for mental distress raises the question of what and how much the public understands about psychiatry, clinical psychology, and mental health services, as well as how these professionals are regarded by the public. Usually psychologists are regarded more positively than psychiatrists,[17] and prevailing members of the public prefer primary care physicians and lay counselors for assistance with mental distress.[18] Another humbling finding for psychiatrists was that public attitudes for drug treatments in mental distress are often unpopular, even viewing medications as, at worst, dangerous, or at best, marginally different from non-evidence-based treatments like diet or vitamins.[19] Ironically, psychopharmacology is perceived as toxic and dangerous on the one hand, and insignificant and ineffectual on the other. Such widespread contradictions in public opinion imply profound lack of knowledge across the board. Psychologists and psychological treatments fare much better in the public's view in these studies.

I have omitted many findings in mental health literacy, including topics like what to do when confronting a mentally ill individual who needs assistance,[20] and studies of how and where to seek help for mental distress. Collectively, Jorm and his colleagues' work around the world is of unparalleled public health importance. Regardless of how powerful our treatments are, if people don't know to access them, or even resist accessing them because of ignorance, distrust, bad experience, or prejudice against the mental health system, we have significantly failed in our mission. As we shall see shortly, the picture for crime literacy and for public understanding of mentally disordered offenders is at least equally, and perhaps more, grim.

7.1.2.2 Crime literacy

> There has always been too much crime. Virtually every generation since the founding of the Nation and before has felt itself threatened by the spectre of rising crime and violence.[21]

Like the specialized field of mental health literacy, the field of 'crime literacy' or perhaps more accurately 'criminology literacy' is also a relatively small one. Table 7.2 compares hits with these various 'literacies' on Google Scholar versus Google Web in July 2013.[22] One may read these data as a crude measure of public interest in the fields. 'Health literacy' is used as a comparison.

These data suggest that interest in these fields dwindles dramatically as one moves from mental health literacy to crime and criminology literacy. If public interest in mental health literacy is low, then public interest in crime literacy is nil. I will only be able to briefly review the literature on crime literacy.

Table 7.2 Comparison of Hits on Google Scholar and Google Web on Literacy Topics

Topic	# Hits, Google Scholar	# Hits, Google Web
'Health literacy'	53,700	1.53 million
'Mental health literacy'	3,660	59,800
'Crime literacy'	70	5,620
'Criminology literacy'	3	94

Searches performed 10 July 2013.

Ironically, the largest volume on research relevant to crime literacy is situated in social science studies of media presentations of crime and criminals—a discussion to follow.

Frequency of crime. The University of Albany offers a valuable 'Sourcebook of Criminal Justice Statistics Online',[23] and the US Bureau of Justice Statistics offers a similar service.[24] The most recent data as of this writing, on public attitudes toward the level of crime in the United States can be viewed in the notes to this chapter.[25] The data are shown in Table 7.3. Briefly, these data compare Gallup data from 1989– 2011 in response to the question, 'Is there more crime in the U.S. than there was a year ago, or less?'

The prevailing thrust of the data shows that public opinion reflects persisting beliefs that crime is increasing compared to the prior year. The single exception in this data set is 2001, when even then the 'more' and 'less' categories are nearly equal, 41% to 43%.

In comparing this set of data to a related question, 'Is there more crime in your area than there was a year ago, or less?', the Sourcebook has collected US data for 1972–2011.[26] Consider the crime rate data from the comparable time frame to Table 7.3's public attitudes data. The data here show less confidence and are more evenly distributed among the more/less/same/don't know-refused categories. For brief comparison purposes, the endorsements for 'more' ranged in selected years

Table 7.3 US Public Attitudes toward Level of Crime Selected Years, 1989–2011

Research question: 'Is there more crime in the U.S. than there was a year ago, or less?'

	More	Less	Same	DK/Refused
1989	84%	5%	5%	6%
1990	84	3	7	6
1992	89	3	4	4
1993	87	4	5	4
1996	71	15	8	6
1997	64	25	6	5
1998	52	35	8	5
2000	47	41	7	5
2001	41	43	10	6
2002	62	21	11	6
2003	60	25	11	4
2004	53	28	14	5
2005	67	21	9	3
2006	68	16	8	8
2007	71	14	8	6
2008	67	15	9	9
2009	74	15	6	5
2010	66	17	8	9
2011	68	17	8	8

from a low of 26% in 2001, and high of 54% in 1981 and 1992. Of interest here is the contrast with the global versus local data. National crime as an abstract concept is perceived as rising, but when considering one's local situation, the perceptions are more benign.

Was crime, in fact, on the rise during these years? The question is simple, but the science is complex. Simply tracking police reports can be misleading because, as noted in Chapter 6, crime victims often do not report crimes. To address this limitation, efforts to track criminal offenses like the National Crime Victimization Survey[27] have been created to directly poll the public for violent and property crime frequencies. Similarly, private polling organizations like Gallup have long surveyed the public about crime trends, as noted above. US Census data can also be an excellent source of crime report data, because of the comprehensiveness of their data collection. Using these more rigorous approaches, Tonry (2011a) succinctly summarizes violent versus property crime rates over the past 25 years (see also Zimring 2006).

> . . . there is no reasonable doubt that crime rates have long been falling and have fallen a lot. This is shown by police data on reported crimes, by U.S. Bureau of the Census data on crimes reported to interviewers by victims, and by medical records on admissions to emergency rooms of hospitals. The same thing is happening in all the major English-speaking countries and in most or all Western European countries—as shown by their police victimization, and medical data systems.[28]

The US Bureau of Justice Statistics data from 1960–2008 for total violent crime (murder, nonnegligent manslaughter, rape, robbery, and aggravated assault) and property crime (burglary, larceny, and motor vehicle theft) show that offenses per 100,000 people peaked over that period around 1991–1993 (with murder peaking at 10.2/100,000 in 1980 and 9.8/100,000 in 1991). After about 1992 a steady decline has followed for both violent and property crime to the present day, leading Zimring to dub this phenomenon 'The Great American Crime Decline'.[29] The 2008 murder rate per 100,000, for instance was 5.4, a low only rivaled by the 4.0–5.0 rates in the early 1960s.[30] As noted above, the US changes were quite similar across industrialized Western countries over the same period.

The reasons for the decline in crime rates over the late-twentieth and early twenty-first century period makes for a very interesting and complex topic, which unfortunately is not sufficiently relevant to my purposes here to review. However, interested readers can read more about the reasons in Zimring (2006) and Tonry (2007, 2011a).

Other aspects of crime. Public perceptions are not just unrealistically pessimistic about crime rates. Public opinion can also be misled pessimistically about criminal justice procedures. For example, the public, until very recently, tends to view sentencing practices, in general, as being too lenient and soft on offenders. However, when members of the public are placed into simulated jury settings, or educated about judicial procedures, public judgments about appropriate sentencing closely match those of actual sentences given by judges.[31] Beginning in 2011, public and bipartisan political discourse finally began to reconsider harsh sentencing and prison reform in response to a spiraling problem of excessive incarceration in the United States.[32] In the later discussion of media presentations of crime/mental illness, additional examples of distorted public viewpoints will be discussed. At this point, I should consider public understanding of mentally ill offenders.

7.1.3 Public understanding of mentally ill offenders

The public tends to believe the mentally ill as a group are more dangerous than the general population. This generalization will be considered in more detail in the stigma section below. Studies specifically addressing the public perception of mentally ill offenders are few. Moreover, studies and recent reviews may be decades old—though the consistency of the results suggests things haven't changed much over the past 50 years.

Classic reviews by Nunnally[33] and Rabkin[34] established the nearly universal distrust of mentally ill individuals on the part of the US public in the mid-twentieth century. In an often-cited study from the 1970s, Steadman and Cocozza[35] reported on a public attitude survey on mentally ill people, criminals, and the 'criminally insane' in a random sample of 145 households in Albany, New York, in 1975. Among their findings was a doubling of fear-of ratings among the public for the criminally insane (61%) versus the mentally ill in general (29%).[36] In a semantic-differential component of their study, comparing 'most people', 'mental patient', and 'criminally insane patient', both the latter groups were rated more dangerous, more harmful, more violent, more tense, less in self-control, more 'bad' (e.g., evil), more unpredictable, more mysterious, more ignorant, more aggressive, and more sexually driven. These descriptors reconstruct a quite negative stereotypical picture consistent with the media depictions discussed later in this chapter. Differences in these areas between the mentally ill versus criminally insane group were nonsignificant, except for (curiously) the perception that mentally ill people had a higher sex drive than criminally insane individuals. More fearful responses in the public toward the patients tended to correlate with more media exposure, a theme that will be discussed more in the section on media effects. In a similar study conducted statewide in New York, Steadman and Cocozza[37] found similar findings and made similar conclusions.

Hartwell[38] reviewed the life trajectories for offenders who had dual-diagnosis (e.g., a serious mental disorder (SMD) and a substance abuse disorder). The literature supported the conclusions that 'triple-stigma' people were more likely to serve sentences for substance abuse, to be homeless after release, to violate probation, and to reoffend. Her study could not address the chicken-or-egg question, whether the poorer outcomes generated the stigma, or the stigma generated the poor outcomes. While there was no public opinion component to her review, she describes public services barriers to this group of patients.

7.1.3.1 Attitudes toward the insanity defense

A more indirect consideration of the literature examining public attitudes toward mentally ill offenders can be examined through research on public attitudes toward the insanity defense. As reflected in a flurry of publications following the 1982 acquittal of John Hinckley, Jr. on grounds of insanity, the public outcry about alleged abuses of the insanity defense multiplied. Hinckley's trial for an attempted assassination of then-President Ronald Reagan was sensational, and as the research to follow showed, was a trigger for mobilizing negative public attitudes toward the insanity defense, or 'not guilty by reason of insanity' (NGRI). The distinguished law scholar and past American Psychiatric Association Manfred Guttmacher awardee, Alexander Brooks, argued for elimination of the NGRI defense in 1985.[39] Brooks's discussion of NGRI was joined, pro and con, by a number of scholars in the 1980s.[40]

Just as there was a burst of scholarly opinion about NGRI in the mid-1980s and early 1990s, a similar burst of research followed on public opinion about NGRI and, to a lesser extent, the role of forensic psychiatry in the criminal courts. A 1978 panel of New York prosecuting and defense attorneys believed the American Law Institute (ALI) insanity guidelines were poorly done; a 1980 Illinois study of 129 psychiatric respondents found only 16% supported Illinois' use of the ALI standard, the majority of these psychiatrists believing that insanity defense is overutilized[41]. Similar results were found in a Wyoming survey[42]. A 1983 study by Jeffrey and Pasewark[43] surveyed a mix of community residents and introductory psychology students, finding 92% thought NGRI was used excessively, and 89% believed offenders escape responsibility for crimes by invoking NGRI. After being informed of the actual use of, and acquittal rate of NGRI, agreement with these perspectives diminished to 52 and 42% respectively. In a reprise of his and others' earlier work on public opinion of NGRI, Pasewark (1986) reviewed public opinion survey research on the topic. Characterizing the studies as making generally negative conclusions about NGRI in the public's view, 87% of respondents believed that NGRI was overused; 69% believed NGRI should not be used in criminal cases.[44]

In terms of the actual rates of use and success (acquittal) using NGRI, Pasewark acknowledges that the data are limited and difficult to obtain. His conclusion for this review was: 'From the information currently available, it would appear that (1) the plea is seldom made; (2) the rate at which the pleas is used varies widely among states and even within the counties of a given state; and (3) once entered, the success rate for the plea varies among jurisdictions, for presently unknown reasons.'[45]

Valerie Hans performed a survey study of public attitudes toward NGRI in the 1980s. A random sample of 434 members of the public in New Castle County, Delaware were interviewed via telephone about the NGRI in general and the Hinckley case in particular. The telephone interviews had a refusal rate of approximately 5% (the refusal data was inconsistently collected by the panel of interviewers). Of the respondents 87.1% believed 'the insanity defense is a loophole that allows too many guilty people to go free.'[46] However, the public understanding of NGRI was poor, as interviews found only 1 of the 434 respondents could give 'a reasonably good approximation of the Model Penal Code definition of legal insanity'.[47] Interestingly, the authors also found that a majority of the public recommended both treatment and punishment for John Hinckley in a component of the study that addressed attitudes explicitly about the Hinckley case. In a follow-up 1986 review of studies about public opinion toward NGRI, Hans[48] noted studies supported that the majority of the public do not believe that NGRI acquittees are, in fact, insane. She also described a significant minority of the public who believe that genuinely mentally ill subjects should be punished for crimes regardless.

A more recent review by Henry Steadman's group[49] verifies the strong public opposition to the defense. Over half of the public believe, across studies, that the NGRI defense is overused and about half believe it should be abolished. Again noting the public confusion about the defense, Silver et al. note that the 1978 Steadman and Cocozza[50] paper in which the public identified, as the two most common examples of NGRI, two well-publicized murderers, Robert Garrow and Charles Manson. However, neither offender had been found NGRI and both had been convicted and sentenced for murder! The authors also reiterated the notion that the public finds the NGRI defense a 'loophole' and that NGRI acquittees go 'scot-free'.[51] In the empirical research portion of this same publication, the authors sampled nearly a million cases of felony indictments for NGRI from 1976–1985, based on collected data in eight states totaling 49 counties. For the public opinion comparison data, the authors used Pasewark and Seidenzahl's (1979) study.[52] Table 7.4 is adapted from Silver et al. and shows the comparison data, from public perception to 'actual' data.

The Silver et al. data about actual use of the NGRI offense introduce the crucial comparison: Public attitudes are one thing, but what about the facts on the frequency

Table 7.4 Silver et al. (1994) Comparison of Public Perception versus Actual Use of NGRI

		Public	Actual
A.	Use of the insanity defense		
	% of felony indictments resulting in an insanity plea	37	0.9
	% of insanity pleas resulting in acquittal	44	26
B.	Disposition of insanity acquittees		
	% of insanity acquittees sent to a mental hospital	50.6	84.7
	% of insanity acquittees set free	25.6	15.3
	Conditional release		11.6
	Outpatient		2.6
	Release		1.1
C.	Length of confinement of insanity acquittees (years)		
	All crimes	21.8	32.5
	Murder		76.4

Adapted from Silver et al. (1994, p. 67).

of use of the NGRI defense, and how often it is successful? This question turns out to be difficult to answer. No national statistics are available; NGRI is delivered not by federal courts but by state ones. Within the states, data on the frequency of NGRI in (for instance) murder cases are at best intermittently kept, much less the court decisions following.[53] A handful of empirical studies from the 1980s and 1990s are still the most cited in the literature.

A 1978 survey by Steadman and colleagues, based on a mail solicitation of all 50 states and the federal prison system, that for 1978 nationwide there were 1554 persons acquitted by NGRI.[54] The variability among states was enormous, and the average per state was 31. Steadman and colleagues estimated that these represented, considering the prison and jail populations of the time, that prisoners outnumbered NGRI acquittees by a factor of 150×.

Another study by Callahan and colleagues from 1991 examined county court dockets by hand, following out the frequency and outcomes of NGRI pleas in eight states. Pleas of NGRI in this study accounted for 1% of all felony cases. Of those, only 26% were successful pleas, that is, only 26% of the defendants were found NGRI. In summary, these data suggest that approximately 0.25%, or 1 in 400 insanity pleas are successful.[55] A third study from this group[56] using this data set above found an inverse relationship between how often the NGRI defense was invoked and its success rate.

What correlates with a successful NGRI defense? For the Cirincione study, the demographic of a single woman with a high school diploma was more likely to succeed than individuals falling outside of this demographic. Other positive predictors included prior mental illness hospitalizations, a prior relationship of victim and defendant, and no prior arrests or incarcerations. In the 1983 Steadman et al. study, three factors discriminated successful NGRI defenses: youth (aged between 25 and 39 years), having greater than five prior hospitalizations for mental illness, and a clinical finding of 'insanity' by the courtroom psychiatrist.

A review by Borum and Fulero[57] summarizes then-current knowledge of NGRI: (1) the defense is raised in less than 1% of felony cases. (2) When pleaded, the overall chances of a successful NGRI plea are about one in four. (3) NGRI in murder cases occurred about one-third as often as felony cases. (4) NGRI acquittees are confined (hospital, prison) as long or longer than defendants convicted on similar charges. (5). NGRI acquittees are no more likely to reoffend than offenders convicted with similar offenses.

A second specialized area of research into mentally ill offenders concerns the special attention given to sex offenders, who often, perhaps usually, have various kinds of psychiatric comorbidities. As a legal, clinical, or criminological category, the sex offender label represents a fuzzy and psychiatrically diverse population. The sex offender, an individual who commits a 'sexual' crime, may be an otherwise 'normal' 17-year-old boy who had consensual sex with his 15-year-old girlfriend; a person with a serious mental illness like Schizophrenia or Bipolar Disorder; a veteran or motor accident victim with a significant brain injury; an elderly individual with Alzheimer's or another dementia; an individual with a paraphilic disorder like

Pedophilic Disorder; or an individual like Jeffrey Dahmer whose psychopathology spans multiple psychiatric categories yet because of the comorbidities, is typical of none of the component disorders.[58] In Dahmer's case, he had alcohol dependence, a necrophilia, a likely Autism Spectrum Disorder, and various neuropsychological functional impairments.[59] Such phenomenological diversity makes the 'sex offender' a clinically useless concept in psychiatric settings, as it spans normal people in unfortunate circumstances, to people with a variety of psychopathologies, on through to rare but horrifically incomprehensible murderers.[60]

The 'sex offender' may be the most despised minority in the United States, though no direct scientific data exist to establish this trope.[61] However, sex offenders have a remarkable number of social policies and public behaviors directed against them, that comparable violent offenders do not. Among these are laws that establish public registries for them after conviction, require community notification of their arrival following release, and regulate their residency in proximity to children.[62] Such laws do not exist for other violent offenders. The severe reaction of the public to sex offenders is well documented.[63] Public attitudes to treatment of sex offenders is favorable, as long as they are also in prison.[64] Harris and Socia[65] tested the label of sex offender in an experimental design in comparison to 'neutral' descriptions, finding that the sex offender label correlated with negative appraisals. Multiple studies have documented that the public overestimates the probability of relapse in sex offenders, their unresponsiveness to treatment, and the prevalence of their crimes.[66]

7.2 Understanding public attitudes toward mental illness and crime

In the prior survey and summary of public views about mental illness and criminality, I have noted that the public's understanding of these phenomena are poor, and quite disjunctive with the science. Of crucial importance is an attempt to understand these misunderstandings and ignorance. After this introduction, I consider the reasons why public attitudes are negative regarding criminality/mental illness.

In considering the mental health literacy (MHL) literature, a fair assessment would be that the mental health professions, as well as educators, have failed in their efforts to educate the public about mental health and mental illness. Is this failure to educate the public simply another example of failures of health literacy in general? That is, is MHL just another subgroup of an overall poor health literacy?

This turns out to be a difficult question to answer in any precise way, because the kind of data generated for 'health literacy' (HL) research differs substantively from the MHL literature. Importantly, the best HL literature typically utilizes a standardized assessment rubric, and report distributions of HL in relative terms (e.g., high, medium, and low), and in the case of perhaps the premier study, the National Assessment for Health Literacy (NAAL)[67] grades the public's HL in terms of Below Basic, Basic, Intermediate, and Proficient. According to this study, 14% of US adults have Below Basic HL, and 22% have Basic levels. Moreover, these studies address confounding factors not addressed consistently in the aforementioned MHL literature. These include confounders such as overall verbal and mathematical literacy, health-related impairments that compromise literacy (e.g., impaired vision in old age, educational level, among others). For instance, according to the NAAL study, overall or general literacy scores were 14% and 29% for Below Basic and Basic, respectively. These data suggest that particularly for Below Basic HL, poor HL is often a manifestation of poor general literacy. As another example, Gazmararian and colleagues[68] tested 3260 new Medicare enrollees aged 65 to 69 years using the Short Test of Functional Health Literacy in Adults. They found 33.9% of English-speaking and 53.9% of Spanish-speaking respondents had inadequate or marginal HL.

Given the high rates of low general literacy, and the additional estimates of Below Basic and Basic HL totaling 43% in the NAAL study, I think it is reasonable to say that a strong relationship exists between general literacy, HL, and MHL, though these relationships might primarily apply at the lower levels of all the 'literacies'. Saying much more than this would be more speculative.[69]

The following subsections address the association between crime and mental illness in two ways, collectively illuminating the negative public perceptions of the VMDR. The first considers the science which has addressed the question of whether mental illness is associated with criminal behavior. The second subsection considers the powerful effect of media portrayals of mental illness and crime. The third examines the theory behind these findings. For this latter section, I'll review others' work as well as provide some if my own thinking on this issue.

7.2.1 Empirical associations of crime & mental illness

After discussion of the stigma, misinformation, and public distrust of the mentally ill, I should compare the actual state of scientific knowledge about the association of crime and mental illness. These studies can be organized, roughly, into three groups: (1) offense rates comparing mentally ill people with the general population, (2) indirect associations of crime and mental illness, and (3) explanatory studies of relationships between crime and mental illness. Most of the studies on crime-mental illness relationships focus on violent crime, though not all. Furthermore, the majority of studies consider major, severe mental disorders rather than 'any psychiatric disorder'. I will try to keep these distinctions clear when relevant. Moreover, almost nothing is known about the relationship between petty/misdemeanor crimes (as opposed to felony crimes) and mental illness when compared to rates in the general population. In this section I present several summary studies and reviews that answer the general questions. Following this, I provide some endnotes that list particular studies of relevance, grouped by my three approaches to the research question.

7.2.1.1 Offense rates between the mentally ill and the general population

Heather Stuart, writing on behalf of the World Psychiatric Association and the National Center for Crisis Management, provides an overview of the relationship between violence and mental illness.[70] The focus on violence rather than crime has to do with the greater valence of public interest and fear, as well as greater ramifications for stigma and discrimination against the mentally ill and the mentally ill offender. Stuart's major conclusions from the research of the prior 20 years is that major mental disorders do present a small increase in risk of violent offending in comparison to the general population, and this risk is significantly increased if there is substance abuse co-occurring with a major mental disorder. Indeed, she notes that the major predictors of violent offending are not mental illnesses but the collected factors of youth, male gender, lower socioeconomic class, and substance abuse. She notes that studies strongly support that people with major mental disorders are at more risk of being *victims* of violent crime than perpetrators of violent crime. People comorbid with substance abuse disorders and major mental illnesses account for about 70% of violent crimes perpetrated by the broader group of people with major mental illness. She notes that the most important violence prevention strategies are early identification and treatment of comorbid mentally ill and substance-abusing people.

Focusing explicitly on the relationship between schizophrenia and violence, Seena Fazel and colleagues published a systematic review and meta-analysis in 2009.[71] Based upon 20 individual studies and a pooled subject number of over 18,000, they calculated odds ratios pooling them with random-effects statistical models. Their conclusions were that schizophrenia was a risk factor for violent offending, particularly homicide. However, as with earlier notations, the risk of violent offending was consistently compounded by substance abuse as a powerful cofactor. These general findings were confirmed in a more recent review focusing on violence and schizophrenia and substance abuse by Rund in 2018.

Writing in the *New England Journal of Medicine* in 2006, Richard Friedman briefly reviews the links between mental illness and violence.[72] He notes that a survey of a subgroup of 7000 subjects within the National Institute of Mental Health (NIMH) Epidemiological Catchment Area Study (http://www.icpsr.umich.edu/icpsrweb/ICPSR/studies/6153) were found to be two to three times more likely to be assaultive than the general population—here 'assaultive' meant using a weapon such as a gun or knife in a fight, being involved in more than one fight involving blows, involving people other than partner or spouse. Here the lifetime prevalence of assaultiveness among the seriously mentally ill was 16%, compared with the 7% rate among those without mental disorders. Friedman is circumspect to note that most people with serious mental illness are not violent, and because serious mental illness is a relatively uncommon condition (e.g., approximately 1% of the population has schizophrenia) the actual incremental risk is small. Overall, the attributable risk he estimated as 3%–5% over the general population. He compares the 2–3× risk with serious mental illness (SMI) alone versus the 7× risk of people with drug and/or alcohol use disorders without major mental illness. Moreover, other factors combine to shape the violence risk in SMI, such as homelessness, being violently victimized oneself, and poor medical health. Once these variables are controlled, the 1-year risk for violence falls only slightly above the risk for the general population.

These assessments have not changed much in 20 years. Writing in 1996, John Monahan and Jean Arnold in their report *Violence by People with Mental Illness: A Consensus Statement by Advocates and Researchers* note:

> . . . the results of several recent large-scale research projects conclude that only a weak association between mental disorders and violence exists in the community. Serious violence by people with major mental disorders appears concentrated in a small fraction of the total number, and especially in those who use alcohol and other drugs. Mental disorders—in sharp contrast to alcohol and drug abuse—account for a minuscule portion of the violence that afflicts American society.[73]

Interested readers may wish to consider the additional studies in this endnote.[74]

7.2.1.2 Associations

Reviewing the question of violence and SMI from a different angle, this section considers statistical associations between various subpopulations of those with mental disorders and/or criminal offenses, and different sites of measurement for these comparisons. Regarding the former, for example, we'll consider the risk of reoffending in released offenders with and without mental illness. Regarding the latter, for instance, we'll consider the probability of reoffending for people who ever sought mental health services.

All of these studies have significant limitations because of selection biases and difficult-to-control-for confounding variables. I will briefly note some illustrative examples of these limitations as I discuss the studies. While association studies of this type can be very helpful for addressing questions and problems in the particular subpopulation of interest, they are of limited value in addressing my broader question of the causal relationships between crime and SMI.

Using a random sample of 650 inmates out of 2972 men in penitentiaries in Quebec in 1988, Hodgins & Côté[75] compared rates of major mental disorder and Antisocial Personality Disorder (ASPD) in inmates with those with no history of major mental disorder as assessed by the Diagnostic Interview Schedule. They were interested in whether inmates with mental disorders would have a history of more convictions and more violent crimes than nondisordered inmates. They found that there was no significant difference in mentally ill offenders (n = 107) and nondisordered inmates (n = 349) in their criminal careers.[76] However, the investigators also considered the combination of major mental disorder plus antisocial personality on criminal careers in disordered versus nondisordered participants. Here they found an association for the inmates with both mental disorder and ASPD for nonviolent, but not violent, crime. They believed this indicated that the combination of ASPD with major mental disorder represented a distinct subgroup of criminal offenders. Of course, the study conclusions are limited by their nonrandom sample skewed by nearly 30% of their selected participants either refusing or unable to participate. In a later study,[77] Hodgins's group studied 178 severely ill subjects imprisoned for violence, to examine differentiating features using multivariate profile analyses. One group, the smallest, was characterized as having violent propensities when under the influence of delusions or hallucinations. A second group, an antisocial group, had a history of violence over their lifespan. A third group, the institutional violence cluster, exhibited random outbursts of violence toward no individual in particular, and largely while institutionalized. The last, and largest group were convicts who claimed to never engage in violent behavior, despite having been convicted of a violent crime. The veracity of this group's claims could not be evaluated within the scope of the study. Of interest, the Hodgins group noted these characteristics are worthy of further study and might suggest differential treatment/rehabilitative approaches.

In a related vein, Matejkowski and colleagues[78] examined a cohort of 1588 US adults with histories of mental health service use for Major Depression (n = 1398) and Bipolar Disorder (n = 190). They asked these subjects about any criminal history as captured by a single query about whether they had been arrested in their lifetime. The authors found that 30% of these subjects were positive for a criminal history. The problem with this study is the lack of a control group of comparable individuals without Major Depression or Bipolar Disorder. The lifetime risk of arrest of adults is difficult to study, though estimates indicate that for men the lifetime risk for any criminal arrest is from 25% to 50%.[79] Keep in mind that for this study and these latter studies the criterion was 'arrest', not conviction or guilt—thus what seems to be a high number in the general population (25%–50%) is less so because arrests are logically a bigger number than conviction rates. Nevertheless, it appears reasonable to conclude from this study that people with Major Depression and Bipolar Disorder have arrest records not much different from the general population.

In her 1993 study, Ellen Hochstedler Steury drew a random sample of court records for felony and misdemeanor defendants over a 5-year period (1981–1985) in Milwaukee, Wisconsin, eliminating duplicate sampling of defendants with more than one offense.[80] She ended up with 4921 unique felony defendants and

5411 unique misdemeanor defendants. She then hand-searched the admission re-cords (over the same time period) of the local Milwaukee public psychiatric fa-cility to identify the entire set of defendants who received mental health care over the same period. She then compared the risk of defendant status with and without mental illness.

Steury did not address the potential for psychiatric admission to other Milwaukee mental health facilities, including general hospitals or private institutions. So her study is confounded by a potential under-capture of defendants who received inpa-tient psychiatric treatment outside of her target public institution. Nevertheless, she found that for both felony and misdemeanor offenses, the mentally ill defendants were 4× the risk of being a defendant compared to the Milwaukee general popula-tion. Because of the potential for noncaptured patient/defendants to receive care in other facilities, her stated risk may be an underestimate.

The National Epidemiologic Survey on Alcohol and Related Conditions (NESARC) was a very large, nationally representative survey which queried about mental disorder, substance abuse, and violence from 2001–2005.[81] Two papers have analyzed the relationships between NESARC data to the relationship between SMI and violence in the community in a 12-month period. Elbogen and Johnson[82] concluded that SMI was unrelated statistically to community violence unless co-occurring substance abuse was involved. However, in a later paper by Van Dorn and colleagues,[83] the authors disputed the earlier conclusions by Elbogen and Johnson on statistical grounds (of which I am not competent to evaluate). Van Dorn and colleagues used a 'causal modeling' rubric in their evaluation of the data and found that SMI was associated with 3.5× additional risk of violence over the 12-month period, which was worsened to approximately 12× risk when substance abuse was involved. They concluded that the incremental risk of violence with SMI was statistically significant albeit modest in power. They also noted their analysis of the NESARC data was more consistent with that of the Swanson et al 1990 data from the National Epidemiological Catchment Area study discussed earlier in this chapter.

Fazel and Grann,[84] using comprehensive national registers for all hospital admis-sions and criminal convictions in Sweden, considered violent crimes over a 13-year period (1988–2000), and sorted the total and those committed by people with severe mental illness. The violent crime rate overall for that period was 45/1000 people. Of those, 2.4/1000 were attributable to people with severe mental illness. This cor-responded to a population-attributable risk of 5.2%[85] or that patients with severe mental illness commit 1 in 20 violent crimes. The contribution of men to this sta-tistic was prevailingly large compared to women (female patients committing 0.6/1000 violent crimes).

Whiting, Lichtenstein and Fazel reviewed research on associations of individual mental disorders and violence in a 2020 Lancet Psychiatry review.[86] They found 2–4× absolute risk of violence in people with diagnosed psychiatric disorders compared to undiagnosed; this being a review article the definitions of 'violence' and what counted as a psychiatric disorder varied by study. Personality disorders and substance abuse, alone and in combination, increased absolute rates of offending over 5–10 years, over and above that of other disorders.

Collectively, these and previously discussed studies establish a significant association between mental illness and violence after controlling for multiple variables, including age, alcohol and drug use, gender, marital status, neighborhood base rates of violence, prior psychiatric hospital treatment, psychosocial stressors, social support, socioeconomic status, and urban versus rural setting.[87] However, these studies did not address the confound that both violence and mental illness share very similar risk factors. These are important confounds, in that without controlling for other criminogenic conditions, the causal power of mental illness in criminality cannot be approached. In an effort to address this, Silver et al.,[88] using a retrospective longitudinal design, considered whether criminal inmates with a mental health treatment history were more likely to have been convicted of homicide and assault as their most recent offense. They controlled for prior violent behavior among other confounds mentioned above. They found that inmates with a psychiatric treatment history were more frequently associated with sexual and violent crimes than other types of crimes. However, as the authors note, the study is limited in generalizability because of the inability to compare inmates with nonoffenders as well as with the general population.

7.2.1.3 Theory and explanation

So far, we have considered the 'what' regarding violent crime and mental disorders. With this section we turn to the 'whys'. A number of investigators have considered the reasons for the modest association of violence with SMI. This subsection considers some of this work. First, I turn to the question of psychosocial factors that predict, correlate, or otherwise covary with offending by the mentally ill.

In 1939, a British psychiatrist and mathematician, Lionel Penrose (father of the noted contemporary British physicist Roger Penrose), published a study that supported his hypothesis, that an inverse relationship existed between the number of hospital beds in a society and its incarceration rates.[89] He theorized that if one reduced the confinement in one domain, the other will increase. Since then, a number of papers have examined this thesis, and the results are mixed. In contemporary times, where alternatives to incarceration as well as hospitalization are common (e.g., halfway houses, compulsory outpatient treatment, and residential care), and economic factors drive both hospitalization and incarceration rates, confounds in evaluating the Penrose hypothesis are abundant.[90] The Penrose hypothesis formalizes the belief of many in the US mental health field that the deinstitutionalization of the chronic mentally ill in the 1960s contributed to the current US crisis in homeless mentally ill, on one hand, and the crisis of incarcerated mentally ill people, on the other. This idea of social drift from medical/

hospital settings for the mentally ill, to penal settings, has been dubbed the 'crim-inalization' of the mentally ill.[91]

In a 2016 systematic review and meta-analysis of 171 studies of the relationships between homelessness, incarceration, and mental illness, Winkler et al.[92] found a strong correlation between shrinking numbers of psychiatric beds and increasing numbers of people in prison with mental disorders. Noting that with contemporary outpatient care, more effective treatments and community supports, shrinking hos-pital bed numbers do not necessarily indicate shrinking investment in mental health care. In their conclusions, they note:

> Together, these factors suggest that Penrose's hydraulic hypothesis could be stated more precisely as the idea that criminality and homelessness increase as efficacious public in-vestment into mental health decreases. Further research is needed to examine this refined hypothesis.[93]

What remains of the Penrose hypothesis, however, is concern that confinements for mentally ill people may not be ethically justified, if indeed treatments are unavail-able. Throughout the research the motif persists that the ill should not be jailed, nor the criminal be hospitalized.

In his review of (primarily) the sociology literature on crime and mental ill-ness relationships, Markowitz notes that 'Homelessness is an important pathway to incarceration of the mentally ill.'[94] About a third of homeless individuals qualify for a diagnosis of serious mental disorder, and when substance abuse is added, about 75% of the homeless population in the United States have a 'dual diagnosis'. The challenges of measuring the role of homelessness in the MI-crime relation-ship is very difficult—the variability of services, outpatient, inpatient, residential, probation-related, for example, all make the mapping of these relationships very complex.

Using a logistic regression analysis, Hawthorne and colleagues[95] examined 39,463 patient records from the San Diego County public mental health system, along with 4544 matching incarceration records from the county jail system for 2005–2006. They examined the records for a number of sociodemographic, clinical, and social factors to compute what were predictors of incarceration and reincarceration. They found that 11.5% of the patients were incarcerated over the 1-year period. As might be expected from the preceding discussions in this chapter, a co-occurring substance abuse disorder was the most robust predictor of incarceration, closely followed by homelessness status. While acknowledging that clinical diagnosis in the public sector system may not be as accurate as research-based rating scale diagnosis, nev-ertheless the diagnoses of Schizophrenia and Bipolar Disorder were also significant predictors of incarceration. Interestingly, another statistically significant correlate ($p < .001$) was length of stay in jail of greater than 3 days. That is, staying in jail longer was a predictor of reoffending. (This could mean, among other interpretations, that length of stay was proportionate to historically hardened offenders, or the oppo-site, that length of stay was a hardening influence for future criminal activity.) The sociodemographic factors of age, gender, insurance status, race/ethnicity, and prior felony conviction were all nonsignificant. What the remaining significant variable was, which was protective (e.g., inversely related to incarceration) was placement into 'adaptive services' (e.g., outpatient treatment or case management).

Examining psychosocial predictors from a different angle, Stephanie Hartwell and colleagues[96] followed a cohort of 1438 people treated for mental disorders during their incarceration. Following discharge from prison, they examined which psy-chosocial factors correlated with 'intensity' of offending (e.g., number of arrests) following discharge from prison. As might be expected from a prison-population sample, half of the subjects had juvenile justice records, and 77% had at least one prior incarceration. Upon release, almost half were on parole or probation. Approximately 46% of the subjects were reincarcerated over the 2-year follow-up period. Statistically significant protective factors against reincarceration included older age, parole (but not probation), and histories of drug arrests and crimes against people. Risk factors included male gender, prior incarcerations, African-American race, but not a juvenile justice record. The authors note this study is different from prior studies of postdischarge arrest in that the outcome variable was intensity (or frequency) of arrests, instead of a single instance or more of rearrest. The study was also limited in lacking suitable comparison groups.

A review of psychosocial predictors of offending by the mentally ill should include meta-analyses, especially useful in getting a bigger picture of the risk factors.

Bonta and colleagues[97] performed a meta-analysis of predictors of offending by the mentally ill, using 64 independent samples and examining 74 predictor vari-ables. The latter divided into four domains: personal demographic, criminal history, deviant lifestyle, and clinical factors. The most frequent and powerful predictors for general offending (as opposed to violent offending) emerged from the criminal his-tory domain, where all the variables were predictors: number of juvenile convictions, number of adult conventions, nonviolent criminal history, escape history, [poor] in-stitutional adjustment, and the first offense being violent. Youth, male, and single marital status were strong predictors as well, consistent with prior studies. Other than ASPD, other mental disorders were not related, or in the case of psychosis, in-versely related to reoffending. Among the 'deviant lifestyle' variables, family prob-lems and substance abuse were also related.

For violent offending, the criminal history and personal demographic factors were duplicated as for general offending. ASPD and shorter stays in the hospital were related to violent offending, though mood disorders and psychotic disorders were not, the latter again being inversely related to reoffending. The authors con-cluded that criminal history variables and personal demographic variables were more important predictors than diagnosis of mental disorder, substance abuse excluded.

Inspired by the Bonta et al. study, Phillips et al.[98] focused on demographic, criminal history, and clinical factors in a UK cohort. Because they did a retrospective chart review study, 'deviant lifestyle' factors were not collected, because these variables were not reliably recorded in their data sources. They followed 315 dischargees from a single hospital for a minimum of 2 years. They used survival analyses to compute differences between groups because of the variable periods of follow-up. Of their subjects, 115, a little more than a third, reoffended over the study period. Of these, a little over half had at least one violent offense, and a little under half committed a general offense. Their statistical analysis indicated no difference in the predictor variables between those violent and nonviolent reoffenders. Regarding differences in predictors for offenders versus nonoffenders, there were no significant differences between the groups for ethnicity, gender, and marital status. However, those with a diagnosis of Personality Disorder offended significantly more than those with mental illness or mental impairment. However, this effect disappeared when frequency of prior offenses was factored in the analysis. This study also affirmed the weakness of clinical factors in predicting reoffending, taking criminal history factors as much more useful.

In summary, in regard to psychosocial explanations of violence in the setting of mental illness, a few conclusions can be drawn. (1) As with the discussion of factors associated with violence in mental disorders, male gender, youth, poverty, antisocial behavior by parents, prior criminal record, and substance abuse are all important contributors. (2) Other than ASPD and substance abuse disorders, and the concept of psychopathy (discussed below), psychiatric diagnostic categories do not seem to correlate tightly with criminal conduct. (3) Homelessness may be a factor, but it is confounded by the above factors, which are more powerful. The picture that is painted by these psychosocial predictors is that mentally ill offenders (much like nonmentally ill offenders) have early psychosocial deprivation, abuse, associated with early antisocial behavior, which is amplified over time, especially once the young offender gets into the US criminal justice system (so-called hardening of criminal behavior). These psychosocial factors set the stage for biological contributions to the causal nexus, which will be sketched below. Of significance here for the VMDR is that psychosocial risk factors are shared for both criminal offending and developing a mental disorder, point to a potential to address both sets of risks in policymaking.

Many of the relevant biological factors in the crime-mental illness association have been discussed in preceding sections. The key challenge in understanding the biology of mentally ill offenders is disentangling the pathways to particular mental disorders from the pathways to criminal behavior. These, as I've already noted, share many common factors. I think it is fair to say from the beginning that the literature has little to say about causal theories for the mentally ill offender. One reason is the one already stated—the associated risk factors between mental illness and criminality are largely shared. A second reason is that the biology of criminality and mental disorders is poorly understood. A third reason—an epidemiological one—is that both criminality and mental disorders (even limited to just severe mental disorders) are all common conditions, so by chance alone large numbers of people will have both conditions. Moreover, some unknown proportion of those with both conditions will have causal interrelationships that foment antisocial behavior, as well as have interrelationships that inhibit one or another.

With these caveats in mind, let's consider some of the recent and interesting biological factors associated with (particularly) criminal behavior.

A huge body of literature surrounds Robert Hare's contemporary concept of psychopathy, establishing, I believe, very strong evidence that psychopathic individuals, at minimum, have substantive neuroanatomic, neurohormonal, neurophysiological, and neuropsychological differences from the general population. This literature is too big to review here, but a few recommended sources can be viewed in this endnote.[99] Of course, not all mentally ill offenders meet rigorous diagnostic criteria for psychopathy or ASPD.[100]

The literature connecting biological factors to criminality, particularly violent criminality, is also substantial, so I will briefly discuss some key studies and reviews. Harris et al.[101] examined three factors previously identified to be related to criminal violence: neurodevelopmental insults, psychopathy, and antisocial parenting. Analyzing variables related to a sample of 868 violent offender inmates in a maximum-security psychiatric hospital, they found that the three factors clustered into two groups, both sharing the antisocial parenting factor: one involving neurodevelopmental insults plus antisocial parenting, the other being psychopathy plus antisocial parenting.

In a recent review, Peskin and et al.[102] identified six neurobiological factors which give people a predisposition to crime. These included:

1. Genetic factors, based upon heritability estimates for antisocial behavior and gene/environmental interactions.
2. Deficits in frontal, temporal, and subcortical brain regions in criminal and antisocial populations.
3. Adult criminal/antisocial populations have deficits in frontal, temporal, and subcortical brain regions.
4. Autonomic undersarousal and hyporesponsivity (e.g., low resting heart rate) are predictors of later criminality.
5. Antisocial individuals have imbalances between neurohormonal regulation of the fear/stress response, on the one hand, and reward-seeking/dominant behavior, on the other.
6. Additional research on neurodevelopmental factors identified predictors of criminal behavior over the lifespan by prenatal nicotine and ethanol exposure, birth complications, and minor physical anomalies.

All of these factors are probabilistic, and none are definitive in predicting criminality in isolation.

In a 2014 *Nature Reviews Neuroscience* article, introducing the discipline of 'neurocriminology', Glenn and Raine[103] review the growing body of literature supporting a 'neurobiological basis'[104] for criminal behavior and violence. First considering *genetic studies*, they identify over 100 behavioral genetics studies that collectively attribute (e.g., through meta-analyses) a heritability for antisocial and aggressive behavior of approximately 40%–60%. However, as with common serious psychiatric disorders like bipolar disorder and schizophrenia, individual alleles, or gene variants, these contributed no more than 5% of the variance for antisocial/aggressive behavior. Simply put, the gene-by-gene contributions were of small individual effect, but the identified genes as a group had powerful effects. In considering *prenatal and perinatal influences*, Raine gives special emphasis to a Danish study, with replications in four other countries, which identified the combination of birth complications and maternal rejection of the child in the first year of life as a strong predictor of violent criminal offending at the age of 34. As noted earlier, birth complications are identified in other studies as associated with aggression, and delinquency and hyperactivity in childhood/adolescence. Again, as noted earlier, poor parenting compounds the risk as does social adversities of various kinds. A consistent predictor of adult violent offending, also noted by Harris et al. above, is maternal consumption of nicotine and ethanol during pregnancy. Elevated serum lead levels in juveniles (often as a result of exposure to lead-containing paint in impoverished, older neighborhoods) has repeatedly been identified as a predictor of aggressivity in later life, as has malnutrition in infancy. In identifying *neurohormonal factors* such as low childhood cortisol levels, and higher serum testosterone levels in adolescents and adults are associated with criminal aggression. *Psychophysiological studies* have identified, as perhaps the most robust correlate, resting heart rate as inversely related to criminality. That is, as heart rate is lower in populations, the more likely is antisocial behavior. This finding has been replicated many times, in both child/adolescent and adult populations, controlling for multiple confounding variables. However, an absolute heart rate value (such as lower than 60 beats per minute) has not been determined, because individual variability over time is significant, and other confounds (e.g., smoking, medications) are common in populations of interest. So, the significant finding here is not absolute values of heart rate, but rather, the inverse, dimensional relationship of resting heart rate and antisocial behavior. Other physiologic measures associated with increased risk of criminality include decreased skin conductance and slow-frequency electroencephalographic activity. Children and adolescents who have difficulty learning associations between neutral cues and painful or otherwise aversive stimuli are at higher risk of offending. Related measures such as electrodermal fear conditioning are also less robust in future offenders. These findings suggest deficits in learning from aversive experiences.

Regarding *brain imaging studies*, the most robust correlate of antisocial and violent behavior is reduced frontal lobe functioning. More specifically, the most vivid effects were in the dorsolateral prefrontal cortex, anterior cingulate cortex, and orbitofrontal cortex. Analogously, head injuries in presumably normal individuals are associated with postinjury disinhibited antisocial behaviors. Individuals who exhibit deliberative, calculated antisocial activities tend to have small size/volume of their amygdala, while impulsively aggressive individuals have increased amygdala reactivity. A Swedish study of over 200,000 people with traumatic brain injury found their risk for violent crime increased threefold.[105] The amygdala is involved in emotion processing, and emotional reactivity and autonomic processes related to emotions.

In a more recent study, Meijers et al.[106] were interested in digging deeper into the question of violence and brain function. Noting the recent reviews of prefrontal impairments in violent offenders,[107] they were interested comparing prefrontal impairments in violent versus nonviolent offenders. Examining 130 incarcerated offenders (without major mental disorders) in Amsterdam with a variety of neuropsychological instruments, they found that violent offenders were more impaired than nonviolent offenders on the stop-signal task, a measure of response inhibition and located prefrontally. They interpreted this finding in support of their hypothesis that violent offenders would have greater prefrontal impairments.

Collectively these findings suggest that biological abnormalities are very commonly associated with criminal and antisocial behavior, particularly violent behavior; this literature continues to proliferate.[108] Having reviewed the evidence about the factors involved with criminal offending, I now turn to the contribution of popular media contributions to the stigma and public concern about mental illnesses as dangerous.

7.2.2 Media portrayals of crime & mental illness

Those of us who have spent more than a few hours viewing popular films, television, online media, and newspapers can very likely identify multiple examples of negative or stigmatizing portrayals of mental illness in the popular media. Adding criminality to pop-media portrayals amplifies the negative images. These portrayals range from superhero (and supervillain) movies and comics to news coverage of mass shootings to television sitcoms and police procedurals to news accounts of the latest school shooting. A contrast case makes this vivid: What was particularly remarkable about Mahershala Ali's Best Supporting Actor Academy Award in 2017 for *Moonlight* was that his character, an urban African-American drug dealer who takes a homeless child under his wing, undermines two stereotypes, the ruthless pusher and the selfless caretaker, to create a truly multidimensional and nuanced character.

Such complex portrayals are generally absent from depictions of the mentally ill, much less those with criminal propensities.

This section will discuss variations on media portrayals of our items of interest: crime, mental illness, and both together. As a bit of a 'spoiler', what will emerge in this discussion is substantial documentation of negative media portrayals of crime/mental illness. What is less clear, especially in more recent studies, is what role such portrayals actually play in shaping public viewpoints about crime/mental illness, much less the VMDR. That is, while it may be evident in casual observation that media portrayals influence public perception, actually providing research evidence that demonstrates that media portrayals are causally potent, turns out to be challenging and infrequently accomplished. Moreover, the questions about media influence are bilateral. The media are interested in sales and public appeal, thus media makers share an important stake in appealing and 'selling' to the public. What sells depends upon what the public demand is. Thus, the public may play as much a role in shaping negative images of crime/mental illness, as the media plays in delivering what the public wants,[109] which may well be negative images.

That said, a 1990 survey from the Robert Wood Johnson Foundation found that media reports are the most common source of public information about mental illness.[110] Teasing apart the questions of whether media shapes public opinion, or does public opinion shape media content, remains a fundamental challenge for media studies.[111] So the prevailing conclusions of this section, of widespread negative portrayals of criminal and mentally ill people, should be considered in light of this 'chicken or egg' question. Regardless, a safe conclusion is that criminal and/or mentally ill people do have a significant public image problem in that negative images still prevail.

Social scientists as well as clinicians have had interest in the media portrayal of mentally ill people for over 50 years. J. C. Nunnally's groundbreaking *Popular Conceptions of Mental Health*[112] compared mental health expert characterizations with that of the lay public, finding widely divergent viewpoints between the two groups, the latter being pervasively negative. The contemporary elder statesman of research into mental illness in popular media is Otto F. Wahl, Ph.D., Professor of Psychology at the University of Hartford. In a series of studies, reviews, and catalogues since the 1970s, Wahl has documented, relentlessly, the negative portrayals of people with mental illness in popular media whether in film, television, literature, or social media. Wahl's 1992 review of several dozen studies going back to the 1950s concludes:

> . . . media portrayals of mental illness are inaccurate and unfavorable. Bizarre symptoms and more serious psychotic disorders are emphasized. Mentally ill persons presented in the mass media are typically social and occupational failures and possess a number of undesirable character traits, including a propensity for violence. The fears of mental health

advocates that media portrayals may perpetuate negative perceptions of mental illness thus appear to be well-founded.[113]

More recent studies and reviews confirm these negative portrayals. Stout and colleagues[114] in 2004 reviewed the literature since 1990, and in their conclusions, identified gaps in knowledge. They examined 33 international studies which addressed film, television, print, and online media sources. A few of the studies included children's media. The prevailing picture from these studies was that media portrayals most commonly presented mentally ill people as ranging from dangerous to sexualized to uncaring—even in children's media. (However, Slopen et al.[115] found that news stories for children were more likely to provide accurate information about mental illness than adult coverage.) A few studies considered media portrayals of psychiatrists, which commonly were also stereotypical and negative. Gabbard and Gabbard[116] provided ten negative stereotypes (e.g., 'libidinous lecher', 'eccentric buffoon', and 'unempathic coldfish') of psychiatrists out of approximately 300 films reviewed.[117] Stout et al also considered studies which attempted to establish causal relationships between portrayals and public views. The designs of the studies reviewed were variable—ranging from correlational studies, surveys about media influence on one's thinking, and pre- and posttesting of public opinion around media events involving mental illness, considering measures such as 'social distance'—the idea that a person would, or would not, want to be around and have personal connections to a mentally ill person.

These studies, while indicative but not conclusive, supported attributions of media influence. Stout and colleagues also considered a handful of small-scale experimental studies which were supportive of a causal effect of negative media attention. Moreover, a few of these also indicated that education about mental illness was not effective in actually changing attitudes and social distance measurements regarding mentally ill people; indeed, providing biomedical/genetic explanations for mental illness tended to worsen stigmatizing attitudes (mentioned earlier in the section on MHL). In a final section on positive portrayals in the media, a consistent confound was the problem of 'newsworthiness' tending to slant even the most balanced of journalistic accounts of mental illnesses. Stout and colleagues concluded by recommending identifying gaps in the research: the aforementioned gaps in causal relationships between portrayals and attitudes, the collective effects of multiple media 'diets', and the use of media as a source of change in public attitudes.

Stuart, in a 2006 review,[118] echoed many of these themes, but only in more recent years has substantive effort been made to demonstrate causal effects of negative (and positive) media attention to public attitudes about mental illness and criminality.

McGinty, Webster, and Barry,[119] in a 2013 paper, performed an experimental study within the context of a large sample of members of the public ($n = 1797$), built into the context of the social science surveys funded by the National Science Foundation's program 'Time-Sharing Experiments for the Social Sciences'. The authors compared responses about attitudes toward mentally ill people, the latter randomized into four groups: a no-intervention group, and three groups assigned to read one of three news stories before the survey. The news stories varied in content, one involving a mass shooting by a mentally ill person, a second involving the same mass shooting but a call for gun restrictions, and a third involving the same mass shooting but with a proposal to ban large-magazine firearms. Outcome measures involved the previously mentioned social distance measures, as well as perceived dangerousness of people with mental illness, and support for gun restrictions for the mentally ill person. The findings indicated that the mass shooting story significantly increased negative attitudes toward the mentally ill, as well as generated support for gun restriction policies. The latter, however, had no effect on attitudes toward the ill. In a 2016 paper by McGinty's group,[120] a random sample of 400 news stories about mental illness was examined over the 1994–2014 time period. Across the study period, the most frequently mentioned topic across the study period was violence (55% of the stories), with second place going to any topic focusing on mental illness treatment. Only 14% described recovery or successful treatment. During the second decade of the sample, stories about mass shootings by mentally ill people were more prominent than the first decade (e.g., 1995–2005). The authors noted that these frequencies far exceed the actual rates of violence among those people with mental illness.

In a 2015 paper by Nina Barbieri and Nadine Connell,[121] the authors reported a study comparing content analyses of news stories of school shootings in the United States and Germany. While media reports focused on individuals as causes in school shootings, German accounts were more likely to call for state-sponsored changes compared to US media reports.

Ma and Ma[122] provided a current review aimed at educators in considering media influence. Finding many of the same findings regarding negative portrayals in the media, they included more recent social media studies. However, they note that some particular disorders have trends toward more neutral or even positive portrayals, in journalistic as well as fictional media. An example of the latter is the positive response of viewers to the Adrian Monk character who is afflicted with Obsessive-Compulsive Disorder in the TV police procedural series *Monk* from 2002–2009. They conclude that progress is being made in balancing reporting, especially in magazine publications. Evidence is mounting for 'cultivation theory',[123] relating that TV effects multiply proportionately to the amount of TV consumed. Thus, news, entertainment, and advertising all may be relevant in balancing the portrayals of mentally ill people. Notable about the effect of advertising is Haverhals and Lang's study,[124] suggesting more positive responses to mentally ill people as viewers saw more direct-to-consumer advertising for psychotropic medication. Also on the positive side, so-called 'entertainment-education "EE"' programs have been found to be useful for other stigmatized conditions such as HIV.[125] These programs insert a scene, and episode, or turn in a storyline to educate, raise awareness, or otherwise influence behavior in viewers.

Media studies of the portrayal of mental illness are limited in their scope and methodological limitations, but several strong conclusions can be drawn. Media portrayals appear in many guises, from advertising, print, broadcast, digital, and social media. These portrayals, while still largely negative and stigmatizing, have also shown that the depiction of mentally ill individuals in dramatic and ordinary life situations can buffer negative attitudes and reduce stigma. Little is known empirically about the effects of media portrayals of mentally ill offenders, but the existing literature does not paint an optimistic picture about these doubly stigmatizing conditions.

7.3 Conclusions

The public's view of the dangerousness of mentally ill people is complex, as this chapter illustrates. Similarly, the scientific assessment of the dangerousness of mentally ill people, including mentally ill criminal offenders, is complex as well. A few firm conclusions can be drawn, nonetheless. First, the public is influenced strongly by news, entertainment, and social media accounts of people with severe mental disorders. Most of this media influence is negative; leading to common public views of people with severe mental disorders as more dangerous, perhaps far more dangerous, than the science indicates. Little is known about public attitudes toward more minor psychiatric illnesses, and scientific understandings of these conditions. Second, the public tends to stigmatize people with severe mental illness, criminal offenders, and mentally ill offenders, and antistigma campaigns have been of limited impact. The public overestimates the dangerousness of each of these groups and has limited insight into social determinants of these conditions. Instead, these individuals' actions are framed as individual responsibility as a prevailing framework of understanding. The public is often, perhaps typically, unaware of the multiple vectors of influence that shape ill and criminal behavior. Third, these attitudes are part of a general sociological phenomenon of 'negative news', that is, what counts as newsworthy, as well as of entertainment interest, are items which are most shocking, offensive, scary, or otherwise negative. In the realm of people who offend and have mental disorders, images of violent psychopathic individuals, as well as unpredictably violent individuals, such as school or mass shooters, prevail in media imagery. Fourth, the robust scientific finding that mentally ill individuals are more likely to be victims of crime than perpetrators is unappreciated in the public sphere. Fifth, these attitudes are underwritten by inadequate health, mental health, and crime literacy, in turn likely framed by deficiencies in basic education in the social sciences.[126]

These conclusions describe barriers to addressing policy concerning the VMDR. They betray uninformed perspectives that lead to unsympathetic attitudes toward both patients and offenders. Progress in humane reforms relevant to the VMDR will depend upon improvements in formative education as well as in ongoing adult public education. This education effort is especially relevant at the level of public policy development. However, a deeper analysis is needed to understand the challenges, which leads to the next chapter.

Notes

1. Hirsch (1983, 1985).
2. Hirsch (1987).
3. Hirsch (1983, p. 163).
4. Interested readers who want to know more about the controversies about cultural literacy in education might start with; Bernstein (1988); Christenbury (1989); Edwards (1984); Hallinan (2010); Hirsch (1983, 1985); Mullican (1991); Schuster (1989); Smith (1988).
5. For more about the concept of health literacy, see Nutbeam (2000) and Kutner, Greenburg, Jin, & Paulsen (2006).
6. Jorm (2012 p. 1); see also Jorm (1997 p. 182).
7. See Jorm (2012) for a recent review.
8. Wang et al. (2007).
9. See Ibrahim (2005). Survival analysis is a statistical technique used to track the time to the occurrence of particular events. In the case here, the event of interest is treatment seeking. See https://community.amstat.org/northeasternillinoischapter/events/past-events/new-item/new-item2 for a detailed discussion of survival analysis.
10. Jorm (2000, 2012).
11. Gulliver, Griffiths,& Christensen (2010).
12. ibid, p. 5, Table 1.
13. Thompson, Issakidis, & Hunt (2008); see also Lauber et al. (2003).
14. Jorm (2012, p. 2).
15. Sadler (2007) notes that mental illness is often experienced as part of a 'personal self' where existential themes (e.g., anxiety, sadness, and lack of directedness) blend into mental illness, leading to a blurring of the self/illness distinction.
16. See Burns & Rapee (2006); Jorm (2012); Jorm & Wright (2007).
17. Jorm (2012); see also Jorm, Christensen, & Griffiths (2006); Jorm & Wright (2007).
18. Jorm (2012).
19. See for instance Dahlberg et al. (2008); Jorm et al. (2005); Kovess-Masfety et al. (2007); Jorm et al. (1997); Lauber et al. (2001); Riedel-Heller et al. (2005); Wang et al. (2007).
20. What we do when people need mental health assistance Jorm (2012) calls 'mental health first aid'.
21. See Barkan & Bryjak (2011).
22. For those few who do not know the difference, Google surveys all web documents, while Google Scholar focuses on academic or scholarly references only.
23. http://www.albany.edu/sourcebook/tost_2.html#2_n.
24. http://www.bjs.gov/index.cfm?ty=pbse&sid=46.
25. http://www.albany.edu/sourcebook/pdf/t2332011.pdf.
26. http://www.albany.edu/sourcebook/pdf/t2352011.pdf.

27. http://www.bjs.gov/index.cfm?ty=dcdetail&iid=245. See also Morgan & Thompson (2021); Rennison (2002).

28. Tonry (2011 p. 7); see also Zimring (2006).

29. Zimring (2006). See also Chapter 6 for more data on crime rates after 2010.

30. http://albany.edu/sourcebook/csv/t31062008.csv.

31. Cuthbertson (2013).

32. See Gingrich & Nolan (2011); Leonard (2015); Mauer (2011).

33. Nunnally (1961).

34. Rabkin (1972, 1974).

35. Steadman & Cocozza (1977).

36. ibid, pp. 525–526.

37. Steadman & Cocozza (1978).

38. Hartwell (2004).

39. Brooks (1985).

40. See for example Bloechl et al. (2007); Fingarette (1976); Geis & Meier (1985); Gross (1985); Hamilton (1986); Hans (1986); Hans & Slater (1983); Moran (1985); Morse (1985); Resnick (1986); Slater & Hans (1984). In the literature review for this chapter, it was remarkable that scholarly interest in the 'insanity defense' waned considerably after the Hinckley-associated peak in the mid-1980s to early 1990s.

41. See the Chapter 6 discussion of the ALI standard (Section 6.1.1.2).

42. Pasewark (1986).

43. ibid, p. 103.

44. Pasewark (1986).

45. ibid, p. 104.

46. Hans & Slater (1983, quotation p. 207).

47. ibid.

48. Hans (1986).

49. Silver et al. (1994).

50. Steadman & Cocozza (1978).

51. Silver et al. (1994, p. 65).

52. Pasewark & Seidenzahl (1979).

53. Pasewark (1986).

54. Steadman & Braff (1983).

55. Callahan et al. (1991).

56. Cirincione et al. (1995).

57. Borum & Fulero (1999).

58. Berlin, Saleh, & Malin (2009).

59. Silva et al. (2002).

60. Foucault (1999) describes the human 'monster' as an entity whose 'existence and form is not only a violation of the laws of society but also a violation of the laws of nature. Its very existence is a breach of the law at both levels. . . .The monster combines the impossible and the forbidden' (pp. 55–56).

61. Nevertheless, see Greer & Jewkes (2005); Tewkesbury (2005); Viki et al. (2012), Wikipedia 2002.

62. See Burchfield & Mingus (2008); Schiavone & Jeglic (2009); Tewksbury (2005); Tewlsbury & Lees (2006).

63. See Quinn, Forsyth, & Mullen-Quinn (2004).

64. Brown (1999).

65. Harris & Socia (2016).

66. Burchfield & Mingus (2008); Harris & Socia (2016); Mancini & Budd (2016); Schiavone & Jeglic (2009).

67. Kutner, Greenberg, Jin, Paulsen, & White (2006).
68. Gazmararian, Baker, Williams et al. (1999).
69. See Pleasant (2013) for an international overview of health literacy.
70. Stuart (2003). See also Maniglio (2009) regarding the increased probabilities of the mentally ill being victimized.
71. Fazel et al. (2009). See also Rund (2018).
72. Friedman (2006).
73. Monahan & Arnold (1996, p. 70).
74. Belfrage (1998); Brennan et al. (2000); Choe et al. (2008); Fazel & Grann (2006); Fazel et al. (2010); Fazel et al. (2011);); Flynn et al. (2021); Furokawa (2015); Harris & Lurigio (2007); Hodgins (1995); Labrum et al. (2021); Lichtenstein et al. (2012); Markowitz (2010); Silver et al. (2008); Steadman & Felson (1984); Steadman et al. (1998); Steadman et al. (1999); Swanson et al. (2002); Swanson et al. (2006); Timonen et al. (2002); Van Dorn et al. (2012).
75. Hodgins & Côté (1993).
76. A substantial number of inmates sampled refused to participate, hence the discrepancy between the total number of participants and the number sampled from prison records.
77. Joyal et al. (2011).
78. Matejkowski et al. (2014).
79. Tillman (1987). See also *The President's Commission on Law Enforcement and Administration of Justice. The Challenge of Crime in a Free Society* (1967).
80. Steury (1993).
81. Hasin & Grant (2015).
82. Elbogen & Johnson (2009).
83. Van Dorn et al. (2012).
84. Fazel & Grann (2006).
85. ibid, p. 1397.
86. Whiting, Lichtenstein, & Fazel (2020).
87. Silver et al. (2008).
88. ibid.
89. Penrose (1939).
90. See Ceccherini-Nelli & Priebe (2007); Lamb (2015).
91. Engel & Silver (2001); Teplin (1984).
92. Winkler et al. (2016).
93. ibid, p. 426.
94. Markowitz (2011, p. 37).
95. Hawthorne et al. (2012). See also Putkonen et al. (2004); Tengström et al. (2004).
96. Hartwell et al. (2016).
97. Bonta et al. (1998).
98. Phillips et al. (2005).
99. See Blair (2010); Buckholz et al. (2010); Fine & Kennett (2004); Haji (2010); Hare, Neumann, & Widiger (2012); Hillis (2014); Kotler & McMahon (2005); Tengstrom et al. (2004); Vidal, Skeem & Camp (2010); Yang et al. (2009).
100. See for instance Gray et al. (2003); Tengstrom et al. (2004); Putkonen et al. (2004).
101. Harris et al. (2001).
102. Peskin et al. (2012).
103. Glenn & Raine (2014).
104. ibid, p. 54.
105. Fazel et al. (2011).
106. Meijers et al. (2017).
107. Cruz Castro-Rodrigues, & Barbosa (2020); Morgan & Lilienfeld (2000); Ogilvie et al. (2011).

108. For additional, more recent reviews of the biosocial etiologies of criminality, see Barnes, Raine, & Farrington (2020); Choy et al. (2019); Kahhale (2022); Ling, Umbach, & Raine (2019).
109. Birkbeck (2014). See also Steadman (1981).
110. DYG Inc. (1990).
111. Birkbeck (2014). See also Barak (1994); Collins (2014); Cross (2004); Gkotskis et al. (2016); Greer & Jewkes (2005); Hollis et al. (2017); Jewkes (2015); Oliver (2003); Olstead (2002); Reiner (2007); Sieff (2003).
112. Nunnally (1961). See also Rabkin (1972).
113. Wahl (1992 p. 348). See also Wahl (1997).
114. Stout et al. (2004).
115. Slopen et al. (2007).
116. Gabbard & Gabbard (1992).
117. Discussed in Stout et al. (2004, p. 553).
118. Stuart (2006).
119. McGinty, Webster, & Barry (2013).
120. McGinty et al. (2016). See also Thornicroft et al. (2013).
121. Barbieri & Connell (2015).
122. Ma (2017).
123. ibid, p. 101.
124. Haverhals & Lang (2004).
125. Schouten et al. (2014).
126. See Lin (2013); Osler & Starkey (2006); Oulton et al. (2004); Ross (2004); Sadler (2022).

8

Deepening the analysis of the vice/mental disorder relationship

Cancel my subscription to the resurrection
Send my credentials to the house of detentions
—The Doors, 'When the Music's Over'

Vice and Psychiatric Diagnosis. John Z. Sadler, Oxford University Press. © Oxford University Press 2024.
DOI: 10.1093/oso/9780198876830.003.0008

In this chapter, I use some of the conceptual tools developed in previous chapters to reformulate an approach to the vice/mental disorder relationship (VMDR). The first section considers the importance of folk-metaphysical assumptions in the VMDR. The second section revisits and rethinks the four exemplar models of the VMDR. The third section then formulates and defends a fifth model, the rehabilitation model. This material then sets the stage for the concluding Chapter 9, where I consider many of the conceptual, ethical, and practical problems of the VMDR in light of a rehabilitation model and the practical and structural changes this new model implies.

8.1 Revisiting the significance of folk-metaphysical assumptions in the VMDR

In Chapter 3, Section 3.6.1, I introduced the idea of folk-metaphysical assumptions and briefly stated their role in shaping diagnostic categories in the *Diagnostic and Statistical Manual of Mental Disorders* (DSM). For this section I elaborate on the concepts of folk metaphysics (FM) and folk-metaphysical assumptions as a keener understanding of these ideas is crucial to my reformulation of the VMDR. It turns out that understanding folk-metaphysical assumptions underlying the VMDR illuminates many of the peculiarities of the VMDR identified in prior chapters. Moreover, this discussion should also provide some philosophical insights into a number of related conceptual problems or ambiguities in the philosophy of psychiatry. These latter issues will be further developed prescriptively in the last chapter.

This section proceeds in three steps. (1) After describing what I mean by folk metaphysics, (2) I briefly discuss some key examples of folk-metaphysical assumptions that appear in mental health and psychiatric discourse relevant to the VMDR, including those of the psychiatric sciences. In this regard, I revisit, very briefly, the development of these exemplar Western folk-metaphysical assumptions which were introduced in Chapters 4 and 5. (3) I then take these exemplar folk-metaphysical assumptions and show how they are embedded in several controversies in VMDR-relevant psychiatric practice, research, and the philosophy of psychiatry.

8.1.1 What are folk metaphysics and their assumptions?

As a preliminary to my discussion of folk-metaphysical assumptions, I want to call the reader's attention to important differences in how we, as people in ordinary life, in contrast to philosophers, engage with the world. In our ordinary, day-to-day lives, we are engaged (nonphilosophically) in an unreflective, perhaps naive way. That is, we make countless assumptions about how the world works, and why people do the things they do, immersed as we are in the flow of everyday life. We assume the sun will indeed rise tomorrow morning, that the clothing that was behind my closet door yesterday will, more or less, still be there today; that my wife's curtness to me this evening was because she had a bad day at work; and so forth. The philosopher Edmund Husserl called this kind of accepting, uncritical engagement with our everyday experience the 'natural attitude'.[1]

However, philosophers, in doing their philosophical work, suspend this naive regard of the world. When doing philosophy, they reflect upon, among other things, the reasons why things are one way rather than some other way, what assumptions we hold about human nature and existence, how we can secure credible knowledge, and how we might find the right way to live. Engaging in this thinking and questioning is to philosophize, and a key way to philosophize is to search for and describe 'metaphysical assumptions'. These kinds of assumptions we hold in our everyday engagement with the world, assumptions that, when not philosophizing, everyone takes for granted. In taking these everyday assumptions for granted, we are able to function effectively and efficiently in our day-to-day lives. Philosophy makes time, however, to call these everyday assumptions into question—assumptions I will call 'folk-metaphysical' assumptions.

An analogy may help in understanding folk-metaphysical assumptions. In the analytic philosophy of mind, philosophers have explored how people in ordinary life make sense of *human behavior*—this latter now commonly called 'folk psychology'. While much has been written about folk psychology, a substantive engagement with this literature would digress from my particular interests here. Here, I mention the folk psychology concept in philosophy of mind as an analogy, as a conceptual stepping-stone, in describing what I call 'folk metaphysics or (FM)', which might be thought of as the foundations of folk psychology. For this comparison, I provide a standard-reference description of folk psychology below. I intend the analogy, however limited, to be indicative, because my folk-metaphysical concept is more difficult to describe, and inferential in its character.

Ian Ravenscroft, in his *Stanford Encyclopedia of Philosophy* entry[2] on folk psychology, describes three senses of the term. Only one of them is relevant for my purposes here. Ravenscroft attributes this notion of folk psychology to philosopher David Lewis. Lewis describes folk psychology as a psychological theory made up of 'platitudes about the mind's function held by ordinary people'. Folk psychology in this sense is identified as how ordinary people inquire about, or understand, why we do the things we do. To explain our behavior, people present accounts (involving various of Lewis's platitudes) of themselves or others using concepts like meaning, emotions, goals, objectives, purposes, stories, and reasons. This latter array of psychological concepts, along with their particular examples, constitute Lewis's set of platitudes about the mind's function. These meaning-making categories in ordinary language are the stuff of folk psychology.

Folk psychology in this sense is an *observable* because if you want to know people's folk-psychological beliefs, you can simply ask them, for example, Why did Donald Trump appeal to so many American voters? or Why did you keep drinking excessively after your driving-while-intoxicated arrest? People will respond in terms of emotions, goals, objectives, or reasons—the terms of Lewis's folk psychology. The 'folk' refers to the likelihood that people will respond, generally, in commonsense language, not the technical language of science (unless, of course, they are scientists, which will be considered later). However, responding in commonsense language is also to acknowledge that scientific knowledge and language can be assimilated into the cultures of commonsense discourse, which then leads to the complexities of folk versus scientific psychology as these discourses intermingle and become more complex.

The concept of FM, on the other hand, is a distinct philosophical concept apart from folk psychology because it describes not psychology but metaphysics, and more specifically, metaphysical assumptions. Like folk psychology, FM are concerned with platitudes, but in the latter case, platitudes about the *nature of reality* held by ordinary people. These metaphysical platitudes are assumed, and rarely explicit—indeed, often so taken for granted that they often lurk, unmentioned and assumed, as the building-blocks for the reasons, beliefs, and attitudes of folk psychology. Unlike discovering precepts of folk psychology through simply asking someone, the presentations of FM are rarely evident to the nonphilosopher through simple inquiry, rather, they have to be *inferred* as assumptions. I define folk metaphysics as:

> The summary cultural assumptions, held by groups of people, about the nature of reality and existence, what it means to be human, how we know things, and the sources of the good.

From this definition, I claim that FM represent a distinct realm of thought, encompassing, for instance, the fundamental assumptions about the nature of reality—apart from simple rationales for human behavior (e.g., folk psychology). For convenience, I will heretofore refer to these four aspects of metaphysics—(1) the nature of reality and existence, (2) what it means to be human, (3) how we know things, and (4) the sources of the good—as the 'metaphysical domain', which can be considered under either the folk-metaphysical or a philosophical metaphysics lens. Referring to a metaphysical domain is to say that philosophers, when doing philosophy within the metaphysical domain as philosophers, do so in a typically philosophical, reflective fashion, while ordinary people, when acting within the metaphysical domain, typically do so in a folk, commonsensical, nonreflective, nonanalytical way. In describing FM, I will contrast it with philosophical metaphysics (PM) in discussions to follow. In other words, once we take the metaphysical domain as a 'space' of reflection and consideration, we step out of the folk-metaphysical 'stance' and enter the philosophical stance.

As cultural assumptions, FM may be relative to cultural groups and interact with the intersectionality of individual members of a cultural group. That is, folk-metaphysical assumptions are often broadly shared, but do not have to be, and may differ in their expression through personal and public history, culture, regionality, and ethnicity.

I identify 11 interrelated features of FM. These features distinguish FM from philosophical metaphysics (PM) which are the inquiries and discussions in the metaphysical domain performed through formal philosophizing.

8.1.2 Contrasting folk metaphysics (FM) and philosophical metaphysics (PM)

In contrast to PM, FM are:

1. **Unsystematic**. FM, as taken for granted, provide no systematic accounts of the metaphysical domain. As assumed, folk-metaphysical assumptions are rarely, if ever, considered how they fit together. Contradictions abound and are tolerated easily. For example, within the folk-metaphysical standpoint, we typically are not bothered by the contradiction between our actions being directed by 'free will' on the one hand, and being influenced by environmental circumstances, on the other. Both ideas are assumed, accepted, and acted upon in ordinary living. In contrast to the unsystematic feature of FM, some philosophical metaphysicians, exhibiting systematic thinking, may question the compatibility of free will and determinism. Even 'compatibilist' philosophers who are untroubled by free will and determinism taken together, provide careful philosophical reasons why, providing a philosophical-metaphysical account of this problem. The philosopher doing PM does not assume compatibility between free will and determinism, as might a person within the folk-metaphysical standpoint.

2. **Naive**. The assumptions of FM, as noted earlier, are taken for granted in everyday life, and rarely questioned. In day-to-day life, we skip along our paths, like children, without considering the nature of reality, the sources of the good, and the means to knowledge, for example. If folk-metaphysical assumptions are questioned, this is done through serious philosophizing, which of course most people, even philosophers, don't do in the midst of the hurly-burly of daily living. Occasionally, exceptional experiences (e.g., mystical experience, psychological trauma, and some mental illnesses like psychosis) disrupt our taken-for-granted folk-metaphysical assumptions, and prompt us to reconsider our ideas about reality, the good, and our place in the world, for example. While exceptional experiences is a topic worth exploring, it's not relevant to my discussion here.

3. **Partially and variably shared among peoples**. While many folk-metaphysical assumptions are shared, many can, and do, differ across cultures. For example, many cultures may agree that a person occupying the same body over time is the same person, but cultural groups may disagree about whether the

individual or the family is the center of moral considerations. Even within cultures, diversity of folk-metaphysical assumptions are common, such as the diversity of assumptions about the nature of a God or gods.

4. **Anthropological.** Related to the above, FM are culture-laden—anthropological—while PM aspire to universality and independence from cultural assumptions, traditions, and entailments. Philosophical metaphysicians talk about 'essences', 'invariants', 'existentials', 'apodicticity', and 'universals', for example. I say 'aspire' toward universality to acknowledge the difficulty in transcending one's metaphysical standpoint to transcend culture and history.

5. **Normatively powerful.** Folk-metaphysical assumptions are 'lived-by' or normatively powerful. This means that people's core values or ultimate concerns are intertwined with folk-metaphysical assumptions and lived out in accordance with such FM-framed ultimate concerns, in the conduct of their everyday life. Consequently, they build their lives around these folk-metaphysical assumptions. For example, the scientist who lives-by the folk-metaphysical assumption of a law-governed mechanistic universe may strongly oppose, and be disturbed by, claims to the contrary, such as the earth being only 5000 years old. The fundamentalist Christian may strongly oppose biological evolution, and its mechanistic metaphysics, as evolution contradicts her lived-by scriptural beliefs about the Creation. For if scripture falters with Creation under evolution science, then what reliability and credibility of scripture is left for the Christian's life path?[3]

6. **Institutionally imbricated.** Social, cultural, and political institutions depend upon assumptions about the metaphysical domain and build their institutions around them.[4] A relevant example to be discussed later is the assumption of free will and individual responsibility for actions, concepts which we can recognize from Chapter 6 as folk-metaphysical assumptions in Western criminal law. These folk-metaphysical assumptions are 'imbricated' into criminal law institutions: their structures, policies, and procedures, providing structural integrity for criminal law around a shared, deeply assumed, metaphysical account of reality and human nature.

7. **Underwrite the sciences.** Because all sciences require metaphysical-domain assumptions about such things as the nature of reality and being, and how to secure genuine or credible knowledge, the sciences are built upon and practiced in accordance with folk-metaphysical assumptions, as implied in the earlier example of the scientist. The scientist does not have conclusive proof of the mechanistic nature of the universe, the latter is an assumption which enables her to do her work. Relevant to our discussions later, FM underwrite both folk- and scientific psychologies and biologies by providing fundamental folk-metaphysical assumptions for research to build upon.

8. **Commonsensical and intuitively evident.** More than just a naive unquestioning in Point 2 above, folk-metaphysical assumptions are not typically

treated with active skepticism, analysis, or suspension-of-belief (as in PM), but rather actively defended as self-evident common sense, something that 'everyone knows' and which sensible people do not question. (Alas, philosophy is not for everyone.) Even in philosophical practice, philosophers may appeal to 'ordinary intuitions' in developing metaphysical arguments. The problem with the latter, as Ladyman et al.[5] have reviewed, is that science has repeatedly demonstrated the occasional unreliability and even falsity of 'ordinary intuitions.'

9. **Everyone uses** (folk-metaphysical assumptions). Folk-metaphysical assumptions are required for the smooth conduct of everyday life, and hence everyone uses them. Folk-metaphysical assumptions have practical utility, which philosophical-metaphysical assumptions, at least in ordinary, everyday living, do not. How reality works is taken for granted, and decisions based upon folk-metaphysical assumptions permit our practical, everyday engagement with the world. A person who aims to act routinely based upon a systematic philosophical-metaphysical account would likely find himself immobilized by analysis and end up in psychiatric care!

10. **Philosophers may question them.** Often, in PM, philosophers may question folk-metaphysical assumptions. However, because of the aforementioned features like their normative power, their habitual embeddedness as assumptions, and their self-evident, commonsensical nature, even philosophers may fail to question their own folk-metaphysical assumptions. For example, Descartes had difficulty suspending his assumptions about the Christian God in developing his formal metaphysics; indeed, the assumption of God's existence and characteristics became interwoven, as a given, into his philosophical methods and metaphysics.[6]

11. **Deeply assumed in ordinary conduct.** FM are phenomena rarely referred to by anyone, so deeply embedded are they in ordinary human affairs. The prior ten features summate to shape the deeply taken-for-grantedness of folk-metaphysical assumptions, making them essentially invisible or undetectable in ordinary, nonreflective engagement with the world.

8.1.3 Expressions of folk-metaphysical assumptions

With this background, I can provide some additional examples of *expressions* of folk-metaphysical beliefs. I focus on 'expressions' because, as assumptions, folk-metaphysical assumptions can, as noted earlier, only be inferred, not observed directly, or solicited by query. For example, the shoplifter, when caught, does not say 'I feel guilty about my act because I am a free-will compatibilist and guilt is a derivative of that metaphysical standpoint.' (e.g., a philosophical-metaphysical expression). Rather, the person simply says, 'I feel guilty about stealing.' (a folk-metaphysical expression about responsibility for his choice.)

The following examples depict the derivative nature of folk-metaphysical assumptions; they are expressed through beliefs and claims about self and world. The examples are then contrasted, in parentheses, with alternative metaphysical assumptions. Neither position within my contrast cases is 'right'; all assumptions have limits because they are assumptions, not inviolate metaphysical certitude. On to sample expressions of FM, chosen for their later relevance to understanding the VMDR:

A. The Lord is my Savior. (A derivative belief based on the folk-metaphysical assumption there is a God. This claim of Lord as Savior makes no conventional sense without a belief in God.)

B. Everything has a cause. (A derivative claim based on the folk-metaphysical assumption of an ordered universe. The statement would make no sense without the folk-metaphysical assumptions of (as two examples) a natural mechanistic universe or a Homeric one controlled by the gods.)

C. People can freely choose for themselves. (This folk-metaphysical belief makes sense only if one assumptively disqualifies or ignores contrary evidence.)

D. I alone am responsible for my salvation. (A derivative belief based upon the folk-metaphysical assumptions that post-death salvation exists, and that only individual persons can qualify. Conventional Christian believers cannot obtain Christian salvation on a group plan, only by *individual* faith and acceptance of the Lord God.)

E. A metaphysics of mind/brain must conform to my intuitions. (A derivative folk-metaphysical claim based upon the assumption that my intuitions are indubitable. Science often provides powerful evidence to the contrary.)

F. Electrons are real. (A derivative folk-metaphysical claim based on the assumption of scientific realism, the view that theoretical, unobservable, and sedimented scientific concepts concretely exist and contribute to the true fabric of reality.)

8.1.4 Philosophical metaphysics contrasted with folk metaphysics

PM differ from FM in having a specific set of aspirations, in contrast to the nonaspirational FM, whose assumptions are practical and taken for granted. These aspirations are, for the most part, not controversial and are descriptive of philosophical inquiry as a field or practice. For example, some examples of philosophical-metaphysical aspirations might include:

1. To provide a systematic account.
2. To provide a scholarly, rigorous, and comprehensive account.
3. To be credible, or even reflect truths.
4. To be culture-independent, not culture-relative.

Moreover, PM exhibit certain characteristics or behavior not exhibited by FM. Some descriptive examples include these:

PM tends to:

1. Be abstract in language and concepts.
2. Have limited practical applications in everyday life.
3. NOT be imbricated into institutions, and if so, by happenstance cultural assimilation (e.g., Cartesian dualism in psychology).

Having discussed the concept of FM, and some common folk-metaphysical assumptions in the Western world, I turn now to why they are important in psychiatry and the VMDR, aided by a review-sketch of their historical origins. I should note that, for the most part, our folk-metaphysical assumptions function quite well in our day-to-day lives, providing for efficient and effective practical engagement with the world. As one might imagine, when called into question with commonly accepted views about common sense, such as the nature of reality and the validity of one's personal life path, challenges to folk-metaphysical assumptions are accompanied by controversy and personal resistance. Such is the case with my examples from psychiatry in a later section.

8.2 Madness, morality, and the Enlightenment Split

I now can begin to spell out the payoff for understanding folk-metaphysical assumptions in the face of the problems in the VMDR. Many examples are possible of how the analysis of folk-metaphysical assumptions could be of value in the philosophy of psychiatry. In earlier publications, I described what I called then 'ontological values'[7] and how they manifested in the structure and categories of the Diagnostic and Statistical Manual of Mental Disorders (DSMs).[8] What I meant by 'ontological values' were values which were tied to particular ontological assumptions about the world, including what today I would describe as values tied to various folk-metaphysical assumptions in the ontological (component of the metaphysical) domain.

This book has considered how particular kinds of values—vice—have played into DSM concepts and categories. Recognition of the vice-laden disorders in the DSM then leads to questions around why some categories in the DSMs are frankly vice-laden, while others are not, and perhaps equally important, how vice-laden mental disorder categories developed in history. In considering these latter questions, I discovered the importance of folk-metaphysical assumptions in writing the history chapters of this book. At this point, I emphasize some examples of folk-metaphysical assumptions that are relevant to understanding the intellectual history of vice-laden mental disorders. These provide concrete examples of the utility of the analysis of folk-metaphysical assumptions in psychiatric controversy.

So, given the project on vice-laden mental disorders, my examples of the relevance of FM to philosophy of psychiatry will be cast in terms of the folk-metaphysical assumptions of criminal law, on the one hand, and the folk-metaphysical assumptions of psychiatry, on the other. I think the incompatibilities with the FM of these two fields is most broadly and clearly described in this short passage from Stephen Morse, a psychologist, attorney, and scholar at the University of Pennsylvania:

> The law's concept of a person is as a practical reasoning, rule-following being, most of whose legally relevant movements must be understood in terms of beliefs, desires, and intentions.[9]

Morse's 'concept of the person' fits transparently into a folk psychology rubric. However, I would aver, folk-metaphysical assumptions are intertwined through statements like: 'Hinckley shot Reagan in order to impress Jodie Foster.' 'Mr. Jones robbed the hospital pharmacy because his child would die without the medication he couldn't afford.' 'He killed his wife in a jealous rage because of her affair with Bob.' In each of these examples, the actions of the protagonist are explained in terms of reasons, intentions, desires, and beliefs. These folk-psychological concepts are embedded in a larger account of human nature, as implied by Morse' use of 'the concept of a person' in the law (e.g., an informal account of human nature and being). (Note that Morse uses metaphysical language: the 'concept' of the person, not the 'psychology' of the person, as in folk psychology.) The specifics of this larger account of human nature, the FM, will be discussed shortly.

Morse connects this 'concept of a person' to two competing views about human action:

> When one asks about human action, 'why did she do that?' two distinct types of answers may therefore be given. The reason-giving explanation accounts for human behavior as a product of intentions that arise from the desires and beliefs of the agent. The second type of explanation treats human behavior as simply one more bit of the phenomena of the universe, subject to the same natural, physical laws that explain all phenomena.[10]

What Morse calls the 'reason-giving explanation' of folk psychology, I claim is underwritten by a set of folk-metaphysical assumptions that are imbricated into Western common and criminal law and discussed at length in Chapters 4, 5, and 6, and exemplified in public minds in Chapter 7. These folk-metaphysical assumptions of criminal law include the ideas of (1) *free will*, that individuals can, by and large, choose their actions; (2) that people are *individually responsible* for their own choices, as opposed to those of other people, external forces, the community, or society (heretofore called 'personal responsibility' for brevity); and (3) that people get their 'just *deserts*'; that is, they should get what is due to them, either positive (good) or negative (bad) (e.g., in the case of wrongdoing, punishment).

Remember that Morse then contrasted this reason-giving explanation within the law with that of natural-scientific explanations of the behavior. I interpret Morse here to mean that the second kind of explanation is of a causal-mechanical kind of the natural and some of the human or behavioral sciences. To frame this in my own terms, the implication is that the second kind of explanation given by the sciences employs a different set of folk-metaphysical assumptions, those of the natural and the social sciences. Some examples of these folk-metaphysical assumptions include: (1) the universe, including human behavior, while complex, is orderly and has a discoverable structure; (2) part of the order of the universe is that causal relationships exist, that is, one set of events can lead to additional events in an orderly fashion: (3) and that human actions are not simply matters of choice, but rather the end result of extremely complex-causal relationships involving many partial determinants internal and external to the human organism. I summarily refer to this second set of folk-metaphysical assumptions the 'complex-multicausal account'.[11] A quick look at (3) of this latter account suggests that the complex-multicausal (CMC) folk-metaphysical account of the sciences may have difficulties in compatibility with the reason-giving account of the law, which is Morse's conclusion, albeit not stated in the FM terminology I use here.

As a more specific example, the conflict of 'free will' concepts with CMC FM is a root of philosophical-metaphysical and philosophy of science debates about the existence, meaning, or structure of 'free will', and derivatively, the concept of moral responsibility. A colossal formal-philosophical literature has emerged from these conflicts[12] which I cannot review here, but simply call to attention.

Morse intends, as do I, to point out that scientific psychology and psychiatry present polymorphous combinations of the reason-giving (RG) folk-metaphysical account, as in law, as well as, and even simultaneously with, the CMC-folk-metaphysical account. This mixing-up of RG (Abrahamic FM) and CMC-folk-metaphysical accounts leads to confusing contradictions and ambiguities. That is, contemporary psychiatry (and clinical psychology as well) mixes up its folk-metaphysical assumptions. Remember, folk-metaphysical assumptions are unsystematic and naive, so in everyday life pose few to no difficulties with contradictions. For example, the hierarchically organized, multilevel, up- and down-regulated, multiconnected, subsystem-laden accounts of neuroscience's explanations of human behavior (e.g., Schaffner (1993)[13] or the Research Domain Criteria (RDoC) scheme[14]) mix well with the CMC-folk-metaphysical account. Freudian psychoanalytic theories of human behavior postulate human actions based upon intentional, RG actions of the ego, along with potentially conflicting irrational causal drives of the id, and inhibitory, habitual constraints of the superego. The tripartite causation described by Freud thus combines folk-metaphysical elements of both the reasons-giving RG account as well as a CMC account, here phrased in terms of deterministic, hydraulic-like vector metaphors between id, ego, and superego. In biological psychiatry the severe mental disorders are considered primarily under a CMC-folk-metaphysical account; but personality disorders often are not, and are considered under a developmental, reasons-giving account based (e.g.) in psychodynamic theory or cognitive-behavioral theory, where the patient has learned maladaptive habitual ways of thinking and acting.[15] In sum, psychology and psychiatry are content (most of the time), from the folk-metaphysical standpoint, of mixing free-will accounts of human behavior and personal responsibility with deterministic CMC accounts.

Before providing more concrete examples of how the CMC-folk-metaphysical account and the reasons-giving folk-metaphysical account play out in philosophy of psychiatry, it may be clarifying to provide a brief historical reframing and synthesis of how these discrepancies in folk-metaphysical worldviews came about. The review-sketch is based upon numerous sources, most importantly, the historical backgrounds of Chapters 4, 5, and 6, which detailed the development of morality and 'madness'. However, the illuminating intellectual histories of Martin and Barresi (2006); Porter (2003); Seidentop (2014); and Thomson (1993) were also key.[16] The framing of this history in terms of FM assumptions, however, is my own.

As many historians of Western medicine and psychiatry/madness have described, prior to the fifteenth century, historical assumptions about the nature of madness centered on supernatural accounts: madness was a manifestation of supernatural interventions by gods and demons, or tests or punishments by the gods.[17] Later in the Christian Medieval era, the Roman Catholic Church, as well as Judaism and Islam elsewhere, the folk-metaphysical assumptions of these Abrahamic religions concerning free will, individual responsibility for salvation or its equivalents, and desert underwrote then-contemporary ideas about madness and morality. The earlier Chapters 4 through 7 provide abundant evidence of the cultural sedimentation and saturation of these folk-metaphysical assumptions in the contemporary West.

Figure 8.1 picks up these historical accounts in the medieval era and beyond. The figure frames the folk-metaphysical assumptions of the respective eras in four terms: views of the nature of madness and its social controls, and views of wrongdoing and its social controls. In the mid- to late-medieval era, views of madness were framed in the aforementioned terms of demon-possession, or tests or punishments from the Abrahamic God. During this period the vectors of social control were primarily the Church and community; the former using education, spiritual interventions (e.g., confession, atonement, prayer, and exorcism) and threats (e.g., excommunications, eternal damnation). The latter (community) often resorted to public humiliations such as the stocks, or expulsions, but often, compassion and tolerant care were provided, with and without Church sanction.

In terms of wrongdoing (the contemporary concept of crime had yet to develop during the medieval centuries in Europe), the Biblical concept of sin dominated thinking, rooted again in the ancient Abrahamic religious metaphysics of individual responsibility, free will, and desert. In this era, Christian and Islamic sin encompassed what today we would call criminal conduct (e.g., sin against others), as well as contemporary legal but immoral conduct (e.g., ordinary lying), and occasionally immoral thoughts as well (e.g., coveting thy neighbor's wife). For Judaism the notion of sin is more complicated; the Christian notion of original sin doesn't apply, and

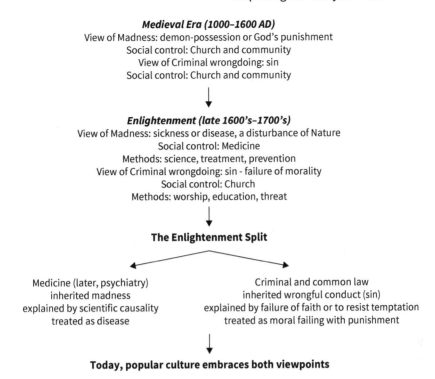

Medieval Era (1000–1600 AD)
View of Madness: demon-possession or God's punishment
Social control: Church and community
View of Criminal wrongdoing: sin
Social control: Church and community

Enlightenment (late 1600's–1700's)
View of Madness: sickness or disease, a disturbance of Nature
Social control: Medicine
Methods: science, treatment, prevention
View of Criminal wrongdoing: sin - failure of morality
Social control: Church
Methods: worship, education, threat

The Enlightenment Split

Medicine (later, psychiatry)
inherited madness
explained by scientific causality
treated as disease

Criminal and common law
inherited wrongful conduct (sin)
explained by failure of faith or to resist temptation
treated as moral failing with punishment

Today, popular culture embraces both viewpoints

Figure 8.1 The Enlightenment Split

Judaic sin is typically neither a contributor to spiritual death toward damnation (as in Christianity) nor an affront to Allah's will (as in Islam). Rather, Judaic sin is an expected, human failing to choose good over evil, grounded in free will.[18] Regardless of these variations around sin in Abrahamic traditions, the themes of free will, individual responsibility, and just deserts persist and prevail in framing accounts of wrongdoing. The social controls of the time were similar to those for madness; however, madness was exceptional: everyone was a sinner, but not everyone was mad.

By the Enlightenment(s) of the 1600s–1700s (multiple regional-cultural trends with these themes arose in Europe and the Americas), the educated, mostly wealthy and male intellectuals of the time began to introduce metaphysical-domain ideas into Western culture, originally in the voice of PM, but ultimately filtering down into folk-metaphysical assumptions. (In this regard, Cartesian dualism is a prominent example.) In the frames of madness and its social control, madness progressively came to be recast as a malady, a disease or illness, while wrongdoing, whether sinful or criminal, retained its morally problematic content. Correspondingly, the social control of 'madness', now redefined as 'mental disease' or 'illness', came to be managed by physicians, and the later 'alienists' and then 'psychiatrists', while the social control of wrongdoing was retained by religious teachings, punishments, and threats. Increasingly, the new concept of social wrongdoing—crime—came to be regulated by the evolving Western common and criminal law. As this Enlightenment Split grew in Western Europe, the management of mental illness/madness came to be dominated by the emerging scientific medicine. Regarding the management of sin, personal wrongdoing, and evil thinking, these behaviors continued to be managed by religion, while the evolving concept of crime (i.e., wrongful actions against others) increasingly came to be regulated by common and criminal law and its trappings—what today we would call the criminal justice system of courts, lawyers, law, criminal procedures, jails, and prisons.[19]

What was transformational with the Enlightenment Split was the social segregation of madness-deviance from Church/community regulation, and instead, the movement of madness-deviance toward science, medicine, and treatment of illness: psychopathology. Science and medical technology came to dominate the social control of madness, while religion and law continued to dominate the methods, using Abrahamic folk-metaphysical assumptions regarding the social control of sin/wrongdoing and crime. On the medicine/psychiatry side, this split was accompanied by distinctive sets of metaphysical assumptions, grounded in the secularizing metaphysical philosophies of Kant, Descartes, Locke, Hegel, and Hobbes, as well as theorists of the New Science like Francis Bacon, and in medicine, Thomas Sydenham.[20] Religion and law retained the Abrahamic folk-metaphysical assumptions. Thus, the dueling folk-metaphysical assumptions of psychiatry/medicine and law/religion came to cultural prominence in the West.

The secularizing trends for medicine and the sciences led to what I have called the CMC-folk-metaphysical account of disease, with its distinctive sets of assumptions apart from concepts like free will, individual responsibility, and desert.[21] Instead, mental illness came to be viewed as the end result of complex-causal pathways emerging from abnormal bodies, abnormal upbringing, and/or abnormal environments—hence a complex multicausal account based on naturalistic metaphysical assumptions, mechanistic organization of human biology, normative assumptions, and complex-causal interactions with person and environment, as well as the individual persons in their historical developments. These assumptions occupy psychiatry as I've noted already.[22] Secularist philosophy of science and medicine then developed new conceptual issues—such as defining 'abnormality' and 'normality' and understanding disease in terms compatible with CMC-folk-metaphysical accounts.[23]

So the Enlightenment Split set up the conditions for the increasing divisions between medicine and psychiatry regarding madness or mental illness, and Church/Law conceptions of madness, sin, and crime. Medicine, and later, psychiatry, inherited madness as its domain: explaining it by scientific causality and treating it as disease. Nineteenth-century formulations of psychopathology centered on Enlightenment era faculty psychologies which split the mind into cognition, affection, and conation—with morality left to religion and the spiritual realm. Criminal and common law inherited wrongful conduct that infringed upon others (the social order), while religion retained much of its domain of addressing sin—personal wrongdoing in thought and actions. Through the emerging post-Enlightenment criminal justice system and the waning, yet still potent, religious institutions, post-Enlightenment wrongful social actions could still be treated, like sin, as moral failings subject to education, threat, and punishment as individually responsible conduct.

Of course, in the meantime all kinds of events were unfolding in social history as noted in Chapters 4 and 5, not the least of which was the scientific treatment of diseases; the growth of cities and industrialization, moving more and more people into congested communities and out of the farms, forests, and fields. Such social movement was accompanied by growing alienation from traditions and mores; leading to peculiarly modern afflictions, such as 'neurosis'.[24]

In the context of these changes in culture, (the appearance of 'modernism') came the seeds of cultural pluralism and diversity which introduce growing levels of metaphysical-domain complexity. These phenomena have mingled folk-metaphysical assumptions in complex ways. Notable also was the Renaissance and Reformation, and the dispersal of new religious communities around the world, through increased travel and immigration which were among the drivers of cultural pluralism as we know it today. The Enlightenment ideas of complex multicausality for diseases, including mental disorders, increasingly spread in higher and even elementary education, where these ideas confronted variations of Abrahamic faith traditions which had evolved in degrees of orthodoxy, differentiated into countless sects and denominations, further diversifying the interpretations of religious texts.

Today, we have a multicultural pluralistic environment in which elements of the Enlightenment Split live on in the academy of sciences and humanities, while the Abrahamic concepts of free will, individual responsibility, and desert persist and are imbricated into Abrahamic religious institutions as well as Western common and criminal law. Hence, the folk-metaphysical assumptions of complex multicausal science/medicine and Church/law live on in countless adumbrations and variations in contemporary Western culture, driving cultural conflicts from the Science Wars and Culture Wars to contemporary, granular conflicts about immunization, spanking children, teaching evolutionary biology, pandemic control, and abortion.

8.3 Some manifestations of folk-metaphysical conflict in the VMDR

The protean manifestations of these two strong traditions are likely countless. I mention a few in this paragraph and then describe more particular psychiatric examples in paragraphs to follow. Westerners today commonly maintain at least two elemental folk-metaphysical identities. One set of these are driven by the academy—the complex of universities and intellectual culture, PM, and contemporary science. The other is driven by the folk-metaphysical assumptions presented by Abrahamic monotheistic religions, and other folk beliefs, a featured example being Morse's 'concepts of the person' in criminal law and psychiatry. So popular culture reflects countless variations on these traditions and their variations, resulting in the 'Culture Wars' or 'Science Wars' around matters like evolution, the birth of the universe, vaccination, and in psychiatry, issues around criminal responsibility and the 'insanity defense'.[25]

Morality concepts following the Enlightenment era were split off, by and large, from the new science, and in the twentieth century, Western psychology. Not until much later, until the late-twentieth century, did psychology, neurobiology, and other social sciences become interested in morality, whether socially or naturally. A new 'moral psychology' emerged as the centerpiece of these studies in neuroscience, psychology, social science, and philosophy. Despite these new developments, Enlightenment faculty psychology has persisted into the present DSMs, as Jennifer Radden and others have pointed out.[26] As will be discussed below, compared to pre-Enlightenment FM, Western culture now depicts a fragmented, inchoate set of assumptions and responses to the metaphysical domain, leading to sharp disagreements and obscure misunderstandings. Let's consider some specific examples.

8.3.1 The social response to crime & mental illness

The conflicts between CMC-folk-metaphysical assumptions and Abrahamic religious folk-metaphysical assumptions play out in our societal responses to criminal behavior and mental illness. For example, Western psychiatry treats 'serious mental disorders' like Schizophrenia and Bipolar Disorder under a CMC-folk-metaphysical account, viewing misconduct as CMC manifestations of disease. On the other hand, Western psychiatry also regards vice-laden mental disorders like the personality disorders, addictions, paraphilias, Conduct Disorder, and Intermittent Explosive Disorder as responsible individual conduct, aligned with Abrahamic folk-metaphysical assumptions. The courts invoke criminal excuse more often for the former, compared to the latter.[27]

The following are particularly vivid examples. In 2003 the American Psychiatric Association issued an official statement claiming DSM-IV Pedophilia was both a criminal behavior *and* a mental disorder.[28] The situation of the insanity defense, the idea that a mentally disordered offender should be excused from conviction 'not guilty by reason of insanity' (NGRI), straddles both folk-metaphysical realms: major mental illness undergirded by CMC-folk-metaphysical assumptions, combined with criminal responsibility as imbricated in the Abrahamic folk-metaphysical assumptions of criminal courts. Some categories of mental disorder (e.g., psychotic disorders) are eligible for NGRI acquittals, while others, including paraphilias and personality disorders, are generally not eligible for NGRI.[29] No wonder psychiatrists and criminal attorneys have so much trouble understanding each other! Finally, the legacy of just deserts lives on in the prevailing model of criminal justice in the United States and UK today: the 'retributive' justice model, which focuses on punishment for responsible misdeeds, as opposed to a CMC-folk-metaphysical derived criminal reform, rehabilitation, restorative justice, or even treatment models advocated by scientific criminology as well as correctional psychiatry.[30]

8.3.2 Public attitudes about mental illness

Chapter 7 considered the mental health literacy research program, led by scholars like Jorm,[31] Gulliver et al.,[32] Wang et al.,[33] Angermeyer and Dietrich,[34] and Pescosolido,[35] who have repeatedly demonstrated, on an international basis, poor public understandings of mental illness. Highlights from their research and reviews cited above indicate that many, perhaps most people don't recognize the symptoms of significant mental illness in themselves or others. Moreover, laypersons in mental distress delay professional help-seeking in terms of years and even decades rather than weeks or months. When the lay public does seek assistance, they often prefer family, friends, and ministers over medical or mental health professionals. Significantly, majorities of laypersons prefer to be self-reliant and view their mental distress as their own fault, implying more compatibility of these public attitudes and beliefs with the Abrahamic folk-metaphysical assumptions of individual responsibility, free will, and desert over the more complex medical/psychiatric CMC account.

8.3.3 Mentally ill and nonmentally ill offenders

In recent years the news media has increasingly covered the problem of incarcerating mentally ill offenders. In 2006, the US Bureau of Justice Statistics (USBJS) noted that 705,600 prisoners in state prisons had concurrent psychotic, mood, and anxiety disorders, and the figures for Federal prisons and local jails were 78,000 and 479,000, respectively.[36] A USBJS report in 2017, based on 2011–2012 data, noted that 37% of prisoners had been told by a mental health professional that they had a mental disorder. For US jails, the figure was 44%.[37] Today, the 'socially deviant' can be simultaneously served by the juvenile justice system, the adult criminal justice system, schools for the intellectually disabled, and public and private mental health institutions.[38] At the same time, the United States has increasingly recognized the expanding problem of the homeless mentally ill in the decades following 'deinstitutionalization' in the 1960s.[39] Consider, for example, an intellectually disabled young adult offender with a psychotic disorder. The simultaneous presence of redundant and inadequate services points to the incoherent and inchoate admixture of Abrahamic and CMC-folk-metaphysical assumptions which 'underwrite' these social welfare efforts. Concisely, our current social welfare efforts educate, punish, treat, rehabilitate, and seclude, a mash-up of both folk-metaphysical traditions.

8.3.4 Other key debates in the philosophy of psychiatry relevant to the VMDR

Implied in much of the above are topics in the philosophy of psychiatry. One is our central question of 'vice-laden' mental disorders being appropriate to psychiatric diagnosis and practice. The folk-metaphysical tension here is between the entailments of Abrahamic folk-metaphysical assumptions (e.g., making for *wrongful* behaviors) and the entailments of CMC-folk-metaphysical assumptions (e.g., multicausal maladaptive behaviors). As another example, much has been written on medicalization in psychiatry; and some authors[40] breaking away from the conceptions of criminality as evil and wrongful (under Abrahamic folk-metaphysical assumptions), and instead presenting criminality as a disease or disorder (under the CMC-folk-metaphysical assumptions).

My final examples are drawn from select moments in the intellectual or conceptual history of psychiatry. The historians Margo Horn and Kathleen Jones[41] independently describe the development of contemporary child and adolescent psychiatry as an outgrowth of physicians and mental health professional's effort to address the early to mid-twentieth-century problem of juvenile delinquency, discussed here in Chapter 5. That is, child psychiatry was built to address crime by minors, taking on criminality and bad behavior, in practical effect, as a mental disorder. This was the childhood context of the 'mad-versus-bad' debate generated vigorously by Thomas Szasz in the latter half of the twentieth century, and still discussed in the philosophy of psychiatry.[42]

These examples are but a few of the many which can be brought to bear upon conceptual issues in psychiatry. I offer the concept of FM and their associated assumptions as an analytic tool for new approaches to old social problems. However, considering the interplay of FM and PM in discourses is not a mere academic exercise. As was presented above through the examples of the VMDR, the holding of metaphysical assumptions cashes out in terms of real stakes and real outcomes regarding mental health policy and patient care. In the former, an Abrahamic metaphysics of free will, individual responsibility, and desert lends itself well to the legacy of a punitive, retributive criminal justice system, one which marginalizes offender rehabilitation and treatment of mental illness. The fracture of the moral away from medicine and the institutional imbrication of moral wrongfulness in the criminal justice system means that biobehavioral, complex-causal understandings of criminality are marginalized. Only very recently has public interest in serious efforts toward criminal rehabilitation been discussed in the public sphere.[43] For still-another example of how metaphysical assumptions drive social policy, research funding for criminology and related US social sciences are relegated to the National Science Foundation, an agency whose funding is dwarfed by the National Institutes of Health. In 2017, the total budget for the National Science Foundation (all non-healthcare-related sciences, from Astronomy to Zoology) was 7.964 billion, while funding for the National Institutes of Health (all health related science) was $33.1 billion.[44] For the National Institute of Mental Health, *all* mental health related funding the FY 2017 budget was 1.5 billion.[45] For NSF, *all* social, behavioral, and economic sciences budget for FY 2017 was $288.77 million dollars.[46] Of course, criminological research is a *subset* of this latter funding, and one which is not easily ascertained with current data. Our knowledge of criminality and the VMDR is crippled by these funding inequities, likely reflecting rigid Abrahamic folk-metaphysical prejudices about offenders and offending.

Moreover, the investment of medieval Abrahamic FM in criminal law constitutes the metaphysical background for, and enables, the criminal law dilemmas of the NGRI defense (Chapter 6, Section 6.1.1; Chapter 7, Section 7.1.3), the ambiguous status of the mentally ill offender (mad and/or bad?; Chapter 7, Section 7.1.3), dual-agency dilemmas in forensic testimony (Doctor? Punisher?) (Chapter 6, Section 6.1.1.1), and the failure of rehabilitation-focused criminal justice interventions to gain traction in the United States (Chapter 6, Section 6.1.1.1).[47]

Abrahamic FM lingers as the metaphysical substructure for the most common conceptual issues in psychiatry. Patients' choices are dichotomized into freely chosen or not freely chosen, leading people with personality disorders to be 'blame-worthy'[48] on the one hand, but psychiatry also sees psychopathological behavior as nonblameworthy: constrained, even compelled, by complex multicausal factors, as well, as any reading of a contemporary psychiatric science journal will illustrate.

The tool of the analysis of metaphysical assumptions, like the philosophy of psychiatry generally, is not a panacea for social ills concerning mental health. What it does do, like the analysis of values in mental health, is provide a description of the relevant concepts and assumptions to consider about improving the field and clarifying ambiguities and controversies. Like the analysis of values, an understanding of metaphysical assumptions and their 'laden-ness' in discourses enables us to discuss and perhaps decide which metaphysical assumptions lead us to an account of mental health which consistently advances human flourishing. Some particulars of a transformational viewpoint will be discussed in the next sections and the next, final, chapter.

8.4 Revisiting the four accounts of the VMDR

In Sections 3.6.3 through 3.6.6 of Chapter 3, I introduced four idealized accounts of the VMDR. The details of these accounts can be reviewed in those sections, and in Sadler (2019).[49] For my purposes here, I review briefly what each of these four accounts are, as well as recount briefly the social and mental health profession's problems perpetrated by each account or standpoint. This review and critique then lead to Section 8.3 of this chapter, which provides an alternative account of the VMDR, and introduces some of the key advantages and challenges facing such an account. This account, in combination with an appreciation of the social, cultural, and political significance of selected folk-metaphysical assumptions from the prior section, sets the stage for Chapter 9 and its discussion of granular ways to address the manifold difficulties associated with the VMDR.

8.4.1 The coincidental account

The coincidental account, you may remember, refers to events or features associated with a person with a mental disorder, but are assumed to be unrelated to the mental disorder—definitionally or causally. In Chapter 3, Section 3.6.3, I offered the example of a person with mania wearing Mardi Gras headgear. In this setting, we typically do not incorporate Mardi Gras headgear into the definition or concept of mania, nor do we attribute Mardi Gras headgear as a contributing cause of mania. Instead, we see a manic person wearing Mardi Gras headgear as a coincidental feature, even though it might well be a coincidental feature which is often observed each year in March in New Orleans. The trouble with the coincidental account is that it may be mistaken in any cause-effect relationship. We should be alert to co-occurrences which may be significant. For example, we might observe that flight attendants with bipolar disorder have more frequent bouts of mania when they have irregular flight schedules and, therefore, irregular sleep-wake cycles, and disruptions of their circadian rhythms. It would be a mistake to attribute this set of observations to simple coincidence.[50]

8.4.2 The medicalization account

The idea of medicalization is to cast human problems as medical problems.[51] Regarding the VMDR, the medicalization account means that social deviance exhibiting wrongful or immoral conduct does not differ in any substantive way within a complex-causal naturalistic metaphysics than a disease/medical account; vicious conduct is causally influenced as is mentally disordered conduct. As will be discussed in more detail later, what underlies the distinctive cultural framework of vicious conduct is the folk-metaphysical 'Enlightenment Split' which delegated wrongful and criminal conduct to a distinct metaphysical domain framed by Abrahamic folk-metaphysical assumptions. Other mental faculties of the time (i.e., cognition, affection, and conation) were assimilated by psychiatry and medicine within the emerging complex-causal FM of the new sciences. As I noted in Chapter 3, Adriane Raine, the neurocriminologist, has been instrumental in challenging, in effect, the Abrahamic folk-metaphysical formulation of criminal misconduct by treating criminality as just another set of human behaviors and experiences subject to his 'biosocial' scientific inquiry. As a neurocriminologist holding complex-causal, science-friendly metaphysical assumptions, Raine doesn't view immorality or criminality as metaphysically distinct from diseases and conventional mental disorders. Criminality may well be as 'disordered' as depression or schizophrenia.

8.4.3 The moralization account

In contrast to Raineian complex-causal FM, which view disease, disorder, and criminality as just three categories of human behavior and experience, the moralization account takes a contrary, but not quite opposite approach: social deviance which infringes upon other people (broadly, immorality and crime) should be addressed by nonmedical social institutions: the education system, religious institutions, and the criminal justice system. This is in large part Thomas Szasz's view, as discussed in Chapter 3 and in my prior work.[52] From the standpoint of FM, the moralization account valorizes the Abrahamic metaphysics of free will, personal responsibility, individualism, and just desert, also discussed in Chapter 3. In this sense, the moralization account emerges from the other side of the Enlightenment Split: from the Abrahamic religious traditions (and mostly the Christian tradition by the 1800s in Euro-American societies) which shape contemporary religious morality and salvation, and Western criminal law, as discussed earlier.

8.4.4 The mixed account

So the mixed VMDR account, to review prior discussion, is a combination of the prior three, constituting the prevailing account in Western psychiatry and mental health care. As the predominant account, I should reiterate that it is not an explicitly endorsed viewpoint (i.e., the mixed account is assumed), but an account which is revealed through examining actual practices and discourse in the mental health field. In prior chapters I have documented many examples—to name a few:

- Conflicts around the insanity defense and mentally disordered offenders as diseased and irresponsible versus mentally disordered offenders as responsible and deserving of punishment.
- Pedophilic Disorder as criminality and as a mental disorder.
- The corruption of medical morality in forensic psychiatry by the charge to participate in criminal trials with the potential for punishment (in service to the State, not patients).
- Conflicts between courtroom reasoning about culpability versus clinical reasoning using complex multifactorial causality.
- And of course, psychiatric diagnostic categories that are vice-laden, such as Antisocial Personality Disorder, Conduct Disorder, Kleptomania, victimizing paraphilias, and Intermittent Explosive Disorder.

From this brief review, I can now turn to a fifth idealized model of the VMDR, which I will argue resolves many of the original problems which inspired this book. Readers who wish to review the various problems associated with the above four accounts should review Chapter 2 and perhaps 3; recounting these arguments again would needlessly prolong this chapter.

8.5 A rehabilitation account of the VMDR

Immediately the reader may wonder why I am proposing a rehabilitation account as my favored approach to the manifold puzzles of the VMDR. Moreover, another question arises about how my rehabilitation account resembles and is distinct from other rehabilitation accounts. In order to make a strong case for my own rehabilitation account of the VMDR, a first step should be to clarify what a VMDR rehabilitation account means. One might surmise, and accurately so, that a VMDR rehabilitation account might resemble criminal rehabilitation practices, on the one hand, and psychiatric rehabilitation practices, on the other. However, I am aiming my VMDR rehabilitation account not at just mental health practice, and not just for criminal justice practice, but something of a unique synthesis, which I call simply 'rehabilitation'. First steps first, so. . . .

8.5.1 What is criminal rehabilitation?

Like many social processes, 'rehabilitation' in the criminal justice field has a history, and with that history, protean meanings of the term. For this section, I examine what 'criminal rehabilitation' means through the lens of a historian of the field, and then turn to a very recent philosophical account. Then I sort these accounts in the context of the split in folk-metaphysical assumptions between the law/criminal justice fields (e.g., the Abrahamic folk-metaphysical assumptions) and the CMC-folk-metaphysical account. We'll see these clarifications are important in understanding my 'rehabilitation' account of the VMDR, further elaborated later in the chapter and in the concluding chapter.

Edgardo Rotman, a historian of rehabilitation, notes that the term connotes both an action and a process, as in 'going through' rehabilitation, but also a state of the person, as in an offender being rehabilitated.[53] However, in reading his text, *Beyond Punishment*,[54] I noticed that Rotman is not just a historian, but an advocate of criminal rehabilitation. Early in his book, through giving a basic definition, he in effect advocates for a position vis-a-vis criminal justice/political ethics:

> Rehabilitation, according to modern standards, can be defined tentatively and broadly as a right to an opportunity to return to (or remain in) society with an improved chance of being a useful citizen and staying out of prison; the term may also be used to denote the actions of the state or private institutions in extending this opportunity. The definition

thus embraces *both the offender's rights* and the government's policies. (1990, p. 3, emphasis mine)[55]

Rotman places the citizenship of the criminal offender (citizenship broadly used here to denote the offender as a human subject of the state) here, and in Rotman's account, at the center of the considerations of what rehabilitation is. For Rotman, containment of the offender to protect the public (either through deterrence or incapacitation), and punishment proper (the two other core functions of the criminal justice system), have little to do with rehabilitation. Only rehabilitation should be the state's response to criminal offenders.[56]

Rotman goes on to delineate what such rights might include in a fully rehabilitative approach to criminal justice:

> Rehabilitation in prisons comprises educational opportunities; vocational training; justly remunerated work; medical, psychological, and psychiatric treatment in an adequate environment; maintenance of family and community links; a safe, fair, and healthy prison environment; postrelease support; elimination of hindrances to reinstatement in the community; and the various services directed to meeting the imprisoned offender's physical, intellectual, social, and spiritual needs, as compatible with incarceration.[57]

Rotman acknowledges that such practices can and should extend out of the prison environment *per se* and into postrelease, community environments so the offender can integrate, prosper, and not reoffend. Moreover, Rotman offers legitimate worry about which moral value-laden practices are to be imposed by society through the criminal justice rehabilitative process, keeping in mind the history of abuses of prisoners in US and world history. He grounds his moral account of rehabilitation by framing rehabilitative practices as enhancing human freedom, eschewing particular religious or political ideologies, and instead aiming the offender at personal responsibility and self-determination; the 'inner freedom' of the individual. Such rehabilitated individuals would be freer from the restrictions of psychological and environmental determinants of offending.

From this brief summary, the reader may recognize the elements of Abrahamic FM undergirding Rotman's account; the restoration implied in this account is directed at the offender's expanding free will and personal responsibility for actions. He summarizes: '. . . a new rehabilitative model should aim toward awakening the personal experience of social responsibility.'[58] While still Abrahamic in its metaphysics, Rotman's account moves away from an Old-Testament vengeful, punitive God toward, perhaps, the love and forgiveness of the New Testament's Jesus.

Philosophers of law have examined what 'rehabilitation' means as well, often linking it to political ethics of penal punishments. Stephen Sverdlik[59] in his thoughtful review and critical discussion of the 'reform theory' of punishment in criminal justice, observes that (and in contrast to Rotman) criminal punishment theory was rooted in the concept of 'reform'. According to Sverdlik, the central theme of these accounts, ranging from Plato to Hegel, Bentham, A. C. Ewing, and beyond, is that punishment provokes offenders to change their ways and become better citizens; much like, as Herbert Morris would have it, parents punishing their children generate moral improvements in them. Sverdlik finds various inconsistencies and faults of logic in philosophical accounts of the role of punishment in criminal justice. While I find his discussion illuminating, such detail is not germane to my discussion here. What is of particular interest in Sverdlik's analysis of influential law philosopher Anthony Duff. In the latter's quote that criminal punishment is 'a species of secular penance',[60] Duff situates punishment in the metaphysics of desert, even using a religious metaphor of penance. Indeed, the language of Christian repentance, penance, and etymological reference to the administration of sacraments for sins committed, all point to the folk-metaphysical Abrahamic roots of punishment-based criminal justice in Duff and similar authors.

In contrast to Rotman's historical perspective, Forsberg and Douglas[61] writing from a contemporary philosophy of law perspective, consider the question of defining 'criminal rehabilitation' (CR) in a recent paper. Their aim is to provide a taxonomy for understanding and comparing what they find as a family of concepts. They frame their comparisons of CR in terms of aims and means. As apropos to their law interests, they want to clarify CR concepts so as to facilitate good policy around CR. While not all aspects of their discussion are relevant to my interests, the varieties of concepts of CR they identify deepens our understanding of the CR mission as documented in the literature.

The authors describe five conceptions of CR: (1) rehabilitation as antirecidivism, (2) rehabilitation as harm reduction, (3) rehabilitation as therapy, (4) rehabilitation as moral improvement, and (5) rehabilitation as restoration. I'll describe, briefly, each next.

8.5.1.1 Rehabilitation as antirecidivism
Forsberg and Douglas define this conception as:

> An intervention *I* administered by a criminal justice system to offender *O* in response to *O*'s offence is an instance of rehabilitation just in case (1) it is intended to reduce the likelihood that *O* will re-offend, (2) other than by reducing *O*'s capacity to reoffend, disincentivising re-offending by *O*, or incentivising non-offending by *O*.[62]

In this treatment, CR is aimed at reducing reoffending. The authors note this version of CR may well be an enabling objective, advancing more superordinate goals like protecting the public. They further specify that this version of CR involves particular means to the goal of reducing recidivism, and they specifically exclude incapacitation and disincentivizing schemes as part of this definition. Instead, they suggest that the antirecidivist position focuses more on the individual's 'intrinsic dispositions'.[63] We'll see shortly how modifying an offender's intrinsic dispositions cashes out in actual criminal-rehabilitative practices.

8.5.1.2 Rehabilitation as harm reduction

For this conception, the authors provide this definition:

> An intervention *I* administered by a criminal justice system to offender *O* in response to *O*'s offence is an instance of rehabilitation just in case (1) it is intended to prevent harmful conduct *by O* (restricted to the kinds of harms that are legitimately the business of the criminal law), (2) other than by reducing *O*'s capacity to engage in such conduct, disincentivising such conduct by *O*, or to incentivising less harmful conduct by *O*.[64]

Like CR as antirecidivism, CR as harm reduction can also be an enabling objective for more superordinate goals like protecting the public. Note that Forsberg and Douglas specify that particular kinds of harms are relevant to this CR approach—that is, those conventionally concerned with criminal law. Other kinds of harms, such as ordinary immoral actions like being unfaithful to one's spouse, fudging your tax returns, or failing to honor a commitment to a friend may not be harm-reduction foci of CR practices. The authors also note that harms perpetrated by the offender that are too-far distant in time from the convicted offense may not fit into the harm-reduction approach. They provide the example of a murderer's prior tax fraud as an unlikely target of harm-reduction CR.

8.5.1.3 Rehabilitation as therapy

For this third version of CR, the authors provide this definition:

> An intervention *I* administered by a criminal justice system to offender *O* in response to *O*'s offence is an instance of rehabilitation just in case it is intended to cure or ameliorate a mental deficit in *O* that is understood by the intervener (1) to have causally contributed to *O*'s past offence(s), or (2) to predispose *O* to further offending.[65]

The authors specify that 'mental deficit' as used here can either mean a mental disorder as conceived by psychiatry and the mental health field, or a 'defect in the capacities relevant for criminal responsibility'.[66] The former they view as a psychiatric understanding, and the latter a forensic understanding. They note that mental disorders don't necessarily diminish rational capacities, nor do impairments in rational capacities necessarily constitute a mental disorder. Again, this CR as therapy account may represent an enabling objective to other goals of CR.

So, the idea is that CR as therapy involves treatment in a conventional medical sense, or techniques associated with CR proper, including, for example, punishment as a 'treatment' for encouraging a change in one's conduct.

This version of CR is of particular interest for this book, as it addresses the VMDR, and invokes the 'enlightenment split' of folk-metaphysical assumptions discussed earlier. The offender conceived as suffering from a mental disorder contributing to criminal conduct, invokes the CMC set of complex multicausality folk-metaphysical assumptions, while the 'mental deficit' capacity account invokes the Abrahamic folk-metaphysical assumptions of (specifically) free will and personal/criminal responsibility in criminal law.

The author's mention of Jean Hampton[67] vividly illustrates this:

> Jean Hampton distinguishes her moral education theory of punishment from rehabilitative views by noting that her theory 'does not perceive punishment as a way of treating a "sick" person for a mental disease, but rather as a way of sending a moral message to a person who has acted immorally and who is to be held responsible for her actions'.[68]

Here the sharp distinction in criminal law between morality and disease is evident. However, if one sets aside the Abrahamic folk-metaphysical standpoint, rejecting punishment not just as ineffective therapy but rather promulgating harm on the person to be rehabilitated, one is left with the conclusions that disordered and immoral/criminal conduct are ultimately behaviors to be understood and explained by science, behaviors harmful to self or others are to be managed, treated, and indeed, rehabilitated.

8.5.1.4 Rehabilitation as moral improvement

The fourth iteration of CR according to Forsberg and Douglas reads:

> An intervention *I* administered by a criminal justice system to offender *O* in response to *O*'s offence is an instance of rehabilitation just in case it is intended to morally improve *O*.[69]

The authors note that this version nests a number of theories, stratagems, and practices undergirded by a variety of ways of describing 'moral improvement'. These descriptions include, but are not limited to, assisting offenders in adopting more ethically justified moral beliefs, the inculcation of various moral virtues, reframing motives in ethical directions, or simply training offenders into competence or facility with desirable moral actions. We'll see below that many of the prevailing practices of CR today, ones that have empirical science efficacy credentials, frame many of their activities similarly, though contemporary CR practices generally eschew the 'moral improvement' term and instead frame their aims in terms of 'prosocial' attitudes, responses, and behaviors. Because this approach is more 'normatively thick'[70] than the preceding CR approaches, the authors note that Duff (2001) insists that the moral improvements be limited to those relevant to the perpetrator's crimes.[71]

8.5.1.5 Rehabilitation as restoration

For the fifth and final version of the CR concept, Forsberg and Douglas offer this:

> An intervention *I* administered by a criminal justice system to offender *O* in response to *O*'s offence is an instance of rehabilitation just in case it is intended to restore *O*'s moral or social relationships or standing.[72]

This version addresses the idea that rehabilitation aims to restore the offender to a moral and/or practical status within the society and community. In this sense it reflects restorative justice models discussed in Chapter 6, Section 6.3.4. Forsberg and Douglas analogize this formulation as akin to paying compensatory damages in tort law, though only through financial means. However, other forms of making restorations exist, such as restoring social bonds in family, friends, and/or community. In the strictly moral arena, restoration may involve, for example, community service, repairing property, or making some other material or labor correction to the offense. Like the broader concept of restorative justice, the variety of rehabilitation typically involves a repairing relationship with the victim(s) of crimes, recognizing material or personal losses, as well as the insult to the victim's social rights or privileges. Concluding their discussion, the authors note John Braithwaite and Philip Pettit's notion of restoring 'dominion'.[73]

In looking over these five aspects of CR, one can readily recognize the overlap and fuzzy boundaries between them, recognized by Forsberg and Douglas and part of the motivation for sorting out these aspects for their clarifying discussions of rehabilitation law to follow. In comparing their work to Rotman's, whose work Forsberg and Douglas seem to be unaware, we can recognize many elements of each of the five versions of CR in Rotman's account. However, an important stipulation here is Rotman leaves no room for punishment and containment of offenders as 'rehabilitation', seeing the CR as solely a function of moving offenders toward meeting their 'physical, intellectual, social, and spiritual needs'.[74] The holistic, encompassing view of Rotman, coupled with the meticulous distinctions about rehabilitation from Forsberg and Douglas, together give a rich picture of the visions of CR, and potentialities to be developed. With this broad perspective, we can turn to examining today's practices of CR.

8.5.2 The practice of criminal rehabilitation

Having explained the goals of CR, an understanding, however basic, of the particulars of CR (sometimes referred to as 'correctional treatment') is warranted. A perspective of criminal/correctional rehabilitation is needed especially to compare and contrast to psychiatric rehabilitation procedures, to follow shortly. The most influential practice model of CR of the past 25 years, the Risk-Need-Responsivity (RNR) model, was formulated in the 1990s by Don Andrews, James Bonta, Paul Gendreau, and colleagues.[75] Since its initial articulation, it has been implemented and tested, generating hundreds of publications and thousands of citations in the past 25 years, having been applied to a wide variety of correctional settings and target populations.[76]

The RNR model, as the name implies, is based on three principles. The *risk* principle states that interventions should be directed to individuals who are at a moderate and especially high risk to reoffend. The *need* principle states that rehabilitation interventions should be directed toward empirically identified, recognized risk factors that lead to reoffending. These risk factors are sometimes called 'crimino-genic needs'. The *responsivity* principle states that the rehabilitative intervention or treatment must be capable or, better yet, empirically demonstrated, to change one or more criminogenic needs—that is, diminish or remove the risk factors for re-offending. I should note that the RNR model is agnostic about particular foci or methods of intervention. Criminogenic needs may be social, environmental, internal-psychological, or historical; thus, while appearing to be a Forsberg and Douglas recidivism-reduction model, in practice the RNR model is an amalgam of the CR approaches described by Forsberg and Douglas.

The *Risk* principle arose out of criminological studies that showed that individuals who committed minor offenses, if diverted or sentenced to noncustodial sentences, were very unlikely to recidivate, that is, commit more crimes. Indeed, the research indicated that tougher sentences, rather than reducing recidivism, actually increased it—likely through the 'hardening' process discussed earlier, relating to traumatic adult incarceration experiences and abusive juvenile custodial settings, combined with learning of new criminal 'skills' and connections while in confinement. Aiming rehabilitation efforts toward high-risk offenders was both more likely to be effective in reducing recidivism and reducing costs, through withholding unneeded, or even toxic, services to low-risk individuals.

A key recognition from this group's research was that informal, 'clinical' judg-ments of individuals at high and low risk proved to be difficult and unreliable. This led investigators to develop the Level of Service Inventory (LSI), a test instrument that identified recidivism risk accurately through actuarial statistics.[77] The LSI has been since updated and configured for various subpopulations as well. Case manage-ment plans can then be tailored to general, as well as particular risk factors, leading to 'tailored', localized rehabilitation programs that subsequently were more likely to be effective. However, a gap often exists between the identification of criminogenic risk factors and the availability and skill in implementing such tailored treatments in the RNR framework. Those implementing RNR-guided case management plans need substantive training—an assurance that research protocols might provide but may not be readily available in real-world correctional settings in geographic and ec-onomically diverse (e.g., underfunded) correctional settings.

'Criminogenic needs' as deficit-based, changeable risk factors then suggest the *Need* principle. Regarding criminogenic needs, space permits discussion of the so-called Big Four.[78] Criminogenic risk factors can be 'static' (e.g., unchangeable), such as gender (e.g., men are far more likely to offend than women) or 'dynamic' (e.g., changeable), such as 'antisocial attitudes' or deprived, dangerous neighbor-hoods. If antisocial attitudes can be changed though treatment/rehabilitation into prosocial attitudes, then 'antisocial attitudes' is a dynamic risk factor and a target of intervention.

These dynamic risk factors are termed 'criminogenic needs' as well, to signify that they represent deficits in an offender's skill set requiring treatment or other interventions to move toward prosocial behaviors. Andrews and Bonta's Big Four dynamic risk factors are the most powerful and, therefore, the most important: (1) antisocial cognitions, (2) antisocial associates, (3) an antisocial personality pattern (such as 'impulsivity'), and (4) a history of antisocial behavior. Notably, a history of antisocial behavior might suggest a static factor, as history cannot be changed. However, as viewed by Andrews and Bonta, one's history is continuous and unfolding, and the offender can learn new prosocial behaviors in response to history's old responses. For example, offenders may learn new ways to respond to high-risk situations or learn self-efficacy cognitive strategies to avoid playing out the 'old scripts' of past antisocial behavior. One can recognize the potential for antisocial personality pattern change when addressing these cognitive strategies.[79] While the Big Four are central targets of intervention, Andrews and Bonta also identify four more important criminogenic needs. Adding these to the Big Four, makes for a 'Central Eight'. The remaining factors of the Central Eight are (5) family/marital conflict, (6) difficulties with schooling or work functioning, (7) neglect of [prosocial] leisure/recreation, and (8) substance abuse. These risk factors/criminogenic needs then inform granular therapies and rehabilitative activities tailored to the particular person's repertoire of skill and attitude deficits.[80] I should note that addressing the Central Eight leads de facto to the multidimensional profile of a flourishing citizen, envisioned above by Rotman as a rehabilitative ideal. So while the RNR model of rehabilitation may seem 'negativistic' by focusing on deficits, the net effect of a well-run RNR program is the kind of flourishing Rotman envisioned and to which we all aspire, through meaningful work, play, citizenship, and love/family.

The *Responsivity* principle then emphasizes that efforts to reduce recidivism through focused, tailored interventions in addressing the criminogenic needs identified in a particular client. This resonates with mental health/medical clinicians through the standard practice of matching treatment to a holistic, individualized 'diagnosis' and treatment plan. The historical problem with corrections is that little effort was directed to particular criminogenic needs of individuals (e.g., 'diagnosis' was ignored) and everyone got the same treatment (e.g., incarceration, uniform education programs). Probation and parole provide a kind of monitoring of the individual, but monitoring is not interventional, and not tailored to particular needs of the individual. Indeed, Andrews and Gendreau[81] developed an instrument to help correctional programs in following the RNR principles and self-assess their programs: The Correctional Program Assessment Inventory (CPAI), is an eight-scale, 141-item instrument that measures organizational culture, program implementation and maintenance, management and staff characteristics, client risk/need practices, program characteristics, core correctional practices, interagency communication, and evaluation.[82] While research into CPAI is robust, the work has demonstrated efficacy on subscales and, therefore, in focused, limited applications. Unfortunately, data on broad application and impact in real-world correctional settings remain limited.[83] What is clear from the existing research, however, is that the CPAI is a powerful predictive instrument: higher-scoring institutions have lower recidivism rates than low-scoring institutions.[84]

Looking back on Rotman's ideal of rehabilitation, one might wonder about the role of spiritual needs in the RNR application, which appears to be neglected. This has been an area of recent interest in CR research.[85] Moreover, debate has emerged about the negativism of the RNR model and its deficit orientation, leading some theorists and commentators to advocate for an alternative model, the Good Lives Model (GLM) of offender rehabilitation, based in part on the strength-based orientation of positive psychology, the latter discussed in earlier chapters.[86] So far, the GLM model has often been used in youth-correctional and sex-offender settings, with some success.[87] However, a recent review by Zeccola et al.[88] concluded that the GLM model just doesn't yet have enough evidence to compare efficacy with the RNR model. Often, correctional programs make efforts to 'integrate' the two approaches.[89]

In conclusion, the concept of CR, while having many synonyms (e.g., reform, corrections, and reintegration) shares the commonality of social actions aimed at enabling the offender to return to society without repeat offending, and preferably, as a fully integrated, productive, and flourishing citizen. The debates on CR center around the best means to this general end. I will draw upon these debates later in developing my own special sense of a rehabilitation model for the VMDR. However, next in line in terms of concepts is considering 'psychiatric (or mental health) rehabilitation'.

8.5.3 What is psychiatric rehabilitation?

William A. Anthony might be considered the dean of American psychiatric rehabilitation. Anthony traces the origins of psychiatric rehabilitation to the moral therapy movement (discussed in Chapter 5, Section 5.3), later through the inclusion of psychiatric patients into public vocational rehabilitation programs, the emergence of community mental health as a movement in the 1960s, and congealing around the psychosocial rehabilitation movement and promulgation of skills training of various kinds.[90] Anthony and colleagues[91] in their introduction to a psychiatric rehabilitation text provide a brief definition:

> The mission of the field of psychiatric rehabilitation is to help persons with long-term psychiatric disabilities increase their functioning so that they are successful and satisfied in the environments of their choice, with the least amount of ongoing professional intervention. (p. 2, internal citation omitted)

This straightforward mission statement belies the substantial discussion and debate around psychiatric rehabilitation. Drawing from Cnaan et al.'s 15 principles of psychosocial rehabilitation from 1988,[92] Corrigan[93] sketches an influential 'integrated, structural model' of psychiatric rehabilitation. He describes four dimensions: (1)

rehabilitation goals, (2) strategies that yield change, (3) settings in which psychiatric rehabilitation occurs, and (4) roles of providers.

Corrigan's vision of rehabilitation goals has six facets. *Inclusion* refers to the ability of clients to participate fully in the everyday community activities such as housing, work, recreation, and interpersonal relationships. *Opportunity* is required to enable other facets of rehabilitation such as inclusion. Opportunity requires addressing the barriers to inclusion such as stigma, ignorance about mental illness, and prejudice. *Independence* point to the manner in which other goals are met (e.g., without undue reliance on others). Clinicians who assist clients in gaining independence recognize that a crucial component is *Empowerment*. This goal of empowerment includes instilling a sense of self-respect in the client, as well as the ability to engage the community barriers to achieving the client's life goals. *Recovery* means that people can control their symptoms and compensate for personal limitations imposed by their illness. Recovery also means that the rehabilitated people recognize their limitations and that such limitations don't necessarily prevent the person from achieving many life goals. The last facet, *Quality of Life*, is a characteristic of living akin to the idea of human flourishing. Not limited to the satisfaction of basic needs like housing, food, and work, but also social and spiritual engagements with other people, institutions, and projects. Psychiatric rehabilitation institutions and practices then implement various enabling activities which aim at fulfilling these goals. These practices include more traditional psychiatric activities like diagnosing and treating symptoms, but extend beyond these to include goal setting, cognitive rehabilitation, family education and support, vocational education and training, social and interpersonal skills training, and 'transfer training', which assures that skills and capabilities learning in one setting (e.g., the rehabilitation facility) are generalized and implemented in other settings (e.g., home, workplace). Moreover, the settings of these activities may be institutional, residential, vocational, and recreational.

Despite substantive contributions to effective psychiatric rehabilitation from US clinicians and researchers, and a strong evidence base for efficacy, less than 5% of people with severe mental disorders receive high-quality psychiatric rehabilitation.[94] The reasons for this lack of implementation of psychiatric rehabilitation are complex and will be taken up later in elaborating my own version of a rehabilitation account for the VMDR, and again in the last chapter.

8.5.4 A rehabilitation account for the VMDR

I can sketch out a rehabilitation account (RA) for the VMDR. The sketch should include a description and goals of such an account; how it relates to the 'competing' accounts of the VMDR, the similarities, differences, and synergisms of the CR and mental health rehabilitation endeavors, and how such an account relates to current and future social welfare practices. I wish to sketch a 'vision' of the RA for the

VMDR, recognizing that substantive conceptual, social, professional, and political changes would be needed—all these discussed more in Chapter 9.

The four accounts for the VMDR I have described in previous chapters—the coincidental, the medicalization, the moralization, and the mixed accounts—all have differences in how the accounts operate and what aspects of the VMDR are addressed. The coincidental account is descriptive of a particular way causal relationships operate when encountering vice and mental illness phenomena together. The coincidental account describes a largely noncausal, accidental relationship between vice and mental disorder when correspondences between these two sets of phenomena occur. Truly coincidental relationships between vice and mental disorders are of marginal interest for a book that seeks to understand noncoincidental, causally related relationships between vice and mental disorder. The medicalization and moralization accounts, however, describe VMDR phenomena in metaphysical terms that frame our understandings of the phenomena. For the medicalization account, the VMDR is situated within the folk-metaphysical varieties of complex multicausal relationships which the sciences seek to make sense of (hence references to CMC accounts). The moralization account, in contrast, reflects the Abrahamic FM of free will, individualism, responsibility, and desert and comprehends these relationships with corresponding moral/ethical terms. While not exclusive in practice, the medicalization and moralization accounts differ in emphasis; the former interested in understanding, explanation, prediction, and sometimes, control, while the latter are primarily interested in control, protection, and sometimes, salvation. Both accounts aim at improving the human condition, in their own ways. The mixed account combines, informally, the other three accounts in irregular and sometimes unpredictable or contradictory ways.

8.5.4.1 How the RA relates to other VMDR accounts

The RA for the VMDR presented here combines elements of the other four accounts, with some important exceptions and additional properties and goals. First, the RA as formulated here is not focused on coincidental relationships but rather aims to *deliberate upon* and *develop* vice-mental disorder relationships in society and culture that *contribute to human flourishing*. So my RA account here is normative and ultimately prescriptive in intent—aiming at how vice and mental illnesses should be handled in a society that flourishes.[95] The RA shares a commitment to a CMC-FM, using science and technique to advance flourishing for the public at large, for the criminal offender, for the mentally ill person, and especially for the mentally ill offender. The RA also shares, with the moralization account, a strong, deliberate commitment to aiming RA work toward ethical ends and human flourishing, but within a metaphysically secular (CMC) and philosophical framework that eschews punishment in its varieties as a rehabilitative tool. The addition of a 'philosophical framework' is crucial here because a diversity of viewpoints and values address the question of how to build flourishing societies. Philosophy is needed to provide metaphysical and practical frameworks on which to build, downstream, rehabilitative efforts for the

VMDR. As will be described and shown in Chapter 9, much philosophical as well as practical and empirical work remains to be done to develop an RA approach to the VMDR.[96] So the RA approach to the VMDR explicitly embraces the CMC-folk-metaphysical approach to explanation and understanding in the sciences, as well as a democratic, deliberative discourse about how the RA/VMDR work contributes to human flourishing, with human rights and humanistic-care assurances. The commitment to deliberation and discourse in the RA distinguishes it from the informal, haphazard mixed account, which unfortunately dominates the cultural and professional mental health landscape today. The RA proposed here is envisioned as a social policy deliberative process continuously under development, assessment, revision, and improvement. This self-regulation of the RA applies to both local, on-the-ground applications, such as exemplified by the CPAI instrument discussed earlier, to government-level deliberative-democratic policy, monitoring, and regulation to minimize abuses and promote humane efficacy. The recognition and appreciation of the determinative power of folk-metaphysical assumptions, in how we think about social welfare, also distinguishes the RA approach from the others.

8.5.4.2 Overlapping goals and values in extant criminal and mental health rehabilitation

Having just read about the goals and values of CR and mental health rehabilitation, the reader can probably identify several shared elements: (1) integration into society as a fully functioning citizen, (2) assistance with social resources required to flourish (e.g., housing, jobs, human connections, and spiritual practices), (3) development of focused skills required to avoid social seclusion (e.g., hospitalization, incarceration), (4) reducing stigma and boosting social engagement, and (5) invigorating the client with empowering social connections, opportunities, rights, and responsibilities. I summarize the shared values as (a) a person-centered orientation, (b) citizenship, (c) social attachments, (d) conscientious freedoms, and (e) expanding personal versatility and resilience.[97] These goals and values, as shared between criminal and psychiatric rehabilitation, are easy to endorse for the RA.

Some aspects of psychiatric and CR, however, are NOT shared, or at most weakly shared, and, indeed, each field could learn from the other: an objective of my RA for the VMDR. I consider several distinctions for each field next.

8.5.4.3 Relative emphasis on individual tailoring of care

After decades, even centuries, of providing one-size-fits-all CR, and relative failures to reduce reoffending, the arrival of a rehabilitation-over-punishment criminal justice vision has been sorely needed. As depicted by the RNR and Good Lives models this work has consolidated around fundamental principles, practices, and outcome assessment tools that explicitly emphasize tailoring efforts to particular, unique individuals. My reading of the psychiatric rehabilitation literature, on the other hand, suggests less consensus on the principles, practice, and outcome assessment within a shared 'person-centered' rubric of implementation.[98] While much greater attention is needed for the history behind these differences, a brief consideration of the history presented for each rehabilitation tradition provides a modicum of understanding. The current dominance of the RNR and GL models for CR was a reaction to the 'nothing works' rhetoric of the latter twentieth century criminal justice field discussed previously. Focused and rigorous work was needed (and still is) to overcome the cynicism bred regarding CR in the larger political and public sphere in the United States, from the late-twentieth century to present. The public's lack of sympathy, or even overt hostility, toward criminal offenders has contributed to this stasis. These public attitudes, as noted in Chapter 7, have been driven by decades of sensationalistic news coverage and stigmatizing media representation. For psychiatric rehabilitation, its pressures and social vectors were of a different kind. Embedded in the United States with states-based legal regulation, a fragmented and incoherent health care system serving partially overlapping populations and sectors (e.g., privately insured care, state-funded public sector care, Veterans Administration-based care, and boutique fee-for-service care), and economic and political pressures to contain costs, the values of efficiency and mass-scale service delivery have prevailed, overwhelmingly, over the micromanagement of individual cases. These pressures then encouraged group-based programs, standard treatment protocols, rigid criteria for admissions, and segregated disorder-focused programs, in an effort to mitigate the conflicts between personalized care and the efficiencies of program-scaling for cost savings. The aforementioned fragmentation of US social welfare services mentioned previously also impedes true person-based care. Collectively, these socioeconomic vectors erect substantial barriers to true person-centered care.[99]

8.5.4.4 Emphasis on differential sets of personal traits and diagnostic categories

That CR and psychiatric rehabilitation (PR) address divergent, but too-often overlapping social problems (as with crimes committed by a mentally ill offender or homelessness/vagrancy, to mention two examples) implies that discrepant sorts of rehabilitative needs will be encountered. The prevailing models of CR focus on individual psychological traits (e.g., antisocial attitudes, impulsivity) as individually based criminogenic needs, for instance, while PR has prevailingly focused on the severely and persistently ill people with psychotic and/or mood disorders. Both rehabilitative efforts have focused, arguably, on the people with the greatest social and personal need, as well as those which pose the most adverse burden on the public and the taxpayer. However, the potential for 'comorbidities' of other kinds of psychological conditions, handicaps, and special needs, multiply the challenges to individually tailored rehabilitation. These are further complicated by mixing in different sorts of legal and ethical challenges (e.g., capacity to consent, probation/parole requirements, various kinds of compelled mental health treatment, and form of payment for services). If CR is to admit clients with mental disorders, then facets of these conditions must be assimilated into tailored CR efforts. Consider, for example, the efforts to address psychological trauma in the CR population, contributing to high risk for violent offenses.[100] These efforts are substantive and address just one comorbid condition, albeit an important and pervasive one. I've already mentioned in earlier chapters the greater risk of violent victimization of mentally ill people, so the burden of rehabilitating people with severe or persistent mental disorders with trauma 'added' is a shared challenge for CR. Needless to say, other comorbidities are abundant.

8.5.4.5 Differential criteria of 'success' or 'efficacy'

In the case of CR, the base goal seems established as reducing recidivism or reoffending. Interestingly, the RNR and GL models seem to spin off many of the ideals of Rotmanian CR through the processes of reducing recidivism. This is to say that by developing prosocial skills, reducing impulsivity, re-engaging with family and community, and rekindling citizenship, for example, the CR effort is fostering the overall flourishing envisioned by Rotman (and me) as well. I could describe this as a *flourishing cascade*: through rehabilitative attention to criminogenic needs one in effect initiates a feed-forward cascade aimed, in the ideal, at overall human flourishing. I'm confident that PR has similar aims, and perhaps the base goal of preventing rehospitalization (or arrest!) serves as a first step toward a flourishing cascade for severely and persistently ill people (e.g., recovery). The particulars of how each tradition capitalizes on achieving these base goals and provoking a flourishing cascade are too complex and unfeasible for me to address here.[101] However, the establishment of intermediate steps beyond these base goals is needed as the research develops. For both fields, the efforts continue to develop consensus within each field for evidence-based program evaluation and assessment.

8.5.4.6 Contrasting moral perspectives

Emerging from Abrahamic versus complex-causal folk-metaphysical assumptions, public and professional attitudes toward CR and PR have moral assessments attached. Substantial portions of the population differ in their moral beliefs and attitudes about the personal responsibility of people who commit crimes, as well as their moral beliefs and attitudes about people who have severe and persistent mental disorders. These moral perspectives get imbricated into policy and the net effects can be revealed by how rehabilitative care for CR and PR are funded. As is usually the case with understanding social-system priorities and values, one should follow the money. PR is primarily funded through private, state, and Federal insurance mechanisms, as well as taxpayer-supported programs for uninsured or underinsured individuals, such as state public sector mental health programs. CR is funded through Federal and state tax-supported criminal justice programs. Both can benefit from grant support for focused programs and research, but these are temporary. Because of these profoundly different funding streams, an integrated CMC rehabilitative model of social welfare for mentally ill, mentally ill offenders, and ordinary criminal offenders poses steep challenges for public policy in the United States. That these funding streams are rooted in strongly held mad-versus-bad moral perspectives within Abrahamic folk-metaphysical assumptions means that a unifying social welfare CMC account of the VMDR is a very tall order. Such challenges in moral attitudes, much less metaphysical assumptions about the criminal offender and the mentally ill person will require a gradualist approach in public policy, likely starting with developing programs for the mentally ill offender—a ripe and rewarding ground for integrating the two rehabilitative approaches on a much smaller social welfare scale.

8.5.4.7 Field-specific and special problems

The practical needs to implement an RA model that integrates the best of both CR and PR, is daunting in a broad vision, and also poses smaller albeit important challenges. First, I shall consider some of the big-picture issues, then consider some of the granular challenges faced by this integrated effort.

To integrate CR and PR into a unique new RA entity, a fundamental issue is the lack of administrative integration and communications permissions in order to deliver coherent, effective, humane, and efficient services. Analogous to the realization that US Intelligence agencies were unprepared for a coordinated homeland terrorist attack like 9/11, private and governmental social welfare services for criminal justice, juvenile justice, youth and adult mental health services, intellectual disability services, domestic violence, and elder care are hampered by their isolation and lack of communication and coordination described in my opening chapters. We will continue to have simultaneously redundant and negligent services without investment in a unified social welfare information system which parses services and tracks movement across specialty systems of care and rehabilitation. Consider, as a particularly complex, but not-uncommon example of a person with an intellectual disability, a bipolar mood disorder, and a history of sex offenses. The medical treatment of the individual on mood-stabilizing medications would be essential, including monitoring for safety and adherence. The monitoring task in particular may be more difficult in the setting of a significant intellectual disability. An RNR/GL approach to address unique criminogenic needs will need collaboration and assistance in adapting these methods to an individual with an intellectual disability. Feasibility constraints would likely lead to use of virtual care delivery, preferably video-based, as widespread mental health expertise is concentrated in cities, while many criminal justice facilities are located in rural areas and small towns and cities. None of this integration and coordination would be possible without a social welfare information system. The latter, of course, would have to address privacy and confidentiality concerns, as well as provide security assurances and formulations to avoid compromises of the civil liberties of the individual. Information system design with insights from philosophy and ethics will be required, much like what was encountered with US Homeland Security efforts.[102] Indeed, such a clearinghouse may be a good first-effort target for development, and the integration provided could potentially make an early impact in improved care, reduced recidivism, and even the saving of lives, as the information barriers of the kind encountered with the case of Seung-Hui Cho in

Chapter 1 could be reduced. On the other hand, big-data related, and artificial intelligence uses to predict, in particular, criminal malfeasance raise substantive ethical and civil liberties concerns.[103]

8.5.4.8 Rejection of punishment as a component of criminal justice

This element of the RA for the VMDR has been alluded to in earlier chapters and has been extensively argued in the law, criminal justice, and philosophy literature.[104] Here, the RA specifically excludes punishment as part of its account; this does not mean that incarceration is necessarily excluded, but it does mean that the punitive elements of incarceration should be minimized. Along with extensive research in criminology and penology, discussed in Chapter 6, demonstrating the lack of efficacy of punishment strategies in preventing reoffending (and hardly contributing to the flourishing of the offender). Incarceration in the RA only serves to incapacitate the person who (at the time of evaluation) cannot be adequately rehabilitated or treated. Incapacitation through incarceration or other means, then, in this setting, serves to protect the public from dangerous offenders who presently cannot be rehabilitated. This said, the fact is that incapacitation constitutes a significant restriction on an individual's freedom, so a punitive element in incapacitated/incarcerated individuals is unavoidable. However, an RA offers much more in services of a humane nature, while minimizing the role of punishment to this kind of restriction of freedom.

8.5.4.9 New roles for forensic psychiatry and criminology

With the relative elimination of punishment in the criminal justice system, the medical-ethical conflict between participating in punishment hearings and 'do-no-harm' conflicts for physician-psychiatrists are reduced. This assumes, of course—falsely—that punishment in the criminal justice system will be minimized overnight. This of course will not happen in immediate future. In the meantime, as discussed in Chapter 6, the role of the forensic psychiatrist in expert testimony in determinations of guilt will conflict with the medical ethic of *do no harm*, and therefore, in my view, cannot be justified ethically. Who then should advise the court about matters of competency to stand trial, or provide an expert basis for an insanity defense? What I suggested earlier in Chapter 6 was the relatively new subfield in criminology, 'forensic criminology' (FC). As I would like to see the field develop, FC involves criminological expertise to be discussed in more detail below, but also includes expertise on the traditional roles of forensic psychiatrists as expert witnesses (e.g., evaluation of competency to stand trial, evaluation of criminal defendants for the NGRI 'insanity' defense, and related topics having to do with the relationship of mental illnesses to criminal concerns). This 'vision' of FC so far has not gained traction in the United States. However, two recent textbooks from outside the United States on 'FC' provide an orientation to the field as it exists in the United Kingdom and Australia.[105] In both the Australian and UK visions for the field, the forensic criminologist participates in a criminal procedure through lending expertise on the science of the genesis of crime, criminal investigations, managing evidence and other investigative material, informing the crime scene examination with its scientific basis, and forensic testimony in the courtroom around these and other topics. The idea of the FC as an expert in the role of mental illness in criminal offenses is not one that is prominent, at least in my reading of the field, however. That said, this role is what I have in mind for the forensic criminologist of the future. Indeed, after all the discussion of criminogenic needs and the psychology of offending that has preoccupied CR theorists, it is a short path to consider the role of various psychopathologies and illnesses in criminal offending. This expertise could then serve the role of expert testimony on standard courtroom tasks for criminal defendants (e.g., assessing competency to stand trial, determining retrospective mental states of the defendant, and assessing eligibility for NGRI (insanity) defenses). Because forensic criminologists are agents of the court and the criminal justice process, they would have no ethical conflict with participation, even with all the conviction potential for punishing and harming the defendant. In summary, I'm proposing that these roles as expert witness to criminal courts be assumed by forensic criminologists, taking psychiatrists out of the criminal courtroom, and returning them to patient care, whether criminal or law abiding.

What might the FC contribute to the current role of the correctional psychiatrist involved in the diagnosis and treatment of prisoners? I believe it would richly complement their therapeutic and rehabilitative role, even in the absence of the full adoption of a rehabilitative orientation to criminal justice and penology.

Why? Currently, many correctional psychiatrists are subject to participating in parole hearings and the advancement of privileges within the prison. Such participation compromises their objectivity, in that the treatment role binds them to benefit giving; complicating their judgment about matters like parole eligibility.[106] Moreover, participating in parole hearings compromises the therapeutic alliance through providing a motivation for the prisoner to dissemble or manipulate in the treatment/rehabilitative relationship in order to present a parole-friendly appearance to the clinician. In short, prisoners present what they want the psychiatrists to see and hear, rather than fully engaging in the rehabilitation relationship toward authentic ends.

This concludes my sketch of the RA for the VMDR. With this material in place, the concluding Chapter 9 fully explores the implications and lessons learned from my analysis.

Notes

1. Natanson (1973).
2. Ravenscroft (2010).
3. In my 2005 book, *Values and Psychiatric Diagnosis*, I described different kinds of values involved in the DSM psychiatric classification system. One of these was 'ontological' values, which I described as deeply presupposed, tightly held assumptions about the nature of reality and existence. An example of an ontological assumption in the recent DSMs was 'individualism', in that mental

disorders were assumed to afflict individual persons, and not be social or family problems—the latter proposed by some schools of family therapy. Another ontological assumption which has generated some interest in the literature to follow was 'hyponarrativity': Hauptman (2015); Hoffman (2015); Tekin (2014); Tekin & Mosko (2015); Varga (2014). DSM hyponarrativity described the manual's eschewing of narrative understandings of psychopathology—that people's illnesses were 'storied', embedded in life histories and sociocultural circumstances. Instead, DSM categories were based on indicative features—symptoms and signs of illness. In the case of Abrahamic FM assumptions being challenged by CMC metaphysics, one can recognize how tenaciously the respective groups may hold them.

4. Hampsher-Monk (1992); Kymlicka (1992); Plucknett ([1956] 2010).
5. Ladyman et al. (2007). See also Ross et al. (2006).
6. See Hatfield (1979); for a contrary view, see Rocca (2005).
7. See Sadler (1997, 2005) and note 3 above.
8. APA (2013).
9. Morse (1998, p. 339).
10. ibid, p. 338.
11. Note that the CMC account does not endorse a particular theory of multicausal relationships, a task which has occupied philosophy of science for decades. Rather, the CMC account is intended to encompass a variety of specific views about the nature of complex-causal relationships, all sharing the FM assumptions described here for the CMC account. The Abrahamic FM assumptions likewise encompass the otherwise distinctive traditions of Christianity, Judaism, and Islam.
12. See for instance Caruso (2012); Dilman (1999); Glannon (2015); Shaw, Pereboom, & Caruso (2019); Waller (2011, 2015, 2017).
13. Schaffner (1993).
14. Cuthbert & Insel (2013).
15. Of potential interest is DSM-5's movement of Personality Disorders into a nosological equivalent basis to other mental disorders, rather than having them set off as a separate axis in a multiaxial diagnostic systems as in DSMs III through IV-TR. APA (1980, 1987, 1994, 2000, 2013).
16. Martin & Barresi (2006); Porter (2003); Seidentop (2014); Thomson (1993).
17. Porter (2002, 2003).
18. Quinn (2000), pp. 831–832.
19. Kelly (1992); Plucknett ([1956] 2010); Sadler (2013a); Seidentop (2014) Thomson (1993); see also Chapters 5 and 6.
20. Bacon, Jardine, & Silverthorne (2000); Porter (2003).
21. Remember the CMC FM is a family of related accounts sharing particular characteristics, a generic term linked to various scientific causal-explanatory approaches.
22. See Schaffner (1993, 2016) for an extensive elaboration of complex-causal human sciences. Note also these causal accounts were framed by human interests in health, safety, and related values.
23. Bolton (2008); Fulford (1989); Porter (2002); Sadler (2005).
24. Porter (2002, 2004).
25. Chapman & Ciment (2015).
26. Radden (1994, 1996). I might note that the RDoC initiative in the US NIMH may marginalize faculty psychology even further, see note 14.
27. Morse (1998). See also Morse (2002, 2008).
28. APA (2003).
29. Slovenko (2002).
30. Adshead & Sarkar (2005).
31. Jorm (2012).
32. Gulliver et al. (2010).
33. Wang et al. (2007).

34. Angermeyer & Dietrich (2006).
35. Pescosolido (2013).
36. US Bureau of Justice Statistics (2006). https://bjs.ojp.gov/library/publications/mental-health-probl ems-prison-and-jail-inmates.
37. US Bureau of Justice Statistics, 2017. https://bjs.ojp.gov/library/publications/indicators-mental-health-problems-reported-prisoners-and-jail-inmates-2011. See also NICIC: Mentally ill persons in corrections. http://nicic.gov/mentalillness.
38. Sadler (2013a). See also Chapter 4.
39. Talbott (2004).
40. See for instance Raine (2013). See also Choy et al (2019).
41. Horn (1989); Jones (1999).
42. See for instance Bolton (2008); Haldipur, Knoll, & Luft (2019); Sadler (2014).
43. See for instance https://www.fastcompany.com/90528312/heres-how-we-get-to-a-world-where-we-don't-need-prisons-at-all; https://www.csmonitor.com/USA/Justice/2020/0914/Can-Amer ica-move-beyond-mass-incarceration-audio.
44. See https://www.hhs.gov/about/budget/fy2017/budget-in-brief/nih/index.html and https://www. nsf.gov/about/budget/fy2017/.
45. https://www.nimh.nih.gov/about/budget/fy-2017-budget-congressional-justification.shtml.
46. https://www.nsf.gov/about/budget/fy2017/pdf/22_fy2017.pdf.
47. See Tonry (2017) for a special-issue journal discussion.
48. See Pickard (2011) for a critical analysis, as well as Lacey & Pickard (2019).
49. Sadler (2019). For a formative discussion of some of these ideas, see Sadler (2008).
50. Gold & Kinrys (2019).
51. Conrad (2007); Sadler et al. (2009).
52. Sadler (2019).
53. Rotman (1990).
54. ibid.
55. ibid, p. 3.
56. The arguments for, and against, punishment and retributivist criminal justice have occupied philosophers for millennia, and social scientists and jurists for centuries. For this note, I sketch most briefly the arguments against punishment and retributivism and provide citations for those who wish to read more into the issue. The discussions warrant a book in themselves! As I was assembling these brief notes, I was gratified to see that the arguments against punishment/retributivism can be neatly organized into topics matching key Abrahamic folk-metaphysical assumptions, which in effect reads as a kind of replication of my own work by a bundle of independent scholars addressing piecemeal elements in their critiques. In his introduction to an anthology on theories of criminal punishment (Tonry 2011a), Michael Tonry provides a summary overture to a common theme about punishment: 'Utilitarians disparaged retributivism as vindictiveness disguised in pretty words and retributivists disparaged utilitarians as amoral, insensitive to human rights and prepared if need be to punish innocents to prevent crime' (2011a, p. 3). One thread of retributivist critique could be characterized as the 'epistemic' critique. Epistemic critiques hold that because the determination of key elements for justified punishment, such as moral/criminal responsibility, free will, and desert, are difficult to determine or 'know', to punish by policy is to perpetuate intolerable frequencies of misplaced, unjustified punishments (see Jeppson (2021) for a review and critique). Other scholars attack the foundational arms of retributivism directly: rejections of free will, based on various arguments, undermine requirements for responsibility and desert; see the collection by Shaw, Pereboom, & Caruso (2019). Others dismantle the notion of moral and criminal responsibility: see Waller (2011, 2015, 2017). While still others critique the concepts of blameworthiness and desert: see Hanna (2019); Kelly (2021). For a historical context, see Trinkaus (1949). So that summarizes ever-so-briefly the philosophical critiques. What does the empirical science show?

Perhaps most disconcerting is the research by social scientists about the impact of punishment and retributivism. Criminologists find that punishment not only doesn't work in preventing reoffending, that instead it often increases the likelihood of reoffending: see the reviews in Weisburd, Farrington, & Gill (2016). Social scientists investigating the effects of parental incarceration on families find that children grow up to more likely end up with delinquency and/or have mental disorders: see the reviews by Besemer & Murray (2016) and Poehlmann-Tynan, Runion, Weymouth, & Burnson (2019). As for prisoners themselves, they not only are more likely to offend again, but re-enter a world with a response repertoire suitable to prison life and not citizenship, with mental disorder sequelae and discrimination barriers regarding employment and other economic opportunities: see review by Kazemian & Walker (2019).

57. Rotman (1990, p. 3).
58. ibid, p. 8.
59. Sverdlik (2014).
60. Sverdlik (2014, p. 623), quoting Duff (2001 pp. xviii–xix). See also Duff (2018).
61. Forsberg & Douglas (2020).
62. ibid, p. 110.
63. ibid, p. 110.
64. ibid, pp. 110–111.
65. ibid, p. 112.
66. ibid.
67. Hampton (1984).
68. Hampton (1984, pp. 214–215), quoted in Fosberg & Douglas (2020 p. 112).
69. Forsberg & Douglas (2020, p. 113).
70. 'Normatively thick' here means, in my interpretation, that these accounts and practices are based upon particular viewpoints about the moral goodness of the particular prosocial attitude and behavior under consideration. In that sense they are more value-laden in that they presuppose a particular range of morally justified practices within a good society.
71. This standard of matching moral improvement efforts to crime set warrants further discussion, but from my clinical perspective, this proposal poses a practically unfeasible demand based upon a naive and scientifically bereft atomistic psychology of wrongdoing. I pity the poor souls who would try to implement such a daunting task!
72. Forsberg & Douglas (2020, p. 116).
73. 'Dominion' concerns an internal change in one's psychological-moral state of mind, manifested by remorse and a willingness to receive psychotherapy, training, or other forms of counseling of a prosocial nature. See Braithwaite & Pettit (1990).
74. Rotman (1990, p. 3).
75. See for instance Andrews (1995); Andrews & Bonta (2010); Farringer et al. (2021); Gendreau, Little, & Goggin (1996).
76. A Google Scholar search on the 'RNR Model' yields over 4000 hits, as of mid-April 2022.
77. See Smith, Cullen, & Latessa (2009); Vose, Cullen, & Smith (2008).
78. Andrews & Bonta (2010); Cullen & Gilbert (2013).
79. Psychiatry has long been pessimistic about the treatment of personality disorders in general and Antisocial Personality Disorders in particular (Roy & Tyrer 2001), reminiscent of the 'nothing works' popular appraisal of CR in the late-twentieth century. However, a new generation of cognitive-behavioral theorists are using cognitive-behavioral therapy to treat personality disorders with empirically validated successes: see review by Beck, Broder, & Hindman (2016).
80. Bonta & Andrews (2016).
81. Gendreau & Andrews (1996).
82. Duriez et al. (2018).
83. Campbell et al. (2018).

84. Gannon et al. (2019); Lowenkamp, Latessa, & Smith (2006).

85. Mowen, Boman, & Stansfield (2018); Stansfield et al. (2020); Ziv (2017).

86. Ward (2010); Ward, Collie, & Bourke (2009); Ward, Mann, & Gannon (2007).

87. Fortune (2018); Harkins et al. (2012); Looman & Abracen (2013).

88. Zeccola, Kelty, & Boer (2021).

89. Wilson & Yates (2009).

90. Anthony & Liberman (1986).

91. Anthony, Cohen, Farkas, & Gagne (2002).

92. Cnaan et al. (1988).

93. Corrigan (2003).

94. Bond & Drake (2017); Nemec & Mullen (2017).

95. Of the many philosophical accounts of eudaimonia, well-being, and 'human flourishing' out there, I am most favorable to Amitai Etizioni's version described in his short book *Happiness is the Wrong Metric* (2018). Very briefly, Etzioni views three components to flourishing: the hedonic aspect, focusing on happiness or pleasure; the meaningfulness aspect, which reflects values greater than oneself; and the 'affirmational' aspect, which has to do with living by morally or ethically good actions. Each is required; none in isolation are sufficient. See also Shanafelt (2009).

96. A primary goal of this book is to stimulate philosophical and empirical work to address human flourishing through deliberative considerations of the various aspects of the VMDR.

97. I am grateful for the unpublished work done on this topic by Saira Bhatti MD and Theresa de Freitas MD during their philosophy of psychiatry elective with me during the last year of their residency at UT Southwestern, 2019–2020. Their work is a significant contribution to this section, but of course, any hare-brained ideas are my fault. For a recent discussion of rehabilitation treatment for people with multiple impairments, see Winance & Bertrand (2022).

98. See Vita & Barlati (2019).

99. While aimed at understanding the socioeconomic placement of the DSM diagnostic manuals, Sadler (2013b) provides bird's-eye view of economic forces influencing US mental health care, including PR.

100. Fritzon et al. (2021); Levenson & Willis (2019).

101. Vita & Barlati (2019).

102. Chen et al. (2008).

103. Surden (2020); Tate & Zabinski (2004).

104. Caruso (2012); Dilman (1999); Glannon (2015); Shaw, Pereboom, & Caruso (2019); Waller (2011, 2015, 2017). See also Garland (1993) and (2002) for detailed analyses of punishment in society.

105. Petherick, Turvey, & Ferguson (2009); Williams (2014).

106. Bronnimann (2020); Verdun Jones (2000).

9

Forty theses: Conclusions, implications, and prescriptions

Conventions blind us.

9.1 Overview of conclusions

As I had suggested in the opening pages, as this book developed it assumed the shape of a mystery story for me—mystery nonfiction, we might say, and academic nonfiction to boot. The mystery was relatively straightforward to state: Why do some categories of mental disorders involve value judgments of immorality and criminality, while others do not? Even more briefly: what is the relationship between mental disorders and vice behaviors? As I began studying the relevant materials, component questions emerged. Like a detective in crime fiction, I drifted from one line of evidence to another, often with only an intuitive understanding of the relevance of this or that finding. Like a documentarian, I assembled what I thought

Vice and Psychiatric Diagnosis. John Z. Sadler, Oxford University Press. © Oxford University Press 2024.
DOI: 10.1093/oso/9780198876830.003.0009

were relevant materials (in my case, ideas and sources) from many traditions and disciplines, so that this book formed a multidimensional 'case record' that could assist other detectives in re-examining and rethinking my analysis. In my chasing of clues, I often faced blind alleys, red herrings, and rabbit-holes.[1] I had to make difficult choices about curtailing this or that line of investigation. Also like the mystery story, door-opening revelations at various stages of the investigation uncovered even bigger considerations. The vice/mental disorder relationship (VMDR) became an entry-point or window into broader quandaries in the social role of psychiatry, interprofessional relationships, criminal justice policy and practice, the ethics of forensic psychiatry, and social welfare theory and practice. In keeping with the detective metaphor, I plotted the evidence and history in graphics, and I traced connections between clues and began to see patterns and common themes, leading to the potential culprit and the climax of the story.

However, my culprit was not a person but a pervasive, powerful, and inconsistent set of assumptions about how key aspects of reality are organized in Western culture and our collective minds. The denouement, begun in the prior chapter and followed through with this one, resolves many elements of the initial mystery. (However, like true crime and crime fiction alike, every facet of the mystery may not be solved. . . .) With any luck, this mystery story will unleash a new generation of library- and Google Scholar-bound gumshoes interested in the ongoing questions and mysteries associated with VMDR and its ramifications. Indeed, the following theses raise new tasks, research questions, and directions for action that demand their own detailed treatments. Unfortunately, such treatments I cannot provide here, however much I want to inspire and provoke them.

My prevailing conclusion: The peculiar bundle of contradictions which describes the current VMDR is, in large part, a cultural artifact of prevailing conflicts and incompatibilities between complex multicausal (CMC) scientific metaphysical assumptions and Abrahamic folk-metaphysical assumptions. These conflicts of assumptions manifest themselves in contrasting views of reality, pertaining to the classification of psychopathology, the practice of forensic/correctional psychiatry, to criminal law, to criminal justice and penology, and even to other social welfare institutions like care of mentally ill and intellectually disabled people, and juvenile justice concerns. Additionally, I should not underestimate their importance in shaping public understanding of mental illness, crime, punishment, and criminal justice. In recognizing, and preferring, CMC folk-metaphysical assumptions over the Abrahamic ones, some broad corollaries may be derived, pointing toward formal and cultural changes in institutions and practices—some changes being subtle, with others more dramatic.

Vicious conduct may, or may not, be disordered. In the former it should be investigated, characterized, with treatments developed, tested, and implemented. In the latter account, nondisordered vice conditions should be treated as a challenge for civil societies to develop effective and just social welfare responses. These general conclusions and prescriptions are not complete. An important conclusion points to the considerable empirical and philosophical work remaining to be done if the medieval schism between vice and mental disorder is to be recast into a more humane science and practice of human welfare for all. In this latter sense, my conclusions point toward new tasks in implementation. Psychiatry, after all, cannot avoid imposing certain kinds of values, including moral ones, on patient relationships and their sciences. The question is which ones are preferable, which permissible, and which are impermissible. Similar concerns about proper values should inform clinical and correctional practices.

Any denouement would be incomplete, however, without closer views about what happens to the protagonists. In my nonfiction mystery story, the remainder of this chapter will be considering what happens to the 'protagonists', the latter being, in my case, the practices, ideas, people, and institutions involved in the VMDR. The protagonists are us.

My telling of a nonfiction mystery story is my way to encourage the reader to read the whole book and witness the development of these ideas—to not skip to the conclusions. Finding out whodunit before reading a crime novel is to lose much of the interest and pleasure in reading the book. More importantly, the preceding chapters depict the evidence and reasoning which generated these summary conclusions. They survey our cultural practices and make the case for how pervasive Abrahamic metaphysical assumptions are. In my 'whatdunit', the credibility of my conclusions resides in the journey of wading through the evidence and arguments. Taking a reader on this journey of discovery is to share the intrigue I enjoyed in doing this work, as well as making the conclusions more credible. I believe many of my conclusions will be controversial in that I am challenging long-established elements of major institutions and their associated practices. I also challenge standard ways of thinking about mental illness, criminality, immorality, and their interactions. Reframing culture is difficult, humility necessary, and clarity essential.

What underlies such potential controversy is the frequent absence of the social structures that provide humane rehabilitation, on the one hand, and powerful fears that reform will leave holes in public protections from crime, on the other. These fears are legitimate—I hold them myself. However, their realization is not inevitable, as my discussion to follow will indicate.

In our current era of divisive discourse, I can anticipate some of the distortions of my views, and fatal predictions in response to them: that I want to let criminals go 'scot-free', that I want to destroy forensic psychiatry, that dangerous criminals will be wandering the streets, that mental health will be tarnished further in the public eye by being lumped with criminality, among others. I address these objections, misunderstandings, fears, and misgivings in the pages to follow.

I should remind readers of the pervasive and rigid character of folk-metaphysical assumptions discussed in Chapter 8 and earlier in my book *Values and Psychiatric Diagnosis*.[2] Folk-metaphysical assumptions may be the most powerful assumptions we carry, structuring our thinking in countless ways. Metaphysical assumptions, along with their related 'ontological values',[3] are the building blocks of our life choices. Recall my example of the difficulty the scientist has when asked to relinquish her belief in a mechanistic universe, or the resistance of the Christian fundamentalist to abandoning the notions of salvation, just deserts, or personal responsibility. As I pointed out in *Values and Psychiatric Diagnosis*, one cannot change one's ontological values (and specifically, one's folk-metaphysical assumptions) like a suit of clothes. The labor of rethinking folk-metaphysical assumptions took me a long time to practice and inhabit. Every old-school problem had to be rethought, and every cognitive reflex questioned. However, when practiced and habituated, I found I can not only tolerate the new suit of clothes, but can recognize they fit better than ever. I was wrong about not being able to change one's ontological suit of clothes. You can, but it takes lots of practice.

In thinking through the implications of mental health and criminal justice institutions solely under CMC folk-metaphysical assumptions, I recognized that some of my implications and prescriptions would require huge reforms in our conventional ways of doing things for mentally ill and immoral/criminal behaviors. I didn't want to avoid the big-ideas or 'vision' implied by my analysis, but also wanted to recognize that incremental changes—small changes—which would be more likely to be accomplished in the near term. Moreover, the recommendations and prescriptions to follow often had a tacit sequential logic: some steps should be taken first, to pave the way for later, bigger, steps.

To respond to this insight, I have adopted a two-phase approach to the potential impact of this work: identify some recommendations as 'transitional' and others as 'ideal'. (In advance I admit not all of my notions sort themselves neatly into these two categories.) As another organizational principle, I've framed my sections to follow according to particular domains of implementation and impact: the role of philosophy, implications for law and criminal justice, implications for particular diagnostic categories in *Diagnostic and Statistical Manual of Mental Disorders* (DSM)-5, to mention a few. Topics overlapping in these domains are common however, so I have provided frequent cross-references.

In these sections that address various facets of my implications/recommendations, I mentioned above the convention of 'ideal' and 'transitional' steps and goals. 'Ideal' refers to the summative vision of VMDR reform, involving multiple transformations of ways of thinking and accompanying development of policies and practices. Ideal recommendations are likely to require upheavals and restructuring of the relevant institutions. 'Transitional' refers to smaller, incremental steps, ones which can be implemented now, toward VMDR reforms which are better suited to earlier, easier, less radical implementation. Transitional steps, with stakeholders willing, are unlikely to require upheavals of institutions, but initiate smaller positive changes on a shorter timescale. They also enable inhabiting new metaphysical assumptions in smaller, more digestible steps. I present my conclusions, implications, and prescriptions as 40 theses, each then considered as Ideal (I) or Transitional (T).

Before I proceed to the next section, I note that my conclusions and prescriptions are not complete. I repeat, much empirical and philosophical work remains yet to be done, if the medieval schism between vice and mental disorder is to be set aside toward a more humane science and practice of human welfare. Now I develop this denouement toward wider conclusions, implications, and prescriptions.

9.2 Clarifying 'punishment'

In prior chapters I have discussed the ethics of punishment in the criminal justice system, as well as alternatives to punishment in other models of justice, such as restorative justice, community justice, as well as Native American and Aboriginal approaches to justice. In formulating my '40 theses' to follow, I recognized that I needed to clarify my use of the 'punishment' concept, as it figures largely into several of the theses to follow. Moreover, the concept has a long and complex history in the criminal law and criminal justice literature, making it particularly important for me to clarify how I'm using the punishment concept in my conclusions and recommendations to follow.

In his chapter on 'Punishment' in the *Oxford Handbook of Crime and Criminal Justice*,[4] Michael Tonry eloquently sketches out the multiple meanings and functions of this term in Western criminal law. I summarize and paraphrase some of Tonry's points here to acquaint the reader with the complexity of such a familiar word:

- punishment as a deterrent to future offending
- punishment as retribution to the offender for wrongs done to others
- punishment as a practical tool in promoting law-abiding behavior in citizens
- punishment as a stimulant to moral growth in the offender
- punishment as part of a system for maximizing social happiness through crime prevention
- punishment as a method to enforce social norms
- criminal punishment as an economic aid to communities through corrections services
- punishment as an expression of social values, fears, and standards
- criminal punishment as a rhetorical device used by politicians to persuade voters to favor them
- punishment as a social apparatus to appease victims' sense of violation, loss, or need for vengeance

Other meanings and functions are possible, of course.

The primary sense of 'punishment' I oppose on an ethical basis, and would like to reform, has to do with the retributional, or what I consider the vengeance elements. These elements form the core of punishment as just desert in Abrahamic folk-metaphysical assumptions. Many clues point to this conclusion throughout the book, so for many my viewpoint should not be too surprising. My primary rationale for rejecting retributional punishment is ethical; finding it hard to justify the rectification of moral wrongs through committing more moral wrongs: harming others. Harming others is as fundamental a moral wrong as we have, as repeatedly discussed in Chapter 4's historical considerations of morality.

My secondary rationales for rejecting retributional punishment are practical. Punishment-as-inflicting-harm is ineffective in deterring reoffending; indeed, the evidence more powerfully supports that retributional punishment *provokes* reoffending.[5] Not only do punishments like incarceration provoke reoffending, retributional punishment perpetuates ongoing crime in later generations and families.[6] This should not be surprising; violence, after all, perpetuates more violence— see Chapter 4 and the world histories of war. The social toxicity of retributive vengeance would seem to undercut multiple-other functions of punishment: promoting law-abiding behavior, stimulating moral growth, maximizing social happiness through the *failure* to prevent crime, and to enforce social norms. The practical inefficacy as well as moral offense of retributional punishment has been reviewed in prior chapters as well as other authors and reviews.[7]

In the upcoming theses below, and with the recognition of the complexities at hand, I should discuss how the multiplex concept of punishment fits into my conclusions and recommendations. To this end I articulate two meanings of punishment for my purposes: for simplicity's sake I'll call the two versions 'maxi-punishment' and 'mini-punishment'. I might have called them 'intentional punishment' and 'contingent punishment' respectively, for reasons that will be evident below, but the intentional vs. contingent language is technical and possibly misleading. My descriptions here also reflect not a dichotomy, but more accurately extremes on a continuum, where 'maxi-' implies the most severe harms, and 'mini-' involves the minimization of harms (as well as the maximization of humane rehabilitation).

The maxi-/mini- language also recognizes that 'punishment' is in the eye of the beholder, as I'll indicate shortly.

'Maxi-punishment' designates retributional, deliberate harms issued to an offender with the goal of hurting and causing misery to the recipient.[8] Maxi-punishment includes incarceration in all its harm-engendering forms and variations, from solitary confinement to conventional jail cells, to banal political neglect of prison staffing, services, and civil order, leading in the extreme to chaotic and dangerous environments. Maxi-punishment has more to do with toxic impact on the offender than on set or setting.[9] The environments of incarceration in particular compound harms for prisoners, as well as for staff, who then aim for the most expedient means of behavior controls of inmates; often escalating punitiveness. Maxi-punishments as in incarceration can include gestural efforts at rehabilitation like including libraries and training for work responsibilities, but these are dwarfed in impact by the punitive aspects of the complete imprisonment experience. Maxi-punishments are not limited to incarcerations however, as other constraints on liberty, psychological and economic stress on families of offenders, loss of rights and privileges, and social exclusion and discrimination as a parolee, or even ex-convict, may count as maxi-punishments. Considerations of 'proportionality' (to the level of the offense) may find their way into maxi-punishments, but the goal of inflicting harm and misery on the offender differs only in severity.

Regarding 'mini-punishment', or perhaps 'contingent punishment', this refers to the punitive aspects of humane, rehabilitative treatment for offenders with or without mental disorders. Ignoring the punitive potential of the State's (court's) compelling actions upon offenders would be naive, requiring an acknowledgment that well-intended rehabilitation efforts may nevertheless be experienced as punitive. The contingent punishment experienced by offenders in the face of compelled rehabilitation must be considered and conscientiously attended to. I mentioned earlier that what is punitive for people is often in the eye of the beholder: a court-ordered requirement for community service may be experienced by some people as punishment, while others may view it as an opportunity, with many other meanings possible and likely. In nonforensic, adult psychiatry, the occasion of an involuntary treatment order filed by the treating clinician and the court may be viewed by some patients as punitive, or be viewed as lifesaving by others, while still others may recognize both aspects in their complexity. Some involuntarily treated patients may well change their minds about their 'commitment' or 'detention' depending on the quality of their treatment, their treatment response, and overall outcome.[10] Compelled humane rehabilitation is still compelled, and still eligible for resentment, resistance, and suffering.

The promise of alternative justice models, involving restorative, community, therapeutic jurisprudence, or other methods may offer more humane procedures, reducing the 'mini-punishment' collateral harm. In the ideal, the contingent aspects of punishment—'mini-punishment'—should be minimized, as the name suggests. Work in this direction should continue.

In thinking through the implications of mental health and criminal justice institutions solely under CMC folk-metaphysical assumptions, I recognized that some of my implications and prescriptions would require huge reforms in our conventional ways of doing things for mentally ill and immoral/criminal behaviors. I didn't want to avoid the big-ideas or 'vision' implied by my analysis, but also wanted to recognize that incremental changes—small changes—are more likely to be accomplished in the short term. Moreover, the recommendations and prescriptions to follow here often had an implied sequential logic: some steps should be taken first, to pave the way for later, bigger, steps.

To respond to this insight, I mentioned a two-phase approach to the potential impact of this work: identify some recommendations as 'transitional' and others as 'ideal'. (In advance I admit not all of my notions sort themselves neatly into these two categories.) As another organizational principle, I've organized my sections below according to particular domains of implementation and impact: the role of philosophy, implications for law and criminal justice, implications for particular diagnostic categories in DSM-5, to mention a few. Topics overlapping in these domains are common however, so I have provided frequent cross-references.

In these sections which address various facets of my implications/recommendations, I mentioned above the convention of 'ideal' and 'transitional' steps and goals.

'Ideal' refers to the summative vision of VMDR reform, involving multiple transformations of ways of thinking and accompanying development of policies and practices. Ideal recommendations are likely to require upheavals and restructuring of the relevant institutions. 'Transitional' refers to smaller, incremental steps, ones which can be implemented now, toward VMDR reform which are better suited to earlier, easier, less radical implementation. Transitional steps, with stakeholders willing, are unlikely to require upheavals of institutions, but initiate smaller positive changes on a shorter timescale. They also enable inhabiting new metaphysical assumptions in smaller, more digestible steps. I present my conclusions, implications, and prescriptions as 40 theses, each then considered as Ideal (I) or Transitional (T).

Before I proceed to the next section, I note that my conclusions and prescriptions are not complete. A frequent and, therefore, major conclusion is empirical and philosophical work, and much remains to be done if the medieval schism between vice and mental disorder is to be set aside toward a more humane science and practice of human welfare. Now I develop more this denouement toward wider conclusions, implications, and prescriptions.

9.3 Forty theses

The number of these conclusions and recommendations are pragmatic, and as one can determine, partially overlapping as implications in one domain may have implications in other domains.

9.3.1 The role of philosophy

Thesis 1: *The identification and analysis of folk-metaphysical assumptions can shed light on the framing of scientific categories, law, public policy, and professional policy.* (T) This major conclusion was elaborated at length in Chapter 8, and I should not recount those arguments here. The identification of folk-metaphysical assumptions lends itself to social science research, 'experimental philosophy', and philosophy proper. The analysis of folk-metaphysical assumptions provides opportunities for philosophical discoveries as well. In the case of this book and this work, when I began, I did not anticipate the concept and importance of folk-metaphysical assumptions, nor did I anticipate how they would render comprehensible the manifold cultural and historical trappings of the vice-mental disorder relationship. The reading of and formulating a history of relationships between morality and madness was key to this discovery, and these unfolding developments can be followed in Chapters 4 and 5. Similarly, the analysis of the goals of medicine and criminal law in Chapter 6, and especially Section 6.1.1, was also a crucial component of these insights. The quite-different modes of reasoning in medicine and criminal procedure reflect the conceptual power of differing folk-metaphysical assumptions. As a philosophical task, the analysis of folk-metaphysical assumptions/implications is transitional in that it enables clarification and comprehension of other problems and ramifications described in the book, as well as summarized in many of the theses below.

Thesis 2: *Exploring the boundaries of ordinary misconduct versus disordered misconduct should be assimilated into the philosophy of psychiatry in the same way as exploring the boundaries between ordinary and disordered anxiety, cognition, mood, and substance use, have been part of the philosophy of psychiatry intellectual project.* (T) This conclusion is a logical extension of a key insight from this book: If psychopathology is to be understood as disturbances of various functions or 'faculties' of the mind/brain, the exclusion of morality from its aegis should end, and disturbances of morality should be assimilated fully into the field as with other mind/brain functions and faculties. Chapters 4 and 5 describe the historical marginalizing of morality as a faculty, as well as the confusing and paradoxical consequences of this marginalization in persisting categories like psychopathy, homicidal insanity, antisocial personality disorder, kleptomania, among others. This thesis is transitional in that work on psychopathologies of morality could begin immediately—and have already done so with extensive research on (particularly) psychopathy. The results would forge new understandings of older, 'classical' diagnostic categories, and remove the socio-historically rigid constraints around the idea of disordered immorality and criminality. The admission of morality as a psychological phenomenon can inform novel neural-pathway approaches to psychopathology as well, such as those sketched by the Research Domain Criteria (RDoC) framework.[11] This thesis poses a substantive set of conceptual tasks for the philosophy of psychiatry, that of distinguishing disordered vice from nondisordered vice, with ramifications for untold potential categories of vicious behavior. Fortunately, philosophy of psychiatry has worked on distinguishing disordered behavior and experience from normative/diverse experience for many years, and this work could be considered a major thread in the field.[12] One aspect has been developing decision rules or concepts to distinguish mental disorders from ordinary experience in the broadest sense, manifested, for example, in the post-DSM-III era through formulating a 'definition of mental disorder'.[13] Another aspect of this work is distinguishing normative psychological experience from psychopathological experience: such as the distinction between ordinary sadness and a depressive disorder,[14] ordinary anxiety from pathological anxiety, or ordinary shoplifting from kleptomania.[15] A third aspect of this work has to do with identifying thresholds for the transition from ordinary human experience to pathological human experience, as illustrated in recent years by the debate around the relationship between grief and depressive disorders,[16] or the transition between normal dissociation and psychotic experience to pathological experiences.[17]

Stated differently, once the exclusion of vice 'experience' is recognized and reversed, and the concept of disordered vice is admitted into the domain of medical psychopathology, a broad set of analogous philosophical tasks open up. Namely, these tasks involve sorting ordinary vice from pathological, disordered vice—the sorting out of particular conditions regarding their normal or pathological status.

While analogous, the project of sorting out disordered from nondisordered vice brings some novel challenges, as well as some relevant history. The relevant history is supplied by the struggles around categories like Attention-Deficit Hyperactivity Disorder, addiction, psychopathy, antisocial personality disorder, klepto- and pyromania, and Intermittent Explosive Disorder, among others. These conditions as vice-laden disorders were laid out in Chapter 2. These vice-laden disorders and their status as mental disorders offer lessons for other, to-be-considered, vice-laden conditions as candidates for the status of 'mental disorder'.

These conditions also offer lessons about the sociocultural context in which clinicians, nosologists, and scientists must deal with, such has the conspicuous underfunding of research on vice-laden disorders like paraphilias in particular, and criminality/immoral conduct in general, on the other. Along with this, recognizing pathological vice means grappling with the 'insanity defense'/not-guilty-by-reason-of-insanity (NGRI) considerations again, especially when this work is transitional, and the criminal law/justice system is still stuck in Abrahamic folk metaphysics and punitive retributive justice models.

My last consideration for this thesis is the novel challenge posed in distinguishing normal versus disordered vice. These distinctions are required for the formalizing of candidate conditions for vice-related mental disorders. Outside of the small number of vice-laden DSM conditions identified in this book, the discussion of potential vice-laden conditions discussed in Chapter 3 becomes more relevant. Spurious as well as serious proposals for vice-laden categories like 'White-collar insider-trading disorder', 'serial killer disorder', and 'pathological bias' beg to be reformulated and reconsidered, along with a potential raft of previously inconceivable vicious conditions yet to be recognized and described. As mentioned earlier, the refinements of disorder-nondisorder philosophical inquiry, developed by the field over the past 30 years,[18] give us a head-start on this new domain of psychopathology. This work has made advances in sorting out poor-quality, invalid, and/or half-baked categories of psychopathology, and the methods of analysis developed can be applied to vice-laden categories. The vice-laden category endeavor is also transitional and sets the stage for scientific studies to consider the validity of proposed disorders, as well as placing such conditions into the complete scientific research matrix of explanation and prediction. Endophenotype and biotype research as in the RDoC research framework could follow. Treatment, rehabilitation, and prevention would develop, benefiting not just mental health but criminology and crime prevention. As this multifaceted work progresses, it could well contribute to the policy argument for reforming correctional and criminal justice systems into more humane, rehabilitative directions as described in Chapter 8.

Thesis 3: *Philosophy should develop spectrum or graded accounts of blameworthiness/wrongful action for moral and criminal offenses.* (T) Critical challenges to concepts of 'free will' take on higher stakes when revisited in the context of the reform of psychiatry and criminal justice. Rethinking, or even rejections of, free will concepts and moral/criminal responsibility,[19] as well as concepts like 'evil'[20] in terms friendly to CMC metaphysical assumptions, are gaining interest and momentum in philosophy. These primary sources offer insights applicable to the challenges of vice-laden disorders in the philosophy of psychiatry. Setting aside the assumptions related to free will and moral/criminal responsibility enables the raising of new questions about how we should regard and treat people who act wrongfully.

Under CMC accounts, people act wrongfully under complex interactions with environment, personal history, and personal biological endowment. The expanding understanding of random or quantum-level neuromolecular events in the brain may shed light on the perception of 'free will' and the handling of vicious conduct, normal or disordered.[21] The conformations of these complex-causal interactions between environment, history, and biology might be called 'attribution matrices' to convey the respective balance of causal constraints and choice options under various wrongful action scenarios.

With this shift away from conventional free will/responsibility concepts, we quickly recognize that not all wrongful acts are the same; they vary by social impact (from trivial to horrific), as well as vary in the phenomenology of their implementation, conventionally described as 'impulsive', 'deliberate', 'accidental', 'reflex', and 'negligent' actions, for example. The phenomenology of vice is a wide-open domain to be explored as it has with conventional psychopathology. The language and concepts associated with wrongful actions are already rich, and we can recognize that nuanced accounts of related concepts like 'blame' are fruitful, a good example being Hanna Pickard's work.[22] Causality theory as well could contribute to these formulations. The shift from all-or-none concepts of responsibility which dominate current Abrahamic criminal law in the West can be rethought through graded, perhaps even 'spectrum', weighted, or dimensional accounts of human wrongful action (e.g., the attribution matrix mentioned earlier). The philosophy of psychiatry, along with the challenge of vice-laden disorders, and the distinction between disordered and normative vicious actions, provide a fecund ground for test cases of the new free-will-free philosophies. This transitional work, these spectrum, circumflex, or differentiated accounts of wrongful action, may, and should, inform public policy and law in the future.

Thesis 4: *The mad-versus-bad debate should disappear as an artifact of the cultural confusions regarding the CMC and Abrahamic FM accounts of the person.*(T) The Abrahamic accounts, (through their persisting cultural prominence in spite of the development of complex-causal reasoning in philosophy and science), have posed substantial cultural hurdles to the inclusion of morality as a medical focus of interest. The 'mad-versus-bad' debate[23] has a long history in the philosophy of psychiatry. The debate was whether or not a particular mental condition was medical or moral. Crystallized in many ways by Thomas Szasz's *The Myth of Mental Illness*; Szasz declared that mental illness was a myth because it was not grounded in existing pathological accounts of disease.[24] Szasz's twentieth-century work collapsed the dichotomy between mad conduct and bad conduct through an endorsement of a then-contemporary standard of medical tissue and cell pathology, all discussed in Chapter 8 and in Sadler.[25] Szasz wanted wrongful conduct, whether mad or bad, to be handled by institutions like the criminal justice system, education, and religion. Only *bona fide* diseases, with pathological somatic findings, warranted medical interventions.

In contrast, my account collapses the mad-versus-bad debate in a different way. If we set aside Abrahamic metaphysical assumptions and admit vice behavior as just another kind of human problems worthy of scientific understanding, treatment, and prevention, then 'bad' points to domains of experience and behavior that can be pathological like any other domain. The historical stigma and neglect by medicine and psychiatry can be corrected through a collaborative paradigm between psychiatry, the social sciences, neuroscience, criminology, and 'neurocriminology'.[26] 'Mad' and 'bad' collapse into a single group of problematic human experiences and behaviors. The sciences provide room for explaining pathological vice as well as explaining ordinary vice. This thinking can be developed as a transitional step through the philosophical work described in preceding paragraphs. Reforming the culture-at-large in these directions, however, remains a big, daunting ideal.

9.3.2 Implications and recommendations for the mental health professions

Thesis 5: *Complex multicausal folk-metaphysical assumptions should prevail in psychiatric theorizing and empirical science, case formulation, and treatment planning, replacing Abrahamic folk-metaphysical assumptions.* (I) The centuries-long persistence of Abrahamic metaphysical assumptions in medicine, law, and public culture has generated multiple barriers to efficient, effective, and humane social welfare efforts, as discussed in my introductory chapters. Setting aside Abrahamic folk-metaphysical assumptions is a not a matter of them being metaphysically incorrect, but because they generate theory, practice, and policy that are pragmatically ineffective, even self-defeating. (Regarding the latter, the best example is incarceration leading to hardening of criminal behaviors and the intergenerational perpetuation of antisocial conduct in families of prisoners.) The Abrahamic barriers and failing policies are discussed throughout the book, in both broad, general terms (e.g., the seeming random appearance of current vice-laden categories, the tension between punitive retribution-based criminal justice and humane rehabilitative criminal justice)[27] as well as smaller, granular applications and problems (e.g., criminal responsibility, the NGRI defense).[28] The splitting of social welfare services into (criminal justice/penal) and clinical/rehabilitative has created services that are both intrusive and neglectful, expensive and ineffective, and redundant and chaotic.[29] Structuring social welfare services on CMC metaphysical assumptions provides the foundation for undoing these flaws and building services that are holistic, coherent, humane, scientifically robust, and more effective. Healthcare trainees should be trained and socialized into viewing immoral or antisocial behavior as potential manifestations of disorder, if present, or manifestations of complex sociobiological causation, if nondisordered.

Finally, the thrust of psychiatric and criminological research should shift away from sorting people based on nonmoral and moral behaviors. When antisocial behavior is involved, the thrust should shift toward explaining, predicting, and rehabilitating problematic behaviors and thinking that endanger the patient and the public.

This goal has elements of the ideal as well as the transitional. The transition from the confounding of mental health care by Abrahamic FM assumptions can be addressed one disorder at a time, one set of treatment/rehabilitation principles at a time, in one locale and practitioner domain at a time, and in these senses pose transitional steps. In law/criminal justice, transitions are already emerging, as Western criminal law and services explore restorative justice models, therapeutic jurisprudence practices, diversion of offenders into mental health services,[30] and mental health crisis services, all of which may involve productive collaborations with psychiatry and other mental health services. Taken collectively and on a broad scale—mental health at large working in synchrony with criminal justice services at large—constitutes the hard-won ideal through the reform of one local policy and practice at a time.

Thesis 6: *Behavioral syndromes involving criminality and wrongful conduct should be assimilated into the aegis of psychiatry research and practice.* (I) This thesis is the mental health counterpart to Thesis 2 in the 'role of philosophy' section above. The task for psychiatry should be to refine existing vice-laden categories, using the same standards of rigor as for other mental disorders.[31] Similarly, psychiatry, aided by the philosophy of psychiatry, should consider, explore, and perform research relevant to distinguishing ordinary vice from disordered vice, mentioned in Thesis 2. Collaboration and exchange between psychiatry/mental health and criminology, and related fields, would augment and accelerate progress, as well as open up new horizons for novel treatment/rehabilitation strategies for particular vice-laden disorders. Basic, translational and clinical neuroscience, criminology, psychology, and other social sciences, as always, should feed these developments in clinical and services research.

Thesis 7: *Criminality (and immorality) should be public health concerns, and psychiatry, along with the social and biological sciences, should contribute to the prevention and reform of criminal offending and the promotion of prosocial flourishing.* (T) In recent years the relationships between public health concerns and crime have been recognized as even more complex than before. The 2021 media and politicians' deliberate spread of COVID-19 misinformation, conspiracy theories, and preposterous treatment claims[32] proliferated through escalating US COVID deaths exceeding one million. To my eyes, such misconduct is both immoral and clinically harmful to the public, but is such behavior criminal? Criminal gun violence in its various forms constitutes one of the major causes of death in the United States, and the United States is the leader in gun violence in Western countries.[33] These two examples alone represent hundreds of thousands of deaths associated with immorality (deliberate social deceit about life-saving public health concerns) and criminality (gun violence). The contribution of mental disorders, recognized and unrecognized, to these public health trends is unknown. Given the novelty of the distinction between normal and pathological vice, the contributions of each to our current situation is also unknown. However, these contributions should be revealed through grant research support, and public health interventions for such widespread, vicious conduct. Relevant policy should be developed and implemented as a consequence of these understandings and commitments.

Thesis 8: *Psychiatry, as well as forensic criminology, should be accountable to the polity as to what counts as prosocial, virtuous, and vicious behavior in their research and treatment programs.* (T) This thesis is a cautionary one, in that the history of psychiatry is rife with examples of 'psychiatric abuse' (e.g., the use of psychiatry to impose unjustified, nondemocratic political power, oppress minorities, silence political opposition, and exploit the vulnerable). Opening the door to vice-laden disorders associated with criminality offers a new potential for politically motivated psychiatric abuse. This concern contributes to my earlier comment that my analysis assumes, even depends upon, a liberal democratic society with human rights, civil liberties, and rule of law intact. That said, I would be naive to assume such an ideal State exists; hence the need for continuous involvement and accountability to the polity in developing psychiatric categories and conditions, as well as their treatment. Psychiatry cannot avoid imposing certain kinds of values, including moral ones, on patient relationships. The question is which ones are permissible, and which aren't, and if in fact such values are implemented in actual practices.

More concretely, in 2004 Bill Fulford and I recommended that patients and their families be involved in developing the DSMs,[34] and the DSM-5 process opened up a mechanism for 'outsider' input,[35] though without any transparent public mechanism for making use of such input. It was, however, a first step, and a good second one would be to generate accountability mechanisms, and a third would be for psychiatric nosologists to formalize review of social science and philosophical literature addressing the ethics of developing DSM or other categories of mental disorders, especially when vice-laden.

Thesis 9: *Psychiatry should reinvigorate its past tradition of aiding in criminal justice reform and the reform of criminal offenders, as well as invigorate its efforts to study and treat psychopathologies of moral conduct.* (T) The proliferation of twenty-first century crimes like mass shootings, hate crimes, cyberbullying, and other cybercrimes should provoke substantial portions of the public to support scientific research addressing the social, developmental, and biological propensities of individuals committing such crimes. Psychiatry, clinical psychology, criminology, and other social sciences should lead collaboratively in this effort.

9.3.3 Implications and recommendations for law and social policy

Thesis 10: *Meaningful and ethical handling of the VMDR requires a substantive civil society, with effective democratic governance, rule of law, social justice, and civil liberties like freedom of press, religion, and speech.* (I) As the lead-off recommendation in this section, I acknowledge this as an aspirational, and unachieved, ideal over the centuries of the human race, as evident from Chapters 4 and 5. That said, all societies vary in degree in living up to these ideals. We might think of adherence to these ideals as a dimension: more, or less, instead of an either/or state of affairs.

The closest and most substantive empirical measurement effort for these multiplex ideals might be the World Justice Project (WJP).[36] The WJP is a nonpartisan international group that conducts huge surveys that evaluate over 100 countries and jurisdictions on a number of aspects of human freedoms, rule of law, and effectiveness of government, summarized through their Rule of Law Index (RLI). The RLI has a careful and consistent methodological structure, large sample base, and empirical rigor. The Index rates these countries around four Universal Principles (accountability, just laws, open government, accessible and impartial dispute resolution), each of which is broken down into multiple component dimensions. The RLI is a tool in assessing how one's country is doing in reference to these democratic ideals. The RLI offers summary overall scores and ranks the countries accordingly. These are of interest for our purposes as a reference toward outstanding institutions and practices in particular countries. In addressing the changes I propose, these countries potentially offer exemplar practices in dealing with the vice-mental disorder relationship, and for this potential the RLI is of interest as a tool in identifying countries and cultures that model humane mental health and criminal justice practices.

In the 2020 report, my country, the United States, ranked twenty-first globally, with the United Kingdom thirteenth, Australia eleventh, Canada nineth, and New Zealand seventh. Compare these English-speaking countries to the top-ranking countries: Denmark first; Norway second; Finland third; Sweden fourth; and the Netherlands fifth. What these Northern European countries are doing differently, and better, regarding the social welfare of mentally ill people and criminal offenders would be of keen interest—though one I cannot elaborate in the concluding section of a very long book.

However, some clues to these approaches are contained in prior chapters. Consider the discussion of Swedish philosopher Lennart Nordenfelt's account of social welfare in Chapter 6, Section 6.1.1.1. Nordenfelt's notion of social welfare is broad, assimilating medicine as well as US-conventional social welfare services as contributing to a holistic 'ability of persons'.[37] Other sources of reform ideas are described in Chapter 6, Section 6.3.1, particular restorative justice models. Examining the mental health and criminal justice practices of these leading RLI nations would be a great project.

Thesis 11: *Criminal justice legislation must address protection of the public but not at the expense of rehabilitation and restoration of the offender, mentally ill or not, to prosocial citizenship.* (I) A crucial distinction emerging from the investment in CMC metaphysical assumptions is that the protection of the public can be disconnected from the intentional punishment and vengeance-oriented justice meted out in most of our current US institutions.[38] I refer again to Scandinavian countries with their low violent crime rates[39] associated with their shorter sentences and more humane prison settings. This thesis could be a transitional one with a collective will to make piecemeal reform of particular laws and institutions, which could be implemented right away.

Not all violent criminal offenders, mentally ill or not, can be treated and rehabilitated effectively. The task for the sciences is to identify personal and institutional factors limiting rehabilitation efficacy, as much as the task is to continuously improve treatments and rehabilitation procedures. However, for those untreatable and/or unable to be rehabilitated, the public must be protected. Protection of the public needn't be punitive for offenders or potential offenders. Public protection should minimize punitive elements, as incarceration or other kinds of seclusion from the public, however humanely designed, exact their own psycho-emotional toll through the isolation of the offender from other people, family, culture, and engagement with the world at large. This emotional toll is illustrated through the revelatory case discussions in Gwen Adshead's and Eileen Horne's *The Devil You Know: Stories of Human Cruelty and Compassion*,[40] where violent offenders are humanized without diluting any of the horror of their actions.

Thesis 12: A nonpunitive, rehabilitative criminal justice system and criminal court obviates the need for an insanity defense. (I) As discussed earlier, the need for rehabilitation, as well as its implementation, does not require a declaration of moral/criminal responsibility or blameworthiness. Subsequently, what matters most is the *actus reus*: did the person commit the criminal act? My version of *mens rea*, or intentional wrongdoing, is framed by the *attribution* of fault or culpability by the defendant. This is to say, the defendant must be found to have committed the criminal act (actus reus) through action or inaction (e.g., negligence). Recall my introductory discussion of the 'punishment' concept at the beginning of this chapter. There I discussed the distinction between wrongdoing and blameworthiness. Wrongdoing is the failure to respect laws and the intentional disregard of laws. Blameworthiness, in its criminal law sense, entails Abrahamic FM assumptions around individual responsibility and just desert. Criminal intent as wrongdoing is required to establish that a crime was committed, but blameworthiness is unnecessary for this assessment. The CMC 'causal' role of the offender in the commission of the crime (as wrongdoing) is crucial, however, to the planning of rehabilitation to preventively intervene with the causal vectors which lead to the offending. The CMC causal role of the offender's wrongdoing also serves as a component of the restorations made to victims of wrongdoing, but not as the sole component. Recall the discussion of restoration and prevention as analogous to the medical handling of medical errors; where an error is viewed not in the context of a single, blameworthy individual, but a *system* failure with requires correction of multiple causal vectors—a 'rehabilitation' of the system. Guilty verdicts would depend upon judgements of intentional wrongdoing but would not depend upon the defendant's 'blameworthiness'. However, the convicted offenders' state of mind would be always of interest in the later rehabilitative efforts. For example, if the offender's intent was motivated in response to a delusion, then certainly the delusional state is relevant to rehabilitation. If the offender's intent was motivated by a racist grudge against the victim, that too would be relevant to rehabilitation. Relevant causal vectors pertinent to both offenders' actions would be relevant to rehabilitation too. Quality rehabilitation requires planning in accordance with the patient's capabilities as well as limitations, as well as understanding the causal nexus of the criminal event.

These steps can be transitional and can progress at the pace set by development of rehabilitation-oriented criminal justice systems. Our actions, criminal, mentally ill, or otherwise, are multiply shaped by complex-causal networks, which dissipate the need to assess personal responsibility and blameworthiness. Such non-singular causation of any behavior, including criminal behavior, shifts the burden away from assessing blameworthiness, and redirects court procedure toward rehabilitation planning for the antisocial conduct.

Stated a little differently, my treatment here of *mens rea* specifies it as a failure to respect the law; followed by the determination of the *actus reus*—whether or not the defendant committed the wrongful action. The relevance of the state of mind of the convicted offender shifts away from the court and toward the systemic rehabilitative planning and efforts to restore the victims and move the offender toward prosocial citizenship.

The latter raises the question about the procedure following the court-determined determination of guilt. Without punitive sentencing, the court must appeal to the rehabilitative sciences to recommend the appropriate course of rehabilitation to restore the offender to prosocial citizenship. Sentencing in this context shifts away from a court's or judge's conventionally retributive sentencing rules and determinations, and instead challenges rehabilitative therapeutics and planning. In this context the concept of 'sentencing' loses its traditional meaning. The law will need to determine mechanisms for transitioning the offender into rehabilitation, and such mechanisms may be extralegal and dependent upon the science of the era.

At first glance, such rehabilitation planning may sound complex and burdensome, but such rehabilitation planning is similar to many, already-existing criminal justice alternatives discussed in Chapter 6, such as therapeutic jurisprudence, mental health diversion, innovative probation services, and formal restorative and community justice procedures. On the mental health side, treatment/rehabilitation models to consider, adapt, and revise already exist. Clinicians already make assessments of the potential for treatment benefit/rehabilitation through ordinary clinical assessment, and, if warranted, involuntary treatment procedures and subsequent treatment planning.

In earlier chapters I discussed the variability between jurisdictions regarding which mental disorders are eligible for involuntary treatment. While details may vary, a general statement applies where patients with certain kinds of psychopathology are judged more likely to benefit from involuntary treatment than patients with other kinds of psychopathology. Some patients are deemed unlikely to benefit from involuntary treatment, even if eligible by diagnostic category, and are considered for other dispositions, including incarceration to protect the public if they are convicted offenders. Rigorous science is needed to provide ethically justifiable involuntary interventions, and equally rigorous public oversight to prevent abuses.

While this kind of prognostic sorting is common regarding involuntary treatment, I don't wish to imply that such sorting schemes are simple, adequate, and cannot be improved upon. Involuntary treatment remains a procedure with weak scientific evidence as to its efficacy.[41] Indeed, a rethinking of involuntary participation in a broader rehabilitative approach is needed. Too often this sorting of eligibility for involuntary treatment is driven by political posturing, vengeance urges, and sensational fear-mongering by politicians, pop culture, and the media. Dispositions of mentally ill offenders is wildly inconsistent across jurisdictions. The wish to punish some mentally ill offenders like those with paraphilic disorders and Intermittent Explosive Disorder (IED), while others, such as people with psychotic illness, are allegedly more forgivable and eligible for NGRI, is enacted variably in various jurisdictions in the United States.[42] Under a CMC metaphysical understanding, such sorting can be done for scientific, pragmatic, and efficacy purposes not through moralizing about who deserves punishment (e.g., just deserts).

These inconsistencies fade under a CMC bottom-up metaphysics of VMDR. For example, people with psychotic illness, pedophilic offenders, and other sex offenders would receive rehabilitative treatment, keyed to the individual's needs, in keeping with psychiatric and criminological rehabilitative methods. Setting aside the determinative Abrahamic metaphysics of individual responsibility, just deserts, and free will means that the distinctions between punishment-eligible offenders and punishment-ineligible offenders evaporate, because every offender is 'ineligible' for maxi-punishment as the latter is not offered. Reciprocally, every offender is in principle eligible for treatment/rehabilitation unless the science cannot deliver it. In the latter case, humane protective custody, restorative procedures, or other less-severe constraints are alternatives. The final 'problem' that disappears, as mentioned earlier, is the insanity defense (the NGRI defense), and its attached mad-versus-bad deliberations. Involuntary seclusion and behavioral control may be needed for offenders in order to protect the public but should be nonpunitive and therapeutic/rehabilitative in orientation. Offenders receive humane care, and the public retains protection from dangerous people.

Thesis 13: *Both mental health and crime prevention require a public health approach.* (T) Criminal justice and penal reform should aim at reducing criminogenic social drivers in such a public health approach. Of course, rehabilitation and treatment of mental and substance abuse disorders, and other conditions commonly associated with wrongful conduct, can be addressed as crime prevention too. Currently operative political drivers that escalate charges and sentences—to be 'tough on crime'—should be replaced by toughness on criminogenic social conditions, long a focus of criminology, public health, and developmental psychology and psychiatry (not to overlook social welfare generally). Identification of etiological vectors and processes have made great strides over the past 25 years, as discussed in Chapter 6. Incentives and funding should also support mental health diversion, probation support, mental health courts, community treatments for mentally ill offenders, and humane means to protect the public from offenders undergoing rehabilitation, as well as offenders who cannot be rehabilitated.

Thesis 14: *Replace punishment- and vengeance-oriented retributive criminal justice with non-traumatizing, restorative and other alternative justice models.* (T) This transitional, incremental thesis perhaps is implied in all of the above, but these options discussed in Chapter 6 should be stated explicitly for completeness' sake. Indeed, many jurisdictions are already exploring these alternatives, as described in Chapter 6.

Thesis 15: *Western democracies need a comprehensive vision of social welfare services that are smoothly integrated, cost-effective, and humane, unifying the missions of mental health care, criminal rehabilitation, intellectual disability, juvenile justice, homelessness, poverty, and substance abuse care.* (I) This thesis is frankly idealistic in the current US political climate, though comprehensive social welfare, and 'welfare states' are thriving in some parts of Europe.[43] Indeed, the notion of the 'welfare state' has negative connotations for large portions of the US polity; though often based on distortions and misinformation about countries with substantive and broad commitments to social welfare.[44] Research on models of social welfare and their integration are ongoing, and I mention a few references here.[45] In Chapter 6 I noted the fragmented character of US social welfare services, divisively administered among the states and subject to results which were both intrusive and negligent. Such fragmentation of social care demands that the threads of social welfare addressing both criminality and mental illness be brought together into a streamlined and more effective system. The generative role of CMC metaphysics in this regard is to break down the identified punitive, marginalized, and inequitable judgments framed through Abrahamic responsibility and just deserts concepts. Then, consolidate our efforts toward all people as equally worthy and deserving of opportunities for flourishing.

Thesis 16: *Not every immoral or criminal action need be considered a manifestation of a disorder or disease, but wrongful actions should be addressed by the biological and social sciences, philosophy, and public policy fields in an effort to find frameworks, analyses, and evidence that enhance the polity's social welfare and the flourishing of all individuals in a society.* (T) A version of this ideal is stated earlier in Thesis 6, but it warrants explicit mention here when considered in the law and public policy sphere.

Thesis 17: *Preventive detention laws, rarely justified, should never be used in the absence of substantive, adequately funded, effective social welfare programs, crime prevention programs, and adequate public-sector mental health and substance abuse care. Otherwise, they may constitute state-sanctioned persecutory discrimination of people with mental disorders.* (T) In addition to restricting civil liberties for people who have not yet committed a crime, preventive detention laws imply a potential for thought-crimes and legislating morality, discussed in Chapter 5. Law should continue to eschew thought-crimes, and criminal offenses should continue to be confined to behavior actually committed. Antisocial actions or behavior should remain the focus of criminal law, considering the complex scientific causality of antisocial behavior.

Preventive detention, moreover, can be a poor substitute for adequately funded and effective social welfare services. Often it can be politically appealing in that it shifts costs and responsibilities to underfunded programs while giving the appearance of protecting the public. Preventive detention in the absence of good social care literally demonizes people while neglecting their health, education, and welfare. Such laws may also constitute state-sanctioned, morally offensive discrimination against the targeted population.

Thesis 18: *Health, civic, and social studies in public education should provide (particularly) secondary education students with the background knowledge, skills, character education, and critical thinking to evaluate social science and public policy proposals for mental illness and crime.* (T) Variously called civics, civic education, citizenship education, and social studies, this portion of citizen education has been, unfortunately, controversial in recent decades, though the controversy both reaches into what the substance of civics education should be, and its role vis-a-vis other public education topics. This is a deep topic unto itself, and I encourage readers to examine some of the recommended literature.[46] This background is needed to aid students in understanding vice-mental disorder relationships without the accompanying blaming, stigma, and punitive attitudes. Moreover, citizenship education can aid in orienting the polity to a solution-orientation rather than fostering a lowest common denominator citizen culture of blame, hate, and vengeance as promulgated through social and popular media as in the current (2022) cultural moment.[47]

Thesis 19: *Criminal justice reform should address vigorous attention to restoration efforts for victims, including attending to victims' mental health and recovery.* (T) As discussed in Chapter 6, Section 6.3.1.2, restorative justice is not solely aimed at offenders, but 'restoration' also applies to victims of crime. As noted earlier, resistance to restorative justice and criminal justice reform often manifests as vindictive resentment aimed at offenders, often with *lex talionis* sentiments. Perhaps the best counter to this opposition is vigorous attention to restorations for victims of crime, as well as their families. Clinical, psychological, and criminological science likely has much to offer here. Just as clinicians attend to family stress and burden, so should victims of crime be so attended.

Thesis 20: *The overcrowding of penal and criminal justice institutions must be avoided.* (T) The history of both criminal justice and mental health institutions has shown—repeatedly—that overcrowding dismantles rehabilitative and treatment objectives, diminishing humane care and sabotaging efficacy of outcomes, all discussed in Chapters 5 and 6. Addressing overcrowding, with suitable political will, may immediately improve outcomes.

9.3.4 Implications and recommendations for the field of psychopathology

Thesis 21: *Antisocial, criminal, and immoral behaviors should be eligible for mental disorder status by the same criteria as any other professionally recognized mental disorder*. (T) As implied in earlier theses, this thesis is so fundamental for psycho-pathology it warrants explicit statement. As a consequence of Abrahamic folk-metaphysical assumptions, antisocial and immoral conduct has been broken off from prevailing concepts in psychopathology, warranting special consideration and study rather than routine consideration and study. With its past segregation into re-ligious and legal institutions (see Chapters 4 and 5), morality became a psychological function in large part lost to psychopathological inquiry. Only in recent decades has research, most notably on psychopathy, noted in Chapter 5, Section 5.8.2, generated substantial psychopathological interest in this condition as a disorder of morality rather than an evil or sinful condition of free and healthy choice. This recommen-dation for psychopathologists means that the field should distinguish normal from disordered morality in all its manifestations.[48]

Regarding disorder status for vicious conditions, the problems and responses are much the same. While substantial discussion in the literature revolves around par-ticulars,[49] what constitutes a mental disorder has consolidated around a core set of stipulations. A condition to be a disorder involves a behavior pattern or syndrome, some distress or impairment, as well as being harmful or socially disvalued. These are the minimum conditions. These distinctions shouldn't depend upon holding particular moral beliefs or exhibiting particular moral contents. In a simple sense, I mentioned the earlier distinction between ordinary shoplifting and Kleptomania. The Kleptomania diagnosis requires more than just occasional shoplifting.

For a more complicated example, psychopathologists and epidemiologists con-sidered whether religious extremism as manifested in jihadist Muslim terrorist ac-tions should be considered mental illness in the wake of the 9/11 attacks.[50] (More contemporaneously, we might consider white-supremacist terrorism in the United States.) In these discussions, jihadism in itself wasn't considered a mental disorder, though could be (though not necessarily so) associated with other, common, rec-ognized mental disorders. Under my discussion of the prevailing accounts of the VMDR in Chapter 8, Section 8.4, perhaps the relationship between religious and other forms of extremism fits the 'coincidental' account best. As another example, we might recall the discussion and analysis of pathological bias from Chapter 3, Section 3.3.2.2. What has not been explored, under the new lens of CMC metaphys-ical assumptions, is implied by the name 'pathological bias'. The implication is that a 'normal' bias exists and distinguishing that from pathological bias would be essential to the credibility of the latter disorder concept.

A related issue comes up in deliberations on the official DSM definition of mental disorder, appearing in DSM-III forward.[51] The DSM authors want to avoid a defini-tion of mental disorder which confuses mental illness with a conflict between an in-dividual and society. This is understandable, as the diagnosis of mental illness should not be politicized or be subject to the whims of the State. The DSM authors want to differentiate conflicts between an individual and society in order to separate mental illness from sociopolitical issues like (e.g.) antishoplifting laws, hate crimes, and ji-hadism.[52] Differentiating between disordered conflicts between the individual and society and nondisordered sociopolitical conflicts between the individual and society, however, has been, and will likely continue to be, difficult and contentious to do in some cases.[53] Therefore, investigating such concerns should be the provenance of the philosophy of psychiatry/mental health, the social sciences, as well as law and social welfare policy.

A second corollary to this thesis, again related to the foregoing, is this: Criminal and immoral conduct, when related to mental disorders, should be critically examined regarding whether such conduct is a core feature of the disorder, instead of only an associated feature. As discussed in Chapter 3, Section 3.4 and 3.5, psychopathological symptoms which are 'loud', and monosymptomatic 'syndromes' may well represent contingent rather than essential features, making for unreliable and invalid categories. This is illustrated by the case of Conduct Disorder (Chapter 2, Section 2.2.2) and in some of my prior work.[54] Phenomenological psychopathology[55] and etiological studies can assist in differentiating the core features from incidental and consequent features of disorders.

A third corollary to this thesis is that the holistic appraisal of the patient (diagnosis) should be augmented to appraise the moral capacities of the patient, as reflected in the ethical implications of the patient's conduct, as well as considering the patient's criminal history, if any, as a domain containing valuable clinical information. Too often in conventional psychiatry, the criminal history defaults to an arrest history, reducing a complex life experience to points on a calendar. Diagnosis as holistic appraisal is discussed in Chapter 3, Section 3.1.1, and this section provides guidance about avoiding premature closure and cursory diagnostic practices.

Each of these reform efforts in this thesis are transitional and could be implemented immediately.

Thesis 22: *As with current trends in understanding the etiologies of psychopathologies, investigations into biopsychosocial, complex multicausal factors for immoral and criminal conduct should continue and be robustly funded and expanded with social 'savings' from criminal justice and penal reform.* (I) The key to this thesis is the 'robustly funded' element. The research funding in criminology, represented in the United States by a small proportion of the National Science Foundation's awards portfolio (see nsf.gov/about/budget) which is in turn dwarfed by the research funding for psychiatric illnesses, represented in the United States by the National Institute for Mental Health (nimh.nih.gov/about/budget/fy-2020-budget-congressional-justification), which is in turn dwarfed by all the other categorical Institutes of the National Institutes of Health (nih.gov/about-nih/what-we-do/budget).

One of my preferred methods for understanding the priorities and values of organizations is by 'following the money'. Clearly the priority of understanding and preventing crime is a low priority in our governmentally funded research institutions. While mental health research fares far better, both budgets suffer in comparison to most medical research priorities. We can understand these budget priorities in many ways, but I would insert the blaming, vengeance-laden cultural legacy of Abrahamic folk-metaphysical assumptions into these understandings of policy priorities. Instead of revenge and punishment we need scientific explanation, prevention, and effective rehabilitation strategies. In 2022 even a bitterly divided, hyper-partisan US Congress could appreciate the futility and waste of the highest incarceration rate in the world.[56] Perhaps the time is right to commit a lot more money on prevention, rehabilitation, and prosocial recovery.

Thesis 23: *DSM-style and other categories of mental disorder of the future should consider moral conduct as a relevant mental function like cognition, conation, and affection, and be subject to disorder status based on the same conceptual and empirical criteria as the other, nonmoral mental disorders.* (T) Following the release of DSM-5 in 2013, the professional discussion regarding diagnosis and classification of psychopathology shifted significantly, with rising criticism within neuroscience, psychiatry, and clinical psychology.[57] A primary concern for this DSM discussion was this: the manual was increasingly irrelevant, even misleading, in supporting basic, translational, and clinical neuroscience etiological studies, inspiring advanced alternative nosologies like HiTOP.[58] The huge US NIMH RDoC initiative, the latter being a multilevel theoretical infrastructure for funding research into mental disorders[59] arose in part out of dissatisfaction with the DSMs as providing constructs for etiological science. These initiatives could transform psychiatric clinical diagnostic practices away from the psychological function-driven, syndrome-based, classical structure of psychopathology that preceded the DSMs.[60] I mention this recent DSM history to frame the dependence of these research theoretical structures for psychiatric nosology on Abrahamic folk-metaphysical assumptions. Whether psychopathology is considered under a framework of psychological dimensions or complex interactions of neural pathways and subsystems, the clinical/practical use of such concepts could still be embedded in Abrahamic folk-metaphysical frameworks when applied to our current social world of clinical practice where vice behaviors are marginalized presumptively as non-clinical. Regarding the VMDR, the attraction of the RDoC framework consists in its friendliness or suitability for utilizing CMC folk-metaphysical assumptions into our fundamental understanding of psychopathology—however broadly or narrowly the field is construed. Such formalizing of CMC FM assumptions would naturally, and should, involve considering impairments in the function of morality as part and parcel of the investigation of complex-causal networks. Such work would abandon more 'traditional' (e.g., Abrahamic) formulations of psychological functions. If RDoC style neuropsychiatric research prevails in shaping future conceptions of psychopathology, the scope of research funding infrastructure should include disturbances in moral thinking and conduct using the RDoC scientific architecture and making potential contributions to the clarification of normal versus disordered vice. In conclusion then, this thesis recommends incorporating moral and nonmoral psychological functions in the investigations of present and future theoretical structures for psychiatric research.

Thesis 24: *Psychopathologists and nosologists will need to transform the philosophy of disorder status into a central consideration, rather than a marginal one.* Starting in the 1990s, the then-developing philosophy of psychiatry 'movement' took on psychopathology and psychiatric classification as central themes to be explored. In the ensuing decades the literature in these fields has exploded, generating new insights into such problems as defining mental disorders, distinguishing normative from pathological mental states and functioning, the clarification of value judgments and entailments in disorder categories, and describing psychopathological phenomena in precise and revealing detail.[61] When embracing the metaphysical assumptions of the CMC type, the opportunities and needs for new research are huge. The need for this work in mainstream clinical and nosological scientific research will never be greater, as the ethical stakes in admitting morality-based psychopathology will be proportionately large. Chapter 3, Section 3, only scratched the surface in exploring the philosophical/conceptual issues of assigning vice-laden behaviors the status of 'disorder'. The stakes range from distinguishing normal from pathological vice in ordinary practice, to addressing human participants' protections in clinical research, to developing social policy consequent to revising our concepts of what counts as a mental disorder.

Thesis 25: *Criminology should partner with psychiatry as clinical psychology has done.* (T) Readers of Chapter 5 learned about the collaboration between psychiatry and what became clinical psychology in the mid-twentieth century. Clinical psychologists (as well as clinical social workers and others) assumed crucial tasks in the emerging mental health division of labor and institutional infrastructures as the mental health field organized and grew. Psychiatrists, with their medical training, were neither trained nor well-suited to these tasks: psychometrics—psychological testing, the development and delivery of psychologically based therapies (notably but not limited to the various psychotherapies), as well as adding their own nonbiomedical perspectives to mental health scientific research. Ever since, psychiatry and clinical psychology have been partners and occasional rivals in mental health care development and delivery.

With disorders of morality and vice no longer excluded from the realm of mental illness, criminology becomes a natural partner under CMC folk-metaphysical assumptions. This is a transitional but nonetheless ambitious thesis in that the nascent field of forensic criminology would need to develop and expand to engage criminological research and knowledge with the challenges of vice-related psychopathology. This vision for forensic criminology was discussed in Chapter 8. Just as psychiatry will need to expand in understanding the contributions of criminology and corrections science to this new domain of psychopathology, so would criminologists need to engage more with the mental health disciplines. Perhaps the development of psychiatry and clinical psychology as collaborators and partners could serve as a model.

Thesis 26: *Vice and mental disorder studies should be embedded in intersectional identities.* (T) Psychiatric categories, including vice-laden ones, should be subject to ongoing social justice analysis; race, gender, and class studies, and political discourse, and not considered just the domain of the traditional human sciences and the mental health professions.[62] The embeddedness of race, gender, and class power structures discussed in Chapter 5 offer lessons about how the mental health field and criminal justice fields have failed to address power inequities in society. Assimilating vice-related disorders into the mental health arena opens up new potential for discrimination and exploitation of non-white people, as has been demonstrated in recent years regarding policing; sexual harassment; anti-Black, Asian, Muslim, and Hispanic violence, as well as domestic violence.[63] The interplay of power relations associated with various identity descriptors (e.g., gender, race, offender, and mentally ill) makes for complex policy and practice challenges. I believe the proposal for integrated social welfare discussed in Thesis 15 makes intersectional VMDR studies and policy both feasible and crucial.[64]

9.3.5 Implications for particular disorders in DSM-5

Thesis 27: *Dismantle the silos and broaden social welfare efforts.* (I) If we accept that criminal/immoral conduct is subject to being disordered and criminal justice shifts toward nonpunitive rehabilitation and public protection, then the insanity defense debate disappears, as does the need for a differential social welfare response. If all antisocial conduct is subject to rehabilitation, then the silos of adult and juvenile criminal justice/mental illness/intellectual disability disappear and the focus on restoration of prosocial and healthy conduct becomes the overall goal for social welfare institutions. As an ideal, this is a long-term aspiration.

Thesis 28: *The Clinical Significance Criterion (CSC) helps in distinguishing disorder from nondisordered behavior whether vice-laden or not.* (T) Just as the clinical significance criterion[65] may be used to differentiate sexual diversity from sexual disorders (through the identification of distress and disability), the CSC may be considered as a conceptual tool in differentiating ordinary misconduct from disordered conduct. The motive for the CSC was to address the problem of false-positive diagnosis (e.g., diagnosing an individual as mentally ill when they are, in fact, not). The false-positive problem is an example of the broader problem in distinguishing between people who may behave differently, or are neurodiverse, but are not mentally ill. By requiring personal distress and/or disability as a criterion for having a mental disorder, the DSM architects hope to reduce false positives and identify only people who were impaired by their condition. While useful in many cases, Cooper[66] discusses the many limitations of this conceptual tool. In my context here, the CSC retains its importance in that distress and impairment become the markers of need for rehabilitation. Impairment extends to difficulties in conforming one's behavior to the law; criminal court dispositions must by necessity become more 'welfarist' than punitive. We might expect that the CSC can be helpful in distinguishing disordered from nondisordered vice as well, considered below with the discussion of paraphilic conditions and disorders.

Thesis 29: *Pedophilic and victimizing paraphilias should receive special attention regarding the determination of disorder status.* (T) In Chapter 2, Section 2.2.6, I discussed the complicated history and diagnostic status of the DSM 'victimizing' paraphilic disorders. The 'victimizing' designation meant that the disorder typically entailed imposing nonconsensual, undesired, harmful behavior on others. DSM-5 made the useful distinction between nonoffending sexual diversity (e.g., Pedophilia), and Pedophilic Disorder, which included sexual offending against minors and distress/disability on the part of the patient, drawing from the CSC.

Pedophilic disorder in DSM-5 provides an interesting challenge to the rethought VMDR. In separating out the victimizing and, therefore, vicious, element by making offending definitive for a disorder, Pedophilic Disorder is unique in separating criminal vice from private 'sexual diversity' experience, though between consenting adults.[67] However, should pedophilic people be expected to simply not have sex with their preferred erotic interests? The pedophile community points out we don't expect heteronormative or homonormative sex offenders to abstain from sex, but we expect pedophiles to. On the other hand, we do expect hetero- and homonormative adults to abstain from rape. Collectively, these issues remain problematic.

Chapter 2, Section 2.2.5.1, provides a discussion of the problematic status of assessing whether an impulsive act violates norms. In that section I argued that judgments of impulsive aggression (in IED) are exercises in practical ethics given the myriad situations and contextual determinants involved. Whether an individual meets social expectations, legal requirements, and other norms are also exercises in practical ethics concerning adults with pedophilic interests, also potentially impulsive (as well as deliberate) in nature. In our culture, while pedophilic adults are not required to be celibate, they are required not to abuse children.[68]

Failure to do so should be recognized as a deviation from a norm as socially repugnant and extreme for the vast majority of the public. Such violation of children by pedophilic offenders, assuming it represents a credible disorder, warrants study and treatment/rehabilitation, as well as protection of the public.[69] However, current policy regarding pedophilic and other sex offenders too often wades deeply into the waters of punishment and vengeance-seeking. Management of sex offenders in a humane manner should also weigh into practical ethics judgments. These practical ethics judgments are comparable to managing the empathic disregard of the psychopath. The psychopathic offender may deviate from a norm so extreme, and at a high social cost, to warrant disorder status and treatment/rehabilitation. Disordered paraphilic behavior that infringes upon nonconsenting others should be subject to treatment and rehabilitation; if no effective management is available, then protecting the public through humane measures is warranted.

Thesis 30: *Make the reduction/elimination of punishment a tool in improving the credibility of research into paraphilic and other highly stigmatized disorders.* (T) Assimilating the paraphilic disorders into the rehabilitative model may diminish the difficulty in diagnosis and discriminating harmless sexual diversity from harmful sexual diversity. As the need of the patient to avoid/minimize symptoms is reduced by the abolition of punitive measures, and the substitution of therapeutic ones, the patient may be freer to reveal useful, veritable information. The incentives to mislead examiners may well diminish, foster more reliable diagnosis, and more effective rehabilitative treatment. Given the culture of stigma, however, this trust by patients may be long in coming.

Thesis 31: *The elimination of punishment and blame may aid in the reduction of stigma for vice-laden disorders.* (I) The vice-laden status of substance use, ADHD, conduct disorders, and emotional dysregulation disorders is a great example of how vice lies within the metaphysical assumptions of the beholder. For religions that forbid substance use/abuse, the addict is a sinner. Disobedient or inattentive children may be viewed as naughty children. For clinicians and scientists committed to CMC accounts, these conditions are simply different problematic behaviors to be addressed through rehabilitation/treatment. Greater understanding may lead to reduced stigma.

Thesis 32: *For vice-laden disorders, replace concepts of 'responsibility' with regulation of extreme behaviors, when applicable.* (T) The case of IED raises issues about the continued need for moral/criminal responsibility assessments and their link to free will notions under Abrahamic folk-metaphysical assumptions. (See Section 2.2.5.1.) The challenges of clinical judgment regarding the thresholds between disordered and normal mental functions extend beyond normal and pathological aggression, to all mental disorders exhibiting pathologies of psychological extremity such as (excessive) anxiety, (excessive) sadness, and (excessive) worry about health, for example. What creates the illusion that IED is special may be the *antisocial* aspect of impulsive aggression, and the *convention* that morality is a forbidden function vis-a-vis determining disorder status. Self-regulation of aggressive impulses is a normative function, just like self-regulation of anxiety or sadness. With a CMC-metaphysics-based rehabilitative approach to IED, one can consider these questions of self-management in treatment/rehabilitation research and planning. The focus is on managing extremities of normal functions, just like we focus on managing excessive anxiety. What is special about IED is assuring public safety during the rehabilitative effort, not whether the patient has 'personal responsibility'.

Thesis 33: *Disconnect conceptually shoddy diagnostic categories from vice-laden diagnostic categories.* (T) Like IED, the other vice-laden impulse control disorders (e.g., Kleptomania, Pyromania, and Gambling Disorder) represent monosymptomatic disorders, and as such, have multiple conceptual problems.[70] Under my proposed 'reforms', treatment and rehabilitation blend together too. Proposed conditions like pathological bias and Intolerant Personality Disorder pose a question of how they should be considered under complex-causal medicalized accounts of vice. The nosological problems with these categories were described in Section 3.3.2, suggesting that wrongful/criminal syndromic behaviors should be evaluated under the same critical considerations as other, nonmoral, kinds of disorders. In this sense, if an Intolerant Personality Disorder category doesn't hold up conceptually or empirically, that should not be because it is vice-laden, but because it is a conceptually- or empirically-shoddy category.

9.3.6 Implications and recommendations for forensic and correctional psychiatry

Thesis 34: *Forensic psychiatry's expert-witness role in criminal trials should end (until a minimally punitive rehabilitative model is widespread).* (I) In Chapter 6 I argued about the untenable ethics of forensic psychiatrists' participation in expert-witness activities, competence to stand trial, and related roles in service to criminal courts. The rationale was simple: no persuasive argument has been offered to undo a physician's obligation to 'do no harm' when the central task is to contribute to determinations of punishment, the latter are by intention harmful. This fundamental premise of medical ethics forbids contributing to a systematized, deliberate process that potentially ends in substantial harm being imposed on an individual- in this case, punishment. If one formulates the situation of criminal activity under CMC assumptions, then the ethical response is rehabilitation and protection of the public, if needed. Because widely available rehabilitation services are not yet available in the United States and elsewhere, psychiatric participation in forensic criminal process cannot be justified ethically. Of course, this thesis is aspirational and ideal at the present moment. How to advise the criminal courts about the role of mental disorders in the postverdict phase is discussed in later theses below.[71]

Thesis 35: *Transformations in forensic psychiatry.* (T) In Chapter 6 I explored the different aspects and activities of the 'forensic psychiatry' field—one consisting of participating in the Court's criminal process, as in expert-witness testimony and assessments of competency to stand trial, and the second consisting in 'correctional' psychiatry, which refers to providing mental health care to prisoners, probationers, and parolees. If forensic psychiatrists no longer provide expert advice in criminal trials, then their role may seem to default to correctional psychiatry, which in principle is compatible with the physician's moral mission of care of the ill and doing no harm.

However, the potential for correctional psychiatrists to be compromised ethically in their professional role persists—as it does for clinical psychiatrists providing usual care in non-correctional settings. Correctional psychiatrists should consider the ethics of participating in parole hearings, as the situation is rife with potential to place the interests of correctional institutions over those of the patient. Similarly, correctional psychiatrists' contributions toward judgments to place inmates into higher- or lower- security environments are similarly rife with potential to permit a patient's interests to be overwhelmed by institutional interests.[72] However, in contrast to criminal court participation as an expert witness, correctional psychiatrists' roles are not defined as secondary to clinical care interests. Rather, correctional psychiatrists face their own sets of ethical challenges posed by their unique setting, as do other psychiatric subspecialists like, for example, geriatricians, child/adolescent specialists, and addictionologists.

The transformation of forensic psychiatry as a field should include not just the loss of participation in criminal procedure as expert witnesses, nor just the movement to corrections-based care, but a new, humane, and exciting direction as well. This direction would begin in the 'sentencing' phase of convicted offenders, under my envisioned minimization of punishment and institution of the rehabilitation model of handling criminal offending. Forensic psychiatrists can instead implement a new role, while no longer participating in harming convicted offenders through convictions leading to punishment. They can engage as friends of the court and the correctional system in planning tailored, individually sensitive rehabilitation plans for the convicted offender, whether mentally ill or not. Their already-extensive experience in working with offenders is a foundation for their transition to this new role; hopefully augmented by forensic criminologists as well. The shift in forensic psychiatry would be toward treatment and rehabilitation planning, implementation, monitoring, and evaluation, thus implementing the vision of an integrated, synergistic criminal and psychiatric/psychological rehabilitation mission.

Thesis 36: *Forensic criminologists should replace psychiatric expert witnesses in criminal court proceedings.* (I) As mentioned earlier, forensic criminologists, without a duty to serve the ill, can provide expert participation in criminal court process, allowing psychiatrists to maintain their loyalty to medical morality and adherence to the principle of 'do no harm'. This aspirational/ideal thesis requires much social change to implement. The training of such forensic criminologists will need to grow from a rare qualification to a standard, widespread one. Such an endeavor could involve decades of development. Ethics guidelines for forensic criminologists are needed, presumably in the context of professional associations for the field. Courts will need to be persuaded of the value of these new specialists in their criminal procedures. Professional rivalries and 'turf' with forensic psychiatrists and forensic psychologists will need to be addressed and resolved. The science and practice of criminal profiling, prediction of future offending, assessment of capacity to stand trial, and correctional behavioral control should shift away from psychiatrists/clinical psychologists and transferred to forensic criminologists. This task will involve not just institutional and administrative change, but generous funding of a research infrastructure to support the field's growth and ongoing provision of quality, humane services.

As implied in this discussion, use of forensic criminologists as a new brand of expert witness is a transitional thesis, assuming the persistence of current retributionist, punishment-oriented criminal justice systems. However, in considering the Ideal of the replacement of retributional criminal justice with restorative/rehabilitative or similar criminal justice models, and robust social commitments to rehabilitation of criminal offenders, mentally disordered or not, then the need for replacement by forensic criminologists may not necessary, nor the need to exclude 'forensic psychiatrists' from criminal procedures. Why? Once criminal justice is no longer oriented toward vengeance and punishment, and toward rehabilitation, the fate of criminal offenders, mentally ill or not, is the same. If found guilty of crimes, they receive rehabilitative treatment with considerations for public protection, if necessary. If the practices of criminal justice are stripped of their vengeful intentions to harm the guilty, then the conflict with do-no-harm medical morality disappears, and physicians can participate fully in criminal procedure, with awareness and care toward ethical challenges that arise within a rehabilitation/treatment orientation.

Thesis 37: *The problematic sorting of categories of psychopathology eligible for, or not eligible for, NGRI defense should dissipate away because of irrelevance of NGRI to criminal justice rehabilitation.* (I) This thesis is ideal in that it presumes the replacement of retributionist models with restorative/rehabilitative models of criminal justice. Under the new CMC FM formulation, the state of mind of the offender is of central interest in rehabilitative planning, after the fact of the determination of guilt. The state of mind of the offender is relevant in treatment selection, rehabilitative interventions, and public safety considerations, which all unfold after the trial. The insanity defense, the NGRI status is unnecessary because the contradictions and obscurity of culpability in criminal intent are obviated. Everyone gets rehabilitation and humane care, and no one gets intentional maxi-punishment. Criminal excuse determinations are unnecessary in the trial phase, only in the postsentencing rehabilitation phase.

9.3.7 Public education about the VMDR

Thesis 38: *Advancing the educational package of mental health literacy, criminology literacy, and knowledge of social welfare services is greatly needed.* (T) As described by Chapter 7 Section 7.1.2, the pitiful record of public understanding of mental illness worldwide is exceeded only by an even-poorer public understanding of criminal behavior and the genesis of crime. The public's level of criminology literacy is far worse than that of mental health literacy, which isn't good either. The literature supports the broad conclusion that public understanding of crime and mental illness is obtained primarily through popular media and entertainments rather than science and formal education. All of these 'literacies' have suffered under the marginalizing of civic education (also known as civics, citizenship education, social studies) in recent decades,[73] itself in need of protection, reform, and improvement. Education on criminality and mental illness will likely require efforts to reduce the demonizing of the criminal offender and boost empathic understanding of the biosocial drivers of criminality and immoral conduct. Advocacy for growth and adoption of relevant educational programs in secondary education is crucial.

Thesis 39: *Neurocriminological and other scientific endeavors to understand criminal behavior are underfunded and warrant much greater research support, which benefits the public as well as would-be offenders.* (T) On the surface, the limited public and private research funding in criminology is an amazing finding—one would think with the prominence of crime as a political topic and public interest, that research would be a top priority for policymakers, grantmakers, and citizens. On the other hand, the conclusions of this book, that vengeance and blame structure our thinking and policymaking regarding crime and criminality, make this finding less surprising.

Unfortunately, concerns about vengeance and punishment consume our political culture and therefore make the marginalizing of criminological science understandable, as one of many political heresies of being 'soft on crime' (see Chapter 6, Section 6.3.1). Other factors likely contribute to this marginalization, such as any research implicating US gun policy in gun violence and local interest in perpetuating prisons as sources of employment, particularly in rural areas, to mention two examples.

Thesis 40: *Mental health and criminology professionals should engage news and entertainment producers about developing entertaining and informative material regarding the VMDR.* (T) Chapter 7's discussion of public responses to media portrayals, both positive and negative, point to the power of popular media in informing, and misinforming, the public about crime and mental illness. Greater engagement by professionals in the earliest phases of journalism and entertainment projects can enhance positive public knowledge and contribute to better public policy. This would not be to 'whitewash' the presentation of these topics, but rather provide accurate, representative, and truly complex portrayals of these difficult social problems. Such attention to complexity and nuance makes for compelling drama.

9.4 Objections and responses

Many will view the above theses as audacious. In this section I consider some likely objections, followed by my responses to said objections.

9.4.1 Objection 1, changing minds

The idea that sufficiently huge members of the public can be swayed to rely upon CMC folk-metaphysical assumptions to effect proposed social changes seems unlikely at best and preposterous at worst.

Response:
Innovations have to start somewhere. Dramatic social change is possible, with history providing many examples, not the least of which are the experiments in democratic governments from 200 years ago. A more recent mental health example is the twenty-first-century recognition and acceptance of nonbinary gender in people. The late-twentieth-century discussions of the then-radical idea that peoples' gender may not be binary (man/woman) had barely surfaced into ordinary public discourse in the West. A Google Scholar search for 'gender nonbinary people' for the 2 centuries 1800–2000 yielded 404 results as June 21, 2022. The same search for the 2-plus decades 2000–2022 yielded 26, 300 results on the same June 21, 2022 date. While the understanding, tolerance, and implications of gender non-binarism are still discussed and debated, the fact of our society having such a discussion is a transition from the unthinkable to ordinary social knowledge. Related matters like gay marriage

and LGBTQ rights have been implemented as well as challenged in recent years. Big change happens.

9.4.2 Objection 2, increasing stigma

Organized psychiatry, such as the American Psychiatric Association, has made tremendous efforts to distinguish mental illness/mental disorders from criminal offending, such as with people who commit mass shootings. Aren't you worried about compounding stigma by including criminal offenders of various sorts under the mental disorder rubric?

Response:
This important objection warrants a response from several angles.

(1) In the ideal, I'm proposing that (e.g.) people committing mass shootings, whether they have a mental disorder or not, receive nonpunitive rehabilitative treatment (or seclusion to protect the public) on a humane basis, as I would with traditionally 'mentally ill' individuals or mentally ill offenders. If CMC folk metaphysics prevails as a cultural trope, then all offenders would not be subject to the kind of stigma we see. People with behavioral problems would get the treatments and rehabilitation they need. Organized psychiatry is worried about mentally ill people being stigmatized and punished for being mentally ill, hence the desire to distinguish the sick (mad) person from the (bad) offender, who is more stigmatized as a wrongdoer. However, these worries are obviated if the offender and the sick person all receive humane treatment, and no one gets punishment. It's all about rising above our reptilian vengeance-oriented proclivities. (2) I understand the motives for organized psychiatry's rhetoric that criminal offenders shouldn't be assumed to be mentally ill. However, the DSM classifies a number of mental disorders which involve criminal or antisocial conduct, such as Conduct Disorder, Antisocial Personality Disorder, Pedophilic Disorder, IED, among others. The simple fact is that psychiatry is already, and arguably, has since its beginnings, been in the business of diagnosing and treating criminal offenders, in wildly inconsistent ways and for puzzling reasons. (These reasons requiring a book like this to sort out.) This self-contradicting rhetoric, while well intended, may confuse the public and policymakers more than clarify matters, because of this double-talk element. As a specific example, and in my view, the issue with individuals committing mass shootings is that we don't know much about them, including whether they have significant psychopathology. Moreover, the United States is singular as a developed nation with a major mass-shooting problem. This suggests other Western nations are doing a far better job in preventing gun violence than us, so perhaps we could learn effective strategies from other developed nations who don't have this problem. What are European nations

and Australia/New Zealand doing that works? In this context, American psychiatry's advocacy should emphasize solutions to gun violence over defining 'mental illness' for the polity. (3) We often hear from ordinary citizens that heinously violent offenders 'have something wrong' with them. Indeed. We should advocate for learning more about these individuals through research and educate the public and policymakers more about the relationships between vice and mental disorders. (4) Yes, I'm worried about compounding stigma, but I believe a coherent, moral, and consistent approach to criminal offending will ultimately reduce stigma for all.

9.4.3 Objection 3, preventive detention

As a corollary to the above, psychiatrists have avoided getting involved in social-protection schemes like preventive detention, especially for high-risk criminal offenders. Aren't you dragging them into this morass?

Response:
Psychiatrists are already involved in preventive detention practices, namely, involuntary hospitalization and treatment, for patients who are thought to be dangerous to themselves or others. The efficacy of these practices remains controversial, but that's a different question. Psychiatrists, I suspect, don't want to get involved in preventive detentions for people who are not currently considered to have mental disorders (e.g., criminal offenders). Psychiatrists have good reasons for this. They are not trained in evaluating, predicting their behavior, and rehabilitating criminal offenders, particularly violent offenders. Moreover, because moral psychopathology has been excluded from Abrahamic science, policy, and practice, psychiatrists are currently ill-prepared for these tasks as wrongful and criminal conduct has been largely excluded from their domain of research, expertise, and practice. Moreover, psychiatrists have few options in becoming expert in these populations at present, because the research base for understanding the VMDR is poor. So yes, a shallow application of new ideas could complicate practice and lead to bad policy. This is always a risk with innovation, and even more so with policymaking. I would support psychiatry resisting further, broader preventive detention practices until our knowledge and service structures are reformed to have rigorous knowledge about the VMDR and provide the humane care I envision.

9.4.4 Objection 4, throwing out narratives and blame

You seem to leave no role for Abrahamic folk-metaphysical assumptions, and their derivative folk-psychological concepts like narrative reasons and blameworthiness. Are these and related ideas to be thrown out?

518 Vice and Psychiatric Diagnosis

Response:
Today, already, the psychological and social sciences, as well as the biomedical sciences, contribute to our discussions about how and why human beings act the way they do. In many cases, the scientific responses operate out of CMC folk-metaphysical assumptions. The CMC sciences have practical limits in everyday discourse, however. The 'reasons-giving' account of our behavior suffices for most of the everyday needs we have for explaining behavior. If I was asked why I left the kitchen without cleaning the dirty dishes last night, I might say 'I forgot to finish cleaning up.' I would not, however, provide a detailed CMC-driven scientific account of the causal vectors—from molecules, neural connections, and my fatigue physiology, to kitchen and distraction variables—at work in that moment. However, when the ethical stakes are high, and the situation complicated, and we need defensible social policy with multifaceted solutions, we should build social policy out of the more complex CMC explanatory nexus. The reasons for preferring one set of FM assumptions over another has to do with the practical needs for the task. Some tasks require a simple solution; others a complex one. H. L. Mencken: 'For every complex problem there is an answer that is clear, simple, and wrong.'[74]

9.4.5 Objection 5, social/organizational crime

A lot of crime out there has little to do with individual actions, and more to do with organizational and social actions, but you don't discuss these. Why?

Response:
That's correct—my treatment in this book is aimed (primarily) at individual violent and property crimes, not organizational or social crimes (such as war crimes). The starting point for *Vice and Psychiatric Diagnosis* was always the individual and is still the case here. How Abrahamic versus CMC folk-metaphysical assumptions structure our response to things like corporate malfeasance, war crimes, and politically motivated disinformation, is a tremendous challenge and an important set of questions for others to take up.

9.4.6 Objection 6, other impacts of the Enlightenment Split

You only focus on the implications of the Enlightenment Split on criminal law and religion, but what about the significance for tort law, corporate law, international law, for example, and other types of law?

Response:
Good question, and it points to the need to explore foreseen and unintended consequences of this work on the impact of differing folk-metaphysical assumptions.

I hope that readers with these concerns will explore the implications of adopting CMC and Abrahamic folk-metaphysical assumptions for these other areas of law.

9.4.7 Objection 7, development of FM assumptions

You hold that the Abrahamic religions—Christianity, Islam, and Judaism—are the source of the notions of free will, individualism, responsibility, and desert, but haven't scholars debated the sources of these concepts going back to ancient philosophy?[75]

Response:
I agree with you about the origins of free will and related concepts. However, my prevailing interest is not about sources, but about social and cultural impact, especially today, and in post-Enlightenment Western history. Our founding cultural lessons about these ideas don't come from history or philosophy classes. From youth forward we learn about them in our religious institutions, our schools, in journalism, in everyday talk, and in entertainment media. These ideas have sedimented into our ordinary cultural beliefs and assumptions, as illustrated in most all of the chapters in this book.

9.4.8 Objection 8, antireligion

You seem to be making a wholesale rejection of (Abrahamic) religion as a cultural force. Are you against religion?

Response:
No. I just think Abrahamic folk-metaphysical assumptions don't work for our problems with crime and mental illness. I don't think the centuries-old folk-metaphysical architecture promulgated by Abrahamic religions through our various subcultures are an effective metaphysical foundation to develop social policies regarding the vice-mental disorder relationship. The moral and spiritual guidance of Abrahamic religions has been, and should continue to be, a resource for people wishing to pursue good and meaningful lives. The metaphysical assumptions culturally imbricated though Abrahamic religions has not served our social policies for the vice-mental disorder relationship well at all. We should move on in this context.

9.4.9 Objection 9, history of psychiatric abuse

The history of psychiatry has its own legacies of abuse, neglect, and trauma. What makes you think merging criminal and psychiatric rehabilitation is going to be better than the status quo?

Response:
Of course, I can't be sure that any of these proposals will in fact result in more humane social welfare. Psychiatry and penology each have their dark periods and shameful legacies. That said, the whole book provides arguments toward the no-punishment ideal. The latter as a prevailing value in psychiatric reform is, to my reading of the history, unprecedented. Moreover, reformulating attitudes toward a no-punishment practice and a CMC understanding of behavior might well mitigate some abuses. Further, the United States can learn from other countries who have already realized a more humane social welfare vision (see Thesis 11 above). We have cause for cautious optimism. However, the potential for bad policy and practice is present in every direction, as we stumble forward in our pursuit of better societies.

9.4.10 Objection 10, psychiatric self-interest

You seem to neglect the implication that your conclusions and recommendations could be viewed as simply serving psychiatry's self-interests in amassing further social power, social control, and profit.

Response:
Granted, for those seeking simple generalizations about complex problems, this criticism could be appealing. However, I think this would be naive and wrongheaded for several reasons and lines of evidence: (1) Psychiatry is, and has been for a long time, a shortage medical specialty.[76] The need in correctional mental health is even greater.[77] The history of psychiatry in Chapter 5 reveals a direct relationship between public support and humane mental health care, as well as the inverse. Today, mental health practitioners don't need more patients or more 'power'. We need more psychiatrists, and more skilled mental health care workers of all varieties. Indeed, the more apt criticism in this domain would be: Where are you going to find all these caregivers? That's a good question, and cause to amplify our existing efforts at recruitment. (2) My proposals directly suggest expanded services by nonpsychiatric professionals, most prominently 'forensic criminologists', but indirectly a massive expansion of rehabilitation specialists of various kinds and skill sets. My proposals are more 'team'-oriented than aggrandizing of psychiatrists and psychiatry per se. Rehabilitation is a team project where big egos should be left behind. (3) Rather than expanding the field of forensic psychiatry, I'm narrowing it to a strong emphasis on correctional psychiatry and later, rehabilitation planning and implementation. My ethics-based recommendations to curtail forensic psychiatry's expert-witness participation in criminal trials is more likely to inspire criticism than applause from my forensic colleagues. This doesn't seem to be a gratuitous expansion of the psychiatric field, but rather, a redefinition and possible contraction.

9.4.11 Objection 11, medicalization

Your recommendations amount to a substantial increase in medicalization, particularly for wrongful conduct of various kinds. Is this increase in medicalization a good thing?

Response:
This question also provokes a complex response. If psychiatry adds categories involving moral psychopathology to its traditional domains, this change will likely result in the medicalizing of some problem behaviors and experiences which would make up new categories of psychopathology. However, one mechanism of medicalization has been the discovery or recognition of new diseases or disorders which are substantively harmful. Sincere, nonexploitative efforts to address the new disorder may well be ethically justifiable. My colleagues and I have discussed the ethics of medicalization in prior work.[78] Ambivalence about medicalization stems from the expansion of health concerns beyond real social needs, or even worse, the social creation of false health needs as a means to sell gratuitous products.[79] Medicalization as a process always deserves ethical reflection and assessment, which I have discussed throughout my conclusions. If medicalization helps people flourish with a favorable balance regarding social cost, then medicalization is a good thing.

9.4.12 Objection 12, dismissal without argument

You seem to be playing fast and loose in dismissing huge parts of the literature in narrative theory and the philosophy of free will and responsibility without much argument. What gives?

Response:
You are correct in noting that I don't engage with philosophical arguments about free will and responsibility, or in the Continental philosophy tradition, about rival discussions of explanation, causation, and understanding, or hermeneutics, whether scientific or narrative. Not only that, I don't give a particular account of complex multicausal explanation, either. Regarding the latter, many rival accounts of multicausal explanation are out there; determining which one(s) should prevail are practical matters depending upon the particular causal questions posed. Moreover, selecting and defending a complex multicausal account for the purposes of the VMDR would be an enormous digression from the main thrust of the book. I do cite sample papers and books regarding these issues and debates.

The misleading part of your question is that I'm 'dismissing' this huge literature. I'm not dismissing this work, but rather, I refer to this literature as sources to be considered in my more general account of the role of folk-metaphysical assumptions in structuring our thinking about things like free will, responsibility, understanding, and explanation. These theories and debates are referenced as embodied in cultural practices like building psychiatric diagnostic categories, discovering the etiology of diseases, or determining criminal responsibility. As a specific example, I don't engage with the analytic philosophy debates about free will and determinism. I don't offer refutations of philosophical traditions, even ones emerging from Abrahamic folk-metaphysical assumptions. Rather, I'm doing a kind of philosophical anthropology, which is examining how debates around free will, personal responsibility, desert, explanation, and understanding reflect cross-cutting cultural assumptions which quietly yet powerfully shape how we think. Indeed, to the degree that philosophy can develop insights into narrative theory, explanation, and understanding, that's all the better for implementing a change in a cultural mind-set that frames and structures our institutions around the VMDR. To extend the philosophical anthropology metaphor, an anthropologist doesn't come to understand cross-cultural concepts and practices through rational argumentation with the endemic population, but rather observes the concepts and practices in use and then infers related assumptions, worldviews, and taken-for-granted practices. In this sense, my work here resembles some elements of ordinary-language philosophy. Rather than examining singular concepts, I'm examining concepts and terms in the larger context of interrelated practices surrounding, for example, 'the insanity defense' or 'culpability'. Then I consider how metaphysical assumptions may shape these practices.

9.4.13 Objection 13, narrative understandings

Don't your conclusions marginalize narrative understandings of criminality and mental disorder? What room is there for a narrative concept of the person?

Response:
What I hope to bring to narrative understandings of criminality, mental illness, and the concept of the person is an awakening of the significance of metaphysical assumptions in shaping our thinking whether narratively or causally. I believe the narrative concept of the person, as a reasons-giving, goal-directed practical approach to navigating our lives, finishes up just fine under my analysis. The analogy I give is an old one, that of Newton's account of mechanics versus relativity or quantum notions of mechanics. The former work just fine for everyday situations and practical engagement with the world, like building buildings which resist collapse or calculating the acceleration of a falling ball of x mass from so many feet up. However, more advanced physics is needed for the motion of light or the neural interactions of molecular-level brain function. Analogously, the utility of narrative concepts of the person depends upon the task at hand, and the book goes to some trouble to sketch out how narrative accounts fail to help us address the vice-mental disorder

relationship in some socially important instances and contexts. The other role of narrative, reasons-giving accounts was mentioned earlier, in that in terms of practical feasibility, the narrative, reasons-giving account is simple, transparent, and almost always reliable in meeting our practical, everyday needs. However, it's often wanting in how to respond to wrongful or criminal conduct.

9.4.14 Objection 14, reducing misrepresentations of self

You claim that moving to a nonpunitive, rehabilitative response to disordered or nondisordered criminal offending will remove an important incentive to misrepresent one's mental state in the criminal justice setting; that is, motives to hide one's psychopathology, or simulate psychopathology toward an NGRI defense. This seems overstated in that offenders can be intractable, and many mental disorders associated with offending, like Antisocial Personality Disorder and Conduct Disorder, specify lying as one of the defining features.

Response:
Your objection bears some merit for the reasons you mention. However, removing one big causal vector for defendant prevarication, namely the threat of severe punishment, seems likely to result in a shifting of a causal equilibrium where dissembling is highly motivated, toward an equilibrium where the benefits are less evident, and honesty more promising, resulting in a net reduction of dissembling. Moreover, the hardening mechanisms of convicted offenders exact a trauma toll which is not quickly rehabilitated, and the manipulativeness, distrust, and desperation resulting from hardening will persist for many individuals even after the system changes. Habitual coping responses to repeated trauma just don't go away overnight, nor do failures of normal human development promulgated by poverty, abuse, trauma, and neglect. Moreover, we know from current mental health care experience that not all patients want psychiatric care or rehabilitation, even ones who need it the most. That will likely always be a given. Given these hard realities, the transition away from a toxic, punitive system and its consequences will not be uniform. However, longer term benefits, like less dissembling by defendants and convicts, can follow with time. Such changes will evolve, nonetheless, if our resolve in reform is strong.

9.5 Afterword

The contemporary times in which this book was completed were full of hardship compounded by many failures of humanity. In finishing up this book project, I had to wonder if this work was ill-timed for publication and release. Plenty of recent events provoke doubts about humanity's resolve, even ability, to pull together and flourish collectively. The climate change crisis has provoked progressively more fires and floods. Public health efforts were compromised in containing the COVID-19 pandemic through the worldwide social media distribution of disinformation and propaganda, contributing to the tragic loss of millions of lives. Social media continues to contribute to our most divisive politics as we struggle collectively to protect truths as well as free speech. Progress in race, gender, class, and other equities have both advanced and regressed. The war in Ukraine, the biggest conflict in Europe since World War II, has threatened, again, a nuclear Armageddon. All of these factors may contribute to a sense of futility in pursuing a better world. That said, hard work fueled by hope is principal in improving our lot. My hope is that this book contributes to that vision.

Notes

1. 'To go down a rabbit-hole' is an English-language idiom that means one is pursuing a hopelessly prolonged inquiry.
2. Sadler (2005).
3. In *Values and Psychiatric Diagnosis* (2005), ontological values were a kind of value having to do with one taken-for-granted assumptions about the nature of being human. In the setting of this book, 'ontological values' are the broader notion where particular folk-metaphysical assumptions reside.
4. Tonry (2011a).
5. See the reviews by Besemer & Murray (2016); Kazemian & Walker (2019); Pereboom (2020), Poehlmann-Tynan et al. (2019); Shrage (2017).
6. Besemer & Murray (2016); Kazemian & Walker (2019); Pereboom (2020); Poehlmann-Tynan et al. (2019); Shrage (2017).
7. Caruso (2020); Jeppsson (2021); Kelly (2021); Shaw, Pereboom, & Caruso 2019; Sverdlik (1988); Tonry (2011a, 2011b); Waller (2020).
8. Akther et al. (2019).
9. Jeppsson's (2021) description of 'harsh punishment' is close to what I'm calling maxi-punishment, but Jeppsson's might be even more severe than I intend.
10. In *Values and Psychiatric Diagnosis* (2005), ontological values were a kind of value having to do with our taken-for-granted assumptions about the nature of being human. In the setting of this book, 'ontological values' are the broader notion where particular folk-metaphysical assumptions reside.
11. Cuthbert & Insel (2013).
12. See for instance Demazeaux & Singy (2015); Kendler & Parnas (2012); Kincaid & Sullivan (2014); Paris & Phillips (2013); Sadler (2002, 2005); Zachar (2014).
13. See Stein et al. (2010).
14. Horwitz & Wakefield (2007).
15. Sadler (2002).
16. Wilkinson (2000).
17. Luhrmann (2011).
18. See note 4.
19. See for instance Caruso (2012, 2013, 2021); Shaw, Pereboom, & Caruso (2019); Waller (2011, 2015, 2017, 2020).
20. Card (2002). I'm grateful to Nancy Potter for introducing me to Card's work.
21. Friston et al. (2006, 2022).

22. Pickard (2011).

23. Fulford et al. (2003).

24. Szasz (1974).

25. Sadler (2019).

26. Berryessa & Raine (2018).

27. See Chapter 6, Section 6.3.1.2.

28. See Chapter 6, Section 6.1.1.2.

29. See Chapter 6, Section 6.3.1.2.

30. See Chapter 6, Section 6.1.1.2.

31. The feeble nosological rigor reflected by vice-laden categories in the DSM is discussed in Chapter 3 and in Sadler (2014) on Conduct Disorder, and in my 2015 work on 'monomanias'.

32. Orso et al. (2020).

33. Abdalla et al. (2021).

34. Sadler & Fulford (2004); Sadler (2005).

35. For a debate about an 'ethical review panel' for DSMs, see the Volume 24, Number 3, issue of *Philosophy, Psychiatry, & Psychology*. A 'philosophical/conceptual review panel', however, is a different story, and could potentially address the conceptual issues in psychiatric classifications through implementing insights from the vigorous 30-year-old literature.

36. www.worldjusticeproject.org.

37. The idea of building other-regarding ethics around 'capabilities' has been pioneered by Martha Nussbaum and Amaryta Sen. For a perspective on this literature, see Nussbaum (2020). For general description, see Robeyns (2021). See Winance & Bertrand (2022) for an exploration of implementing personalized social welfare for people with multiple disabilities.

38. I should remind all that my recommendations in this book are for criminal law, primarily violent and property crime by individuals, and not directed to corporate malfeasance and torts.

39. According to World Bank data, intentional homicide in the United States in 2018 was 5/100k; Norway 0/100k; Sweden, Denmark, the UK, and the Netherlands 1/100k; and Finland 2/100k. http://data.worldbank.org/indicator/VC.IHR.PSRC.P5.

40. Adshead & Horne (2021).

41. Most notably a 2017 Cochrane review by Kisely et al. documenting lack of efficacy for any of the main outcomes: health service use, readmission, mental state, social function, quality of life, homelessness, and satisfaction with care. A weak effect was found for reducing victimization. See also Akther et al. (2019).

42. Lee & Cohen (2021);Testa & West (2010).

43. A recent issue of *Social Policy and Society* addressed sustainable social welfare, and provided a handy reference resource: McGann & Murphy (2022).

44. Barr (2020); Briggs (1961).

45. Manow (2020); Scaratti et al. (2018); Vogel & Theorell (2006).

46. See for instance Kymlicka & Norman (2000); Lin (2015); Ross (2004); Sadler (2022).

47. See Sunstein (2017). A solution-orientation to civic education requires a solution-oriented media as well. See https://www.solutionsjournalism.org/.

48. A significant conceptual issue for the philosophy of psychiatry is this: 'Normal' morality must include all sorts of moral failings, posing the challenge to distinguish normal from disordered morality in the context of 'ordinary' wrongdoing. This may sound daunting, but this may be more due to our lack of psychological, theoretical, and empirical tools in the moral realm. We have theorized about and worked with other psychological capacities (e.g., 'anxiety' or 'sadness/depression') and their disordered versions for many decades.

49. See Bolton (2008) for a book-length review.

50. Mercier et al. (2018); Trimbur et al. (2021).

51. See DSM-5, APA (2013); Stein et al. (2010).

52. Sadler (2005); Stein et al. (2010).

53. Sadler (1997, 2005).

54. See Sadler (2014, 2015).

55. Stanghellini et al. (2019).

56. https://thebipartisanpost.com/all-articles/mass-incarceration-was-a-bipartisan-effort-ending-it-needs-to-be-too, https://www.prisonpolicy.org/ Also: https://www.nytimes.com/2018/12/18/us/politics/senate-criminal-justice-bill.html.

57. See for instance Roehr (2013) for a brief summary.

58. Kotov et al. (2017).

59. See for instance Cuthbert & Insel (2013).

60. Berrios (1996); Radden (1994).

61. See Fulford et al. (2013); Sadler (2005); and Stanghellini et al. (2019) for extensive references and reviews.

62. Bueter (2021).

63. Oexle & Corrigan (2018).

64. See Crenshaw (2017); Nayak (2021).

65. Cooper (2013); First & Wakefield (2013).

66. Cooper (2013); First & Wakefield (2013).

67. Sadler (2013). Notably, simple deviations from heteronormative reproductive coupling have a long history as 'vices' in Abrahamic and other religious traditions, complicating the politics and sociology of rehabilitating, not punishing, paraphilic offenders. See Chapter 5, Section 5.8.7.

68. For an analysis of moral objections against adult-child sex, see Malón (2015). For recent and on-going discussion about pedophilic diagnosis, see Seto (2012, 2022).

69. According to the US Department of Justice Office of Sex Offender Sentencing, Monitoring, Apprehending, Registering, and Tracking, only about 10% of child sexual abuse perpetrators are strangers to the child. About 30% of perpetrators are family members, and the remaining 60% of perpetrators are known to the child but not family members. https://web.archive.org/web/2019031 0222140/https://www.nsopw.gov/en-US/Education/FactsStatistics.

70. See Sadler (2015).

71. I should note that contemporary forensic psychiatrists may be involved as expert witnesses with lawsuit/tort procedure as well as criminal procedure. Given that such civil actions may culminate in 'punitive damages' being awarded (over and above compensation and restoration to injured parties), the problem of physician involvement in punishment-related proceedings extends into torts as well. While this professional-ethics issue is well worth exploring, at this point of concluding a very long book, I will leave this issue as simply raised.

72. Candilis & Huttenbach (2015); Morris & West (2020); Simon, Beckmann, Stone et al. (2020).

73. Fitzgerald et al. (2021); Ross (2004); Sadler (2023). Likewise, mental health literacy also overlaps with health literacy, itself too-often feeble among the public. Conrad & Brendel (2020); Farberman (1997); Mezuk et al. (2021); Nastasi (2004).

74. See Sturmberg (2014) for medicine-relevant aphorisms such as this one from Mencken.

75. Frede (2011).

76. Satiani et al. (2018).

77. Morris & Edwards (2022).

78. Sadler et al. (2009).

79. Conrad (2007). See also Sadler et al. (2009).

Bibliography

—. (1844). *Commonwealth vs. Abner Rogers, Jr.*, 7 Met. 500, 48 Mass. 500, Commonwealth of Massachusetts. http://masscases.com/cases/sjc/48/48mass500.html.

—. (1957). *Report of Committee on Homosexual Offences and Prostitution, Presented to Parliament by the Secretary of State for the Home Department and Secretary of State for Scotland by Command of Her Majesty, Document § 13, 1957* (HO 345/1/1). https://discovery.nationalarchives.gov.uk/details/r/C1386377.

—. (undated). Annotated Justinian Code: Concerning the Composition of a New Code. College of Law George William Hopper Library, University of Wyoming https://www.uwyo.edu/lawlib blume-justinian/ajc-edition-2/books/book1/index.html.

—. (undated). The Code of Hammurabi. https://avalon.law.yale.edu/subject_menus/hammenu.asp.

—. (undated). Oath of Maimonides. https://www.jewishvirtuallibrary.org/oath-of-maimonides.

Abdalla, S. M., Keyes, K. M., & Galea, S. (2021). "A Public Health Approach to Tackling the Role of Culture in Shaping the Gun Violence Epidemic in the United States." *Public Health Reports*, 136(1), 6–9. https://doi:10.1177/0033354920965263

Abelson, E. S. (1989). "The Invention of Kleptomania." *Signs*, 15(1), 123–143. https://doi:10.1086/494567

Adshead, G. (2008). "Vice and Viciousness." *Philosophy, Psychiatry, & Psychology*, 15(1), 23–26. https://doi:10.1353/ppp.0.0158

Adshead, G., & Horne, E. (2021). *The Devil You Know: Stories of Human Cruelty and Compassion.* New York: Simon & Schuster.

Adshead, G., & Sarkar, S. P. (2005). "Justice and Welfare: Two Ethical Paradigms in Forensic Psychiatry." *Australian and New Zealand Journal of Psychiatry*, 39(11-12), 1011–1017. https://doi:10.1080/j.1440-1614.2005.01719.x

Agalaryan, A., & Rouleau, J.-L. (2014). "Paraphilic Coercive Disorder: An Unresolved Issue." *Archives of Sexual Behavior*, 43(7), 1253–1256. https://doi:10.1007/s10508-014-0372-5

Akther, S. F., Molyneaux, E., Stuart, R., Johnson, S., Simpson, A., & Oram, S. (2019). "Patients' Experiences of Assessment and Detention under Mental Health Legislation: Systematic Review and Qualitative Meta-Synthesis." *BJPsych Open*, 5(3), e37. https://doi:10.1192/bjo.2019.19

Alexander, F. G., & Selesnick, S. T. (1966). *The History of Psychiatry: An Evaluation of Psychiatric Thought and Practice from Prehistoric Times to the Present.* New York: Harper and Row.

Alexander, L. (2002). "The Philosophy of Criminal Law." In J. L. Coleman, K. E. Himma, & S. Shapiro (Eds.), *The Oxford Handbook of Jurisprudence and Philosophy of Law* (pp. 815–867). Oxford: Oxford University Press.

Allan, A., Louw, D. A., & Verschoor, T. (1995). "Law and Psychology: A Historical Perspective (1)." *Medicine and Law*, 14(7–8), 671–676.

Allderidge, P. H. (1974). "Criminal Insanity: Bethlem to Broadmoor." *Proceedings of the Royal Society of Medicine*, 67(9), 897–904. https://www.ncbi.nlm.nih.gov/pmc/articles/PMC1645961/

Allyn, D. (1996). "Private Acts/Public Policy: Alfred Kinsey, the American-Law-Institute and the Privatization of American Sexual Morality." *Journal of American Studies*, 30(3), 405–428. https://doi:10.1017/S0021875800024889

American Association of Mental Retardation (AAMR) (2002). *Mental Retardation: Definition, Classification and Systems of Supports (10th ed.).* Washington, DC: American Association of Mental Retardation.

American Academy of Psychiatry and the Law (2005). Ethics Guidelines for the Practice of Forensic Psychiatry. https://www.aapl.org/ethics-guidelines

American Bar Association (1980). *ABA Model Code of Professional Responsibility*. Chicago: ABA Publishing. https://www.americanbar.org/content/dam/aba/administrative/professional_respons ibility/mrpc_migrated/mcpr.pdf

American Law Institute (ALI) (1962). *The Model Penal Code*. Philadelphia: American Law Institute.

American Psychiatric Association, & Committee on Nomenclature and Statistics. (1952). Diagnostic and statistical manual of mental disorders. (DSM-1)

American Psychiatric Association (1968). *Diagnostic and Statistical Manual of Mental Disorders, Second ed. (DSM-II)*. Washington, DC: American Psychiatric Association.

American Psychiatric Association (1974). *Diagnosis and Statistical Manual of Mental Disorders, Second ed. (DSM-II), Seventh Printing*. Washington, DC: American Psychiatric Association.

American Psychiatric Association (1980). *Diagnostic and Statistical Manual of Mental Disorders, Third ed. (DSM-III)*. Washington, DC: American Psychiatric Association.

American Psychiatric Association (1987). *Diagnostic and Statistical Manual of Mental Disorders, Third ed., Revised (DSM-III-R)*. Washington, DC: American Psychiatric Association.

American Psychiatric Association (1994). *Diagnostic and Statistical Manual of Mental Disorders, Fourth ed. (DSM-IV)*. Washington, DC: American Psychiatric Association.

American Psychiatric Association (1999). *Dangerous Sex Offenders: A Task Force Report of the American Psychiatric Association*. Washington, DC: American Psychiatric Association Publishing.

American Psychiatric Association (2000). *Diagnostic and Statistical Manual of Mental Disorders, Fourth ed., Text Revised (DSM-IV-TR)*. Washington, DC: American Psychiatric Association.

American Psychiatric Association (2010). APA DSM-5 Prelude Project. Washington, DC: American Psychiatric Association. www.DSM5.org

American Psychiatric Association, DSM-5 Childhood and Adolescent Disorders Workgroup. (2010). *Justification for Temper Dysregulation Disorder with Dysphoria*. Washington, DC: American Psychiatric Association. www.DSM5.org

American Psychiatric Association (2013). *Diagnostic and Statistical Manual of Mental Disorders (DSM-5®), Fifth ed*. Washington, DC: American Psychiatric Association.

American Psychiatric Association (2003). *American Psychiatric Association Statement: Diagnostic Criteria for Pedophilia (June 17, 2003)*. (Release No. 03-28). Washington, DC: American Psychiatric Association. http://www.psych.org

Andreasen, N. C. (2006). "DSM and the Death of Phenomenology in America: An Example of Unintended Consequences." *Schizophrenia Bulletin, 33*(1), 108–112. https://doi:10.1093/schbul/sbl054

Andrews, D. (1995). "The Psychology of Criminal Conduct and Effective Treatment." In J. McGuire (Ed.), *What Works: Reducing Reoffending: Guidelines from Research and Practice* (pp. 35–62). Oxford: John Wiley & Sons.

Andrews, D. A., & Bonta, J. (2010). *The Psychology of Criminal Conduct, Fifth ed*. New Providence, NJ: Matthew Bender & Co.

Angell, M. (2009). "Drug Companies & Doctors: A Story of Corruption." *The New York Review of Books, 56*(1), 8–12. http://www.nybooks.com/articles/22237

Angermeyer, M. C., & Dietrich, S. (2006). "Public Beliefs About and Attitudes towards People with Mental Illness: A Review of Population Studies." *Acta Psychiatrica Scandinavica, 113*(3), 163–179. https://doi:10.1111/j.1600-0447.2005.00699.x

Anonymous (1883). "Obituary of Hervey B. Wilbur, M.D." *Journal of Mental Science (British Journal of Psychiatry), 29*(126), 322–323. https://doi:10.1192/bjp.29.126.322

Anonymous (1887). "[Review] The Diseases of the Bible (Bennett, Risdon)." *The British Medical Journal, 2*(1406), 1283–1284. http://www.jstor.org/stable/20213878

Anonymous (1897). "Women Who Steal." *British Medical Journal, 1*(1881), 160. http://www.jstor.org stable/20248582

Anthony, W., Cohen, M., Farkas, M., & Gagne, C. (2002). *Psychiatric Rehabilitation, Second ed*. Boston: Boston University Center for Psychiatric Rehabilitation.

Anthony, W. A., & Liberman, R. P. (1986). "The Practice of Psychiatric Rehabilitation: Historical, Conceptual, and Research Base." *Schizophrenia Bulletin, 12*(4), 542–559. https://doi:10.1093/schbul/12.4.542

Appelbaum, P. S. (1997a). "A Theory of Ethics for Forensic Psychiatry." *Journal of the American Academy of Psychiatry and the Law, 25*(3), 233–247.

Appelbaum, P. S. (1997b). "Ethics in Evolution: The Incompatibility of Clinical and Forensic Functions." *American Journal of Psychiatry, 154*(4), 445–446. https://doi:10.1176/ajp.154.4.445

Appelbaum, P. S. (1998). "Dr. Appelbaum Replies." *American Journal of Psychiatry, 155*(4), 576–579. https://doi:10.1176/ajp.155.4.576

Appelbaum, P. S., Lidz, C. W., & Grisso, T. (2004). "Therapeutic Misconception in Clinical Research: Frequency and Risk Factors." *IRB: Ethics & Human Research, 26*(2), 1–8. https://doi:10.2307/3564231

Appelbaum, P. S., Roth, L. H., & Lidz, C. (1982). "The Therapeutic Misconception: Informed Consent in Psychiatric Research." *International Journal of Law and Psychiatry, 5*(3–4), 319–329. https://doi:10.1016/0160-2527(82)90026-7

Appelbaum, P. S., Roth, L. H., Lidz, C. W., Benson, P., & Winslade, W. (1987). "False Hopes and Best Data: Consent to Research and the Therapeutic Misconception." *The Hastings Center Report, 17*(2), 20–24. https://doi:10.2307/3562038

Aquinas, T. (1981). *Summa Theologica*. Translated by Fathers of the English Dominican Province. Notre Dame, IN: Ave Maria Publishers.

Aristotle (1984). "Nicomachean Ethics." In J. Barnes (Ed.), *The Complete Works of Aristotle, the Revised Oxford Translation.*(Popular Culture and Philosophy series) (pp. 1729–1867). Princeton, NJ: Princeton University Press.

Aristotle (2014). *Nicomachean Ethics, Revised ed.* Edited and translated by Roger Crisp. Cambridge: Cambridge University Press.

Arp, R. (Ed.) (2014). *The Devil and Philosophy: The Nature of His Game.* (Popular Culture and Philosophy series). Chicago: Open Court Publishing.

Arrigo, B. A., & Bullock, J. L. (2008). "The Psychological Effects of Solitary Confinement on Prisoners in Supermax Units: Reviewing What We Know and Recommending What Should Change." *International Journal of Offender Therapy and Comparative Criminology, 52*(6), 622–640. https://doi:10.1177/0306624x07309720

Audi, R. (Ed.) (1999). *The Cambridge Dictionary of Philosophy, Second ed.* Cambridge: Cambridge University Press.

Saint Augustine (1992). *Confessions.* Translated by H. Chadwick. New York/Oxford: Oxford University Press.

Saint Augustine (Bishop of Hippo) (1876). *The Confessions.* Translated by J. G. Pilkington. Edinburgh: T. & T. Clark.

Averbach, A. (1957). "Causation: A Medico-Legal Battlefield." *Cleveland State Law Review, 6*(2), 209–226. https://engagedscholarship.csuohio.edu/clevstlrev/vol6/iss2/7/

Bach, B., Markon, K., Simonsen, E., & Krueger, R. F. (2015). "Clinical Utility of the DSM-5 Alternative Model of Personality Disorders: Six Cases from Practice." *Journal of Psychiatric Practice*®, *21*(1), 3–25. https://doi:10.1097/01.pra.0000460618.02805.ef

Bacon, F. (2000). *Francis Bacon: The New Oregon.* Edited by L. Jardine & M. Silverthorne. Cambridge: Cambridge University Press.

Baehr, J. (2006). "Character, Reliability and Virtue Epistemology." *Philosophical Quarterly, 56*(223), 193–212. https://doi:10.1111/j.1467-9213.2006.00437.x

Baker, H. H. (1910). "Private Hearings: Their Advantages and Disadvantages." *Annals of the American Academy of Political and Social Science, 36*(1), 80–84. https://doi:10.1177/000271621003600115

Balkissoon, D. (2013). "Extreme Temper Tantrums May Signal Mood Disorder." *Today's Parent.* https: www.todaysparent.com/kids/extreme-tantrums/

Ball, M. S. (1975). "The Play's the Thing: An Unscientific Reflection on Courts under the Rubric of Theater." *Stanford Law Review, 28*(1), 81–115. https://doi:10.2307/1228228

Balon, R. (2012). "The Debate about Paraphilic Coercive Disorder Is Mostly Ideological and Going Nowhere." *Archives of Sexual Behavior, 41*(3), 535–536. https://doi:10.1007/s10508-011-9892-4

Balon, R. (2017). "Burden of Sexual Dysfunction." *Journal of Sex & Marital Therapy, 43*(1), 49–55. https://doi:10.1080/0092623X.2015.1113597

Bancroft, J. (2004). "Alfred C. Kinsey and the Politics of Sex Research." *Annual Review of Sex Research*, 15(1), 1–39. https://doi:10.1080/10532528.2004.10559818

Banicki, K. (2014). "Positive Psychology on Character Strengths and Virtues. A Disquieting Suggestion." *New Ideas in Psychology, 33*, 21–34. https://doi:10.1016/j.newideapsych.2013.12.001

Banzato, C. E. M. (2004). "Classification in Psychiatry: The Move towards ICD-11 and DSM-V." *Current Opinion in Psychiatry, 17*(6), 497–501. https://doi:10.1097/00001504-200411000-00013

Barak, G. (Ed.) (1994). *Media, Process, and the Social Construction of Crime: Studies in Newsmaking Criminology*. New York: Garland Publishing.

Barbieri, N., & Connell, N. M. (2015). "A Cross-National Assessment of Media Reactions and Blame Finding of Student Perpetrated School Shootings." *American Journal of Criminal Justice, 40*(1), 23–46. https://doi:10.1007/s12103-014-9236-8

Barkan, S. E., & Bryjak, G. J. (2011). "Crime and Justice in American Society." In S. E. Barkan & G. J. Bryjak (Eds.), *Fundamentals of Criminal Justice: A Sociological View, Second ed.* (pp. 2–25). Sudbury, MA: Jones & Bartlett Learning.

Barnes, J. C., Raine, A., & Farrington, D. P. (2022). "The Interaction of Biopsychological and Socio-Environmental Influences on Criminological Outcomes." *Justice Quarterly, 39*(1), 26–50. https://doi:10.1080/07418825.2020.1730425

Baron, R. J. (1990). "Medical Hermeneutics: Where Is the 'Text' We Are Interpreting?" *Theoretical Medicine, 11*(1), 25–28. https://doi:10.1007/BF00489235

Barr, N. (2020). *Economics of the Welfare State* (Sixth ed.). New York: Oxford University Press.

Barratt, E. S., Stanford, M. S., Felthous, A. R., & Kent, T. A. (1997). "The Effects of Phenytoin on Impulsive and Premeditated Aggression: A Controlled Study." *Journal of Clinical Psychopharmacology, 17*(5), 341–349. https://journals.lww.com/psychopharmacology/Fulltext/1997/10000/The_Effects_of_Phenytoin_on_Impulsive_and.2.aspx

Barton, W. E. (1987). *The History and Influence of the American Psychiatric Association*. Washington, DC: American Psychiatric Press.

Baumer, E. P. (2012). Crime trends, in *The Oxford Handbook of Crime and Criminal Justice*, edited by M. Tonry. Oxford: Oxford University Press, pp. 26-59.

Bayer, R. (1981). *Homosexuality and American Psychiatry: The Politics of Diagnosis*. New York: Basic Books.

Bayer, R. (1987). *Homosexuality and American Psychiatry: The Politics of Diagnosis, with a New Afterword on AIDS and Homosexuality*. Princeton, NJ: Princeton University Press.

Bazelon, D. L. (1978). "The Role of the Psychiatrist in the Criminal Justice System." *Bulletin of the American Academy of Psychiatry Law, 6*(2), 139–146. http://jaapl.org/content/6/2/139

Beauchamp, T. L. (Ed.) (1998). *David Hume: An Enquiry Concerning the Principles of Morals*. (The Clarendon ed. of the Works of David Hume series). Oxford: Clarendon Press/Oxford University Press.

Beauchamp, T. L. (2003). "A Defense of the Common Morality." *Kennedy Institute of Ethics Journal, 13*(3), 259–274. https://doi:10.1353/ken.2003.0019

Beauchamp, T. L. (2014). "On Common Morality as Embodied Practice: A Reply to Kukla." *Cambridge Quarterly of Healthcare Ethics, 23*(1), 86–93. https://doi:10.1017/S0963180113000492

Beccaria, C. (1766/1886). *On Crimes and Punishments*. Translated by D. Young. Indianapolis: Hackett Publishing.

Beccaria, C. B. (1767). *An Essay on Crimes and Punishment*. Translator not identified. London: J. Almon. https://oll.libertyfund.org/title/voltaire-an-essay-on-crimes-and-punishments

Beck, J. S., Broder, F., & Hindman, R. (2016). "Frontiers in Cognitive Behaviour Therapy for Personality Disorders." *Behaviour Change, 33*(2), 80–93. https://doi:10.1017/bec.2016.3

Beckett, K. (1997). *Making Crime Pay: Law and Order in Contemporary American Politics*. New York: Oxford University Press.

Beech, A. R., Miner, M. H., & Thornton, D. (2016). "Paraphilias in the DSM-5." *Annual Review of Clinical Psychology, 12*, 383–406. https://doi:10.1146/annurev-clinpsy-021815-093330

Beecher, H. K. (1966). "Ethics and Clinical Research." *New England Journal of Medicine, 274*(24), 1354–1360. https://doi:10.1056/NEJM196606162742405

Behr, E. (2011). *Prohibition: Thirteen Years That Changed America* (9 June 2011 ed.). New York: Arcade Publishing.

Belfrage, H. (1998). "A Ten-Year Follow-up of Criminality in Stockholm Mental Patients: New Evidence for a Relation between Mental Disorder and Crime." *British Journal of Criminology*, 38(1), 145–155. https://doi:10.1093/oxfordjournals.bjc.a014217

Bell, C. (2004). "Racism: A Mental Illness?" *Psychiatric Services*, 55(12), 1343. https://doi:10.1176/appi.ps.55.12.1343

Bell, C. C., & Dunbar, E. (2012). "Racism and Pathological Bias as a Co-Occurring Problem in Diagnosis and Assessment." In T. A. Widiger (Ed.), *The Oxford Handbook of Personality Disorders* (pp. 694–709). New York: Oxford University Press.

Bender, S., Stokes, A., & Gaspaire, S. (2018). "Implications of the Coverage of the DSM-5 in Textbooks on Learning and Teaching of Psychology within Higher Education." *Psychology Teaching Review*, 24(1), 53–58.

Ben-Noun, L. L. (2003). "What Was the Mental Disease That Afflicted King Saul?" *Clinical Case Studies*, 2(4), 270–282. https://doi:10.1177/1534650103256296

Benson, B. A., & Brooks, W. T. (2008). "Aggressive Challenging Behaviour and Intellectual Disability." *Current Opinion in Psychiatry*, 21(5), 454–458. https://doi:10.1097/YCO.0b013e328306a090

Bentham, J. (1787). *Panopticon; or, the Inspection-House: Containing the Idea of a New Principle of Construction Applicable to Any Sort of Establishment, in Which Persons of Any Description Are to Be Kept under Inspection.* Dublin: T. Payne. https://oll.libertyfund.org/title/bowring-the-works-of-jeremy-bentham-vol-4#lf0872-04_head_010

Bentham, J. (1907). *An Introduction to the Principles of Morals and Legislation.* Oxford: Clarendon Press. https: oll.libertyfund.org/title/bentham-an-introduction-to-the-principles-of-morals-and-legislation

Berlin, F. S., Saleh, F. M., & Malin, H. M. (2009). "Mental Illness and Sex Offending." In F. M. Saleh, A. J., Grudzinskas, J. M. Bradford, & D. J. Brodsky (Eds.), *Sex Offenders: Identification, Risk Assessment, Treatment, and Legal Issues* (pp. 119–129). New York: Oxford University Press.

Berman, M. E., & Coccaro, E. F. (1998). "Neurobiologic Correlates of Violence: Relevance to Criminal Responsibility." *Behavioral Sciences & the Law*, 16(3), 303–318. https://doi:10.1002/(SICI)1099-0798(199822)16:3<303::AID-BSL309>3.0.CO;2-C

Berman, M. E., McCloskey, M. S., Fanning, J. R., Schumacher, J. A., & Coccaro, E. F. (2009). "Serotonin Augmentation Reduces Response to Attack in Aggressive Individuals." *Psychological Science*, 20(6), 714–720. https://doi:10.1111/j.1467-9280.2009.02355.x

Berman, M. N. (2013). "Rehabilitating Retributivism." *Law and Philosophy*, 32(1), 83–108. https://doi:10.1007/s10982-012-9146-1

Bernstein, A. (1988). "Cultural Literacy: Process and Content." *Change*, 20(4), 4. https://doi:10.1080/00091383.1988.9939154

Berrios, G. E. (1996). *The History of Mental Symptoms: Descriptive Psychopathology since the Nineteenth Century.* New York: Cambridge University Press.

Berrios, G. E. (2006). "'Mind in General' by Sir Alexander Crichton." *History of Psychiatry*, 17(4), 469–486. https://doi:10.1177/0957154x06071679

Berryessa, C. M., & Raine, A. (2018). Neurocriminology. In A. Brisman, E. Carrabine, & N. South (Eds.), *The Routledge Companion to Criminological Theory and Concepts* (pp. 78–82). New York: Routledge.

Bertram, C. (2020). "Jean Jacques Rousseau." In E. N. Zalta (Ed.), *The Stanford Encyclopedia of Philosophy* (Winter 2020 ed.). Stanford, CA: Metaphysics Research Lab, Stanford University. https://plato.stanford.edu/archives/win2020/entries/rousseau/

Besemer, S., & Murray, J. (2016). "Incarceration and Development of Delinquency." In T. P. Beauchaine & S. P. Hinshaw (Eds.), *The Oxford Handbook of Externalizing Spectrum Disorders* (pp. 323–343). New York: Oxford University Press.

Best, M., Williams, J. M., & Coccaro, E. F. (2002). "Evidence for a Dysfunctional Prefrontal Circuit in Patients with an Impulsive Aggressive Disorder." *Proceedings of the National Academy of Sciences of the United States of America*, 99(12), 8448–8453. https://doi:10.1073/pnas.112604099

Bever, E., & Styers, R. (Eds.) (2018). *Magic in the Modern World: Strategies of Repression and Legitimization.* University Park: Pennsylvania State University Press.

Biddle, B. J. (1986). "Recent Developments in Role Theory." *Annual Review of Sociology, 12,* 67–92. https://doi:10.2307/2083195

Birkbeck, C. (2014). *Media Representations of Crime and Criminal Justice.* In *Oxford Handbooks Online* (pp. 1–13). Oxford: Oxford University Press. https://www.oxfordhandbooks.com/view/10.1093/oxfordhb/9780199935383.001.0001/oxfordhb-9780199935383-e-15

Blackwell, B. (2017). "Barry Blackwell: Corporate Corruption in the Psychopharmaceutical Industry (Revised)." https://www.inhn.org/inhn-projects/controversies/barry-blackwell-corporate-corruption-in-the-psychopharmaceutical-industry-revised

Blader, J. C., & Carlson, G. A. (2007). "Increased Rates of Bipolar Disorder Diagnoses among U.S. Child, Adolescent, and Adult Inpatients, 1996–2004." *Biological Psychiatry, 62*(2), 107–114. https://doi:10.1016/j.biopsych.2006.11.006

Blair, R. J. R. (2010). "Neuroimaging of Psychopathy and Antisocial Behavior: A Targeted Review." *Current Psychiatry Reports, 12,* 76–82. https://doi:1007/s11920-009-0086-x

Blanchard, R. (2010). "The DSM Diagnostic Criteria for Pedophilia." *Archives of Sexual Behavior, 39*(2), 304–316. https://doi:10.1007/s10508-009-9536-0

Blanchard, R. (2013). "A Dissenting Opinion on DSM-5 Pedophilic Disorder." *Archives of Sexual Behavior, 42*(5), 675–678. https://doi:10.1007/s10508-013-0117-x

Blanchard, R., Christensen, B. K., Strong, S. M., Cantor, J. M., Kuban, M. E., Klassen, P., ... Blak, T. (2002). "Retrospective Self-Reports of Childhood Accidents Causing Unconsciousness in Phallometrically Diagnosed Pedophiles." *Archives of Sexual Behavior, 31*(6), 511–526. https://doi:10.1023/A:1020659331965

Blanchard, R., Klassen, P., Dickey, R., Kuban, M. E., & Blak, T. (2001). "Sensitivity and Specificity of the Phallometric Test for Pedophilia in Nonadmitting Sex Offenders." *Psychological Assessment, 13*(1), 118–126. https://doi:10.1037/1040-3590.13.1.118

Blanchard, R., Kuban, M. E., Klassen, P., Dickey, R., Christensen, B. K., Cantor, J. M., & Black, T. (2003). "Self-Reported Head Injuries before and after Age 13 in Pedophilic and Nonpedophilic Males Referred for Clinical Assessment." *Archives of Sexual Behavior, 32*(6), 573–581. https://doi:10.1023/A:1026093612434

Blashfield, R. K. (1982). "Feighner et al., Invisible Colleges, and the Matthew Effect." *Schizophrenia Bulletin, 8*(1), 1–6. https://doi 10.1093/schbul/8.1.1

Blashfield, R. K. (1984). *The Classification of Psychopathology: Neo-Kraepelinian and Quantitative Approaches.* Boston: Springer.

Blashfield, R. K., Keeley, J. W., Flanagan, E. H., & Miles, S. R. (2014). "The Cycle of Classification: DSM-I through DSM-5." *Annual Review of Clinical Psychology, 10*(1), 25–51. https://doi:10.1146/annurev-clinpsy-032813-153639

Blashfield, R. K., & Livesley, W. J. (1991). "Metaphorical Analysis of Psychiatric Classification as a Psychological Test." *Journal of Abnormal Psychology, 100*(3), 262–270. https://doi:10.1037/0021-843X.100.3.262

Blasingame, G. D. (2014). "Practical Strategies for Working with Youth with Intellectual Disabilities Who Have Sexual Behavior Problems." In D. S. Bromberg & W. T. O'Donohue (Eds.), *Toolkit for Working with Juvenile Sex Offenders* (pp. 479–505). San Diego: Academic Press.

Block, J. J. (2008). "Issues for DSM-V: Internet Addiction." *American Journal of Psychiatry, 165*(3), 306–307. https://doi:10.1176/appi.ajp.2007.07101556

Bloechl, A. L., Vitacco, M. J., Neumann, C. S., & Erickson, S. E. (2007). "An Empirical Investigation of Insanity Defense Attitudes: Exploring Factors Related to Bias." *International Journal of Law and Psychiatry, 30*(2), 153–161. https://doi:10.1016/j.ijlp.2006.03.007

Boerjan, M., Bluyssen, S. J. M., Bleichrodt, R. P., van Weel-Baumgarten, E. M., & van Goor, H. (2010). "Work-Related Health Complaints in Surgical Residents and the Influence of Social Support and Job-Related Autonomy." *Medical Education, 44*(8), 835–844. https://doi:10.1111/j.1365-2923.2010.03724.x

Bok, H. (2018). "Baron De Montesquieu, Charles-Louis De Secondat." In E. N. Zalta (Ed.), *The Stanford Encyclopedia of Philosophy* (Winter 2018 ed.). Stanford, CA: Metaphysics Research Lab, Stanford University. https://plato.stanford.edu/archives/win2018/entries montesquieu/

Bolton, D. (2008). *What Is Mental Disorder?: An Essay in Philosophy, Science, and Values.* New York: Oxford University Press.

Bolton, J. (2011a). "Between the Quack and the Fanatic: Movements in Our Self-Belief." *Medicine, Health Care and Philosophy, 14*(3), 281–285. https://doi:10.1007/s11019-011-9313-4

Bolton, J. (2011b). "Aristotle in the Psychiatry Residents' Clinic." *Academic Psychiatry, 35*(5), 298–301. https://doi:10.1176/appi.ap.35.5.298

Bond, G. R., & Drake, R. E. (2017). "New Directions for Psychiatric Rehabilitation in the USA." *Epidemiology and Psychiatric Sciences, 26*(3), 223–227. https://doi:10.1017/s2045796016000834

Bonta, J., & Andrews, D. A. (2016). *The Psychology of Criminal Conduct, Sixth ed.* New York: Routledge.

Bonta, J., Law, M., & Hanson, K. (1998). "The Prediction of Criminal and Violent Recidivism among Mentally Disordered Offenders: A Meta-Analysis." *Psychological Bulletin, 123*(2), 123–142. https://doi:10.1037/0033-2909.123.2.123

Boonin, D. (2008). *The Problem of Punishment.* Cambridge: Cambridge University Press.

Booth, B. D. (2016). "Elderly Sexual Offenders." *Current Psychiatry Reports, 18*(4), 34. https://doi:10.1007/s11920-016-0678-1

Borum, R., & Fulero, S. M. (1999). "Empirical Research on the Insanity Defense and Attempted Reforms: Evidence toward Informed Policy: Erratum." *Law and Human Behavior, 23*(3), 375–394. https://doi:10.1023/A:1022364700424

Bradley, C. M., & Hoffmann, J. L. (1996). "Public Perception, Justice, and the 'Search for Truth' in Criminal Cases." *Southern California Law Review, 69*(4), 1267–1302.

Braithwaite, J. (1999). "Restorative Justice: Assessing Optimistic and Pessimistic Accounts." *Crime and Justice, 25,* 1–127. http://www.jstor.org/stable/1147608

Braithwaite, J., & Pettit, P. (1990). *Not Just Deserts: A Republican Theory of Criminal Justice.* Oxford: Oxford University Press.

Breckinridge, S. P., & Abbott, E. (1912). *The Delinquent Child and the Home.* Chicago: Russell Sage Foundation.

Brendel, D. H. (2006). *Healing Psychiatry: Bridging the Science/Humanism Divide.* Cambridge, MA: MIT Press.

Brennan, P. A., Mednick, S. A., & Hodgins, S. (2000). "Major Mental Disorders and Criminal Violence in a Danish Birth Cohort." *Archives of General Psychiatry, 57*(5), 494–500. https://doi:10.1001/archpsyc.57.5.494

Brennan, T. A. (1987). "Untangling Causation Issues in Law and Medicine: Hazardous Substance Litigation." *Annals of Internal Medicine, 107*(5), 741–747. https://doi:10.7326/0003-4819-107-5-741

Briggs, A. (1961). "The Welfare State in Historical Perspective." *European Journal of Sociology/Archives europeennes de sociologie, 2*(2), 221–258. https://doi:10.1017/S0003975600000412

Brinkley, D. G. (2000). *Rosa Parks: A Life.* New York: Penguin.

Broackes, J. (2005). "David Hume." In T. Honderich (Ed.), *The Oxford Companion to Philosophy, Second ed.* (pp. 403–407). New York/Oxford: Oxford University Press.

Bronnimann, N. (2020). "Remorse in Parole Hearings: An Elusive Concept with Concrete Consequences." *Missouri Law Review, 85*(2), Article 18, 321–356. https://scholarship.law.missouri.edu/mlr/vol85/iss2/18/

Bronson, J., & Berzofsky, M. (2017). *Indicators of Mental Health Problems Reported by Prisoners and Jail Inmates, 2011–2012* (NCJ Number 250612). https://www.ojp.gov/ncjrs/virtual-library abstracts/indicators-mental-health-problems-reported-prisoners-and-jail

Brooks, A. D. (1985). "The Merits of Abolishing the Insanity Defense." *Annals of the American Academy of Political and Social Science, 477*(1), 125–136. https://doi:10.1177/0002716285477001012

Broome, E. C. (1946). "Ezekiel's Abnormal Personality." *Journal of Biblical Literature, 65*(3), 277–292. https://doi:10.2307/3262666

Brown, L. S. (1992). "A Feminist Critique of the Personality Disorders." In L. S. Brown & M. Ballou (Eds.), *Personality and Psychopathology: Feminist Reappraisals* (pp. 206–228). New York: Guilford Press.

Brown, R., Dunn, S., Byrnes, K., Morris, R., Heinrich, P., & Shaw, J. (2009). "Doctors' Stress Responses and Poor Communication Performance in Simulated Bad-News Consultations." *Academic Medicine, 84*(11), 1595–1602. https://doi:10.1097/ACM.0b013e3181baf537

Brown, S. (1999). "Public Attitudes toward the Treatment of Sex Offenders." *Legal and Criminological Psychology, 4*(2), 239–252. https://doi:10.1348/135532599167879

Brülde, B. (2001). "The Goals of Medicine. Towards a Unified Theory." *Health Care Analysis, 9*(1), 1–13. https://doi:10.1023/A:1011385310274

Buckholtz, J. W., Treadway, M. T., Cowan, R. L., Woodward, N. D., Benning, S. D., Li, R., . . . Zald, D. H. (2010). "Mesolimbic Dopamine Reward System Hypersensitivity in Individuals with Psychopathic Traits." *Nature Neuroscience, 13*(4), 419–421. https://doi:10.1038/nn.2510

Bueter, A. (2021). "Public Epistemic Trustworthiness and the Integration of Patients in Psychiatric Classification." *Synthese, 198*(19), 4711–4729. https://doi:10.1007/s11229-018-01913-z

Bulger, R. E., Heitman, E., & Reiser, S. J. (Eds.) (2002). *The Ethical Dimensions of the Biological and Health Sciences, Second ed.* Cambridge: Cambridge University Press.

Bullough, V. L. (1990). The Kinsey Scale in Historical Perspective. In D. P. McWhirter, S. A. Sanders, & J. M. Reinisch (Eds.), *Homosexuality/Heterosexuality: Concepts of Sexual Orientation* (pp. 3–15). New York: Oxford University Press.

Bullough, V. L. (1994a). *Science in the Bedroom: A History of Sex Research.* New York: Basic Books.

Bullough, V. L. (1994b). "The Development of Sexology in the USA in the Early Twentieth Century." In R. Porter & M. Teich (Eds.), *Sexual Knowledge, Sexual Science: The History of Attitudes to Sexuality* (pp. 303–322). Cambridge: Cambridge University Press.

Bullough, V. L. (1998). "Alfred Kinsey and the Kinsey Report: Historical Overview and Lasting Contributions." *The Journal of Sex Research, 35*(2), 127–131. https://doi:10.1080/00224499809551925

Bullough, V. L. (2004). "Sex Will Never Be the Same: The Contributions of Alfred C. Kinsey." *Archives of Sexual Behavior, 33*(3), 277–286. https://doi:10.1023/B:ASEB.0000026627.24993.03

Bullough, V. L. (2006). "The Kinsey Biographies." *Sexuality & Culture, 10*(1), 15–22. https://doi:10.1007/s12119-006-1002-8

Burchfield, K. B., & Mingus, W. (2008). "Not in My Neighborhood: Assessing Registered Sex Offenders' Experiences with Local Social Capital and Social Control." *Criminal Justice and Behavior, 35*(3), 356–374. https://doi:10.1177/0093854807311375

Burns, J. R., & Rapee, R. M. (2006). "Adolescent Mental Health Literacy: Young People's Knowledge of Depression and Help Seeking." *Journal of Adolescence, 29*(2), 225–239. https://doi:10.1016/j.adolescence.2005.05.004

Butera, G. (2010). "Thomas Aquinas and Cognitive Therapy: An Exploration of the Promise of the Thomistic Psychology." *Philosophy, Psychiatry, & Psychology, 17*(4), 347–366. https://doi:10.1353/ppp.2010.0023

Butler, R. W., Braff, D. L., Rausch, J. L., Jenkins, M. A., Sprock, J., & Geyer, M. A. (1990). "Physiological Evidence of Exaggerated Startle Response in a Subgroup of Vietnam Veterans with Combat-Related PTSD." *American Journal of Psychiatry, 147*(10), 1308–1312.

Bynum, B. (2003). "Discarded Diagnoses: Monomania." *The Lancet, 362*(9393), 1425. https://doi:10.1016/S0140-6736(03)14643-0

Calcedo-Barba, A. (2010). "Objectivity and Ethics in Forensic Psychiatry." *Current Opinion in Psychiatry, 23*(5), 447–452. https://doi:10.1097/YCO.0b013e32833cd1e6

Califf, R. M., Zarin, D. A., Kramer, J. M., Sherman, R. E., Aberle, L. H., & Tasneem, A. (2012). Characteristics of clinical trials registered in ClinicalTrials. gov, 2007–2010. *JAMA, 307*(17), 1838–1847.

Callahan, D. (1996). "The Goals of Medicine: Preface." *The Hastings Center Report, 26*(6), 2.

Callahan, L. A., Steadman, H. J., McGreevy, M. A., & Robbins, P. C. (1991). "The Volume and Characteristics of Insanity Defense Pleas: An Eight-State Study." *Bulletin of the American Academy of Psychiatry and the Law, 19*(4), 331–338.

Calvin, J. (1541/2009). *Institutes of the Christian Religion: The First English Version of the 1541 French ed.* Translated by E. A. McKee. Grand Rapids, MI/Cambridge: Wm. B. Eerdmans Publishing.

Camilleri, J. A., & Quinsey, V. L. (2008). "Pedophilia: Assessment and Treatment." In D. R. Laws & W. T. O'Donohue (Eds.), *Sexual Deviance: Theory, Assessment, and Treatment, Second ed.* (pp. 183–212). New York: Guildford Press.

Campbell, C. M., Abboud, M. J., Hamilton, Z. K., vanWormer, J., & Posey, B. (2018). "Evidence-Based or Just Promising? Lessons Learned in Taking Inventory of State Correctional Programming." *Justice Evaluation Journal, 1*(2), 188–214. https://doi:10.1080/24751979.2018.1528849

Campbell, S. M., Ulrich, C. M., & Grady, C. (2016). "A Broader Understanding of Moral Distress." *American Journal of Bioethics, 16*(12), 2–9. https://doi:10.1080/15265161.2016.1239782

Candilis, P. J., & Huttenbach, E. D. (2015). "Ethics in Correctional Mental Health." In R. L. Trestman, K. L. Appelbaum, & J. L. Metzner (Eds.), *Oxford Textbook of Correctional Psychiatry* (pp. 41–45). Oxford: Oxford University Press.

Card, C. (2002). *The Atrocity Paradigm: A Theory of Evil.* Oxford: Oxford University Press.

Cartwright, S. A. (1851). "Report on the Disease of Physical Peculiarities of the Negro." *The New Orleans Medical and Surgical Journal, 7,* 707–708.

Caruso, G. D. (2012). *Free Will and Consciousness: A Determinist Account of the Illusion of Free Will.* Lanham, MD: Lexington Books.

Caruso, G. D. (Ed.) (2013). *Exploring the Illusion of Free Will and Moral Responsibility.* Lanham, MD: Lexington Books.

Caruso, G. D. (2020). "Justice without Retribution: An Epistemic Argument against Retributive Criminal Punishment." *Neuroethics, 13*(1), 13–28. https://doi:10.1007/s12152-018-9357-8

Caruso, G. D. (2021). *Rejecting Retributivism: Free Will, Punishment, and Criminal Justice.* Cambridge: Cambridge University Press.

Catty, J. (2004). "'The Vehicle of Success': Theoretical and Empirical Perspectives on the Therapeutic Alliance in Psychotherapy and Psychiatry." *Psychology and Psychotherapy: Theory, Research and Practice, 77*(2), 255–272. https://doi:10.1348/147608304323112528

Cavadino, M., & Dignan, J. (2006). "Penal Policy and Political Economy." *Criminology & Criminal Justice, 6*(4), 435–456. https://doi:10.1177/1748895806068581

Ceccherini-Nelli, A., & Priebe, S. (2007). "Economic Factors and Psychiatric Hospital Beds–an Analysis of Historical Trends." *International Journal of Social Economics, 34*(11), 788–810. https://doi:10.1108/03068290710826396

Chadwick, H. (Ed.) (1992). *The Treatise on the Apostolic Tradition of St. Hippolytus of Rome: Bishop and Martyr.* London: Routledge.

Chapman, R., & Ciment, J. (Eds.) (2015). *Culture Wars: An Encyclopedia of Issues, Viewpoints and Voices.* New York: Routledge.

Charland, L. C. (2002). "Tuke's Healing Discipline: Commentary on Erica Lilleleht's 'Progress and Power: Exploring the Disciplinary Connections between Moral Treatment and Psychiatric Rehabilitation.'" *Philosophy, Psychiatry, & Psychology, 9*(2), 183–186. https://doi:10.1353/ppp.2003.0023

Charland, L. C. (2004). "A Madness for Identity: Psychiatric Labels, Consumer Autonomy, and the Perils of the Internet." *Philosophy, Psychiatry, & Psychology, 11*(4), 335–349. https://doi:10.1353/ppp.2005.0006

Charland, L. C. (2006). "Moral Nature of the DSM-IV Cluster B Personality Disorders." *Journal of Personality Disorders, 20*(2), 116–125. https://doi:10.1521/pedi.2006.20.2.116

Charland, L. C. (2008). "Alexander Crichton on the Psychopathology of the Passions." *History of Psychiatry, 19*(75, Pt 3), 275–296. https://doi:10.1177/0957154X07078703

Charland, L. C. (2010). "Science and Morals in the Affective Psychopathology of Philippe Pinel." *History of Psychiatry, 21*(1), 38–53. https://doi: 10.1177/0957154X09338334

Chen, H., Reid, E., Sinai, J., Silke, A., & Ganor, B. (Eds.) (2008). *Terrorism Informatics: Knowledge Management and Data Mining for Homeland Security.* New York: Springer Science & Business Media.

Chisolm, M. S., & Lyketsos, C. G. (2012). *Systematic psychiatric evaluation: A step-by-step guide to applying the perspectives of psychiatry.* JHU Press.

Choe, J. Y., Teplin, L. A., & Abram, K. M. (2008). "Perpetration of Violence, Violent Victimization, and Severe Mental Illness: Balancing Public Health Concerns." *Psychiatric Services, 59*(2), 153–164. https://doi:10.1176/appi.ps.59.2.153

Choy, O., Portnoy, J., Raine, A., Remmel, R. J., Schug, R., Tuvblad, C., & Yang, Y. (2019). "Biosocial Influences on Offending across the Life Course." In D. P. Farrington, L. Kazemian, & A. R. Piquero (Eds.), *The Oxford Handbook of Developmental and Life-Course Criminology* (pp. 325–354). New York: Oxford University Press.

Christenbury, L. (1989)." Cultural Literacy: A Terrible Idea Whose Time Has Come." *The English Journal, 78*(1), 14–17. https://doi:10.2307/817980

Chung, M. C., Fulford, K. W. M., & Graham, G. (Eds.) (2007). *Reconceiving Schizophrenia.* Oxford: Oxford University Press.

Ciani, A. S. C., Scarpazza, C., Covelli, V., & Battaglia, U. (2019). "Profiling Acquired Pedophilic Behavior: Retrospective Analysis of 66 Italian Forensic Cases of Pedophilia." *International Journal of Law and Psychiatry, 67*, 101508. https://doi:10.1016/j.ijlp.2019.101508

Cirincione, C., Steadman, H. J., & McGreevy, M. A. (1995). "Rates of Insanity Acquittals and the Factors Associated with Successful Insanity Pleas." *Bulletin of the American Academy of Psychiatry and the Law, 23*(3), 399–409.

Clark, L. A. (2002). "Evaluation and Devaluation in Personality Assessment." In J. Z. Sadler (Ed.), *Descriptions and Prescriptions: Values, Mental Disorders, and the DSMs* (pp. 131–147). Baltimore: Johns Hopkins University Press.

Cleckley, H. (1988). *The Mask of Sanity: An Attempt to Clarify Some Issues about the So-Called Psychopathic Personality* (Fifth ed.: private printing for non-profit educational use). Augusta, GA: Emily S. Cleckley. https://www.gwern.net/docs psychology/1941-cleckley-maskofsanity.pdf

Cleckley, H. M. (1941). *The Mask of Sanity: An Attempt to Reinterpret the So-Called Psychopathic Personality*. St. Louis: Mosby.

Cloninger, C. R. (Ed.) (1999). *Personality and Psychopathology*. Washington, DC: American Psychiatric Press.

Cloninger, C. R. (2004). *Feeling Good: The Science of Well-Being*. New York: Oxford University Press.

Cnaan, R. A., Blankertz, L., Messinger, K. W., & Gardner, J. R. (1988). "Psychosocial Rehabilitation: Toward a Definition." *Psychosocial Rehabilitation Journal, 11*(4), 61–77. https://doi:10.1037/h0099561

Coccaro, E. F. (2000). "Intermittent Explosive Disorder." *Current Psychiatry Reports, 2*(1), 67–71. https://doi:10.1007/s11920-000-0045-z

Coccaro, E. F. (2004). "Intermittent Explosive Disorder and Impulsive Aggression: The Time for Serious Study Is Now." *Current Psychiatry Reports, 6*(1), 1–2.

Coccaro, E. F., & Lee, R. (2010). "Cerebrospinal Fluid 5-Hydroxyindolacetic Acid and Homovanillic Acid: Reciprocal Relationships with Impulsive Aggression in Human Subjects." *Journal of Neural Transmission, 117*(2), 241–248. https://doi:10.1007/s00702-009-0359-x

Coccaro, E. F., Lee, R., & Kavoussi, R. J. (2010a). "Inverse Relationship between Numbers of 5-HT Transporter Binding Sites and Life History of Aggression and Intermittent Explosive Disorder." *Journal of Psychiatric Research, 44*(3), 137–142. https://doi:10.1016/j.jpsychires.2009.07.004

Coccaro, E. F., Lee, R., & Kavoussi, R. J. (2010b). "Aggression, Suicidality, and Intermittent Explosive Disorder: Serotonergic Correlates in Personality Disorder and Healthy Control Subjects." *Neuropsychopharmacology, 35*(2), 435–444. https://doi:10.1038/npp.2009.148

Coccaro, E. F., McCloskey, M. S., Fitzgerald, D. A., & Phan, K. L. (2007). "Amygdala and Orbitofrontal Reactivity to Social Threat in Individuals with Impulsive Aggression." *Biological Psychiatry, 62*(2), 168–178. https://doi:10.1016/j.biopsych.2006.08.024

Coccaro, E. F., Noblett, K. L., & McCloskey, M. S. (2009). "Attributional and Emotional Responses to Socially Ambiguous Cues: Validation of a New Assessment of Social/Emotional Information Processing in Healthy Adults and Impulsive Aggressive Patients." *Journal of Psychiatric Research, 43*(10), 915–925. https://doi:10.1016/j.jpsychires.2009.01.012

Coccaro, E. F., Posternak, M. A., & Zimmerman, M. (2005). "Prevalence and Features of Intermittent Explosive Disorder in a Clinical Setting." *Journal of Clinical Psychiatry, 66*(10), 1221–1227. https://doi:10.4088/JCP.v66n1003

Coccaro, E. F., Schmidt, C. A., Samuels, J. F., & Nestadt, G. (2004). "Lifetime and 1-Month Prevalence Rates of Intermittent Explosive Disorder in a Community Sample." *Journal of Clinical Psychiatry, 65*(6), 820–824. https://doi:10.4088/JCP.v65n0613

Cohen, L. J., Gertmenian-King, E., Kunik, L., Weaver, C., London, E. D., & Galynker, I. (2005). "Personality Measures in Former Heroin Users Receiving Methadone or in Protracted Abstinence from Opiates." *Acta Psychiatrica Scandinavica, 112*(2), 149–158. https://doi:10.1111/j.1600-0447.2005.00546.x

Cohen, L. J., Grebchenko, Y. F., Steinfeld, M., Frenda, S. J., & Galynker, I. I. (2008). "Comparison of Personality Traits in Pedophiles, Abstinent Opiate Addicts, and Healthy Controls: Considering Pedophilia as an Addictive Behavior." *Journal of Nervous and Mental Disease, 196*(11), 829–837. https://doi:10.1097/NMD.0b013e31818b4e3d

Cohen, L. J., McGeoch, P. G., Watras-Gans, S., Acker, S., Poznansky, O., Cullen, K., . . . Galynker, I. (2002). "Personality Impairment in Male Pedophiles." *Journal of Clinical Psychiatry*, *63*(10), 912–919. https://doi:10.4088/JCP.v63n1009

Cohen, L. J., Nikiforov, K., Gans, S., Poznansky, O., McGeoch, P., Weaver, C., . . . Galynker, I. (2002). "Heterosexual Male Perpetrators of Childhood Sexual Abuse: A Preliminary Neuropsychiatric Model." *Psychiatric Quarterly*, *73*(4), 313–336. https://doi:10.1023/A:1020416101092

Cohen, L. J., Watras-Gans, S., McGeoch, P. G., Poznansky, O., Itskovich, Y., Murphy, S., . . . Galynker, I. I. (2002). "Impulsive Personality Traits in Male Pedophiles Versus Healthy Controls: Is Pedophilia an Impulsive-Aggressive Disorder?" *Comprehensive Psychiatry*, *43*(2), 127–134. https://doi:10.1053/comp.2002.30796

Cohen, M. R. (1940). "Moral Aspects of the Criminal Law." *Yale Law Journal*, *49*(6), 987–1026. https://doi:10.2307/792227

Cohen, M. R. (1950). *Reason and Law: Studies in Juristic Philosophy* (First ed.). Glencoe, IL: The Free Press.

Cohen, S. (1973). *Folk Devils and Moral Panics: The Creation of the Mods and Rockers*. London: Paladin.

Cohon, R. (2018). "Hume's Moral Philosophy." In E. N. Zalta (Ed.), *The Stanford Encyclopedia of Philosophy* (Fall 2018 ed.) . Stanford, CA: Metaphysics Research Lab, Stanford University. https://plato.stanford.edu/archives/fall2018/entries/hume-moral/

Coke, E. (1791). *The First Part of the Institutes of the Laws of England: Or, a Commentary upon Littleton*. Dublin: James Moore.

Colaizzi, J. (1989). *Homicidal Insanity, 1800-1985*. Tuscaloosa: University of Alabama Press.

Collins, R. E. (2014). "The Construction of Race and Crime in Canadian Print Media: A 30-Year Analysis." *Criminology & Criminal Justice*, *14*(1), 77–99. https://doi:10.1177/1748895813476874

Confucius. (1971). *Confucian Analects, Great Learning and Doctrine of the Mean*. Translated by J. Legge. New York: Dover Publications.

Connolly, W. E. (1987). *Politics and Ambiguity*. Madison: University of Wisconsin Press.

Connolly, W. E. (1993). *The Terms of Political Discourse, Third ed.* Princeton, NJ: Princeton University Press.

Connolly, W. E. (2017). *Aspirational Fascism: The Struggle for Multifaceted Democracy under Trumpism*. Minneapolis: University of Minnesota Press.

Conrad, P. (2007). *The Medicalization of Society: On the Transformation of Human Conditions into Treatable Disorders*. Baltimore: Johns Hopkins University Press.

Conrad, R. C., & Brendel, R. W. (2020). "Structural Deprioritization and Stigmatization of Mental Health Concerns in the Educational Setting." *The American Journal of Bioethics*, *20*(10), 67–69. https://doi:10.1080/15265161.2020.1806389

Conybeare, F. C. (1898). "The Testament of Solomon." *Jewish Quarterly Review*, *11*(1), 1–45. https://doi:10.2307/1450398

Coogan, M. D. (Ed.) (2001). *The New Oxford Annotated Bible with the Apocrypha, Third ed., New Revised Standard Version*. New York: Oxford University Press.

Coomarasamy, A., & Khan, K. S. (2004). "What Is the Evidence That Postgraduate Teaching in Evidence Based Medicine Changes Anything? A Systematic Review." *British Medical Journal*, *329*(7473), 1017. https://doi:10.1136/bmj.329.7473.1017

Cooper, M. W. (1994). "Is Medicine Hermeneutics All the Way Down?" *Theoretical Medicine*, *15*(2), 149–180. https://doi:10.1007/BF00994023

Cooper, R. (2018). *Diagnosing the Diagnostic and Statistical Manual of Mental Disorders: Fifth ed.* London: Routledge.

Cooper, R. V. (2013) "Avoiding False Positives: Zones of Rarity, the Threshold Problem, and the DSM Clinical Significance Criterion." *Canadian Journal of Psychiatry*, *58*(11), 606–611. https://doi:10.1177/070674371305801105

Copeland, R. (1994). "Medieval Theory and Criticism." In M. Groden & M. Kreiswirth (Eds.), *The Johns Hopkins Guide to Literary Theory and Criticism* (pp. 500–507). Baltimore: Johns Hopkins University Press.

Corrigan, P. W. (2003). "Towards an Integrated, Structural Model of Psychiatric Rehabilitation." *Psychiatric Rehabilitation Journal*, *26*(4), 346–358. https://doi:10.2975/26.2003.346.358

Cortoni, F., Babchishin, K. M., & Rat, C. (2017). "The Proportion of Sexual Offenders Who Are Female Is Higher than Thought: A Meta-Analysis." *Criminal Justice and Behavior, 44*(2), 145–162. https://doi:10.1177/0093854816658923

Covey, H. C. (2005). "Western Christianity's Two Historical Treatments of People with Disabilities or Mental Illness." *Social Science Journal, 42*(1), 107–114. https://doi:10.1016/j.soscij.2004.11.009

Crafa, D., & Nagel, S. K. (2020). "Traces of Culture: The Feedback Loop between Behavior, Brain, and Disorder." *Transcultural Psychiatry, 57*(3), 387–407. https://doi:10.1177/1363461519879515

Crenshaw, K. W. (2017). *On Intersectionality: Essential Writings.* New York: The New Press.

Cronbach, L. J., & Meehl, P. E. (1955). "Construct Validity in Psychological Tests." *Psychological Bulletin, 52*(4), 281–302. https://doi:10.1037/h0040957

Cross, S. (2004). "Visualizing Madness." *Television & New Media, 5*(3), 197–216. https://doi:10.1177/1527476403254001

Cruz, A. R., de Castro-Rodrigues, A., & Barbosa, F. (2020). "Executive Dysfunction, Violence and Aggression." *Aggression and Violent Behavior, 51*, 101380. https://doi:10.1016/j.avb.2020.101380

Cuesta, M. J. L., & Peralta, V. (2001). "Integrating Psychopathological Dimensions in Functional Psychoses: A Hierarchical Approach." *Schizophrenia Research, 52*(3), 215–229. https://doi:10.1016/S0920-9964(00)00190-0

Cullen, F., & Gilbert, K. (2013). *Reaffirming Rehabilitation, Second ed.* New York: Routledge.

Culver, C. M., & Gert, B. (1982). *Philosophy in Medicine: Conceptual and Ethical Issues in Medicine and Psychiatry.* Oxford: Oxford University Press.

Cuthbert, B. N., & Insel, T. R. (2013). "Toward the Future of Psychiatric Diagnosis: The Seven Pillars of RDoC." *BMC Medicine, 11*(1), 1–8, Article: 126. https://doi:10.1186/1741-7015-11-126

Cuthbertson, S. (2013). *Analysis of Complete 'YouBeTheJudge' Website Experiences, #Youbethejudge.* London: Analytical Services, Ministry of Justice, United Kingdom. https://www.gov.uk/government/publications/the-publics-understanding-and-views-of-sentencing-and-the-criminal-justice-system

Dahlberg, K. M., Waern, M., & Runeson, B. (2008). "Mental Health Literacy and Attitudes in a Swedish Community Sample—Investigating the Role of Personal Experience of Mental Health Care." *BMC Public Health, 8*(1), 8. https://doi:10.1186/1471-2458-8-8

Dain, N. (1964). *Concepts of Insanity in the United States, 1789-1865.* New Brunswick, NJ: Rutgers University Press.

Dain, N. (1992). "Madness and the Stigma of Sin in American Christianity." In P. J. Fink & A. Tasman (Eds.), *Stigma and Mental Illness* (pp. 73–84). Washington, DC: American Psychiatric Press.

Dalal, P. K., & Basu, D. (2016). "Twenty Years of Internet Addiction . . . *Quo Vadis?*" *Indian Journal of Psychiatry, 58*(1), 6–11. https://doi:10.4103/0019-5545.174354

Daly, K., & Proietti-Scifoni, G. (2011). "Reparation and Restoration." In M. Tonry (Ed.), *The Oxford Handbook of Crime and Criminal Justice* (The Oxford Handbooks in Criminology and Criminal Justice series) (pp. 207–253). Oxford/New York: Oxford University Press.

Danforth, S. (2011). Learning From Samuel A. Kirk's 16 Versions of Learning Disability: A Rejoinder to Mather and Morris. *Intellectual and Developmental Disabilities, 49*(2), 120–126.

Danforth, S., Slocum, L., & Dunkle, J. (2010). Turning the educability narrative: Samuel A. Kirk at the intersection of learning disability and "mental retardation". *Intellectual and Developmental Disabilities, 48*(3), 180–194.

Daniel, S. L. (1986). "The Patient as Text: A Model of Clinical Hermeneutics." *Theoretical Medicine, 7*(2), 195–210. https://doi:10.1007/BF00489230

Danielou, Alain (Ed. & Trans.) (1994). *The Complete KāMa SūTra: The First Unabridged Modern Translation of the Classic Indian Text by VāTsyāYana.* Rochester, VT: Park Street Press.

Danner, D., & Sagall, E. L. (1977). "Medicolegal Causation: A Source of Professional Misunderstanding." *American Journal of Law & Medicine, 3*(3), 303–308. https://doi:10.1017/s0098858800005244

Davidson, A. I. (2001). *The Emergence of Sexuality: Historical Epistemology and the Formation of Concepts.* Cambridge, MA: Harvard University Press.

Davidson, L. (2003). *Living Outside Mental Illness: Qualitative Studies of Recovery in Schizophrenia* (Qualitative Studies in Psychology series). New York/London: New York University Press.

Davidson, L. (2013). "Cure and Recovery." In K. W. M. Fulford, M. Davies, R. G. T. Gipps, G. Graham, J. Z. Sadler, G. Stanghellini, & T. Thornton (Eds.), *The Oxford Handbook of Philosophy and Psychiatry* (pp. 197–213). Oxford: Oxford University Press.

Davidson, L., & Strauss, J. S. (1992). *Sense of Self in Recovery from Severe Mental Illness. Psychology and Psychotherapy: Theory, Research and Practice*, 65(2), 131–145. https://doi:10.1111/j.2044-8341.1992.tb01693.x

Davis, D. L. (1996). "Cultural Sensitivity and the Sexual Disorders of the DSM-IV: Review and Assessment". In J. E. Mezzich, A. Kleinman, H. Fabrega, & D. L. Parron (Eds.), *Culture and Psychiatric Diagnosis: A DSM-IV Perspective* (pp. 191–208). Washington, DC: American Psychiatric Press.

Davis, D. L. (1998). "The Sexual and Gender Identity Disorders." *Transcultural Psychiatry*, 35(3), 401–412. https://doi:10.1177/136346159803500306

Davis, M., & Elliston, F. A. (Eds.) (1986). *Ethics and the Legal Profession*. Buffalo, NY: Prometheus Books.

de Champs, E. (1999). "The Place of Jeremy Bentham's Theory of Fictions in Eighteenth-Century Linguistic Thought." *Journal of Bentham Studies*, 2(1), 1–28. https://doi:10.14324/111.2045-757X.011

de Pablo, A. G. (1994). "The Medicine of the Soul. The Origin and Development of Thought on the Soul, Diseases of the Soul and Their Treatment, in Medieval and Renaissance Medicine." *History of Psychiatry*, 5(20), 483–516. https://doi:10.1177/0957154X9400502003

Decker, H. S. (2013). *The Making of DSM-III: A Diagnostic Manual's Conquest of American Psychiatry*. New York: Oxford University Press.

DeGrazia, D. (2003). "Common Morality, Coherence, and the Principles of Biomedical Ethics." *Kennedy Institute of Ethics Journal*, 13(3), 219–230. https://doi:10.1353/ken.2003.0020

Dell'Osso, B., Altamura, A. C., Allen, A., Marazziti, D., & Hollander, E. (2006). "Epidemiologic and Clinical Updates on Impulse Control Disorders: A Critical Review." *European Archives of Psychiatry & Clinical Neuroscience*, 256(8), 464–475. https://doi:10.1007/s00406-006-0668-0

Demazeux, S., & Singy, P. (2015). *The DSM-5 in Perspective: Philosophical Reflections on the Psychiatric Babel* (History, Philosophy and Theory of the Life Sciences series). Dordrecht: Springer.

Denyer, N. C. (1995). "Diogenes the Cynic." In T. Honderich (Ed.), *The Oxford Companion to Philosophy* (pp. 201–202). Oxford: Oxford University Press.

Dercum, F. X. (1917). *A Clinical Manual of Mental Diseases*. Philadelphia: Saunders.

Descartes, R. (1909-14/2001). *Discourse on Method*. In C. W. Eliot (Ed.), The Harvard Classics series. New York: P. F. Collier & Son. https://www.bartleby.com/34 1/

Deutsch, A. (1949). *The Mentally Ill in America: A History of Their Care and Treatment from Colonial Times* (Second ed.). New York: Columbia University Press.

Devlin, P. (1965). *The Enforcement of Morals*. London: Oxford University Press.

Dhand, A. (2002). "The Dharma of Ethics, the Ethics of Dharma: Quizzing the Ideals of Hinduism." *Journal of Religious Ethics*, 30(3), 347–372. https://doi:10.1111/1467-9795.00113

Dillaway, H., & Paré, E. (2008). "Locating Mothers: How Cultural Debates about Stay-at-Home versus Working Mothers Define Women and Home." *Journal of Family Issues*, 29(4), 437–464. https://doi:10.1177/0192513X07310309

Dilman, I. (1999). *Free Will: An Historical and Philosophical Introduction*. London: Routledge.

Divakaruni, C. B. (1999). "Mrs. Dutta Writes a Letter." In A. Tan & K. Kenison (Eds.), *The Best American Short Stories, 1999* (pp. 29–48). Boston: Houghton Mifflin.

Dobkin, P. L., & Hutchinson, T. A. (2010). "Primary Prevention for Future Doctors: Promoting Well-Being in Trainees." *Medical Education*, 44(3), 224–226. https://doi:10.1111/j.1365-2923.2009.03613.x

Doley, R., Dickens, G., & Gannon, T. (Eds.) (2015). *The Psychology of Arson: A Practical Guide to Understanding and Managing Deliberate Firesetters*. London: Routledge.

Douglas, J. E., Burgess, A. W., Burgess, A. G., & Ressler, R. K. (Eds.) (2006). *Crime Classification Manual: A Standard System for Investigating and Classifying Violent Crimes, Second ed.* San Francisco: Jossey-Bass.

Driver, J. (1999). "Modesty and Ignorance." *Ethics*, 109(4), 827–834. https://doi:10.1086/233947

Driver, J. (2014). "The History of Utilitarianism." In E. N. Zalta (Ed.), *The Stanford Encyclopedia of Philosophy* (Winter 2014 ed.). Stanford, CA: Metaphysics Research Lab, Stanford University. https://plato.stanford.edu/archives/win2014/entries/utilitarianism-history/

Dubber, M. D. (1999). "Reforming American Penal Law." *Journal of Criminal Law and Criminology (1973-)*, 90(1), 49–108. https://doi:10.2307/1144163

Duff, A. (2001). *Punishment, Communication, and Community*. New York: Oxford University Press.

Duff, R. A. (2013). "Punishment and the Duties of Offenders." *Law and Philosophy*, 32(1), 109–127. https://doi:10.1007/s10982-012-9150-5

Duff, R. A. (2018). *The Realm of Criminal Law*. Oxford: Oxford University Press.

Dunbar, E. (2003). "Symbolic, Relational, and Ideological Signifiers of Bias-Motivated Offenders: Toward a Strategy of Assessment." *American Journal of Orthopsychiatry*, 73(2), 203–211. https://doi:10.1037/0002-9432.73.2.203

Dunbar, E. (2004). "Reconsidering the Clinical Utility of Bias as a Mental Health Problem: Intervention Strategies for Psychotherapy Practice." *Psychotherapy: Theory, Research, Practice, Training*, 41(2), 97–111. https://doi:10.1037/0033-3204.41.2.97

Duriez, S. A., Sullivan, C., Latessa, E. J., & Lovins, L. B. (2018). "The Evolution of Correctional Program Assessment in the Age of Evidence-Based Practices." *Corrections*, 3(2), 119–136. https://doi:10.1080/23774657.2017.1343104

Dworkin, R. (1966). "Lord Devlin and the Enforcement of Morals." *The Yale Law Journal*, 75(6), 986–1005. https://doi:10.2307/794893

Dworkin, R. (1986). *Law's Empire*. Cambridge, MA: Harvard University Press.

Dworkin, R. M. (Ed.) (1977). *The Philosophy of Law*. Oxford: Oxford University Press.

Dwyer, E. (2004). "The State and the Multiply Disadvantaged: The Case of Epilepsy." In S. Noll & J. W. Trent Jr. (Eds.), *Mental Retardation in America: A Historical Reader* (pp. 258–280). New York: New York University Press.

DYG, Inc. (1990). *Public Attitudes toward People with Chronic Mental Illness: Final Report*. Princeton, NJ: Robert Wood Johnson Foundation.

Dyrbye, L. N., Thomas, M. R., Harper, W., Massie Jr, F. S., Power, D. V., Eacker, A., Szydlo, D. W., Novotny P. J., Sloan J. A., & Shanafelt, T. D. (2009). "The Learning Environment and Medical Student Burnout: A Multicentre Study." *Medical Education*, 43(3), 274–282. https://doi:10.1111/j.1365-2923.2008.03282.x

Dyrbye, L. N., Thomas, M. R., Power, D. V., Durning, S., Moutier, C., Massie Jr., F. S., Harper, W., Eacker, A., Sydlow, D. W., Sloan, J. A., & Shanafelt, T. D. (2010). "Burnout and Serious Thoughts of Dropping Out of Medical School: A Multi-Institutional Study." *Academic Medicine*, 85(1), 94–102. https://doi:10.1097/acm.0b013e3181c46aad

Dyshniku, F., Murray, M. E., Fazio, R. L., Lykins, A. D., & Cantor, J. M. (2015). "Minor Physical Anomalies as a Window into the Prenatal Origins of Pedophilia." *Archives of Sexual Behavior*, 44(8), 2151–2159. https://doi:10.1007/s10508-015-0564-7

Eckleberry-Hunt, J., Lick, D., Boura, J., Hunt, R., Balasubramaniam, M., Mulhem, E., & Fisher, C. (2009). "An Exploratory Study of Resident Burnout and Wellness." *Academic Medicine*, 84(2), 269–277. https://doi:10.1097/ACM.0b013e3181938a45

Edwards, A. T. (1984). "Cultural Literacy: What Are Our Goals?" *The English Journal*, 73(4), 71–72. https://doi:10.2307/816593

Eigen, J. P. (1991a). "Delusion in the Courtroom: The Role of Partial Insanity in Early Forensic Testimony." *Medical History*, 35(1), 25–49. https://doi:10.1017/S0025727300053114

Eigen, J. P. (1991b). "Mad-Doctors in the Dock: Forensic Psychiatry's Early Claims to Expert Knowledge." *Transactions and Studies of the College of Physicians of Philadelphia*, 13(4), 445–462.

Eisenberg, J. M. (2001). "What Does Evidence Mean? Can the Law and Medicine Be Reconciled?" *Journal of Health Politics, Policy and Law*, 26(2), 369–381. https://doi:10.1215/03616878-26-2-369

Eisenberg, L. (1986). "Health Care: For Patients or for Profits?" *American Journal of Psychiatry*, 143(8), 1015–1019. https://doi:10.1176/ajp.143.8.1015

Eke, A. W., Seto, M. C., & Williams, J. (2011). "Examining the Criminal History and Future Offending of Child Pornography Offenders: An Extended Prospective Follow-up Study." *Law and Human Behavior*, 35(6), 466–478. https://doi:10.1007/s10979-010-9252-2

Elbogen, E. B., & Johnson, S. C. (2009). "The Intricate Link between Violence and Mental Disorder: Results from the National Epidemiologic Survey on Alcohol and Related Conditions." *Archives of General Psychiatry*, 66(2), 152–161. https://doi:10.1001/archgenpsychiatry.2008.537

Elliott, F. A. (1982). "Neurological Findings in Adult Minimal Brain Dysfunction and the Dyscontrol Syndrome." *Journal of Nervous and Mental Disease*, 170(11), 680–687. https://doi:10.1097/00005053-198211000-00007

Elliott, F. A. (1992). "Violence: The Neurologic Contribution: An Overview." *Archives of Neurology*, *49*(6), 595–603. https://doi:10.1001/archneur.1992.00530300027006

Elstein, A. S., & Schwarz, A. (2002). "Clinical Problem Solving and Diagnostic Decision Making: Selective Review of the Cognitive Literature." *British Medical Journal, 324*(7339), 729–732. https://doi:10.1136/bmj.324.7339.729

Elwyn, G., Frosch, D., Thomson, R., Joseph-Williams, N., Lloyd, A., Kinnersley, P., . . . Barry, M. (2012). "Shared Decision Making: A Model for Clinical Practice." *Journal of General Internal Medicine*, *27*(10), 1361–1367. https://doi:10.1007/s11606-012-2077-6

Emanuel, E. J., Grady, C., Crouch, R. A., Lie, R. K., Miller, F. G., & Wendler, D. D. (Eds.) (2008). "A Selected History of Research with Humans," in the *Oxford Textbook of Clinical Research Ethics* (pp. 9–121). New York: Oxford University Press.

Engel, G. L. (1977). "The Need for a New Medical Model: A Challenge for Biomedicine." *Science*, *196*(4286), 129–136. https://doi:10.1126/science.847460

Engel, G. L. (1980). "The Clinical Application of the Biopsychosocial Model." *American Journal of Psychiatry, 137*(5), 535–544. https://doi:10.1176/ajp.137.5.535

Engel, G. L. (1997). "From Biomedical to Biopsychosocial: Being Scientific in the Human Domain." *Psychosomatics, 38*(6), 521–528. https://doi:10.1016/S0033-3182(97)71396-3

Engel, R. S., & Silver, E. (2001). "Policing Mentally Disordered Suspects: A Re-Examination of the Criminalization Hypothesis." *Criminology, 39*(2), 225–252. https://doi:10.1111/j.1745-9125.2001.tb00922.x

Engelhardt Jr., H. T., & Jotterand, F. (Eds.) (2008). *The Philosophy of Medicine Reborn: A Pellegrino Reader.* Notre Dame, IN: University of Notre Dame Press.

Erasmus, D. (1958). *In Praise of Folly.* Translated by J. Wilson. Ann Arbor: University of Michigan Press. https://www.ccel.org/ccel/erasmus/folly.txt

Erickson, P., & Erickson, S. (2008). *Crime, Punishment, and Mental Illness: Law and the Behavioral Sciences in Conflict.* New Brunswick, NJ: Rutgers University Press.

Esquirol, J.-É. D. (1845). *Mental Maladies: A Treatise on Insanity, First ed. in English.* Translated from French by E. K. Hunt. Philadelphia: Lea and Blanchard. https://wellcomecollection.org/works/krsk78ew

Etzioni, A. (2018). *Happiness Is the Wrong Metric: A Liberal Communitarian Response to Populism.* (Library of Public Policy and Public Administration series, Vol. 11). Cham, Switzerland: Springer.

Ewing, C. P. (1983). "'Dr. Death' and the Case for an Ethical Ban on Psychiatric and Psychological Predictions of Dangerousness in Capital Sentencing Proceedings." *American Journal of Law & Medicine, 8*(4), 407–428. https://doi:10.1017/S0098858800013368

Fairweather, A., & Zagzebski, L. (Eds.) (2001). *Virtue Epistemology: Essays in Epistemic Virtue and Responsibility.* New York: Oxford University Press.

Fan, R. (2002). "Reconstructionist Confucianism and Bioethics: A Note on Moral Difference." In H. T. Engelhardt & L. M. Rasmussen (Eds.), *Bioethics and Moral Content: National Traditions of Health Care Morality* (pp. 281–287). Dordrecht: Kluwer Academic Publishers.

Farberman, R. K. (1997). "Public Attitudes about Psychologists and Mental Health Care: Research to Guide the American Psychological Association Public Education Campaign." *Professional Psychology: Research and Practice, 28*(2), 128–136. https://doi:10.1037/0735-7028.28.2.128

Farringer, A. J., Duriez, S. A., Manchak, S. M., & Sullivan, C. C. (2021). "Adherence to 'What Works': Examining Trends across 14 Years of Correctional Program Assessment." *Corrections, 6*(4), 269–287. https://doi:10.1080/23774657.2019.1659193

Fazel, S., & Baillargeon, J. (2011). "The Health of Prisoners." *The Lancet, 377*(9769), 956–965. https://doi:10.1016/S0140-6736(10)61053-7

Fazel, S., & Grann, M. (2006). "The Population Impact of Severe Mental Illness on Violent Crime." *American Journal of Psychiatry, 163*(8), 1397–1403. https://doi:10.1176/ajp.2006.163.8.1397

Fazel, S., Gulati, G., Linsell, L., Geddes, J. R., & Grann, M. (2009). "Schizophrenia and Violence: Systematic Review and Meta-Analysis." *PLoS Medicine, 6*(8), e1000120. https://doi.org/10.1371/journal.pmed.1000120

Fazel, S., Lichtenstein, P., Grann, M., Goodwin, G. M., & Långström, N. (2010). "Bipolar Disorder and Violent Crime: New Evidence from Population-Based Longitudinal Studies and Systematic Review." *Archives of General Psychiatry, 67*(9), 931–938. https://doi:10.1001/archgenpsychiatry.2010.97

Feldman, M. D., & Eisendrath, S. J. (1996). *The spectrum of factitious disorders (Vol. 40)*. Washington, DC: American Psychiatric Publishing.

Ferguson, S. D., & Coccaro, E. F. (2009). "History of Mild to Moderate Traumatic Brain Injury and Aggression in Physically Healthy Participants with and without Personality Disorder." *Journal of Personality Disorders, 23*(3), 230–239. https://doi:10.1521/pedi.2009.23.3.230

Ferri, E. (1917). *Criminal Sociology*. Edited and translated by J. I. Kelly & J. Lisle. Edited by W. W. Smithers. Boston: Little, Brown, and Company.

FindLaw, legal writers and editors. (2019). "The Insanity Defense among the States." https://www.find law.com/criminal criminal-procedure/the-insanity-defense-among-the-states.html

Fine, C., & Kennett, J. (2004). "Mental Impairment, Moral Understanding and Criminal Responsibility: Psychopathy and the Purposes of Punishment." *International Journal of Law and Psychiatry, 27*(5), 425–443. https://doi:10.1016/j.ijlp.2004.06.005

Fingarette, H. (1976). "Disabilities of Mind and Criminal Responsibility—A Unitary Doctrine." *Columbia Law Review, 76*(2), 236–266. https://doi:10.2307/1121637

First, M. B. (2010). "DSM-5 Proposals for Paraphilias: Suggestions for Reducing False Positives Related to Use of Behavioral Manifestations." *Archives of Sexual Behavior, 39*(6), 1239–1244. https://doi:10.1007/s10508-010-9657-5

First, M. B., & Pincus, H. A. (2002). "The DSM-IV Text Revision: Rationale and Potential Impact on Clinical Practice." *Psychiatric Services, 53*(3), 288–292. https://doi:10.1176/appi.ps.53.3.288

First, M. B., Pincus, H. A., Levine, J. B., Williams, J. B. W., Ustun, B., & Peele, R. (2004). "Clinical Utility as a Criterion for Revising Psychiatric Diagnoses." *American Journal of Psychiatry, 161*(6), 946–954. https://doi:10.1176/appi.ajp.161.6.946

First, M. B., & Wakefield, J. C. (2013). "Diagnostic Criteria as Dysfunction Indicators: Bridging the Chasm between the Definition of Mental Disorder and Diagnostic Criteria for Specific Disorders." *The Canadian Journal of Psychiatry, 58*(12), 663–669. https://doi:10.1177/070674371305801203

Fisher, T. (2014). "Economic Analysis of Criminal Law." In M. D. Dubber & T. Hörnle (Eds.), *The Oxford Handbook of Criminal Law* (pp. 38–58). Oxford: Oxford University Press.

Fitzgerald, J. C., Cohen, A. K., Maker Castro, E., & Pope, A. (2021). "A Systematic Review of the Last Decade of Civic Education Research in the United States." *Peabody Journal of Education, 96*(3), 235–246. https://doi:10.1080/0161956X.2021.1942703

Flannery, D. J., Modzeleski, W., & Kretschmar, J. (2013). "Violence and School Shootings." *Current Psychiatry Reports, 15*(1), Article number: 331. http://dx.doi.org/10.1007/s11920-012-0331-6

Flor-Henry, P., Lang, R. A., Koles, Z. J., & Frenzel, R. R. (1991). "Quantitative EEG Studies of Pedophilia." *International Journal of Psychophysiology, 10*(3), 253–258. https://doi:10.1016/0167-8760(91)90036-W

Flynn, S., Ibrahim, S., Kapur, N., Appleby, L., & Shaw, J. (2021). "Mental Disorder in People Convicted of Homicide: Long-Term National Trends in Rates and Court Outcome." *British Journal of Psychiatry, 218*(4), 210–216. https://doi:10.1192/bjp.2020.94

Follette, W. C., & Houts, A. C. (1996). "Models of Scientific Progress and the Role of Theory in Taxonomy Development: A Case Study of the DSM." *Journal of Consulting and Clinical Psychology, 64*(6), 1120–1132. https://doi:10.1037/0022-006X.64.6.1120

Ford, M. R., & Widiger, T. A. (1989). "Sex Bias in the Diagnosis of Histrionic and Antisocial Personality Disorders." *Journal of Consulting and Clinical Psychology, 57*(2), 301–305. https://doi:10.1037/0022-006X.57.2.301

Forsberg, L., & Douglas, T. (2020). "What Is Criminal Rehabilitation?" *Criminal Law and Philosophy, 16*(1), 103–126. https://doi:10.1007/s11572-020-09547-4

Fortune, C.-A. (2018). "The Good Lives Model: A Strength-Based Approach for Youth Offenders." *Aggression and Violent Behavior, 38*, 21–30. https://doi:10.1016/j.avb.2017.11.003

Foucault, M. (1965). *Madness and Civilization: A History of Insanity in the Age of Reason*. Translated by R. Howard. New York: Pantheon Books.

Foucault, M. (1977). *Discipline and Punish: The Birth of the Prison*. Translated by A. Sheridan. New York: Vintage-Random House.

Foucault, M. (1978). *The History of Sexuality, Volume 1: An Introduction* (First American ed.). Translated by R. Hurley. New York: Pantheon Books.

Foucault, M. (1980). *Power/Knowledge: Selected Interviews and Other Writings, 1972-1977*(First American ed.). Edited by C. Gordon. New York: Pantheon Books.

Foucault, M. (1999). *Abnormal: Lectures at the Collège de France, 1974-1975 (Vol. 1)*. Edited by G. Burchell. Translated and edited by V. Marchetti, A. Salomoni, & A. I. Davidson. New York: Picador.

Foucault, M. (2003). *Abnormal: Lectures at the Collège de France, 1974-1975 (Vol. 2)*. New York: Macmillon.

Foucault, M. (2008). *Psychiatric Power: Lectures at the Collège de France, 1973-1974*. New York: Palgrave Macmillan.

Frances, A. (2010). "The First Draft of DSM-V." *British Medical Journal, 340*, c1168. http://dx.doi.org/10.1136 bmj.c1168

Frances, A. (2013). *Saving Normal: An Insider's Revolt against Out-of-Control Psychiatric Diagnosis, DSM-5, Big Pharma and the Medicalization of Ordinary Life*. New York: William Morrow & Co.

Frances, A., First, M. B., & Pincus, H. A. (1995). *DSM-IV Guidebook*. Washington, DC: American Psychiatric Association.

Frances, A., Sreenivasan, S., & Weinberger, L. E. (2008). "Defining Mental Disorder When It Really Counts: DSM-IV-TR and SVP/SDP Statutes." *Journal of the American Academy of Psychiatry and the Law, 36*(3), 375–384. http://jaapl.org/content/36/3/375.long

Frances, A. J. (1994). "Foreword." In J. Z. Sadler, O. P. Wiggins, & M. A. Schwartz (Eds.), *Philosophical Perspectives on Psychiatric Diagnostic Classification* (Johns Hopkins Series in Psychiatry and Neuroscience) (pp. vii–ix). Baltimore: Johns Hopkins University Press.

Frances, A. J., Widiger, T. A., & Pincus, H. A. (1989). "The Development of DSM-IV." *Archives of General Psychiatry, 46*(4), 373–375. https://doi:10.1001/archpsyc.1989.01810040079012

Francis, A., Widiger, T. A., First, M. B., Pincus, H. A., Tilly, S. M., Miele, G. M., & Davis, W. W. (1991). "DSM-IV: Toward a More Empirical Diagnostic System." *Canadian Psychology / Psychologie canadienne, 32*(2), 171–173. https://doi:10.1037/h0078973

Frankena, W. K. (1973). "The Ethics of Love Conceived as an Ethics of Virtue." *The Journal of Religious Ethics, 1*, 21–36. http://www.jstor.org/stable/40016695

Frede, M. (2011). *A Free Will: Origins of the Notion in Ancient Thought*. Edited by A. A. Long. Berkeley/Los Angeles: University of California Press.

Frick, P. J., & Moffitt, T. E. (2010). *A Proposal to the DSM-V Childhood Disorders and the ADHD and Disruptive Behavior Disorders Work Groups to Include a Specifier to the Diagnosis of Conduct Disorder Based on the Presence of Callous–Unemotional Traits* (pp. 1–36). Washington, DC: American Psychiatric Association.

Friedli, L., & the World Health Organization (2009). *Mental Health, Resilience and Inequalities (No. EU/08/5087203)*. Copenhagen: WHO Regional Office for Europe. https://apps.who.int/iris/handle/10665/107925

Friedman, L. M. (2005). *A History of American Law*. New York: Simon and Schuster.

Friedman, R. A. (2006). "Violence and Mental Illness—How Strong Is the Link?" *New England Journal of Medicine, 355*(20), 2064–2066. https://doi:10.1056/NEJMp068229

Friston, K., Da Costa, L., Sajid, N., Heins, C., Ueltzhöffer, K., Pavliotis, G. A., & Parr, T. (2022). "The Free Energy Principle Made Simpler but Not Too Simple." https://arxiv.org/abs/2201.06387

Friston, K., Kilner, J., & Harrison, L. (2006). "A Free Energy Principle for the Brain." *Journal of Physiology-Paris, 100*(1), 70–87. https://doi:10.1016/j.jphysparis.2006.10.001

Fritzon, K., Miller, S., Bargh, D., Hollows, K., Osborne, A., & Howlett, A. (2021). "Understanding the Relationships between Trauma and Criminogenic Risk Using the Risk-Need-Responsivity Model." *Journal of Aggression, Maltreatment & Trauma, 30*(3), 294–323. https://doi:10.1080/10926771.2020.1806972

Fulford, K. W. M., Davies, M., Gipps, R. G. T., Graham, G., Sadler, J. Z., Stanghellini, G., & Thornton, T. (Eds.) (2013). *The Oxford Handbook of Philosophy and Psychiatry*. Oxford: Oxford University Press.

Fulford, K. W. M. (1989). *Moral Theory and Medical Practice*. Cambridge/New York: Cambridge University Press.

Fulford, K. W. M. (1994). "Ten Principles of Values-Based Medicine (VBM)." In T. Schramme & J. Thome (Eds.), *Philosophy and Psychiatry* (pp. 50–81). Berlin/New York: Walter de Gruyter.

Fulford, K. W. M. (2002). "Report to the Chair of the DSM-VI Task Force from the Editors of Philosophy, Psychiatry, and Psychology, 'Contentious and Noncontentious Evaluative Language in Psychiatric Diagnosis.'" In J. Z. Sadler (Ed.), *Descriptions and Prescriptions: Values, Mental Disorders, and the DSMs* (pp. 323–362). Baltimore: Johns Hopkins University Press.

Fulford, K. W. M. (2005). "Values in Psychiatric Diagnosis: Developments in Policy, Training and Research." *Psychopathology*, *38*(4), 171–176. https://doi:10.1159/000086085

Fulford, K. W. M., Morris, K. J., Sadler, J. Z., & Stanghellini, G. (2003). "Past improbable, future possible: The renaissance in philosophy and psychiatry." In K. W. M. Fulford, K. J. Morris, J. Z. Sadler, & G. Stanghellini (Eds.), *Nature and Narrative: An introduction to the new philosophy of psychiatry* (pp. 1–41). Oxford: Oxford University Press.

Fuller, A. K., Fuller, A. E., & Blashfield, R. K. (1990). "Paraphilic Coercive Disorder." *Journal of Sex Education & Therapy*, *16*(3), 164–171. https://doi:10.1080/01614576.1990.11074988

Gabbard, G. O., & Gabbard, K. (1992). "Cinematic Stereotypes Contributing to the Stigmatization of Psychiatrists." In P. J. Fink & A. Tasman (Eds.), *Stigma and Mental Illness* (pp. 113–126). Washington, DC: American Psychiatric Press.

Gabbe, S., Webb, L. E., Moore, D. E., Harrell Jr, F. E., Spickard Jr, W. A., & Powell Jr, R. (2008). "Burnout in Medical School Deans: An Uncommon Problem." *Academic Medicine*, *83*(5), 476–482. https://doi:10.1097/ACM.0b013e31816bdb96

Gagné-Julien, A.-M. (2021). "Dysfunction and the Definition of Mental Disorder in the DSM." *Philosophy, Psychiatry, & Psychology*, *28*(4), 353–370. https://doi:10.1353/ppp.2021.0055

Galli, V., McElroy, S. L., Soutullo, C. A., Kizer, D., Raute, N., Keck Jr., P. E., & McConville, B. J. (1999). "The Psychiatric Diagnoses of Twenty-Two Adolescents Who Have Sexually Molested Other Children." *Comprehensive Psychiatry*, *40*(2), 85–88. https://doi:10.1016/S0010-440X(99)90110-4

Gamwell, L., & Tomes, N. (1995). *Madness in America: Cultural and Medical Perceptions of Mental Illness before 1914*. Ithaca and London: Cornell University Press.

Gannon, T. A., Olver, M. E., Mallion, J. S., & James, M. (2019). "Does Specialized Psychological Treatment for Offending Reduce Recidivism? A Meta-Analysis Examining Staff and Program Variables as Predictors of Treatment Effectiveness." *Clinical Psychology Review*, *73*, 101752. https://doi.org/10.1016/j.cpr.2019.101752

Gariepy, T. P. (1994). "The Introduction and Acceptance of Listerian Antisepsis in the United States." *Journal of the History of Medicine and Allied Sciences*, *49*(2), 167–206. https://doi:10.1093/jhmas/49.2.167

Garland, D. (1993). *Punishment and Modern society: A study in social theory*. Chicago: University of Chicago Press.

Garland, D. (2002). *The Culture of Control: Crime and Social Order in Contemporary Society*. New York: Oxford University Press.

Garner, B. A. (Ed.) (2004). *Black's Law Dictionary, Eighth ed.* St. Paul, MN: Thomson/West.

Garton, S. (2004). *Histories of Sexuality: Antiquity to Sexual Revolution*. New York: Routledge.

Gazmararian, J. A., Baker, D. W., Williams, M. V., Parker, R. M., Scott, T. L., Green, D. C., . . . Koplan, J. P. (1999). "Health Literacy among Medicare Enrollees in a Managed Care Organization." *JAMA*, *281*(6), 545–551. https://doi:10.1001/jama.281.6.545

Geis, G., & Meier, R. F. (1985). "Abolition of the Insanity Plea in Idaho: A Case Study." *Annals of the American Academy of Political and Social Science*, *477*(1), 72–83. https://doi:10.1177/0002716285477001007

Geller, J. L. (1992a). "Arson in Review: From Profit to Pathology." *Psychiatric Clinics of North America*, *15*(3), 623–645. https://doi:10.1016/S0193-953X(18)30228-4

Geller, J. L. (1992b). "Communicative Arson." *Psychiatric Services*, *43*(1), 76–77. https://doi:10.1176/ps.43.1.76

Geller, J. L. (1992c). "Pathological Firesetting in Adults." *International Journal of Law and Psychiatry*, *15*(3), 283–302. https://doi:10.1016/0160-2527(92)90004-K

Geller, J. L., & Bertsch, G. (1985). "Fire-Setting Behavior in the Histories of a State Hospital Population." *American Journal of Psychiatry*, *142*(4), 464–468. https://doi:10.1176/ajp.142.4.464

Geller, J. L., Erlen, J., & Pinkus, R. L. (1986). "A Historical Appraisal of America's Experience with 'Pyromania'—a Diagnosis in Search of a Disorder." *International Journal of Law and Psychiatry*, 9(2), 201–229. https://doi:10.1016/0160-2527(86)90047-6

Gendreau, P., & Andrews, D. A. (1996). *Correctional Program Assessment Inventory (CPAI)* (Sixth ed.) Saint John, New Brunswick, Canada: University of New Brunswick/Carleton University.

Gendreau, P., Little, T., & Goggin, C. (1996). "A Meta-Analysis of Predictors of Adult Offender Recidivism: What Works!" *Criminology*, 34(4), 575–608. https://doi:10.1111/j.1745-9125.1996.tb01220.x

Gert, B. (2004). *Common Morality: Deciding What to Do*. Oxford/New York: Oxford University Press.

Gert, B. (2005). "Thomas Hobbes." In T. Honderich (Ed.), *The Oxford Companion to Philosophy, New ed.* (pp. 392–396). Oxford: Oxford University Press.

Ghaemi, S. N. (2003). *The Concepts of Psychiatry: A Pluralistic Approach to the Mind and Mental Illness*. Baltimore: Johns Hopkins University Press.

Ghaemi, S. N. (2010). *The Rise and Fall of the Biopsychosocial Model: Reconciling Art and Science in Psychiatry*. Baltimore: Johns Hopkins University Press.

Giannelli, P. C. (1993). "'Junk Science': The Criminal Cases." *Journal of Criminal Law and Criminology*, 84(1), 105–128. https://doi:10.2307/1143887

Gilbert, G. H. (1901). "Demonology in the New Testament." *The Biblical World (1893-1920)*, 18(5), 352–360. https://www.jstor.org/stable/3136751

Gilman, S. L. (1998). "Sibling Incest, Madness, and the 'Jews.'" *Jewish Social Studies*, 4(2), 157–179. http: www.jstor.org/stable/4467524

Gingrich, N., & Nolan, P. (2011). "Prison Reform: A Smart Way for States to Save Money and Lives, Opinion." *Washington Post*, 7 January 2011. http://www.washingtonpost.com/wp-dyn/content/article 2011/01/06/AR2011010604386.html

Gkotsis, G., Oellrich, A., Hubbard, T., Dobson, R., Liakata, M., Velupillai, S., & Dutta, R. (2016). *The Language of Mental Health Problems in Social Media*. Paper presented at the Proceedings of the Third Workshop on Computational Linguistics and Clinical Psychology: From Linguistic Signal to Clinical Reality, pp. 63–73, 16 June 2016, San Diego, CA.

Glannon, W. (Ed.) (2015). *Free Will and the Brain: Neuroscientific, Philosophical, and Legal Perspectives*. Cambridge: Cambridge University Press.

Glenn, A. L., & Raine, A. (2014). "Neurocriminology: Implications for the Punishment, Prediction and Prevention of Criminal Behaviour." *Nature Reviews Neuroscience*, 15(1), 54–63. https://doi:10.1038/nrn3640

Glueck, B. (1916). *Studies in Forensic Psychiatry*. Boston: Little, Brown, and Company. https://jscholarship.library.jhu.edu/bitstream/handle 1774.2/33482/31151024684825.pdf

Goffman, E. (1961). *Asylums: Essays on the Social Situation of Mental Patients and Other Inmates*. Norwell, MA: Doubleday (Anchor).

Gold, A. (2012). "On the Roots of Modern Forensic Psychiatry: Ethics Ramifications." *Journal of the American Academy of Psychiatry and the Law*, 40(2), 246–252. http://jaapl.org/content/40/2/246

Gold, A. K., & Kinrys, G. (2019). "Treating Circadian Rhythm Disruption in Bipolar Disorder." *Current Psychiatry Reports*, 21(3), Article 14. https://doi.org/10.1007/s11920-019-1001-8

Goldman, H. H., & Morrissey, J. P. (1985). "The Alchemy of Mental Health Policy: Homelessness and the Fourth Cycle of Reform." *American Journal of Public Health*, 75(7), 727–731. https://doi:10.2105/ajph.75.7.727

Goldstein, J. (1998). "Professional Knowledge and Professional Self-Interest: The Rise and Fall of Monomania in the 19th-Century France." *International Journal of Law and Psychiatry*, 21(4), 385–396. https://doi:10.1016/S0160-2527(98)00029-6

Goldstein, J. E. (1987). *Console and Classify: The French Psychiatric Profession in the Nineteenth Century*. Cambridge: Cambridge University Press.

Goldstein, J. E. (2001). *Console and Classify: The French Psychiatric Profession in the Nineteenth Century*. Chicago: University of Chicago Press.

Goldstein, J. L., & Godemont, M. M. L. (2003). "The Legend and Lessons of Geel, Belgium: A 1500-Year-Old Legend, a 21st-Century Model." *Community Mental Health Journal*, 39(5), 441–458. https://doi:10.1023/A:1025813003347

Gonaver, W. (2018). *The Peculiar Institution and the Making of Modern Psychiatry, 1840–1880*. Chapel Hill: University of North Carolina Press.

González, J. L. (2010a). *The Story of Christianity, Volume 1: The Early Church to the Dawn of the Reformation*. New York: Harper Collins.

González, J. L. (2010b). *The Story of Christianity, Volume 2: The Reformation to the Present Day*. New York: Harper Collins.

Goodman, J., McElligott, A., & Marks, L. (Eds.) (2003). *Useful Bodies: Humans in the Service of Medical Science in the Twentieth Century*. Baltimore: Johns Hopkins University Press.

Goodey, C. F. (2005). Blockheads, roundheads, pointy heads: Intellectual disability and the brain before modern medicine. *Journal of the History of the Behavioral Sciences, 41*(2), 165–183.

Gordon, N. (1999). "Episodic Dyscontrol Syndrome." *Developmental Medicine & Child Neurology, 41*(11), 786–788. https://doi:10.1017/S0012162299001565

Gorenstein, E. E. (1992). *The Science of Mental Illness*. London: Academic Press.

Goudriaan, A. E., Oosterlaan, J., de Beurs, E., & Van den Brink, W. (2004). "Pathological Gambling: A Comprehensive Review of Biobehavioral Findings." *Neuroscience & Biobehavioral Reviews, 28*(2), 123–141. https://doi:10.1016/j.neubiorev.2004.03.001

Graeber, D., & Wengrow, D. (2021). *The dawn of everything: A new history of humanity*. London: Penguin UK.

Granzig, W. A. (2006). "The Legacy of Alfred C. Kinsey." *Sexuality & Culture, 10*(1), 99–102. https://doi:10.1007/s12119-006-1009-1

Gray, N. S., MacCulloch, M. J., Smith, J., Morris, M., & Snowden, R. J. (2003). "Violence Viewed by Psychopathic Murderers." *Nature, 423*(6939), 497–498. https://doi:10.1038/423497a

Grebchenko, Y., Steinfeld, M., Kaleem, M., Cullen, K., Kunik, L. I., Galynker, I., & Cohen, L. J. (2005). "Personality Profile across Addictive Behavior." *Bridging East West Psychiatry, 3*(1), 11–16.

Greco, J. (1993). "Virtues and Vices of Virtue Epistemology." *Canadian Journal of Philosophy, 23*(3), 413–432. https://www.jstor.org/stable/40231831

Green, R. (2002). "Is Pedophilia a Mental Disorder?" *Archives of Sexual Behavior, 31*(6), 467–471. https://doi:10.1023/a:1020699013309

Greenberg, D. M., Bradford, J. M. W., & Curry, S. (1996). "Are Pedophiles with Aggressive Tendencies More Sexually Violent?" *Journal of the American Academy of Psychiatry and the Law, 24*(2), 225–235. http: jaapl.org/content/24/2/225

Greenberg, S. A., & Shuman, D. W. (1997). "Irreconcilable Conflict between Therapeutic and Forensic Roles." *Professional Psychology: Research and Practice, 28*(1), 50–57. https://doi:10.1037/0735-7028.28.1.50

Greene, J. A. (2007). *Prescribing by Numbers: Drugs and the Definition of Disease*. Baltimore: Johns Hopkins University Press.

Greer, C., & Jewkes, Y. (2005). "Extremes of Otherness: Media Images of Social Exclusion." *Social Justice, 32*(1), 20–31. http://www.jstor.org/stable/29768287

Grinnell, F. (2011). *Everyday Practice of Science: Where Intuition and Passion Meet Objectivity and Logic*. New York: Oxford University Press.

Grisso, T. (1996). "Society's Retributive Response to Juvenile Violence: A Developmental Perspective." *Law and Human Behavior, 20*(3), 229–247. https://doi:10.2307/1393974

Grob, G. N. (1977). "Rediscovering Asylums: The Unhistorical History of the Mental Hospital." *The Hastings Center Report, 7*(4), 33–41. https://doi:10.2307/3560476

Grob, G. N. (1983). *Mental Illness and American Society, 1875-1940*. Princeton, NJ: Princeton University Press.

Grob, G. N. (1991). *From Asylum to Community: Mental Health Policy in Modern America*. Princeton, NJ: Princeton University Press.

Grob, G. N. (1991). "Origins of *DSM-I*: A Study in Appearance and Reality." *American Journal of Psychiatry, 148*(4), 421–431. https://doi:10.1176/ajp.148.4.421

Grob, G. N. (1994). *The Mad among Us: A History of the Care of America's Mentally Ill*. New York: The Free Press.

Grob, G. N. (2008a). "Mental Health Policy in the Liberal State: The Example of the United States." *International Journal of Law and Psychiatry, 31*(2), 89–100. https://doi:10.1016/j.ijlp.2008.02.003

Grob, G. N. (2008b). "The Transformation of American Psychiatry: From Institution to Community, 1800-2000." In E. R. Wallace & J. Gach (Eds.), *History of Psychiatry and Medical Psychology: With an Epilogue on Psychiatry and the Mind-Body Relation* (pp. 533–554). Boston: Springer.

Gross, H. (1985). "Justice and the Insanity Defense." *Annals of the American Academy of Political and Social Science, 477*(1), 96–103. https://doi:10.1177/0002716285477001009

Grossberg, M. (2002). "Changing Conceptions of Child Welfare in the United States, 1820–1935." In M. K. Rosenheim, F. E. Zimring, D. S. Tanenhaus, & B. Dohrn (Eds.), *A Century of Juvenile Justice* (pp. 3–41). Chicago: University of Chicago Press.

Grounds, A. (2001). "Reforming the Mental Health Act." *British Journal of Psychiatry, 179*(5), 387–389. https://doi:10.1192 bjp.179.5.387

Grzywacz, J. G., & Keyes, C. L. M. (2004). "Toward Health Promotion: Physical and Social Behaviors in Complete Health." *American Journal of Health Behavior, 28*(2), 99–111. https://doi:10.5993/AJHB.28.2.1

Guindon, M. H., Green, A. G., & Hanna, F. J. (2003). "Intolerance and Psychopathology: Toward a General Diagnosis for Racism, Sexism, and Homophobia." *American Journal of Orthopsychiatry, 73*(2), 167–176. https://doi:10.1037/0002-9432.73.2.167

Gulliver, A., Griffiths, K. M., & Christensen, H. (2010). "Perceived Barriers and Facilitators to Mental Health Help-Seeking in Young People: A Systematic Review." *BMC Psychiatry, 10*, Article 113. https://doi.org/10.1186/1471-244X-10-113

Gupta, M. (2007). "Does Evidence-Based Medicine Apply to Psychiatry?" *Theoretical Medicine and Bioethics, 28*(2), 103–120. https://doi:10.1007/s11017-007-9029-x

Gupta, M. (2009). "Ethics and Evidence in Psychiatric Practice." *Perspectives in Biology and Medicine, 52*(2), 276–288. https://doi:10.1353/pbm.0.0081

Gupta, M. (2011). "Improved Health or Improved Decision Making? The Ethical Goals of EBM." *Journal of Evaluation in Clinical Practice, 17*(5), 957–963. https://doi:10.1111/j.1365-2753.2011.01743.x

Gupta, M. (2014). *Is Evidence-Based Psychiatry Ethical?* Oxford: Oxford University Press.

Gutheil, T. G., & Appelbaum, P. S. (2000). *Clinical Handbook of Psychiatry and the Law* (Third ed.). Philadelphia: Lippincott Williams & Wilkins.

Gutheil, T. G., Hauser, M., White, M. S., Spruiell, G., & Strasburger, L. H. (2003). "'The Whole Truth' Versus 'the Admissible Truth': An Ethics Dilemma for Expert Witnesses." *Journal of the American Academy of Psychiatry and the Law, 31*(4), 422–427. http://jaapl.org/content/31/4/422

Gutting, G. (1994). "Introduction: Michel Foucault: A User's Manual." In G. Gutting (Ed.), *The Cambridge Companion to Foucault* (pp. 1–27). Cambridge: Cambridge University Press.

Gutting, G. (2001). *French Philosophy in the Twentieth Century.* Cambridge: Cambridge University Press.

Hacsi, T. (1995). "From Indenture to Family Foster Care: A Brief History of Child Placing." *Child Welfare, 74*(1), 162–180.

Hage, P. (1981). "On Male Initiation and Dual Organisation in New Guinea." *Man, 16*(2), 268–275. https://doi:10.2307/2801399

Haji, I. (2010). "Psychopathy, Ethical Perception, and Moral Culpability." *Neuroethics, 3*(2), 135–150. https://doi:10.1007/s12152-009-9049-5

Haldipur, C. V., Knoll IV, J. L., & v.d. Luft, E. (Eds.) (2019). *Thomas Szasz: An Appraisal of His Legacy.* Oxford: Oxford University Press.

Hale, M., Emly, S., & Wilson, G. (1736). *The History of the Pleas of the Crown.* London: Professional Books.

Hale, Sir Matthew, & Emlyn, S. (1736). *Historia Placitorum Coronæ: The History of the Pleas of the Crown, Volume I.* London: E. and R. Nutt, and R. Gosling. https://archive.org/details/historiaplacito r01hale/page/n3/mode/2up

Hall, T. (1970). *Carl Friedrich Gauss: A Biography.* Translated by A. J. Froderberg. Cambridge, MA: MIT Press.

Haller Jr, J. S. (1972). "The Negro and the Southern Physician: A Study of Medical and Racial Attitudes 1800-1860." *Medical History, 16*(3), 238–253. https://doi:10.1017/s0025727300017737

Hallinan, M. T. (2010). "[Review] The Making of Democracy and Our Schools (Hirsch Jr, E.D.)." *Contemporary Sociology: A Journal of Reviews, 39*(4), 454–456. http://www.jstor.org/stable/27857189

Halpern, A. L., Freedman, A. M., & Schoenholtz, J. C. (1998). "Ethics in Forensic Psychiatry." *American Journal of Psychiatry, 155*(4), 575a–576. https://doi:10.1176/ajp.155.4.575a

Hamilton, J. R. (1986). "Insanity Legislation." *Journal of Medical Ethics*, *12*(1), 13–17. https://doi:10.1136/jme.12.1.13

Hampsher-Monk, I. W. (1992). *A History of Modern Political Thought: Major Political Thinkers from Hobbes to Marx*. Oxford: Blackwell.

Hampton, J. (1984). "The Moral Education Theory of Punishment." *Philosophy & Public Affairs*, *13*(3), 208–238. http://www.jstor.org/stable/2265412

Haney, C. (1980). "Psychology and Legal Change: On the Limits of a Factual Jurisprudence." *Law and Human Behavior*, *4*(3), 147–199. https://doi:10.2307/1393639

Hanna, N. (2019). "Hitting Retributivism Where It Hurts." *Criminal Law and Philosophy*, *13*(1), 109–127. https://doi:10.1007 s11572-018-9461-1

Hans, V. P. (1986). "An Analysis of Public Attitudes toward the Insanity Defense." *Criminology*, *24*(2), 393–414. https://doi:10.1111/j.1745-9125.1986.tb01502.x

Hans, V. P., & Slater, D. (1983). "John Hinkley, Jr. and the Insanity Defense: The Public's Verdict." *Public Opinion Quarterly*, *47*(2), 202–212. https://doi:10.1086/268780

Hanson, M. J., & Callahan, D. (Eds.) (2000). *The Goals of Medicine: The Forgotten Issue in Health Care Reform* (Hastings Center Studies in Ethics series). Washington, DC: Georgetown University Press.

Haoka, T., Sasahara, S., Tomotsune, Y., Yoshino, S., Maeno, T., & Matsuzaki, I. (2010). "The Effect of Stress-Related Factors on Mental Health Status among Resident Doctors in Japan." *Medical Education*, *44*(8), 826–834. https://doi:10.1111/j.1365-2923.2010.03725.x

Haque, A. A. (2013). "Retributivism: The Right and the Good." *Law and Philosophy*, *32*(1), 59–82. https://doi:10.1007/s10982-012-9155-0

Hare, R. D., Neumann, C. S., & Widiger, T. A. (2012). "Psychopathy." In T. A. Widiger (Ed.), *The Oxford Handbook of Personality Disorders* (pp. 478–504). New York: Oxford University Press.

Harkins, L., Flak, V. E., Beech, A. R., & Woodhams, J. (2012). "Evaluation of a Community-Based Sex Offender Treatment Program Using a Good Lives Model Approach." *Sexual Abuse*, *24*(6), 519–543. https://doi:10.1177/1079063211429469

Harrelson, W. (1951). "The Idea of Agape in the New Testament." *Journal of Religion*, *31*(3), 169–182. http://www.jstor.org/stable/1197811. Accessed 01/05/2022).

Harris, A., & Lurigio, A. J. (2007). "Mental Illness and Violence: A Brief Review of Research and Assessment Strategies." *Aggression and Violent Behavior*, *12*(5), 542–551. https://doi:10.1016/j.avb.2007.02.008

Harris, A. J., & Socia, K. M. (2016). "What's in a Name? Evaluating the Effects of the 'Sex Offender' Label on Public Opinions and Beliefs." *Sexual Abuse*, *28*(7), 660–678. https://doi:10.1177/107906321 4564391

Harris, G. T., & Rice, M. E. (2006). "Treatment of Psychopathy: A Review of Empirical Findings." In C. J. Patrick (Ed.), *Handbook of Psychopathy* (pp. 555–572). New York: The Guilford Press.

Harris, G. T., Rice, M. E., & Lalumière, M. (2001). "Criminal Violence: The Roles of Psychopathy, Neurodevelopmental Insults, and Antisocial Parenting." *Criminal Justice and Behavior*, *28*(4), 402–426. https://doi:10.1177/009385480102800402

Harris, H. W., & Schaffner, K. F. (1992). "Molecular Genetics, Reductionism, and Disease Concepts in Psychiatry." *The Journal of Medicine and Philosophy*, *17*(2), 127–153. https://doi:10.1093/jmp/17.2.127

Hart, H. L. A. (1963). *Law, Liberty, and Morality*. Palo Alto, CA: Stanford University Press.

Hart, H. L. A., & Green, L. (2012). *The Concept of Law* (Third ed.). Edited by P. A. Bulloch & J. Raz. Oxford: Oxford University Press.

Hart, H. L. A., & Honoré, T. (1985). *Causation in the Law*. Oxford/New York: Oxford University Press.

Hartwell, S. (2004). "Triple Stigma: Persons with Mental Illness and Substance Abuse Problems in the Criminal Justice System." *Criminal Justice Policy Review*, *15*(1), 84–99. https://doi:10.1177/08874 03403255064

Hartwell, S., Fisher, W., Deng, X., Pinals, D. A., & Siegfriedt, J. (2016). "Intensity of Offending Following State Prison Release among Persons Treated for Mental Health Problems While Incarcerated." *Psychiatric Services*, *67*(1), 49–54. https://doi:10.1176/appi.ps.201400417

Hasin, D. S., & Grant, B. F. (2015). "The National Epidemiologic Survey on Alcohol and Related Conditions (NESARC) Waves 1 and 2: Review and Summary of Findings." *Social Psychiatry and Psychiatric Epidemiology*, *50*(11), 1609–1640. https://doi:10.1007/s00127-015-1088-0

Hasin, D. S., O'Brien, C. P., Auriacombe, M., Borges, G., Bucholz, K., Budney, A., . . . Grant, B. F. (2013). "DSM-5 Criteria for Substance Use Disorders: Recommendations and Rationale." *American Journal of Psychiatry, 170*(8), 834–851. https://doi:10.1176/appi.ajp.2013.12060782

Hastings Center. (1996). "The Goals of Medicine: Setting New Priorities." *Hastings Center Report, 26*(6), S1–S27. https://doi:10.1002/j.1552-146X.1996.tb04777.x

Hatfield, G. C. (1979). "Force (God) in Descartes' Physics." *Studies in History and Philosophy of Science Part A, 10*(2), 113–140. https://doi:10.1016/0039-3681(79)90013-X

Hauerwas, S. (1991). *The Peaceable Kingdom: A Primer in Christian Ethics.* South Bend, IN: University of Notre Dame Press.

Hauptman, A. J. (2015). "Weighing Hyponarrativity in the Face of Complex Medical Decision Making." *Philosophy, Psychiatry, & Psychology, 22*(4), 327–331. https://doi:10.1353/ppp.2015.0056

Havens, L. L. (1973). *Approaches to the Mind: Movement of the Psychiatric Schools from Sects toward Science.* Boston: Little, Brown and Company.

Havens, L. L., & Ghaemi, S. N. (2004). *Psychiatric movements: From sects to science.* Livingston, NJ: Transaction Publishers.

Haverhals, L., & Lang, A. (2004). *An Empirical Examination of the Effect of DTC Advertising on Stigma towards Mental Illness.* Paper presented at the Paper presented at the Annual Meeting of International Communication Association, New Orleans, LA. (Conference Paper/Unpublished Manuscript). http://citation.allacademic.com/meta/p112363_index.html

Hawthorne, W. B., Folsom, D. P., Sommerfeld, D. H., Lanouette, N. M., Lewis, M., Aarons, G. A., . . . Jeste, D. V. (2012). "Incarceration among Adults Who Are in the Public Mental Health System: Rates, Risk Factors, and Short-Term Outcomes." *Psychiatric Services, 63*(1), 26–32. https://doi:10.1176/appi.ps.201000505

Hayes, S., & Carpenter, B. (2012). "Out of Time: The Moral Temporality of Sex, Crime and Taboo." *Critical Criminology, 20*(2), 141–152. https://doi:10.1007/s10612-011-9130-3

Healy, B. (2005). "A Medical-Industrial Complex." *U.S. News & World Report, 138*(3), 54. http://diamondskyinc.com/news.asp?sid=2&cid=7&aid=198

Healy, D. (1997). *The Antidepressant Era.* Cambridge, MA: Harvard University Press.

Healy, D. (2002). *The Creation of Psychopharmacology.* Cambridge, MA: Harvard University Press.

Healy, D. (2003). *Let Them Eat Prozac.* Toronto: James Lorimer & Company.

Healy, D. (2004). *The Creation of Psychopharmacology.* Cambridge, MA: Harvard University Press.

Healy, W. (1915). *The Individual Delinquent: A Text-Book of Diagnosis and Prognosis for All Concerned in Understanding Offenders.* Boston: Little, Brown & Co.

Healy, W., & Bronner, A. F. (1926). *Delinquents and Criminals, Their Making and Unmaking: Studies in Two American Cities.* New York: MacMillan Publishing.

Heather, N. (2013). "Is Alcohol Addiction Usefully Called a Disease?" *Philosophy, Psychiatry, & Psychology, 20*(4), 321–324. https://doi:10.1353/ppp.2013.0050

Heinrichs, D. W. (2015). "Model-Based Science and the Ethics of Ongoing Treatment Negotiation." In J. Z. Sadler, K. W. M. Fulford, & W. C. W. van Staden (Eds.), *The Oxford Handbook of Psychiatric Ethics* (pp. 1143–1159). Oxford: Oxford University Press.

Henry, J. (Ed.) (2007) *Dictionary of Medical Biography.* Westport, CT: Greenwood Press.

Hill, J., & Maughan, B. (Eds.) (2001). *Conduct Disorders in Childhood and Adolescence.* New York: Cambridge University Press.

Hill, S. Y. (1985). "The Disease Concept of Alcoholism: A Review." *Drug and Alcohol Dependence, 16*(3), 193–214. https://doi:10.1016/0376-8716(85)90045-6

Hillis, A. E. (2014). "Inability to Empathize: Brain Lesions That Disrupt Sharing and Understanding Another's Emotions." *Brain, 137*(4), 981–997. https://doi:10.1093/brain/awt317

Hippocrates. (1923). *The Art, Loeb Classical Library, Volume II.* Translated by W. H. S. Jones. Cambridge, MA: Harvard University Press.

Hirsch Jr., E. D. (1983). "Cultural Literacy." *American Scholar, 52*(2), 159–169. http://www.jstor.org/stable/41211231

Hirsch Jr., E. D. (1985). "'Cultural Literacy' Doesn't Mean 'Core Curriculum.'" *The English Journal, 74*(6), 47–49. https://doi:10.2307/816894

Hirsch Jr., E. D. (1987). *Cultural Literacy: What Every American Needs to Know.* Boston: Houghton Mifflin Company.

Hobbes, T. (1651). "*Of the Interiour Beginnings of Voluntary Motions Commonly Called the* Passions, and the Speeches by Which They Are Expressed." In *Leviathan.* https://www.gutenberg.org/files/3207 3207-h/3207-h.htmpp

Hobbes, T. (1651). "Of the Natural Condition of Mankind, as Concerning Their Felicity, and Misery, Section the Incommodities of Such a War." In *Leviathan.* https://www.gutenberg.org/files/3207/3207-h 3207-h.htm

Hodgins, S. (1995). "Major Mental Disorder and Crime: An Overview." *Psychology, Crime & Law, 2*(1), 5–17. https://doi:10.1080/10683169508409761

Hodgins, S., & Côté, G. (1993). "The Criminality of Mentally Disordered Offenders." *Criminal Justice and Behavior, 20*(2), 115–129. https://doi:10.1177/0093854893020002001

Hoffman, G. A. (2015). "How Hyponarrativity May Hinder Antidepressants' 'Happy Ending.'" *Philosophy, Psychiatry, & Psychology, 22*(4), 317–321. https://doi:10.1353/ppp.2015.0050

Holden, C. (2010). "Behavioral Addictions Debut in Proposed DSM-V." *Science, 327*(5968), 935. https: doi.org/10.1126/science.327.5968.935

Hollenbach, P. W. (1981). "Jesus, Demoniacs, and Public Authorities: A Socio-Historical Study." *Journal of the American Academy of Religion, 49*(4), 567–588. https://doi:10.1093/jaarel/XLIX.4.567

Hollis, M. E., Downey, S., del Carmen, A., & Dobbs, R. R. (2017). "The Relationship between Media Portrayals and Crime: Perceptions of Fear of Crime among Citizens." *Crime Prevention and Community Safety, 19*(1), 46–60. https://doi:10.1057/s41300-017-0015-6

Hopkins, E. W. (1924). *Ethics of India.* New Haven, CT: Yale University Press.

Hopkins, J. (1990). "Tantric Buddhism, Degeneration or Enhancement: The Viewpoint of a Tibetan Tradition." *Buddhist-Christian Studies, 10,* 87–96. https://doi:10.2307/1390191

Horn, M. (1989). *Before It's Too Late: The Child Guidance Movement in the United States, 1922-1945.* Philadelphia: Temple University Press.

Horwitz, A. V., & Wakefield, J. C. (2007). *The Loss of Sadness: How Psychiatry Transformed Normal Sorrow into Depressive Disorder.* Oxford: Oxford University Press.

Hucker, S., Langevin, R., Wortzman, G., Bain, J., Handy, L., Chambers, J., & Wright, S. (1986). "Neuropsychological Impairment in Pedophiles." *Canadian Journal of Behavioural Science / Revue canadienne des sciences du comportement, 18*(4), 440–448. https://doi:10.1037/h0079965

Huizinga, J. (1954). *The Waning of the Middle Ages: A Study of the Forms of Life, Thought, and Art in France and the Netherlands in the XIVth and XVth Centuries.* Translated by F. J. Hopman. Garden City, NY: Doubleday.

Hume, D. (1605). *A Treatise of Human Nature, Book III: Of Morals.* https:www.gutenberg.org/files/4705/4705-h/4705-h.htm

Humphreys, M. (2008). "Risk, Rights, Recovery: The Twelfth Biennial Report 2005–2007—The Mental Health Act Commission." *International Journal of Mental Health and Capacity Law, 17,* 108–111.

Hunter, R., & Macalpine, I. (1963). *Three Hundred Years of Psychiatry, 1535-1860: A History Presented in Selected English Texts.* London/New York: Oxford University Press.

Hurley, J., & Linsley, P. (2005). "Proposed Changes to the Mental Health Act of England and Wales—Research Investigating the Debate." *Journal of Psychiatric and Mental Health Nursing, 12*(1), 121–123. https://doi:10.1111/j.1365-2850.2004.00810.x

Husak, D. (2010). *The Philosophy of Criminal Law: Selected Essays.* New York: Oxford University Press.

Hutchinson, D. S. (1995). "Ethics." In J. Barnes (Ed.), *The Cambridge Companion to Aristotle* (pp. 195–231). Cambridge: Cambridge University Press.

I.F.R. (1872). "Supreme Judicial Court of New Hampshire." State v. Pike. *The American Law Register (1852-1891), 20*(4), 233–259. https://doi:10.2307/3303702

Ibrahim, J. G. (2005). *Applied Survival Analysis.* Paper presented at the American Statistical Association-Northeast Illinois Chapter: Summer 2005 Workshop, Renaissance Chicago North Shore Hotel. https: community.amstat.org/northeasternillinoischapter/events/past-events/new-item/new-item2

Idov, M. (2013). "The Turn Against Nabokov." *The New Yorker, 27.* https://www.newyorker.com/books page-turner/the-turn-against-nabokov

Insel, T., Cuthbert, B., Garvey, M., Heinssen, R., Pine, D. S., Quinn, K., . . . Wang, P. (2010). "Research Domain Criteria (RDoC): Toward a New Classification Framework for Research on Mental Disorders." *American Journal of Psychiatry, 167*(7), 748–751. https://doi:10.1176/appi.ajp.2010.09091379

Insel, T. R. (2014). "The NIMH Research Domain Criteria (RDoC) Project: Precision Medicine for Psychiatry." *American Journal of Psychiatry, 171*(4), 395–397. https://doi:10.1176/appi. ajp.2014.14020138

Insel, T. R., & Wang, P. S. (2010). "Rethinking Mental Illness." *JAMA, 303*(19), 1970–1971. https:// doi:10.1001/jama.2010.555

Inwood, M. J. (2005). "Enlightenment." In T. Honderich (Ed.), *The Oxford Companion to Philosophy, New ed.* (pp. 252–253). Oxford: Oxford University Press.

Irvine, J. M. (2005). *Disorders of Desire: Sexuality and Gender in Modern American Sexology* (Rev. and expanded ed.). Philadelphia: Temple University Press.

Irwin, T. H. (1992). "Who Discovered the Will?" *Philosophical Perspectives, Vol. 6, Ethics,* 453–473. https://doi:10.2307/2214256

Jablensky, A. (2002). "The Classification of Personality Disorders: Critical Review and Need for Rethinking." *Psychopathology, 35*(2–3), 112–116. https://doi:10.1159/000065129

Jackson, D. (2012 Dec 20). "Biden Pledges 'Action' against Gun Violence." *USA Today,* 20 December 2012. http://www.usatoday.com/story/news/politics/2012/12/20/obama-biden-gun-control-effort-newtown/1782257/ unap

Jackson, S. W. (1983). "Melancholia and Partial Insanity." *Journal of the History of the Behavioral Sciences, 19*(2), 173–184. https://doi:10.1002/1520-6696

Jackson, S. W. (1985). "Acedia the Sin and Its Relationship to Sorrow and Melancholia." In A. Kleinman & B. Good (Eds.), *Culture and Depression: Studies in Anthropology and Cross-Cultural Psychiatry and Affect and Disorder* (pp. 43–62). Berkeley: University of California Press.

James, D. J., & Glaze, L. E. (2006). *Bureau of Justice Statistics Special Report: Mental Health Problems of Prison and Jail Inmates* (NCJ Number: 213600). https://www.ojp.gov/ncjrs/virtual-library abstracts/mental-health-problems-prison-and-jail-inmates

Janssen, D. F. (2013). "Is 'Pedophilia' a Paraphrase of the Incest Taboo? Apropos: Are the Corollaries of Taboo Offered up as Reasons for It?" *Archives of Sexual Behavior, 42*(5), 679–683. https:// doi:10.1007/s10508-013-0131-z

Jarvis, E. (1842). Statistics of insanity in the United States. *The Boston Medical and Surgical Journal, 27*(7), 116–121.

Jaspers, K. (1963/1997a). *General Psychopathology, Volume One.* Translated by J. Hoenig & M. W. Hamilton. Baltimore/London: Johns Hopkins University Press.

Jaspers, K. (1997b). *General Psychopathology, Volume Two.* Translated by J. Hoenig & M. W. Hamilton. Baltimore/London: Johns Hopkins University Press.

Jastrow, M. (1911). "Nergal." In H. Chisholm & F. Hooper (Eds.), *Encyclopedia Britannica* (Eleventh ed., Vol. XIX). (pp. 388–389). New York: Cambridge University Press.

Jellinek, E. M. (1960). *The Disease Concept of Alcoholism.* New Haven, CT: Hillhouse Press.

Jensen, J. V. (1987). "Rhetorical Emphases of Taoism." *Rhetorica: A Journal of the History of Rhetoric, 5*(3), 219–229. https://doi:10.1525/rh.1987.5.3.219

Jeppsson, S. M. I. (2021). "Retributivism, Justification and Credence: The Epistemic Argument Revisited." *Neuroethics, 14*(2), 177–190. https://doi:10.1007/s12152-020-09436-6

Jewkes, Y. (2015). *Media and Crime* (Third ed., Revised ed.). London: Sage.

Johnson, R., & Cureton, A. (2018). "Kant's Moral Philosophy." In E. N. Zalta (Ed.), *The Stanford Encyclopedia of Philosophy* (Spring 2018 ed.). Stanford, CA: Metaphysics Research Lab, Stanford University. https://plato.stanford.edu/archives/spr2018/entries/kant-moral/

Jones, K. W. (1999). *Taming the Troublesome Child: American Families, Child Guidance, and the Limits of Psychiatric Authority.* Cambridge, MA: Harvard University Press.

Jorm, A. F. (2000). "Mental Health Literacy: Public Knowledge and Beliefs about Mental Disorders." *British Journal of Psychiatry, 177*(5), 396–401. https://doi:10.1192/bjp.177.5.396

Jorm, A. F. (2012). "Mental Health Literacy: Empowering the Community to Take Action for Better Mental Health." *American Psychologist, 67*(3), 231–243. https://doi:10.1037/a0025957

Jorm, A. F., Christensen, H., & Griffiths, K. M. (2005). "Public Beliefs about Causes and Risk Factors for Mental Disorders." *Social Psychiatry and Psychiatric Epidemiology, 40*(9), 764–767. https:// doi:10.1007/s00127-005-0940-z

Jorm, A. F., Christensen, H., & Griffiths, K. M. (2006). "Changes in Depression Awareness and Attitudes in Australia: The Impact of Beyondblue: The National Depression Initiative." *Australian and New Zealand Journal of Psychiatry, 40*(1), 42–46. https://doi:10.1111/j.1440-1614.2006.01739.x

Jorm, A. F., Korten, A. E., Jacomb, P. A., Christensen, H., Rodgers, B., & Pollitt, P. (1997). "'Mental Health Literacy': A Survey of the Public's Ability to Recognise Mental Disorders and Their Beliefs About the Effectiveness of Treatment." *Medical Journal of Australia, 166*(4), 182–186. https://doi:10.5694/j.1326-5377.1997.tb140071.x

Jorm, A. F., & Wright, A. (2007). "Beliefs of Young People and Their Parents about the Effectiveness of Interventions for Mental Disorders." *Australian & New Zealand Journal of Psychiatry, 41*(8), 656–666. https://doi:10.1080/00048670701449179

Jotterand, F. (2014). "Questioning the Moral Enhancement Project." *American Journal of Bioethics, 14*(4), 1–3. https://doi:10.1080/15265161.2014.905031

Joyal, C. C., Côté, G., Meloche, J., & Hodgins, S. (2011). "Severe Mental Illness and Aggressive Behavior: On the Importance of Considering Subgroups." *International Journal of Forensic Mental Health, 10*(2), 107–117. https://doi:10.1080/14999013.2011.577136

Kafka, M. P. (1997). "Hypersexual Desire in Males: An Operational Definition and Clinical Implications for Males with Paraphilias and Paraphilia-Related Disorders." *Archives of Sexual Behavior, 26*(5), 505–526. https://doi:10.1023/A:1024507922470

Kafka, M. P. (2003). "Sex Offending and Sexual Appetite: The Clinical and Theoretical Relevance of Hypersexual Desire." *International Journal of Offender Therapy and Comparative Criminology, 47*(4), 439–451. https://doi:10.1177/0306624x03253845

Kafka, M. P. (2010). "Hypersexual Disorder: A Proposed Diagnosis for DSM-V." *Archives of Sexual Behavior, 39*(2), 377–400. https://doi:10.1007/s10508-009-9574-7

Kafka, M. P. (2014). "What Happened to Hypersexual Disorder?" *Archives of Sexual Behavior, 43*(7), 1259–1261. https://doi:10.1007/s10508-014-0326-y

Kafka, M. P., & Hennen, J. (1999). "The Paraphilia-Related Disorders: An Empirical Investigation of Nonparaphilic Hypersexuality Disorders in Outpatient Males." *Journal of Sex & Marital Therapy, 25*(4), 305–319. https://doi:10.1080/00926239908404008

Kafka, M. P., & Hennen, J. (2003). "Hypersexual Desire in Males: Are Males with Paraphilias Different from Males with Paraphilia-Related Disorders?" *Sexual Abuse: A Journal of Research and Treatment, 15*(4), 307–321. https://doi:10.1023/A:1025000227956

Kahhale, I. (2022). "Neural Basis of Antisocial Behaviour." *Nature Reviews Psychology, 1*(3), 129. https://doi:10.1038/s44159-022-00027-1

Kant, I. (1798/2006). *Anthropology from a Pragmatic Point of View.* Translated by R. B. Louden. Translated and edited by R. B. Louden. Cambridge: Cambridge University Press.

Kant, I. (1998). *Groundwork of the Metaphysics of Morals.* Translated by M. J. Gregor. Cambridge/New York: Cambridge University Press.

Kapusta, M. A., & Frank, S. (1977). "The Book of Job and the Modern View of Depression." *Annals of Internal Medicine, 86*(5), 667–672. https://doi:10.7326/0003-4819-86-5-667

Karila, L., Wéry, A., Weinstein, A., Cottencin, O., Petit, A., Reynaud, M., & Billieux, J. (2014). "Sexual Addiction or Hypersexual Disorder: Different Terms for the Same Problem? A Review of the Literature." *Current Pharmaceutical Design, 20*(25), 4012–4020. https://doi:10.2174/13816128113199990619

Kassirer, J. P. (1989). "Diagnostic Reasoning." *Annals of Internal Medicine, 110*(11), 893–900. https://doi:10.7326/0003-4819-110-11-893

Kassirer, J. P., Moskowitz, A. J., Lau, J., & Pauker, S. G. (1987). "Decision Analysis: A Progress Report." *Annals of Internal Medicine, 106*(2), 275–291. https://doi:10.7326/0003-4819-106-2-275

Kazemian, L., & Walker, A. (2019). "Effects of Incarceration." In D. P. Farrington, L. Kazemian, & A. R. Piquero (Eds.), *The Oxford Handbook of Developmental and Life-Course Criminology* (pp. 576–599). New York: Oxford University Press.

Keck, L. E. (1996). "Rethinking 'New Testament Ethics.'" *Journal of Biblical Literature, 115*(1), 3–16. https://doi:10.2307/3266815

Kelly, E. I. (2021). "From Retributive to Restorative Justice." *Criminal Law and Philosophy, 15*(2), 237–247. https://doi:10.1007/s11572-021-09574-9

Kelly, J. M. (1992). *A Short History of Western Legal Theory*. Oxford: Clarendon Press.

Kendell, R. E. (1988). "Diagnostic and Statistical Manual of Mental Disorders (Third ed., Revised (DSM-III-R)" [Book Review]. *American Journal of Psychiatry, 145*(10), 1301–1302.

Kendi, I. X. (2016). *Stamped from the Beginning: The Definitive History of Racist Ideas in America*. New York: Nation Books.

Kendler, K. S. (2008). "Explanatory Models for Psychiatric Illness." *American Journal of Psychiatry, 165*(6), 695–702. https://doi:10.1176/appi.ajp.2008.07071061

Kendler, K. S. (2013). "A History of the DSM-5 Scientific Review Committee." *Psychological Medicine, 43*(9), 1793–1800. https://doi:10.1017/S0033291713001578

Kendler, K. S., & Parnas, J. (Eds.) (2008). *Philosophical Issues in Psychiatry: Explanation, Phenomenology and Nosology*. Baltimore: Johns Hopkins University Press.

Kendler, K. S., & Parnas, J. (Eds.) (2012). *Philosophical Issues in Psychiatry II: Nosology*. (International Perspectives in Philosophy and Psychiatry series). Oxford: Oxford University Press.

Kendler, K. S., Parnas, J., & Zachar, P. (Eds.) (2020). *Levels of Analysis in Psychopathology: Cross-Disciplinary Perspectives*. Cambridge/New York: Cambridge University Press.

Kendler, K. S., & Zachar, P. (Eds.) (2019). *Toward a Philosophical Approach to Psychiatry: The Writings of Kenneth Kendler*. Cambridge: Cambridge Scholars Publishing.

Kendler, K. S., Zachar, P., & Craver, C. (2011). "What Kinds of Things Are Psychiatric Disorders?" *Psychological Medicine, 41*(6), 1143–1150. https://doi:10.1017/S0033291710001844

Kessler, R. C., Chiu, W. T., Demler, O., & Walters, E. E. (2005). "Prevalence, Severity, and Comorbidity of 12-Month DSM-IV Disorders in the National Comorbidity Survey Replication." *Archives of General Psychiatry, 62*(6), 617–627. https://doi:10.1001/archpsyc.62.6.617

Kessler, R. C., Coccaro, E. F., Fava, M., Jaeger, S., Jin, R., & Walters, E. (2006). "The Prevalence and Correlates of DSM-IV Intermittent Explosive Disorder in the National Comorbidity Survey Replication." *Archives of General Psychiatry, 63*(6), 669–678. https://doi:10.1001/archpsyc.63.6.669

Keyes, C. L. M. (2002). "The Mental Health Continuum: From Languishing to Flourishing in Life." *Journal of Health and Social Behavior, 43*(2), 207–222. https://doi:10.2307/3090197

Keyes, C. L. M. (2005). "Mental Illness and/or Mental Health? Investigating Axioms of the Complete State Model of Health." *Journal of Consulting and Clinical Psychology, 73*(3), 539–548. https://doi:10.1037/0022-006x.73.3.539

Keyes, C. L. M. (2007). "Promoting and Protecting Mental Health as Flourishing: A Complementary Strategy for Improving National Mental Health." *American Psychologist, 62*(2), 95–108. https://doi:10.1037/0003-066x.62.2.95

Keyes, C. L. M. (2014). "Happiness, Flourishing, and Life Satisfaction." In W. C. Cockerham, R. Dingwall, & S. R. Quah (Eds.), *The Wiley Blackwell Encyclopedia of Health, Illness, Behavior, and Society* (pp. 747–751). Oxford: John Wiley & Sons.

Keyes, C. L. M., & Grzywacz, J. G. (2005). "Health as a Complete State: The Added Value in Work Performance and Healthcare Costs." *Journal of Occupational and Environmental Medicine, 47*(5), 523–532. https://doi:10.1097/01.jom.0000161737.21198.3a

Khan, K. S., & Coomarasamy, A. (2006). "A Hierarchy of Effective Teaching and Learning to Acquire Competence in Evidenced-Based Medicine." *BMC Medical Education, 6*, Article 59. https://doi.org/10.1186/1472-6920-6-59

Kidd, I. G. (1999). *Posidonius: Volume III, the Translation of the Fragments*. Cambridge: Cambridge University Press.

Kieckhefer R. (2022). *Magic in the Middle Ages*, Third Edition. Cambridge, UK: Cambridge University Press.

Kincaid, H., & Sullivan, J. A. (Eds.) (2014). *Classifying Psychopathology: Mental Kinds and Natural Kinds*. Cambridge, MA: MIT Press.

Kirk, S. A., & Kutchins, H. (1992). *The Selling of DSM-III: The Rhetoric of Science in Psychiatry*. New Brunswick, NJ: Transaction Publishers.

Kirmayer, L. J. (2018). "Ethno- and Cultural Psychiatry." In H. Callan & S. Coleman (Eds.), *The International Encyclopedia of Anthropology* (pp. 1–11). https://doi.org/10.1002/9781118924396.wbiea2362.

Kisely, S. R., Campbell, L. A., & O'Reilly, R. (2017). "Compulsory Community and Involuntary Outpatient Treatment for People with Severe Mental Disorders." *Cochrane Database of Systematic Reviews, 3*, Article CD004408. https://doi.org/10.1002/14651858.CD004408.pub5

Klein, J., & Giglioni, G. (2020). "Francis Bacon." In E. N. Zalta (Ed.), *The Stanford Encyclopedia of Philosophy* (Fall 2020 ed.). Stanford, CA: Metaphysics Research Lab, Stanford University. https://plato.stanford.edu/archives/fall2020/entries/francis-bacon/

Knight, R. A. (2010). "Is a Diagnostic Category for Paraphilic Coercive Disorder Defensible?" *Archives of Sexual Behavior, 39*(2), 419–426. https://doi:10.1007/s10508-009-9571-x

Koob, G. F. (2014). "Neurocircuitry of Alcohol Addiction: Synthesis from Animal Models." In E. V. Sullivan & A. Pfefferbaum (Eds.), *Handbook of Clinical Neurology* (pp. 33–54). New York: Elsevier.

Kor, A., Fogel, Y. A., Reid, R. C., & Potenza, M. N. (2013). "Should Hypersexual Disorder Be Classified as an Addiction?" *Sexual Addiction & Compulsivity, 20*(1–2), 27–47. https://doi:10.1080/10720162.2013.768132

Kotler, J. S., & McMahon, R. J. (2005). "Child Psychopathy: Theories, Measurement, and Relations with the Development and Persistence of Conduct Problems." *Clinical Child and Family Psychology Review, 8*(4), 291–325. https://doi:10.1007/s10567-005-8810-5

Kotov, R., Krueger, R. F., Watson, D., Achenbach, T. M., Althoff, R. R., Bagby, R. M., . . . Zimmerman, M. (2017). "The Hierarchical Taxonomy of Psychopathology (HiTOP): A Dimensional Alternative to Traditional Nosologies." *Journal of Abnormal Psychology, 126*(4), 454–477. https://doi:10.1037/abn0000258

Koutouvidis, N., Marketos, S. G. (1995). "The Contribution of Thomas Sydenham (1624–1689) to the Evolution of Psychiatry." *History of Psychiatry, 6*(24), 513–520. https://doi:10.1177/0957154x9500602408

Kovel, J. (1980). "The American Mental Health Industry." In D. Ingleby (Ed.), *Critical Psychiatry: The Politics of Mental Health* (pp. 72–101). New York: Pantheon.

Kovess-Masfety, V., Saragoussi, D., Sevilla-Dedieu, C., Gilbert, F., Suchocka, A., Arveiller, N., . . . Hardy-Bayle, M.-C. (2007). "What Makes People Decide Who to Turn to When Faced with a Mental Health Problem? Results from a French Survey." *BMC Public Health, 7*, Article 188. https://doi.org/10.1186/1471-2458-7-188

Kraepelin, E. (1904). *Lectures on Clinical Psychiatry* (authorized translation from German) Revised and edited by T. Johnstone. London: Baillière, Tindall and Cox.

Krafft-Ebing, R. v. (1965). *Psychopathia Sexualis: A Medico-Forensic Study* (first unexpurgated ed. in English). New York: Putnam.

Kramer, H., & Sprenger, J. (1487/2009). *Malleus Maleficarum*. Translated and edited by C. S. MacKay. Cambridge: Cambridge University Press.

Kramer, P. D. (1993). *Listening to Prozac: A Psychiatrist Explores Antidepressant Drugs and the Remaking of the Self*. New York: Viking Penguin.

Krueger, R. B., Reed, G. M., First, M. B., Marais, A., Kismodi, E., & Briken, P. (2017). "Proposals for Paraphilic Disorders in the International Classification of Diseases and Related Health Problems, Eleventh Revision (ICD-11)." *Archives of Sexual Behavior, 46*(5), 1529–1545. https://doi:10.1007/s10508-017-0944-2

Kupers, T. A. (1996). "Trauma and Its Sequelae in Male Prisoners: Effects of Confinement, Overcrowding, and Diminished Services." *American Journal of Orthopsychiatry, 66*(2), 189–196. https://doi:10.1037/h0080170

Kurki, L. (2000). "Restorative and Community Justice in the United States." *Crime and Justice, 27*, 235–303. https://doi:10.2307/1147665

Kuss, D. J., Griffiths, M. D., & Pontes, H. M. (2017). "Chaos and Confusion in DSM-5 Diagnosis of Internet Gaming Disorder: Issues, Concerns, and Recommendations for Clarity in the Field." *Journal of Behavioral Addictions, 6*(2), 103–109. https://doi:10.1556/2006.5.2016.062

Kutner, M., Greenburg, E., Jin, Y., & Paulsen, C. (2006). *The Health Literacy of America's Adults: Results from the 2003 National Assessment of Adult Literacy (NCES 2006-483)*. Washington, DC: National Center for Education Statistics (NCES). https://nces.ed.gov/pubs2006/2006483.pdf

Kutz, I. (2000). "Job and His 'Doctors': Bedside Wisdom in the Book of Job." *British Medical Journal, 321*(7276), 1613–1615. https://doi:10.1136/bmj.321.7276.1613

Kymlicka, W. (1990). *Contemporary Political Philosophy: An Introduction*. Oxford: Oxford University Press.

Kymlicka, W., & Norman, W. J. (2000). "Citizenship in Culturally Diverse Societies: Issues, Contexts, Concepts." In W. Kymlicka & W. Norman (Eds.), *Citizenship in Diverse Societies* (pp. 1–43). New York: Oxford University Press.

Labrum, T., Zingman, M. A., Nossel, I., & Dixon, L. (2021). "Violence by Persons with Serious Mental Illness toward Family Caregivers and Other Relatives: A Review." *Harvard Review of Psychiatry*, 29(1), 10–19. https://doi:10.1097/hrp.0000000000000263

Lacey, N., & Pickard, H. (2019). "A Dual-Process Approach to Criminal Law: Victims and the Clinical Model of Responsibility without Blame." *Journal of Political Philosophy*, 27(2), 229–251. https://doi:10.1111/jopp.12160

Ladyman, J., Ross, D., with Spurrett, D., & Collier, J. (2007). *Every Thing Must Go: Metaphysics Naturalized*. Oxford: Oxford University Press.

LaMay, C. L. (1997). "America's Censor: Anthony Comstock and Free Speech." *Communications and the Law*, 19(3), 1–59.

Lamb, H. R. (2015). "Does Deinstitutionalization Cause Criminalization?" The Penrose Hypothesis." *JAMA Psychiatry*, 72(2), 105–106. https://doi:10.1001/jamapsychiatry.2014.2444

Lamb, H. R., & Weinberger, L. E. (1998). "Persons with Severe Mental Illness in Jails and Prisons: A Review." *Psychiatric Services*, 49(4), 483–492. https://doi:10.1176/ps.49.4.483

Lane, C. (2008). *Shyness: How Normal Behavior Became a Sickness*. New Haven, CT: Yale University Press.

Langevin, R. (2006). "Sexual Offenses and Traumatic Brain Injury." *Brain and Cognition*, 60(2), 206–207. https://doi:10.1016/j.bandc.2004.09.018

Langevin, R., & Curnoe, S. (2008). "Are the Mentally Retarded and Learning Disordered Overrepresented among Sex Offenders and Paraphilics?" *International Journal of Offender Therapy and Comparative Criminology*, 52(4), 401–415. https://doi:10.1177/0306624x07305826

Langevin, R., Curnoe, S., & Bain, J. (2000). "A Study of Clerics Who Commit Sexual Offenses: Are They Different from Other Sex Offenders?" *Child Abuse and Neglect*, 24(4), 535–545. https://doi:10.1016/S0145-2134(00)00113-7

Langevin, R., Wortzman, G., Dickey, R., & Wright, P. (1988). "Neuropsychological Impairment in Incest Offenders." *Annals of Sex Research*, 1(3), 401–415. https://doi:10.1177/107906328800100304

Langevin, R., Wortzman, G., Wright, P., & Handy, L. (1989). "Studies of Brain Damage and Dysfunction in Sex Offenders." *Annals of Sex Research*, 2(2), 163–179. https://doi:10.1007/BF00851321

Laqueur, T. W. (1989). "Bodies, Details, and the Humanitarian Narrative." In L. Hunt (Ed.), *The New Cultural History* (pp. 176–204). Berkeley: University of California Press.

Laqueur, T. W. (1990). *Making Sex: Body and Gender from the Greeks to Freud*. Cambridge, MA: Harvard University Press.

Lauber, C., Nordt, C., Falcato, L., & Rössler, W. (2001). "Lay Recommendations on How to Treat Mental Disorders." *Social Psychiatry and Psychiatric Epidemiology*, 36(11), 553–556. https://doi:10.1007/s001270170006

Lauber, C., Nordt, C., Falcato, L., & Rössler, W. (2003). "Do People Recognise Mental Illness? Factors Influencing Mental Health Literacy." *European Archives of Psychiatry and Clinical Neuroscience*, 253(5), 248–251. https://doi:10.1007/s00406-003-0439-0

Lawrence, C. (Ed.) (2007) *Dictionary of Medical Biography* (Vol. 5: S-Z). Westport, CT: Greenwood Press.

Lawrence, D. (1996). "Tantric Argument: The Transfiguration of Philosophical Discourse in the Pratyabhijñā System of Utpaladeva and Abhinavagupta." *Philosophy East and West*, 46(2), 165–204. https://doi:10.2307/1399403

Laws, D. R., & O'Donohue, W. T. (2008). "Introduction: Fundamental Issues in Sexual Deviance." In D. R. Laws & W. T. O'Donohue (Eds.), *Sexual Deviance: Theory, Assessment, and Treatment, Second ed.* (pp. 1–20). New York: Guilford Press.

Laws, D. R., & Ward, T. (2011). *Desistance from Sex Offending: Alternatives to Throwing Away the Keys*. New York: Guilford Press.

Lebow, D. (2019). "Trumpism and the Dialectic of Neoliberal Reason." *Perspectives on Politics*, 17(2), 380–398. https://doi:10.1017/S1537592719000434

Leder, D. (1990). "Clinical Interpretation: The Hermeneutics of Medicine." *Theoretical Medicine, 11*(1), 9–24. https://doi:10.1007/BF00489234

Lee, G., & Cohen, D. (2021). "Incidences of Involuntary Psychiatric Detentions in 25 U.S. States." *Psychiatric Services, 72*(1), 61–68. https://doi:10.1176/appi.ps.201900477

Lee, R., & Coccaro, E. F. (2001). "The Neuropsychopharmacology of Criminality and Aggression." *Canadian Journal of Psychiatry - Revue Canadienne de Psychiatrie, 46*(1), 35–44. https://doi:10.1177/070674370104600106

Lee, R., Ferris, C., Van de Kar, L. D., & Coccaro, E. F. (2009). "Cerebrospinal Fluid Oxytocin, Life History of Aggression, and Personality Disorder." *Psychoneuroendocrinology, 34*(10), 1567–1573. https://doi:10.1016/j.psyneuen.2009.06.002

Lee, R., Kavoussi, R. J., & Coccaro, E. F. (2008). "Placebo-Controlled, Randomized Trial of Fluoxetine in the Treatment of Aggression in Male Intimate Partner Abusers." *International Clinical Psychopharmacology, 23*(6), 337–341. https://doi:10.1097/YIC.0b013e32830fbdd2

Leibenluft, E., Charney, D. S., Towbin, K. E., Bhangoo, R. K., & Pine, D. S. (2003). "Defining Clinical Phenotypes of Juvenile Mania." *American Journal of Psychiatry, 160*(3), 430–437. https://doi:10.1176/appi.ajp.160.3.430

Leibenluft, E., Cohen, P., Gorrindo, T., Brook, J. S., & Price, D. S. (2006). "Chronic Versus Episodic Irritability in Youth: A Community-Based, Longitudinal Study of Clinical and Diagnostic Associations." *Journal of Child and Adolescent Psychopharmacology, 16*(4), 456–466. https://doi:10.1089/cap.2006.16.456

Leichter, H. M. (2003). "'Evil Habits' and 'Personal Choices': Assigning Responsibility for Health in the 20th Century." *Milbank Quarterly, 81*(4), 603–626. https://doi:10.1046/j.0887-378X.2003.00296.x

Lenzner, R. (2008). "Bernie Madoff's $50 Billion Ponzi Scheme." *Forbes,* 12 December 2008. http://www.forbes.com/2008/12/12/madoff-ponzi-hedge-pf-ii-n_rl_1212croesus_inl.html

Leonard, E. B. (2015). *Crime, Inequality, and Power.* London: Routledge.

Leone, S. S., Huibers, M. J. H., Knottnerus, J. A., & Kant, I. (2008). "The Prognosis of Burnout and Prolonged Fatigue in the Working Population: A Comparison." *Journal of Occupational & Environmental Medicine, 50*(10), 1195–1202. https://doi:10.1097/JOM.0b013e31817e7c05

Levenson, J. S., & Willis, G. M. (2019). "Implementing Trauma-Informed Care in Correctional Treatment and Supervision." *Journal of Aggression, Maltreatment & Trauma, 28*(4), 481–501. https://doi:10.1080/10926771.2018.1531959

Lewis, B. (2011). *Narrative Psychiatry: How Stories Can Shape Clinical Practice.* Baltimore: Johns Hopkins University Press.

Lichtenstein, P., Halldner, L., Zetterqvist, J., Sjölander, A., Serlachius, E., Fazel, S., . . . Larsson, H. (2012). "Medication for Attention Deficit–Hyperactivity Disorder and Criminality." *New England Journal of Medicine, 367*(21), 2006–2014. https://doi:10.1056/NEJMoa1203241

Liégeois, A. (1991). "Hidden Philosophy and Theology in Morel's Theory of Degeneration and Nosology." *History of Psychiatry, 2*(8), 419–427. https://doi:10.1177/0957154X9100200805

Lilleleht, E. (2002). "Progress and Power: Exploring the Disciplinary Connections between Moral Treatment and Psychiatric Rehabilitation." *Philosophy, Psychiatry, & Psychology, 9*(2), 167–182. https://doi:10.1353/ppp.2003.0028

Lin, A. (2015). "Citizenship Education in American Schools and Its Role in Developing Civic Engagement: A Review of the Research." *Educational Review, 67*(1), 35–63. https://doi:10.1080/00131911.2013.813440

Lind, E. A., Thibaut, J., & Walker, L. (1973). "Discovery and Presentation of Evidence in Adversary and Nonadversary Proceedings." *Michigan Law Review, 71*(6), 1129–1144. https://doi:10.2307/1287749

Ling, S., Umbach, R., & Raine, A. (2019). "Biological Explanations of Criminal Behavior." *Psychology, Crime & Law, 25*(6), 626–640. https://doi:10.1080/1068316X.2019.1572753

Lippman, M. (2009). *Contemporary Criminal Law: Concepts, Cases, and Controversies* (Second ed.). Thousand Oaks, CA: Sage.

Lippman, M. (2012). "The Drafting and Development of the 1948 Convention on Genocide and the Politics of International Law." In H. van der Wilt, J. Vervliet, G. Sluiter, & J. H. ten Cate (Eds.), *The Genocide Convention: The Legacy of 60 Years* (pp. 15–25). Lieden/Boston: Brill/Marinus Nijhoff Publishers. (Reprinted from: 16 March 2012).

Liptak, A. (2008). "1 in 100 U.S. Adults Behind Bars, New Study Says." *New York Times,* 28 February 2008. https://www.nytimes.com/2008/02/28/us/28cnd-prison.html

Livesley, W. J. (1985a). "The Classification of Personality Disorder: I. The Choice of Category Concept." *Canadian Journal of Psychiatry, 30*(5), 353–358. https://doi:10.1177/070674378503000510

Livesley, W. J. (1985b). "The Classification of Personality Disorder: II. The Problem of Diagnostic Criteria." *Canadian Journal of Psychiatry, 30*(5), 359–362. https://doi:10.1177/070674378503000511

Lock, J. D. (1990). "Some Aspects of Medical Hermeneutics: The Role of Dialectic and Narrative." *Theoretical Medicine, 11*(1), 41–49. https://doi:10.1007/BF00489237

Locke, J. (1689/1824). "Two Treatises of Government." In *The Works of John Locke in Nine Volumes* (Twelfth ed., Vol. 4.) (Original work published 1689). London: Rivington. https://oll.libertyfund.org/title/locke-the-works-of-john-locke-vol-4-economic-writings-and-two-treatises-of-government#Locke_0128-04_523

Locke, J. (1690). *An Essay Concerning Humane Understanding, Volume 1.* https://www.gutenberg.org ebooks/10615. London: Holt-Basset.

Locke, J. A. (1689/1824). "A Letter Concerning Toleration." In *The Works of John Locke in Nine Volumes* (Twelfth ed., Vol. 5). London: Rivington. https://oll.libertyfund.org/title/locke-the-works-vol-5-four-letters-concerning-toleration

Lombroso, C., & (translated by von Borosini, V. (1912). "Crime and Insanity in the Twenty-First Century." *Journal of the American Institute of Criminal Law and Criminology, 3*(1), 57–61. https://doi.org/10.2307/1132846

Longo, D. L., Fauci, A. S., Kasper, D. L., Hauser, S. L., Jameson, J. L., & Loscalzo, J. (Eds.) (2012). *Harrison's Principles of Internal Medicine* (Eighteenth ed.). New York: McGraw-Hill.

Longpré, N., Sims-Knight, J. E., Neumann, C., Guay, J.-P., & Knight, R. A. (2020). "Is Paraphilic Coercion a Different Construct from Sadism or the Lower End of an Agonistic Continuum?" *Journal of Criminal Justice, 71*, Article 101743. https://doi.org/10.1016/j.jcrimjus.2020.101743

Looman, J., & Abracen, J. (2013). "The Risk Need Responsivity Model of Offender Rehabilitation: Is There Really a Need for a Paradigm Shift?" *International Journal of Behavioral Consultation and Therapy, 8*(3–4), 30–36. https://doi:10.1037/h0100980

Lowenkamp, C. T., Latessa, E. J., & Smith, P. (2006). "Does Correctional Program Quality Really Matter? The Impact of Adhering to the Principles of Effective Intervention." *Criminology & Public Policy, 5*(3), 575–594. https://doi:10.1111/j.1745-9133.2006.00388.x

Lucretius (50 BCE). *On the Nature of Things.* Translated by W. E. Leonard. Available from The Internet Classics Archive by Daniel C. Stevenson, Web Atomics. http://classics.mit.edu/Carus/nature_things.html

Luhrmann, T. M. (2011). "Hallucinations and Sensory Overrides." *Annual Review of Anthropology, 40*, 71–85. https://doi:10.1146/annurev-anthro-081309-145819

Luna, E. G. (1999). "The Models of Criminal Procedure." *Buffalo Criminal Law Review, 2*(2), 389–535. https://doi:10.1525/nclr.1999.2.2.389

Lysaker, P., & Lysaker, J. (2008). *Schizophrenia and the Fate of the Self.* (International Perspectives in Philosophy and Psychiatry series). Oxford: Oxford University Press.

Ma, Z. (2017). "How the Media Cover Mental Illnesses: A Review." *Health Education, 117*(1), 90–109. https://doi:10.1108/HE-01-2016-0004

Machiavelli, N. (1998). *The Prince.* W.K. Marriott (transl.) London: Everyman's Library Classics. https://www.gutenberg.org/files/1232/1232-h/1232-h.htm

MacIntyre, A. C. (1998). *A Short History of Ethics: A History of Moral Philosophy from the Homeric Age to the Twentieth Century, Second ed.* London: Routledge & Kegan Paul.

Mackay, C. S. (2009). *The Hammer of Witches: A Complete Translation of the Malleus Maleficarum.* New York: Cambridge University Press

Macy, J. R. (1979). "Dependent Co-Arising: The Distinctiveness of Buddhist Ethics." *Journal of Religious Ethics, 7*(1), 38–52. http://www.jstor.org/stable/40018242

Maier, T. (2003). *Dr. Spock: An American Life.* New York: Basic Books.

Malón, A. (2015). "Adult–Child Sex and the Limits of Liberal Sexual Morality." *Archives of Sexual Behavior, 44*(4), 1071–1083. https://doi:10.1007/s10508-014-0442-8

Mancini, C., & Budd, K. M. (2016). "Is the Public Convinced That 'Nothing Works?' Predictors of Treatment Support for Sex Offenders among Americans." *Crime & Delinquency*, 62(6), 777–799. https://doi:10.1177/0011128715597693

Maniglio, R. (2009). "Severe Mental Illness and Criminal Victimization: A Systematic Review." *Acta Psychiatrica Scandinavica*, 119(3), 180–191. https://doi:10.1111/j.1600-0447.2008.01300.x

Manow, P. (2020). "Models of the Welfare State." In D. Béland, S. Leibfried, K. J. Morgan, H. Obinger, & C. Pierson (Eds.), *The Oxford Handbook of the Welfare State* (pp. 787–803). Oxford: Oxford University Press.

Margolis, J. (1994). "Taxonomic Puzzles." In J. Z. Sadler, O. P. Wiggins, & M. A. Schwartz (Eds.), *Philosophical Perspectives on Psychiatric Diagnostic Classification* (pp. 104–128). Baltimore: Johns Hopkins University Press.

Margulies, D. M., Weintraub, S., Basile, J., Grover, P. J., & Carlson, G. A. (2012). "Will Disruptive Mood Dysregulation Disorder Reduce False Diagnosis of Bipolar Disorder in Children?" *Bipolar Disorders*, 14(5), 488–496. https://doi:10.1111/j.1399-5618.2012.01029.x

Markowitz, F. E. (2011). "Mental Illness, Crime, and Violence: Risk, Context, and Social Control." *Aggression and Violent Behavior*, 16(1), 36–44. https://doi:10.1016/j.avb.2010.10.003

Marshall, W. L. (2014). "Phallometric Assessments of Sexual Interests: An Update." *Current Psychiatry Reports*, 16(1), Article 428. https://doi.org/10.1007/s11920-013-0428-6

Martin, R. (2018). *The Elusive Messiah: A Philosophical Overview of the Quest for the Historical Jesus*. London: Routledge.

Martin, R., & Barresi, J. (2006). *The Rise and Fall of Soul and Self: An Intellectual History of Personal Identity*. New York: Columbia University Press.

Marx, O. M. (2008). "German Romantic Psychiatry." In E. R. Wallace & J. Gach (Eds.), *History of Psychiatry and Medical Psychology* (pp. 313–333). New York: Springer.

Maslach, C., Jackson, S. E., & Leiter, M. P. (1997). "Maslach Burnout Inventory: Third ed." In C. P. Zalaquett & R. J. Wood (Eds.), *Evaluating Stress: A Book of Resources.* (pp. 191–218). Lanham, MD: Scarecrow Education.

Matejkowski, J., Lee, S., & Han, W. (2014). "The Association between Criminal History and Mental Health Service Use among People with Serious Mental Illness." *Psychiatric Quarterly*, 85(1), 9–24. https://doi:10.1007/s11126-013-9266-2

Mather, N., & Morris, R. J. (2011). What Samuel A. Kirk Really Said About Mental Retardation and Learning Disabilities: A Response to Danforth, Slocum, and Dunkle. *Intellectual and Developmental Disabilities*, 49(2), 113-119.

Matheson, S. L., Shepherd, A. M., & Carr, V. J. (2014). "How Much Do We Know About Schizophrenia and How Well Do We Know It? Evidence from the Schizophrenia Library." *Psychological Medicine*, 44(16), 3387–3405. https://doi:10.1017/S0033291714000166

Matthews, E. (2007). *Body-Subjects and Disordered Minds: Treating the 'Whole' Person in Psychiatry*. New York: Oxford University Press.

Mauer, M. (2011). "Addressing Racial Disparities in Incarceration." *Prison Journal*, 91(3_Suppl), 87S–101S. https://doi:10.1177/0032885511415227

Mazar, A. (1992). *Archaeology of the Land of the Bible, Volume I: 10,000–586 B.C.E.* (Reprint ed.). New York: Doubleday.

McClimens, A. (2007). Language, labels and diagnosis: An idiot's guide to learning disability. *Journal of Intellectual Disabilities*, 11(3), 257-266.

McCloskey, M. S., Berman, M. E., Noblett, K. L., & Coccaro, E. F. (2006). "Intermittent Explosive Disorder-Integrated Research Diagnostic Criteria: Convergent and Discriminant Validity." *Journal of Psychiatric Research*, 40(3), 231–242. https://doi:10.1016/j.jpsychires.2005.07.004

McCloskey, M. S., Kleabir, K., Berman, M. E., Chen, E. Y., & Coccaro, E. F. (2010). "Unhealthy Aggression: Intermittent Explosive Disorder and Adverse Physical Health Outcomes." *Health Psychology*, 29(3), 324–332. https://doi:10.1037/a0019072

McCloskey, M. S., New, A. S., Siever, L. J., Goodman, M., Koenigsberg, H. W., Flory, J. D., & Coccaro, E. F. (2009). "Evaluation of Behavioral Impulsivity and Aggression Tasks as Endophenotypes for Borderline Personality Disorder." *Journal of Psychiatric Research*, 43(12), 1036–1048. https://doi:10.1016/j.jpsychires.2009.01.002

McConville, S. (1995). "The Victorian Prison: England, 1865-1965." In N. Morris & D. J. Rothman (Eds.), *The Oxford History of the Prison: The Practice of Punishment in Western Society* (pp. 177–150). New York: Oxford University Press.

McCullough, L. (2007). "Benjamin Rush." In W. F. Bynum & H. Bynum (Eds.), *Dictionary of Medical Biography* (Vol. 4, M-R, pp. 1092–1094).Westport, CT: Greenwood Press.

McDonald, S., & Kretzmann, N. (2000). "Medieval Philosophy." In E. Craig (Ed.), *Concise Routledge Encyclopedia of Philosophy* (pp. 552–560). London: Routledge.

Murphy, M. P., & McGann, M. (2022). Introduction: Towards a sustainable welfare state. *Social Policy and Society, 21*(3), 439–446.

McGinnis, J. (2010). *Avicenna*. New York/Oxford: Oxford University Press.

McGinty, E. E., Kennedy-Hendricks, A., Choksy, S., & Barry, C. L. (2016). "Trends in News Media Coverage of Mental Illness in the United States: 1995–2014." *Health Affairs, 35*(6), 1121–1129. https://doi:10.1377/hlthaff.2016.0011

McGinty, E. E., Webster, D. W., & Barry, C. L. (2013). "Effects of News Media Messages about Mass Shootings on Attitudes toward Persons with Serious Mental Illness and Public Support for Gun Control Policies." *American Journal of Psychiatry, 170*(5), 494–501. https://doi:10.1176/appi.ajp.2013.13010014

McGuire, R., McCabe, R., & Priebe, S. (2001). "Theoretical Frameworks for Understanding and Investigating the Therapeutic Relationship in Psychiatry." *Social Psychiatry and Psychiatric Epidemiology, 36*(11), 557–564. https://doi:10.1007/s001270170007

McHugh, P. R., & Slavney, P. R. (1998). *The Perspectives of Psychiatry* (Second ed.). Baltimore: Johns Hopkins University Press.

McKenzie, J. (1922). *Hindu Ethics: A Historical and Critical Essay*. New York: Humphrey Milford/ Oxford University Press.

Meehl, P. E. (1973). *Psychodiagnosis: Selected Papers*. Minneapolis: University of Minnesota Press.

Meehl, P. E. (1995). "Bootstraps Taxometrics: Solving the Classification Problem in Psychopathology." *American Psychologist, 50*(4), 266–275. https://doi:10.1037/0003-066X.50.4.266

Meeks, W. A. (1986). "Understanding Early Christian Ethics." *Journal of Biblical Literature, 105*(1), 3–11. http://www.jstor.org/stable/3261106

Mehlman, M. J. (2009). *The Price of Perfection: Individualism and Society in the Era of Biomedical Enhancement*. Baltimore: Johns Hopkins University Press.

Meijers, J., Harte, J. M., Meynen, G., & Cuijpers, P. (2017). "Differences in Executive Functioning between Violent and Non-Violent Offenders." *Psychological Medicine, 47*(10), 1784–1793. https://doi:10.1017/S0033291717000241

Mendez, M. F., Chow, T., Ringman, J., Twitchell, G., & Hinkin, C. H. (2000). "Pedophilia and Temporal Lobe Disturbances." *Journal of Neuropsychiatry and Clinical Neuroscience, 12*(1), 71–76. https://doi:10.1176/jnp.12.1.71

Mental Health Act Commission (undated). Website: www.mhac.org.uk

Mercier, B., Norris, A., & Shariff, A. F. (2018). "Muslim Mass Shooters Are Perceived as Less Mentally Ill and More Motivated by Religion." *Psychology of Violence, 8*(6), 772–781. https://doi:10.1037/vio 0000217

Merikangas, K. R., & McClair, V. L. (2012). "Epidemiology of Substance Use Disorders." *Human Genetics, 131*(6), 779–789. https://doi:10.1007/s00439-012-1168-0

Meskell, M. W. (1999). "An American Resolution: The History of Prisons in the United States from 1777 to 1877." *Stanford Law Review, 51*(4), 839–865. https://doi:10.2307/1229442

Meynen, G. (2009). "Should or Should Not Forensic Psychiatrists Think About Free Will?" *Medicine, Health Care and Philosophy, 12*(2), 203–212. https://doi:10.1007/s11019-008-9166-7

Meynen, G. (2010a). "Free Will and Mental Disorder: Exploring the Relationship." *Theoretical Medicine and Bioethics, 31*(6), 429–443. https://doi:10.1007/s11017-010-9158-5

Meynen, G. (2010b). "Free Will and Psychiatric Assessments of Criminal Responsibility: A Parallel with Informed Consent." *Medicine, Health Care and Philosophy, 13*(4), 313–320. https://doi:10.1007/ s11019-010-9250-7

Meynen, G. (2012). "Obsessive-Compulsive Disorder, Free Will, and Control." *Philosophy, Psychiatry, & Psychology, 19*(4), 323–332.

Mezuk, B., Needham, B., Joiner, K., Watkins, D., Stoddard, S., Burgard, S., & Link, B. (2021). "What Elephant? Pedagogical Approaches to Addressing Stigma toward Mental Disorders in Undergraduate Public Health Education." *Pedagogy in Health Promotion, 7*(3), 183–190. https://doi:10.1177/23733 79920922871

Mezzich, J. E. (Ed.) (2002). *Culture and Psychiatric Diagnosis: A DSM-IV® Perspective*. Washington, DC: American Psychiatric Publishing.

Mezzich, J. E. (2007). "Psychiatry for the Person: Articulating Medicine's Science and Humanism." *World Psychiatry, 6*(2), 65–67. (https://www.ncbi.nlm.nih.gov/pmc/articles/PMC2219901/

Mezzich, J. E., Kleinman, A., Fabrega, H., & Parron, D. L. (Eds.) (1996). *Culture and Psychiatric Diagnosis: A DSM-IV® Perspective*. Washington, DC: American Psychiatric Press.

Micale, M. S., & Porter, R. (Eds.) (1994). *Discovering the History of Psychiatry*. New York: Oxford University Press.

Michaud, S. G., & Aynesworth, H. (1999). *The Only Living Witness: The True Story of Serial Sex Killer Ted Bundy*. Irving, TX: Authorlink Press.

Millon, T. (2004). *Masters of the Mind: Exploring the Story of Mental Illness from Ancient Times to the New Millennium, First ed*. Hoboken, NJ: John Wiley & Sons.

Millon, T., & Davis, R. D. (1995). "The Development of Personality Disorders." In D. Cicchetti & D. J. Cohen (Eds.), *Developmental Psychopathology, Volume 2: Risk, Disorder, and Adaption* (pp. 633–676). New York: John Wiley & Sons.

Millon, T., & Davis, R. D. (1998). "Ten Subtypes of Psychopathy." In T. Millon, E. Simonsen, M. Birket-Smith, & R. D. Davis (Eds.), *Psychopathy: Antisocial, Criminal, and Violent Behavior* (pp. 161–170). New York: Guilford Press.

Millon, T., & Klerman, G. L. (Eds.) (1986). *Contemporary Directions in Psychopathology: Toward the DSM-IV*. New York: Guilford Press.

Millon, T., Simonsen, E., & Birket-Smith, M. (1998). "Historical Conceptions of Psychopathy in the United States and Europe." In T. Millon, E. Simonsen, M. Birket-Smith, & R. D. Davis (Eds.), *Psychopathy: Antisocial, Criminal, and Violent Behavior* (pp. 3–31). New York: Guilford Press.

Minkler, M. (1999). "Personal Responsibility for Health? A Review of the Arguments and the Evidence at Century's End." *Health Education & Behavior, 26*(1), 121–141. https://doi:10.1177/10901981990 2600110

Minow, M. (1998). "Between Vengeance and Forgiveness: Feminist Responses to Violent Injustice." *New England Law Review, 32*(4), 967–981.

Mohr, J. C. (1997). "The Origins of Forensic Psychiatry in the United States and the Great Nineteenth-Century Crisis over the Adjudication of Wills." *Journal of the American Academy of Psychiatry and Law, 25*(3), 273–284.

Monahan, J., & Arnold, J. (1996). "Violence by People with Mental Illness: A Consensus Statement by Advocates and Researchers." *Psychiatric Rehabilitation Journal, 19*(4), 67–70. https://doi:10.1037/ h0095420

Monahan, J., & Steadman, H. J. (Eds.) (1996). *Violence and Mental Disorder: Developments in Risk Assessment*. Chicago: University of Chicago Press.

Moncrieff, J. (2003). "The Politics of a New Mental Health Act." *British Journal of Psychiatry, 183*(1), 8–9. https://doi:10.1192/bjp.183.1.8

Monfasani, J. (2000). "Humanism." In E. Craig (Ed.), *Concise Routledge Encyclopedia of Philosophy* (pp. 365–366). London New York: Routledge.

Montesquieu, C. (1748). *The Spirit of the Laws*. Translated by T. Nugent [1752]. Kitchener, ON: Batoche Books. https:socialsciences.mcmaster.ca/~econ/ugcm/3ll3/montesquieu/spiritoflaws.pdf

Mooij, A. (1998). "Kant on Criminal Law and Psychiatry." *International Journal of Law and Psychiatry, 21*(4), 335–341. https://doi:10.1016/S0160-2527(98)00027-2

Moore, M. (2011). "Causation in the Criminal Law." In J. Deigh & D. Dolinko (Eds.), *The Oxford Handbook of Philosophy of Criminal Law* (pp. 168–193). Oxford: Oxford University Press.

Mora, G. (2008). "Renaissance Conceptions and Treatments of Madness." In E. R. Wallace IV & J. Gach (Eds.), *History of Psychiatry and Medical Psychology* (pp. 227–254). New York: Springer.

Moran, P. (2002). "Editorial: Dangerous Severe Personality Disorder Bad Tidings from the UK." *International Journal of Social Psychiatry, 48*(1), 6–10. https://doi:10.1177/002076402128783037

Moran, R. (1985). "The Modern Foundation for the Insanity Defense: The Cases of James Hadfield (1800) and Daniel McNaughtan (1843)." *Annals of the American Academy of Political and Social Science, 477*(1), 31–42. https://doi:10.1177/0002716285477001004

Moreno, C., Laje, G., Blanco, C., Jiang, H., Schmidt, A. B., & Olfson, M. (2007). "National Trends in the Outpatient Diagnosis and Treatment of Bipolar Disorder in Youth." *Archives of General Psychiatry, 64*(9), 1032–1039. https://doi:10.1001/archpsyc.64.9.1032

Morgan, A. B., & Lilienfeld, S. O. (2000). "A Meta-Analytic Review of the Relation between Antisocial Behavior and Neuropsychological Measures of Executive Function." *Clinical Psychology Review, 20*(1), 113–136. https://doi:10.1016/S0272-7358(98)00096-8

Morgan, R. E., & Thompson, A. (2021). *Criminal Victimization, 2020* (NCJ Number 301775). Washington, DC: Bureau of Justice Statistics. https://bjs.ojp.gov/library/publications/criminal-victimization-2020.

Morris, N. (1995). "The Contemporary Prison: 1965-Present." In N. Morris & D. J. Rothman (Eds.), *The Oxford History of the Prison: The Practice of Punishment in Western Society* (pp. 227–259). New York: Oxford University Press.

Morris, N. P., & Edwards, M. L. (2022). "Addressing Shortages of Mental Health Professionals in U.S. Jails and Prisons." *Journal of Correctional Health Care, 28*(4), 209–214. https://doi:10.1089/jchc.21.08.0072

Morris, N. P., & West, S. G. (2020). "Misconceptions about Working in Correctional Psychiatry." *Journal of the American Academy of Psychiatry and the Law, 48*(2), 251–258. https://doi:10.29158/jaapl.003 921-20

Morrissey, J. P., & Goldman, H. H. (1984). "Cycles of Reform in the Care of the Chronically Mentally Ill." *Psychiatric Services, 35*(8), 785–793. https://doi:10.1176/ps.35.8.785

Morse, S. J. (1985). "Retaining a Modified Insanity Defense." *Annals of the American Academy of Political and Social Science, 477*(1), 137–147. https://doi:10.1177/0002716285477001013

Morse, S. J. (1998). "Excusing and the New Excuse Defenses: A Legal and Conceptual Review." In M. Tonry (Ed.), *Crime and Justice: A Review of Research* (pp. 329–406). Chicago: University of Chicago Press.

Morse, S. J. (1999). "Neither Desert nor Disease." *Legal Theory, 5*(3), 265–309. https://doi:10.1017/S1352325299053021

Morse, S. J. (2002). "Uncontrollable Urges and Irrational People." *Virginia Law Review, 88*(5), 1025–1078. https://doi:10.2307/1073996

Morse, S. J. (2008). "Vice, Disorder, Conduct, and Culpability." *Philosophy, Psychiatry, & Psychology, 15*(1), 47–49. https://doi:10.1353/ppp.0.0157

Moser, C. (2001). "Paraphilia: A Critique of a Confused Concept." In P. J. Kleinplatz (Ed.), *New Directions in Sex Therapy: Innovations and Alternatives* (pp. 91–108). Philadelphia: Brunner-Routledge.

Moser, C. (2002). "Are Any of the Paraphilias in the DSM Mental Disorders?" *Archives of Sexual Behavior, 31*, 490–491.

Moser, C. (2009). "When Is an Unusual Sexual Interest a Mental Disorder?" *Archives of Sexual Behavior, 38*(3), 323–325. https://doi:10.1007/s10508-008-9436-8

Moser, C. (2011). "Hypersexual Disorder: Just More Muddled Thinking." *Archives of Sexual Behavior, 40*(2), 227–229. https://doi:10.1007/s10508-010-9690-4

Moser, C. (2018). "Paraphilias and the ICD-11: Progress but Still Logically Inconsistent." *Archives of Sexual Behavior, 47*(4), 825–826. https://doi:10.1007/s10508-017-1141-z

Moser, C., & Kleinplatz, P. J. (2005a). "DSM-IV-TR and the Paraphilias: An Argument for Removal." *Journal of Psychology & Human Sexuality, 17*(3–4), 91–109. https://doi:10.1300/J056v17n03_05

Moser, C., & Kleinplatz, P. J. (2005b). "Does Heterosexuality Belong in the DSM?" *Lesbian & Gay Psychology Review, 6*(3), 261–267.

Mosteller, R. P. (1996). "Syndromes and Politics in Criminal Trials and Evidence Law." *Duke Law Journal, 46*(3), 461–516. https://doi:10.2307/1372940

Mott, S. C. (1987). "The Use of the New Testament for Social Ethics." *Journal of Religious Ethics, 15*(2), 225–260. http://www.jstor.org/stable/40015067

Mowen, T. J., Boman, J. H., & Stansfield, R. (2018). "Uniting Needs, Responses, and Theory During Reentry: The Distinct and Joint Contributions of Peer Influence and Religious/Spiritual Support on Substance Use." *Journal of Offender Rehabilitation*, 57(3–4), 222–240. https://doi:10.1080/10509 674.2017.1400488

Mullican, J. S. (1991). "Cultural Literacy: Whose Culture? Whose Literacy?" *English Education*, 23(4), 244–250. http://www.jstor.org/stable/40172768

Munson, R. (1981). "Why Medicine Cannot Be a Science." *Journal of Medicine and Philosophy*, 6(2), 183–208. https://doi:10.1093/jmp/6.2.183

Murphy, J. G. (2007). "Legal Moralism and Retribution Revisited." *Criminal Law and Philosophy*, 1(1), 5–20. https://doi:10.1007/s11572-006-9000-3

Murphy, M. (2019). "The Natural Law Tradition in Ethics." In E. N. Zalta (Ed.), *The Stanford Encyclopedia of Philosophy* (Summer 2019 ed.). Stanford, CA: Metaphysics Research Lab, Stanford University. https://plato.stanford.edu/archives/sum2019/entries/natural-law-ethics/

Murray-Close, D., Ostrov, J. M., Nelson, D. A., Crick, N. R., & Coccaro, E. F. (2010). "Proactive, Reactive, and Romantic Relational Aggression in Adulthood: Measurement, Predictive Validity, Gender Differences, and Association with Intermittent Explosive Disorder." *Journal of Psychiatric Research*, 44(6), 393–404. https://doi:10.1016/j.jpsychires.2009.09.005

Nabokov, V. (2010). *Lolita*. New York: Vintage/Random House.

Nadelson, T. (1979). "The Munchausen Spectrum: Borderline Character Features." *General Hospital Psychiatry*, 1(1), 11–17. https://doi:10.1016/0163-8343(79)90073-2

Nadler, S. (2020). "Baruch Spinoza." In E. N. Zalta (Ed.), *The Stanford Encyclopedia of Philosophy* (Summer 2020 ed.). Stanford, CA: Metaphysics Research Lab, Stanford University. https://plato.stanford.edu/archives/sum2020/entries/spinoza/

Nanji, A. (1993). "Islamic Ethics." In P. Singer (Ed.), *A Companion to Ethics* (pp. 106–118). Cambridge, MA: Blackwell Publishing.

Nasser, M. (1987). "Psychiatry in Ancient Egypt." *Bulletin of the Royal College of Psychiatrists*, 11(12), 420–422. https://doi:10.1192/pb.11.12.420

Nastasi, B. K. (2004). "Meeting the Challenges of the Future: Integrating Public Health and Public Education for Mental Health Promotion." *Journal of Educational and Psychological Consultation*, 15(3-4), 295–312. https://doi:10.1080/10474412.2004.9669519

Natanson, M. (1973). *Edmund Husserl: Philosopher of Infinite Tasks*. Evanston, IL: Northwestern University Press.

National Advisory Mental Health Council's Workgroup (2010). *From Discovery to Cure: Accelerating the Development of New and Personalized Interventions for Mental Illnesses*. https://www.nimh.nih.gov/sites/default/files/documents/about/advisory-boards-and-groups/namhc/reports/fromdisc overytocure.pdf

National Center on Addiction and Substance Abuse at Columbia University (CASA) (2010). *Behind Bars II Substance Abuse and America's Prison Population* (NCJ Number: 230327). https://www.ojp.gov/ncjrs/virtual-library/abstracts behind-bars-ii-substance-abuse-and-americas-prison-population

National Institute of Corrections Information Center (NICIC) (undated). *Mentally Ill Persons in Corrections*. http://nicic.gov/mentalillness

National Institute of Mental Health (2012). "Daily or Severe Tantrums May Point to Mental Health Issues." *Science News*, 29 August 2012. https://www.nimh.nih.gov/archive/news/2012/daily-or-sev ere-tantrums-may-point-to-mental-health-issues

National Institute of Mental Health (2022). *Mental Health Information: Statistics*. https://www.nimh.nih.gov/health statistics/mental-illness

Nayak, S. (2021). "Intersectionality and Psychotherapy with an Eye to Clinical and Professional Ethics." In M. Trachsel, J. Gaab, N. Biller-Andorno, Ş. Tekin, & J. Z. Sadler (Eds.), *The Oxford Handbook of Psychotherapy Ethics* (pp. 890–903). Oxford: Oxford University Press.

Nederman, C. (2019). "Niccolò Machiavelli." In E. N. Zalta (Ed.), *The Stanford Encyclopedia of Philosophy* (Summer 2019 ed.). Stanford, CA: Metaphysics Research Lab, Stanford University. https://plato.stanford.edu/archives/sum2019/entries/machiavelli/

Nedopil, N. (2009). "The Role of Forensic Psychiatry in Mental Health Systems in Europe." *Criminal Behaviour and Mental Health*, 19(4), 224–234. https://doi:10.1002/cbm.719

Neely, C. T. (1991). "'Documents in Madness': Reading Madness and Gender in Shakespeare's Tragedies and Early Modern Culture." *Shakespeare Quarterly*, 42(3), 315–338. https://doi:10.2307/2870846

Neely, C. T. (2004). *Distracted Subjects: Madness and Gender in Shakespeare and Early Modern Culture*. Cambridge: Cambridge University Press.

Nemec, P. B., & Mullen, M. G. (2017). "The Long Road from Policy to Practice." *Psychiatric Rehabilitation Journal, 40*(2), 260–262. https://doi:10.1037/prj0000265

Nemeroff, C. B., Weinberger, D., Rutter, M., MacMillan, H. L., Bryant, R. A., Wessely, S., . . . Lysaker, P. (2013). "DSM-5: A Collection of Psychiatrist Views on the Changes, Controversies, and Future Directions." *BMC Medicine, 11*. https://doi.org/10.1186/1741-7015-11-202

Nestler, E. J. (2014). "Epigenetic Mechanisms of Drug Addiction." *Neuropharmacology, 76*, 259–268. https://doi:10.1016/j.neuropharm.2013.04.004

Newhauser, R. (Ed.) (2007). *The Seven Deadly Sins: From Communities to Individuals* (Studies in Medieval and Reformation Traditions series). Leiden/Boston: Brill.

Nielsen, K. E. (2012). *A Disability History of the United States*. Boston: Beacon Press.

Niemiec, R. M. (2019). "Finding the Golden Mean: The Overuse, Underuse, and Optimal Use of Character Strengths." *Counselling Psychology Quarterly, 32*(3–4), 453–471. https://doi:10.1080/09515070.2019.1617674

Niemiec, R. M., Shogren, K. A., & Wehmeyer, M. L. (2017). "Character Strengths and Intellectual and Developmental Disability: A Strengths-Based Approach from Positive Psychology." *Education and Training in Autism and Developmental Disabilities, 52*(1), 13–25. https://www.jstor.org/stable/26420372

Noll, S., & Trent Jr., J. W. (Eds.) (2004). *Mental Retardation in America: A Historical Reader*. New York: New York University Press.

Nordenfelt, L. (2000). *Action, Ability and Health: Essays in the Philosophy of Action and Welfare*. Dordrecht: Kluwer Academic Publishers.

Nordenfelt, L. (2001). "On the Goals of Medicine, Health Enhancement and Social Welfare." *Health Care Analysis, 9*(1), 15–23. https://doi:10.1023/A:1011350927112

Nordenfelt, L., & Lindahl, B. I. B. (Eds.) (2012). *Health, Disease, and Causal Explanations in Medicine* (Philosophy of Medicine series, Vol. 16). New York: Springer.

Nozick, R. (1974). *Anarchy, State, and Utopia*. New York: Basic Books.

Nunnally, J. C. (1961). *Popular Conceptions of Mental Health, Their Development and Change*. New York: Holt, Rinehart, & Winston.

Nussbaum, M. C. (1999). *Sex and Social Justice*. New York: Oxford University Press.

Nussbaum, M. C. (2006). *Frontiers of Justice: Disability, Nationality, Species Membership*. Cambridge, MA: Belknap Press.

Nussbaum, M. C. (2013). *Political Emotions: Why Love Matters for Justice*. Cambridge, MA: Harvard University Press.

Nussbaum, M. C. (2019). *The Monarchy of Fear: A Philosopher Looks at Our Political Crisis*. New York: Simon & Schuster.

Nussbaum, M. C. (2020). "The Capabilities Approach and the History of Philosophy." In E. Chiappero-Martinetti, S. Osmani, & M. Qizilbash (Eds.), *The Cambridge Handbook of the Capability Approach* (pp. 13–39). Cambridge: Cambridge University Press.

Nutbeam, D. (2000). "Health Literacy as a Public Health Goal: A Challenge for Contemporary Health Education and Communication Strategies into the 21st Century." *Health Promotion International, 15*(3), 259–267. https://doi:10.1093/heapro/15.3.259

Nye, R. A. (1999). *Sexuality*. Oxford: Oxford University Press.

O'Brien, P. (1983). "The Kleptomania Diagnosis: Bourgeois Women and Theft in Late Nineteenth-Century France." *Journal of Social History, 17*(1), 65–77. https://doi:10.1353/jsh/17.1.65

O'Donohue, W., Regev, L. G., & Hagstrom, A. (2000). "Problems with the DSM-IV Diagnosis of Pedophilia." *Sexual Abuse: A Journal of Research and Treatment, 12*(2), 95–105. https://doi:10.1023/A:1009586023326

Oexle, N., & Corrigan, P. W. (2018). "Understanding Mental Illness Stigma toward Persons with Multiple Stigmatized Conditions: Implications of Intersectionality Theory." *Psychiatric Services, 69*(5), 587–589. https://doi:10.1176/appi.ps.201700312

Ogden, C. K. (1932). *Bentham's Theory of Fictions* (First ed.). New York: Harcourt, Brace and Company.

Ogilvie, J. M., Stewart, A. L., Chan, R. C. K., & Shum, D. H. K. (2011). "Neuropsychological Measures of Executive Function and Antisocial Behavior: A Meta-Analysis." *Criminology, 49*(4), 1063–1107. https://doi:10.1111/j.1745-9125.2011.00252.x

Oliver, M. B. (2003). "African American Men as 'Criminal and Dangerous': Implications of Media Portrayals of Crime on the 'Criminalization' of African American Men." *Journal of African American Studies, 7*(2), 3–18. https://doi:10.1007/s12111-003-1006-5

Olstead, R. (2002). "Contesting the Text: Canadian Media Depictions of the Conflation of Mental Illness and Criminality." *Sociology of Health and Illness, 24*(5), 621–643. https://doi:10.1111/1467-9566.00311

Oosterhuis, H. (2000). *Stepchildren of Nature: Krafft-Ebing, Psychiatry, and the Making of Sexual Identity.* Chicago: University of Chicago Press.

Orso, D., Federici, N., Copetti, R., Vetrugno, L., & Bove, T. (2020). "Infodemic and the Spread of Fake News in the COVID-19-Era." *European Journal of Emergency Medicine, 27*(5), 327–328. https://doi:10.1097/mej.0000000000000713

Orszag, P. R., & Ellis, P. (2007). "The Challenge of Rising Health Care Costs—A View from the Congressional Budget Office." *New England Journal of Medicine, 357*(18), 1793–1795. https://doi:10.1056/NEJMp078190

Osler, A., & Starkey, H. (2006). "Education for Democratic Citizenship: A Review of Research, Policy and Practice 1995–2005." *Research Papers in Education, 21*(4), 433–466. https://doi:10.1080/02671520600942438

Oulton, C., Day, V., Dillon, J., & Grace, M. (2004). "Controversial Issues - Teachers' Attitudes and Practices in the Context of Citizenship Education." *Oxford Review of Education, 30*(4), 489–507. https://doi:10.1080/0305498042000303973

Overholser, W. (1959). "Shakespeare's Psychiatry—And After." *Shakespeare Quarterly, 10*(3), 335–352. https://doi:10.2307/2866854

Packer, H. L. (1964). "Two Models of the Criminal Process." *University of Pennsylvania Law Review, 113*(1), 1–68. https://doi:10.2307/3310562

Packer, H. L. (1968). *The Limits of the Criminal Sanction.* Stanford, CA: Stanford University Press.

Paine, H. L. (1923). "Psychotic Symptoms of Epilepsy." *American Journal of Psychiatry, 79*(4), 713–719. https://doi:10.1176/ajp.79.4.713

Palmer, R. E. (1969). *Hermeneutics: Interpretation Theory in Schleiermacher, Dilthey, Heidegger, and Gadamer.* Evanston, IL: Northwestern University Press.

Paolucci, E. O., & Violato, C. (2004). "A Meta-Analysis of the Published Research on the Affective, Cognitive, and Behavioral Effects of Corporal Punishment." *Journal of Psychology, 138*(3), 197–222. https://doi:10.3200/JRLP.138.3.197-222

Pardo, M. S. (2005). "The Field of Evidence and the Field of Knowledge." *Law and Philosophy, 24*(4), 321–392. https://doi:10.1007/s10982-004-4999-6

Parens, E., & Johnston, J. (2011). "Troubled Children: Diagnosing, Treating, and Attending to Context." *Hastings Center Report, 41*(2), S4–S31. https://doi.org/10.1353/hcr.2011.0032

Paris, J., & Phillips, J. (Eds.) (2013). *Making the DSM-5: Concepts and Controversies.* New York: Springer.

Park, N., & Peterson, C. (2006). "Methodological Issues in Positive Psychology and the Assessment of Character Strengths." In A. D. Ong & M. H. M. van Dulmen (Eds.), *Handbook of Methods in Positive Psychology* (pp. 292–305). New York: Oxford University Press.

Parnas, J., Sass, L. A., & Kendler, K. S. (Eds.) (2008). *Philosophical Issues in Psychiatry: Explanation, Phenomenology, and Nosology.* Baltimore: Johns Hopkins University Press.

Parsons, H. C. (1918). "Effect of the War on the Reformative Probation and Suspended Sentence (Report of Committee "B" of the Institute)." *Journal of Criminal Law and Criminology, 9*(3), 420–424. https://doi:10.2307/1133555

Partridge, G. E. (1930). "Current Conceptions of Psychopathic Personality." *American Journal of Psychiatry, 87*(1), 53–99. https://doi:10.1176/ajp.87.1.53

Pasewark, R. A. (1986). "A Review of Research on the Insanity Defense." *Annals of the American Academy of Political and Social Sciences, 484*(1), 100–114. https://doi:10.1177/0002716286484001008

Pasewark, R. A., & Seidenzahl, D. (1979). "Opinions Concerning the Insanity Plea and Criminality among Mental Patients." *Bulletin of the American Academy of Psychiatry and the Law, 7*(2), 199–204.

Patrick, C. J. (Ed.) (2006). *Handbook of Psychopathy* (First ed.). New York: Guilford Press.

Pellegrino, E. D. (1999). "The Goals and Ends of Medicine: How Are They to Be Defined?" In M. J. Hanson & D. Callahan (Eds.), *The Goals of Medicine: The Forgotten Issue in Health Care Reform* (pp. 55–68). Washington, DC: Georgetown University Press.

Pellegrino, E. D., & Thomasma, D. C. (1981). *A Philosophical Basis of Medical Practice: Toward a Philosophy and Ethic of the Healing Professions*. New York: Oxford University Press.

Penrose, L. S. (1939). "Mental Disease and Crime: Outline of a Comparative Study of European Statistics." *British Journal of Medical Psychology*, *18*(1), 1–15. https://doi:10.1111/j.2044-8341.1939.tb00704.x

Pereboom, D. (2020). "Incapacitation, Reintegration, and Limited General Deterrence." *Neuroethics*, *13*(1), 87–97. https://doi:10.1007/s12152-018-9382-7

Pescosolido, B. A. (2013). "The Public Stigma of Mental Illness: What Do We Think; What Do We Know; What Can We Prove?" *Journal of Health and Social Behavior*, *54*(1), 1–21. https://doi:10.1177/0022146512471197

Peskin, M., Gao, Y., Glenn, A. L., Rudo-Hutt, A., Yang, Y., & Raine, A. (2012). "Biology and Crime." In F. T. Cullen & P. Wilcox (Eds.), *Oxford Handbook of Criminological Theory* (pp. 22–39). New York: Oxford University Press.

Peter, E. (2013). "Advancing the Concept of Moral Distress." *Journal of Bioethical Inquiry*, *10*(3), 293–295. https://doi:10.1007/s11673-013-9471-6

Peternelj-Taylor, C. (2004). "An Exploration of Othering in Forensic Psychiatric and Correctional Nursing." *Canadian Journal of Nursing Research*, *36*(4), 130–146. https://cjnr.archive.mcgill.ca/article/view/1915

Peterson, C., & Seligman, M. E. P. (2004). *Character Strengths and Virtues: A Handbook and Classification*. New York: Oxford University Press.

Petherick, W., Turvey, B. E., & Ferguson, C. E. (Eds.) (2009). *Forensic Criminology*. London: Elsevier Academic Press.

Petry, N. M., Zajac, K., & Ginley, M. K. (2018). "Behavioral Addictions as Mental Disorders: To Be or Not to Be?" *Annual Review of Clinical Psychology*, *14*, 399–423. https://doi:10.1146/annurev-clinpsy-032816-045120

Pettit, P. (2002). "Is Criminal Justice Politically Feasible?" *Buffalo Criminal Law Review*, *5*(2), 427–450. https://doi:10.1525/nclr.2002.5.2.427

Pew Center on the States (2009). *One in 31: The Long Reach of American Corrections*. Washington, DC: The Pew Charitable Trusts. https://www.pewtrusts.org/en/research-and-analysis/reports/2009/03/02/one-in-31-the-long-reach-of-american-corrections

Phillips, H. K., Gray, N. S., MacCulloch, S. I., Taylor, J., Moore, S. C., Huckle, P., & MacCulloch, M. J. (2005). "Risk Assessment in Offenders with Mental Disorders: Relative Efficacy of Personal Demographic, Criminal History, and Clinical Variables." *Journal of Interpersonal Violence*, *20*(7), 833–847. https://doi:10.1177/0886260504272898

Phillips, J. (1996). "Key Concepts: Hermeneutics." *Philosophy, Psychiatry, & Psychology*, *3*(1), 61–69. https://doi:10.1353/ppp.1996.0007

Phillips, J., Frances, A., Cerullo, M. A., Chardavoyne, J., Decker, H. S., First, M. B., . . . Zachar, P. (2012). The six most essential questions in psychiatric diagnosis: a pluralogue part 1: conceptual and definitional issues in psychiatric diagnosis. *Philosophy, Ethics, and Humanities in Medicine*, *7*, 1–29.

Phillips, J., & Sadler, J. Z. (2021). "Evidence, Science, and Ethics in Talk-Based Healing Practices." In M. Trachsel, J. Gaab, N. Biller-Andorno, Ş. Tekin, & J. Z. Sadler (Eds.), *The Oxford Handbook of Psychotherapy Ethic* (pp. 288–310). New York: Oxford University Press.

Pickard, H. (2011). "Responsibility without Blame: Empathy and the Effective Treatment of Personality Disorder." *Philosophy, Psychiatry, & Psychology*, *18*(3), 209–223. https://doi:10.1353/ppp.2011.0032

Pilgrim, D. (2007). "The Survival of Psychiatric Diagnosis." *Social Science & Medicine*, *65*(3), 536–547. https://doi:10.1016/j.socscimed.2007.03.054

Pilgrim, D. (2012). "Lessons from the Mental Health Act Commission for England and Wales: The Limitations of Legalism—Plus-Safeguards." *Journal of Social Policy*, *41*(1), 61–81. https://doi:10.1017/S0047279411000523

Pincus, H. A., Frances, A., Davis, W. W., First, M. B., & Widiger, T. A. (1992). "DSM-IV and New Diagnostic Categories: Holding the Line on Proliferation." *American Journal of Psychiatry, 149*(1), 112–117. https://doi:10.1176/ajp.149.1.112

Pincus, H. A., & McQueen, L. (2002). "The Limits of an Evidence-Based Classification of Mental Disorders." In J. Z. Sadler (Ed.), *Descriptions and Prescriptions: Values, Mental Disorders, and the DSMs* (pp. 9–24). Baltimore: Johns Hopkins University Press.

Pink, T. (2000). "The Will." In E. Craig (Ed.), *The Routledge Encyclopedia of Philosophy* (pp. 929). London/New York: Routledge.

Pizarro, J. M., Stenius, V. M. K., & Pratt, T. C. (2006). "Supermax Prisons: Myths, Realities, and the Politics of Punishment in American Society." *Criminal Justice Policy Review, 17*(1), 6–21. https://doi:10.1177/0887403405275015

Plato (360 BCE). *Phaedrus*. Available from MIT The Internet Classics Archive by Daniel C. Stevenson, Web Atomics. http://classics.mit.edu/Plato/phaedrus.html

Plato (1991). *The Republic: The Complete and Unabridged Jowett Translation*. Translated by B. Jowett. New York: Vintage Books.

Plato (2009). *Phaedo*. Translated by D. Gallop. Oxford: Oxford University Press.

Plato, Phaedrus, tr. Benjamin Jowett, not dated, available online http://classics.mit.edu/Plato/phaedrus.html

Pleasant, A. (2013). "Health Literacy around the World: Part 1. Health Literacy Efforts Outside of the United States." *Health Literacy, 1*, 97–203.

Pleck, E. (1987). *Domestic Tyranny: The Making of Social Policy against Family Violence from Colonial Times to the Present*. New York: Oxford University Press.

Plucknett, T. F. T. (1956/2010). *A Concise History of the Common Law, Fifth ed*. Indianapolis, IN: Liberty Fund. https://oll.libertyfund.org/title/plucknett-a-concise-history-of-the-common-law

Plutarch, L. M. (1894). *Plutarch's Lives*. Translated by A. Aubrey & G. Long. London: George Bell & Sons. https://gutenberg.org/files/14033/14033-h/14033-h.htm#LIFE_OF_SOLON

Pocai, B. (2019). The ICD-11 has been adopted by the World Health Assembly. *World Psychiatry, 18*(3), 371-372.

Poehlmann-Tynan, J., Runion, H., Weymouth, L. A., & Burnson, C. (2019). "Children with Incarcerated Parents." In T. H. Ollendick, S. W. White, & B. A. White (Eds.), *The Oxford Handbook of Clinical Child and Adolescent Psychology* (pp. 511–525). New York: Oxford University Press.

Pollack, S. (1974). "Forensic Psychiatry—A Specialty." *Bulletin of the American Academy of Psychiatry and the Law, 11*(1), 1–6.

Porter, J. P., & Koski, G. (2008). "Regulations for the Protection of Humans in Research in the United States: The Common Rule." In E. J. Emanuel, C. C. Grady, R. A. Crouch, R. K. Lie, F. G. Miller, & D. D. Wendler (Eds.), *The Oxford Textbook of Clinical Research Ethics* (pp. 156–167). New York: Oxford University Press.

Porter, R. (1983). "The Rage of Party: A Glorious Revolution in English Psychiatry?" *Medical History, 27*(1), 35–50. https://doi:10.1017/s0025727300042253

Porter, R. (1999). *The Greatest Benefit to Mankind: A Medical History of Humanity*. New York: W.W. Norton & Company.

Porter, R. (2002). *Madness: A Brief History*. Oxford: Oxford University Press.

Porter, R. (2003). *Flesh in the Age of Reason* (First American ed.). New York: W.W. Norton & Co.

Porter, R. (2004). *Madmen: A Social History of Madhouses, Mad—Doctors & Lunatics*. Stroud: Tempus

Porter, R., & Hall, L. A. (1995). *The Facts of Life: The Creation of Sexual Knowledge in Britain, 1650–1950*. New Haven, CT: Yale University Press.

Porter, R., & Teich, M. (Eds.) (1994). *Sexual Knowledge, Sexual Science: The History of Attitudes to Sexuality*. Cambridge: Cambridge University Press.

Potter, N. N. (Ed.) (2006). *Trauma, Truth and Reconciliation: Healing Damaged Relationships*. Oxford: Oxford University Press.

Potter, N. N. (2009). *Mapping the Edges and the in-Between: A Critical Analysis of Borderline Personality Disorder*. New York: Oxford University Press.

Potter, N. N. (2013). "Moral Evaluations and the Cluster B Personality Disorders." *Philosophy, Psychiatry, & Psychology, 20*(3), 217–219. https://doi:10.1353/ppp.2013.0037

Potter, N. N. (2016). *The Virtue of Defiance and Psychiatric Engagement*. Oxford: Oxford University Press.

Potter, W. (2010). *Deadly Spin: An Insurance Company Insider Speaks out on How Corporate PR Is Killing Health Care and Deceiving Americans*. New York: Bloomsbury Press.

Potter, W., & Penniman, N. (2017). *Nation on the Take: How Big Money Corrupts Our Democracy and What We Can Do About It*. New York: Bloomsbury Press.

Pound, R. (1959). *An Introduction to the Philosophy of Law, Revised ed.* New Haven, CT: Yale University Press.

Prebish, C. S. (1996). Ambiguity and Conflict in the Study of Buddhist Ethics: An Introduction. *The Journal of Religious Ethics*, 24(2), 295–303. https://www.jstor.org/stable/40015211

President's Commission on Law Enforcement and Administration of Justice (1967). *Challenge of Crime in a Free Society*. Washington, DC: U.S. Department of Justice, Office of Justice Programs. https: www.ojp.gov/ncjrs/virtual-library/abstracts/challenge-crime-free-society

Prins, J. T., Hoekstra-Weebers, J. E., Gazendam-Donofrio, S. M., Dillingh, G. S., Bakker, A. B., Huisman, M., . . . van der Heijden, F. M. (2010). "Burnout and Engagement among Resident Doctors in the Netherlands: A National Study." *Medical Education*, 44(3), 236–247. https://doi:10.1111/j.1365-2923.2009.03590.x

ProPublica (2016). https://www.propublica.org/article/the-executive-pay-cap-that-backfired.

Prosono, M. T. (2003). "History of Forensic Psychiatry." In R. Rosner (Ed.), *Principles and Practice of Forensic Psychiatry, Second ed.* (pp. 14–30). Boca Raton, FL: CRC Press.

Pryce, A. (2006). "Let's Talk About Sexual Behavior in the Human Male: Kinsey and the Invention of (Post)Modern Sexualities." *Sexuality & Culture*, 10(1), 63–93. https://doi:10.1007/s12119-006-1007-3

Public Broadcasting System (PBS), US (2002). "State Insanity Defense Laws." *Frontline*. https://www.pbs.org/wgbh/pages frontline/shows/crime/trial/states.html

Putkonen, A., Kotilainen, I., Joyal, C. C., & Tiihonen, J. (2004). "Comorbid Personality Disorders and Substance Use Disorders of Mentally Ill Homicide Offenders: A Structured Clinical Study on Dual and Triple Diagnoses." *Schizophrenia Bulletin*, 30(1), 59–72. https://doi:10.1093/oxfordjournals.schbul.a007068

Putnam, H. (1981). "Fact and Value." In *Reason, Truth and History* (pp. 127–149). New York: Cambridge University Press.

Putnam, H. (1990a). "Beyond the Fact/Value Dichotomy." In J. Conant (Ed.), *Realism with a Human Face* (pp. 135–141). Cambridge, MA: Harvard University Press.

Putnam, H. (1990b). "The Place of Facts in a World of Values." In J. Conant (Ed.), *Realism with a Human Face* (pp. 142–162). Cambridge, MA: Harvard University Press.

Quen, J. M. (1983). "Isaac Ray and the Development of American Psychiatry and the Law." *Psychiatric Clinics of North America*, 6(4), 527–537. https://doi:10.1016/S0193-953X(18)30792-5

Quen, J. M. (1994). "Law and Psychiatry in America over the Past 150 Years." *Psychiatric Services*, 45(10), 1005–1010. https://doi:10.1176/ps.45.10.1005

Quinn, J. F., Forsyth, C. J., & Mullen-Quinn, C. (2004). "Societal Reaction to Sex Offenders: A Review of the Origins and Results of the Myths Surrounding Their Crimes and Treatment Amenability." *Deviant Behavior*, 25(3), 215–232. https://doi:10.1080/01639620490431147

Quinn, M. A., Wilcox, A., Orav, E. J., Bates, D. W., & Simon, S. R. (2009). "The Relationship between Perceived Practice Quality and Quality Improvement Activities and Physician Practice Dissatisfaction, Professional Isolation, and Work-Life Stress." *Medical Care*, 47(8), 924–928. https://doi:10.1097/mlr.0b013e3181a393e4

Quinn, P. L. (2000). "Sin." In E. Craig (Ed.), *Routledge Concise Encyclopedia of Philosophy* (pp. 831–832). London: Routledge.

Quinsey, V. L. (2010). "Coercive Paraphilic Disorder." *Archives of Sexual Behavior*, 39(2), 405–410. https://doi:10.1007/s10508-009-9547-x

Quinsey, V. L. (2012). "Pragmatic and Darwinian Views of the Paraphilias." *Archives of Sexual Behavior*, 41(1), 217–220. https://doi:10.1007/s10508-011-9872-8

Rabkin, J. (1974). "Public Attitudes toward Mental Illness: A Review of the Literature." *Schizophrenia Bulletin*, 1(10), 9–33. https://doi:10.1093/schbul/1.10.9

Rabkin, J. G. (1972). "Opinions about Mental Illness: A Review of the Literature." *Psychological Bulletin*, 77(3), 153–171. https://doi:10.1037/h0032341

Radden, J. (1994). "Recent Criticism of Psychiatric Nosology: A Review." *Philosophy, Psychiatry, & Psychology*, 1(3), 193–200.

Radden, J. (1996). "Lumps and Bumps: Kantian Faculty Psychology, Phrenology, and Twentieth-Century Psychiatric Classification." *Philosophy, Psychiatry, & Psychology*, 3(1), 1–14. https://doi:10.1353/ppp.1996.0008

Radden, J. (Ed.) (2002). *The Nature of Melancholy: From Aristotle to Kristeva*. New York: Oxford University Press.

Radden, J., & Sadler, J. Z. (2010). *The Virtuous Psychiatrist: Character Ethics in Psychiatric Practice*. Oxford/New York: Oxford University Press.

Rafter, N. (2008). *The Criminal Brain: Understanding Biological Theories of Crime*. New York: NYU Press.

Rafter, N. H. (1997a). *Creating Born Criminals*. Urbana: University of Illinois Press.

Rafter, N. H. (1997b). "Psychopathy and the Evolution of Criminological Knowledge." *Theoretical Criminology*, 1(2), 235–259. https://doi:10.1177/1362480697001002004

Raine, A. (2001). "A Reply to Dolan's and Cordess' Reviews of *The Psychopathology of Crime*." *Cognitive Neuropsychiatry*, 6(4), 304–307. https://doi:10.1080/13546800143000078

Raine, A. (2013). *The Psychopathology of Crime: Criminal Behavior as a Clinical Disorder*. Amsterdam: Elsevier.

Ramsey, P. (1950). *Basic Christian Ethics*. New York: Scribner.

Rapley, M., Moncrieff, J., & Dillon, J. (2011). "Carving Nature at Its Joints? DSM and the Medicalization of Everyday Life." In M. Rapley, J. Moncrieff, & J. Dillon (Eds.), *De-Medicalizing Misery: Psychiatry, Psychology and the Human Condition* (pp. 1–9). London: Palgrave Macmillan.

Ratcliffe, M. (2008). *Feelings of Being: Phenomenology, Psychiatry and the Sense of Reality*. New York: Oxford University Press.

Ravenscroft, I. (2010). "Folk Psychology as a Theory." In E. N. Zalta (Ed.), *The Stanford Encyclopedia of Philosophy* (Fall 2010 ed.). Stanford, CA: The Metaphysics Research Lab. http://plato.stanford.edu/archives/fall2010/entries/folkpsych-theory

Rawls, J. (2005). *Political Liberalism, Expanded ed*. New York: Columbia University Press.

Ray, I. (1838). *A Treatise on the Medical Jurisprudence of Insanity* Boston: Little, Brown and Company.

Raymond, N. C., Coleman, E., Ohlerking, F., Christenson, G. A., & Miner, M. (1999). "Psychiatric Comorbidity in Pedophilic Sex Offenders." *American Journal of Psychiatry*, 156(5), 786–788. https://doi:10.1176/ajp.156.5.786

Raynor, P. (2007). "Community Penalties: Probation, 'What Works' and Offender Management." In M. Maguire, R. Morgan, & R. Reiner (Eds.), *The Oxford Handbook of Criminology* (pp. 1061–1099). New York: Oxford University Press.

Regier, D. A., Narrow, W. E., Kuhl, E. A., & Kupfer, D. J. (2009). "The Conceptual Development of DSM-V." *American Journal of Psychiatry*, 166(6), 645–650. https://doi:10.1176/appi.ajp.2009.09020279

Reid, R. C., Carpenter, B. N., Hook, J. N., Garos, S., Manning, J. C., Gilliland, R., . . . Fong, T. (2012). "Report of Findings in a DSM-5 Field Trial for Hypersexual Disorder." *The Journal of Sexual Medicine*, 9(11), 2868–2877. https://doi:10.1111/j.1743-6109.2012.02936.x

Reimer, M. (2013). "Moral Disorder in the DSM-IV?: The Cluster B Personality Disorders." *Philosophy, Psychiatry, & Psychology*, 20(3), 203–215. https://doi:10.1353/ppp.2013.0034

Reiner, R. (2007). "Media-Made Criminality: The Representation of Crime in the Mass Media." In M. Maguire, R. Morgan, & R. Reiner (Eds.), *The Oxford Handbook of Criminology* (Fourth ed.) (pp. 302–337). Oxford: Oxford University Press.

Relman, A. S. (1980). "The New Medical-Industrial Complex." *New England Journal of Medicine*, 303(17), 963–970. https://doi:10.1056/nejm198010233031703

Relman, A. S. (2007). *A Second Opinion: Rescuing America's Health Care*. New York: Public Affairs Books.

Rennison, C. (2002). *National Crime Victimization Survey: Criminal Victimization 2001, Changes 2000-01 with Trends 1993-2001* (NCJ 194610). Washington, DC: US Department of Justice, Bureau of Justice Statistics. https://bjs.ojp.gov/content/pub/pdf/cv01.pdf

Resnick, P. J. (1986). "Perceptions of Psychiatric Testimony: A Historical Perspective on the Hysterical Invective." *Bulletin of the American Academy of Psychiatry and the Law*, 14(3), 203–219.

Resnick, P. J. (2007). "The Andrea Yates Case: Insanity on Trial." *Cleveland State Law Review, 55*(2), 147–156.

Resnik, D. B. (2007). "Responsibility for Health: Personal, Social, and Environmental." *Journal of Medical Ethics, 33*(8), 444–445. https://doi:10.1136/jme.2006.017574

Restak, R. M. (2000). *Mysteries of the Mind.* Washington, DC: National Geographic Society.

Reverby, S. M. (2009). *Examining Tuskegee: The Infamous Syphilis Study and Its Legacy.* Chapel Hill: University of North Carolina Press.

Reynolds III, C. F., Lewis, D. A., Detre, T., Schatzberg, A. F., & Kupfer, D. J. (2009). "The Future of Psychiatry as Clinical Neuroscience." *Academic Medicine, 84*(4), 446–450. https://doi:10.1097/ACM.0b013e31819a8052

Rhodes, R. (2019). "Why Not Common Morality?" *Journal of Medical Ethics, 45*(12), 770–777. https://doi:10.1136/medethics-2019-105621

Rich, B. A., Grimley, M. E., Schmajuk, M., Blair, K. S., Blair, R. J. R., & Leibenluft, E. (2008). "Face Emotion Labeling Deficits in Children with Bipolar Disorder and Severe Mood Dysregulation." *Development and Psychopathology, 20*(2), 529–546. https://doi:10.1017/S0954579408000266

Rich, B. A., Schmajuk, M., Perez-Edgar, K. E., Fox, N. A., Pine, D. S., & Leibenluft, E. (2007). "Different Psychophysiological and Behavioral Responses Elicited by Frustration in Pediatric Bipolar Disorder and Severe Mood Dysregulation." *American Journal of Psychiatry, 164*(2), 309–317. https://doi:10.1176/ajp.2007.164.2.309

Riedel-Heller, S. G., Matschinger, H., & Angermeyer, M. C. (2005). "Mental Disorders—Who and What Might Help?" *Social Psychiatry and Psychiatric Epidemiology, 40*(2), 167–174. https://doi:10.1007/s00127-005-0863-8

Rissmiller, D. J., & Rissmiller, J. H. (2006). "Open Forum: Evolution of the Antipsychiatry Movement into Mental Health Consumerism." *Psychiatric Services, 57*(6), 863–866. https://doi:10.1176/ps.2006.57.6.863

Roach, K. (1999). "Four Models of the Criminal Process." *Journal of Criminal Law and Criminology (1973-), 89*(2), 671–716. https://doi:10.2307/1144140

Robeyns, I. (2021). "The Capability Approach." In G. Berik & E. Kongar (Eds.), *The Routledge Handbook of Feminist Economics* (pp. 72–80). London: Routledge.

Robins, E., & Guze, S. B. (1970). "Establishment of Diagnostic Validity in Psychiatric Illness: Its Application to Schizophrenia." *American Journal of Psychiatry, 126*(7), 983–987. https://doi:10.1176/ajp.126.7.983

Robinson, D. N. (1996). *Wild Beasts and Idle Humours: The Insanity Defense from Antiquity to the Present.* Cambridge, MA: Harvard University Press.

Robitscher, J. (1978). "The Many Faces of Forensic Psychiatry." *Bulletin of the American Academy of Psychiatry and the Law, 6*(2), 209–213.

Rocca, M. D. (2005). "Descartes, the Cartesian Circle, and Epistemology without God." *Philosophy and Phenomenological Research, 70*(1), 1–33. https://doi:10.1111/j.1933-1592.2005.tb00504.x

Rodwin, M. A. (1993). *Medicine, Money, and Morals: Physicians' Conflicts of Interest.* New York: Oxford University Press.

Rodwin, M. A. (2011). *Conflicts of Interest and the Future of Medicine: The United States, France, and Japan.* New York: Oxford University Press.

Roehr, B. (2013). "American Psychiatric Association Explains DSM-5." *British Medical Journal, 346*, f3591. https://doi:10.1136/bmj.f3591

Rogers, A. (2008). *Murder and the Death Penalty in Massachusetts.* Amherst: University of Massachusetts Press.

Rohlf, M. (2020). "Immanuel Kant." In E. N. Zalta (Ed.), *The Stanford Encyclopedia of Philosophy* (Fall 2020 ed.). Stanford, CA: Metaphysics Research Lab, Stanford University. https://plato.stanford.edu/archives/fall2020/entries/kant/

Rosch, E., & Mervis, C. B. (1975). "Family Resemblances: Studies in the Internal Structure of Categories." *Cognitive Psychology, 7*(4), 573–605. https://doi:10.1016/0010-0285(75)90024-9

Rosen, S. (1968). *Plato's Symposium.* New Haven, CT: Yale University Press.

Ross, D., Ladyman, J., Spurrett, D., & Collier, J. (2006). *Every Thing Must Go: Information—Theoretic Structural Realism.* Oxford: Oxford University Press.

Ross, E. W. (2004). "Negotiating the Politics of Citizenship Education." *Political Science & Politics, 37*(2), 249–251. https://doi:10.1017/S1049096504004172

Rotenstein, L. S., Torre, M., Ramos, M. A., Rosales, R. C., Guille, C., Sen, S., & Mata, D. A. (2018). "Prevalence of Burnout among Physicians: A Systematic Review." *JAMA, 320*(11), 1131–1150. https://doi:10.1001/jama.2018.12777

Roth, M. T., & Hoffner Jr., H. A. (1997). *Law Collections from Mesopotamia and Asia Minor* (Vol. 6). Edited by P. Michalowski. Atlanta, GA: Scholars Press.

Rothman, D. J. (1995). "Perfecting the Prison: United States, 1789-1965." In N. Morris & D. J. Rothman (Eds.), *The Oxford History of the Prison: The Practice of Punishment in Western Society* (pp. 111–129). New York: Oxford University Press.

Rothman, D. J. (2002a). *The Discovery of the Asylum Social Order and Disorder in the New Republic.* New York: Routledge.

Rothman, D. J. (2002b). *Conscience and Convenience: The Asylum and Its Alternatives in Progressive America.* New York: Routledge.

Rothman, D. J. (2012). "Consequences of Industry Relationships for Public Health and Medicine." *American Journal of Public Health, 102*(1), 55. https://ajph.aphapublications.org/doi/full/10.2105/AJPH.2011.300507

Rothman, D. J., & Rothman, S. M. (1984). *The Willowbrook Wars: Bringing the Mentally Disabled into the Community.* Piscataway, NJ: Transaction.

Rothman, S. M., & Rothman, D. J. (2003). *The Pursuit of Perfection: The Promise and Perils of Medical Enhancement* (First ed.). New York: Pantheon Books.

Rotman, E. (1990). *Beyond Punishment: A New View on the Rehabilitation of Criminal Offenders.* Westport, CT: Greenwood Press.

Rotman, E. (1995). "The Failure of Reform: United States, 1965-1965." In N. Morris & D. J. Rothman (Eds.), *The Oxford History of the Prison: The Practice of Punishment in Western Society* (pp. 169–197). New York: Oxford University Press.

Rousseau, J.-J. ([1762] 1913). *The Social Contract and Discourses.* Translated by G. D. H. Cole. London/Toronto: J. M. Dent & Sons. https://oll.libertyfund.org title/cole-the-social-contract-and-discourses

Roy, S., & Tyrer, P. (2001). "Treatment of Personality Disorders." *Current Opinion in Psychiatry, 14*(6), 555–558.

Royal College of Psychiatrists, Working Group on the Definition and Treatment of Severe Personality Disorder ([1999] 2002). *Offenders with Personality Disorder: Council Report CR71.* London: Gaskell.

Rund, B. R. (2018). "A Review of Factors Associated with Severe Violence in Schizophrenia." *Nordic Journal of Psychiatry, 72*(8), 561–571. https://doi:10.1080/08039488.2018.1497199

Rush, B. (1839). *An Inquiry into the Influence of Physical Causes upon the Moral Faculty. Delivered before a Meeting of the American Philosophical Society, Held at Philadelphia, on the Twenty-Seventh of February 1786.* Philadelphia: Haswell, Barrington & Haswell.

Rutherford, D. (2019). "Descartes' Ethics." In E. N. Zalta (Ed.), *The Stanford Encyclopedia of Philosophy* (Winter 2019 ed.). Stanford, CA: Metaphysics Research Lab, Stanford University. https://plato.stanford.edu/archives/win2019/entries/descartes-ethics/ Unpaginated.

Sackett, D. L., Richardson, W. S., Rosenberg, W., & Haynes, R. B. (1997). *Evidence-Based Medicine: How to Practice and Teach EBM* (First ed.). New York: Churchill Livingstone.

Sackett, D. L., Rosenberg, W. M. C., Gray, J. A. M., Haynes, R. B., & Richardson, W. S. (1996). "Evidence Based Medicine: What It Is and What It Isn't." *British Medical Journal, 312*(7023), 71–72. https://doi:10.1136/bmj.312.7023.71

Sackett, D. L., Straus, S. E., Richardson, W. S., Rosenberg, W., & Haynes, R. B. (2000). *Evidence-Based Medicine: How to Practice and Teach EBM* (Second ed). Edinburgh/New York: Church-Livingstone.

Sadler, J. Z. (1992). "Eidetic and Empirical Research: A Hermeneutic Complementarity." In M. Spitzer, F. Uehlein, M. A. Schwartz, & C. Mundt (Eds.), *Phenomenology, Language & Schizophrenia* (pp. 103–114). New York: Springer.

Sadler, J. Z. (1997). "Recognizing Values: A Descriptive-Causal Method for Medical/Scientific Discourses." *Journal of Medicine and Philosophy: A Forum for Bioethics and Philosophy of Medicine, 22*(6), 541–565. https://doi:10.1093/jmp 22.6.541

Sadler, J. Z. (2002). "Can We Ever Know About the Past? A Philosophical Consideration of the Assessment of Retrospective States." In R. I. Simon & D. W. Shuman (Eds.), *Retrospective Assessment of Mental States in Litigation: Predicting the Past* (pp. 47–71). Washington, DC: American Psychiatric Publishing, Inc.

Sadler, J. Z. (2004). "Diagnosis and Anti-Diagnosis." In J. Radden (Ed.), *Philosophical Perspectives on Technology and Psychiatry: A Companion* (pp. 163–179). Oxford/New York: Oxford University Press.

Sadler, J. Z. (2005). *Values and Psychiatric Diagnosis.* New York: Oxford University Press.

Sadler, J. Z. (2007). "The Psychiatric Significance of the Personal Self." *Psychiatry: Interpersonal and Biological Processes, 70*(2), 113–129. https://doi:10.1521/psyc.2007.70.2.113

Sadler, J. Z. (2008). "Vice and the Diagnostic Classification of Mental Disorders: A Philosophical Case Conference." *Philosophy, Psychiatry, & Psychology, 15*(1), 1–17. https://doi:10.1353/ppp.0.0152

Sadler, J. Z. (2009). "The Instrument Metaphor, Hyponarrativity, and the Generic Clinician." In J. Phillips (Ed.), *Philosophical Perspectives on Technology and Psychiatry* (pp. 23–33). New York/Oxford: Oxford University Press.

Sadler, J. Z. (2013). "Values in Psychiatric Diagnosis and Classification." In K. W. M. Fulford, M. Davies, R. G. T. Gipps, G. Graham, J. Z. Sadler, G. Stanghellini, & T. Thornton (Eds.), *The Oxford Handbook of Philosophy and Psychiatry* (pp. 753–778). Oxford: Oxford University Press.

Sadler, J. Z. (2013a). "Vice and Mental Disorders." In K. W. M. Fulford, M. Davies, R. Gipps, G. Graham, J. Z. Sadler, G. Stanghellini, & T. Thornton (Eds.), *The Oxford Handbook of Philosophy and Psychiatry* (pp. 451–479). Oxford: Oxford University Press.

Sadler, J. Z. (2013b). "Considering the Economy of DSM Alternatives." In J. Paris & J. Phillips (Eds.), *Making the DSM-5: Concepts and Controversies* (pp. 21–38). New York: Springer.

Sadler, J. Z. (2014). "Conduct Disorder as a Vice-Laden Diagnostic Concept." In C. Perring & L. A. Wells (Eds.), *Diagnostic Dilemmas in Child and Adolescent Psychiatry* (pp. 166–181). Oxford/New York: Oxford University Press.

Sadler, J. Z. (2015). "The Crippling Legacy on Monomanias in DSM-5." In S. Demazeux & P. Singy (Eds.), *The DSM-5 in Perspective: Philosophical Reflections on the Psychiatric Bible* (pp. 141–155). New York: Springer.

Sadler, J. Z. (2019). "Conceptual Models of Normative Content in Mental Disorders." In C. V. Haldipur, J. L. Knoll IV, & E. v.d. Luft (Eds.), *Thomas Szasz: An Appraisal of His Legacy* (pp. 38–51). Oxford: Oxford University Press.

Sadler, J. Z. (2023,). "Values Literacy and Citizenship." In J. J. Stuhr, J. Pawelski, & S. Sidoti (Eds.), *Philosophical Contributions to Human Flourishing* (pp. 213–236). Oxford: Oxford University Press.

Sadler, J. Z., & Agich, G. J. (1995). "Diseases, Functions, Values, and Psychiatric Classification." *Philosophy, Psychiatry, & Psychology, 2*(3), 219–231.

Sadler, J. Z., & Fulford, B. (2004). "Should Patients and Their Families Contribute to the DSM-V Process?" *Psychiatric Services, 55*(2), 133–138. https://doi:10.1176/appi.ps.55.2.133

Sadler, J. Z., & Hulgus, Y. F. (1989). "Hypothesizing and Evidence-Gathering: The Nexus of Understanding." *Family Process, 28*(3), 255–267. https://doi:10.1111/j.1545-5300.1989.00255.x

Sadler, J. Z., & Hulgus, Y. F. (1991). "Clinical Controversy and the Domains of Scientific Evidence." *Family Process, 30*(1), 21–36. https://doi:10.1111/j.1545-5300.1991.00021.x

Sadler, J. Z., & Hulgus, Y. F. (1992). "Clinical Problem Solving and the Biopsychosocial Model." *American Journal of Psychiatry, 149*(10), 1315–1323. https://doi:10.1176/ajp.149.10.1315

Sadler, J. Z., & Hulgus, Y. F. (1994). "Enriching the Psychosocial Content of a Multiaxial Diagnostic System." In J. Z. Sadler, M. A. Schwartz, & O. P. Wiggins (Eds.), *Philosophical Perspectives on Psychiatric Diagnostic Classification* (pp. 261–278). Baltimore: Johns Hopkins University Press.

Sadler, J. Z., Jotterand, F., Lee, S. C., & Inrig, S. (2009). "Can Medicalization Be Good? Situating Medicalization within Bioethics." *Theoretical Medicine Bioethics, 30*(6), 411–425. https://doi:10.1007/s11017-009-9122-4

Salmon, W. C., & Kitcher, P. (Eds.) (1989). *Four Decades of Scientific Explanation.* Minneapolis: University of Minnesota Press.

Samuel-Siegel, D. (2019). "What Is Restorative Justice?" *Richland Public Interest Law Review, 23*(2), 1.

Sanders, N. E., & Lei, V. (2018). "The Role of Prior Information in Inference on the Annualized Rates of Mass Shootings in the United States." *Statistics and Public Policy*, 5(1), 1–8. https://doi:10.1080/2330443X.2018.1448733

Satiani, A., Niedermier, J., Satiani, B., & Svendsen, D. P. (2018). "Projected Workforce of Psychiatrists in the United States: A Population Analysis." *Psychiatric Services*, 69(6), 710–713. https://doi:10.1176/appi.ps.201700344

Saunders, J. B. (2017). "Substance Use and Addictive Disorders in DSM-5 and ICD 10 and the Draft ICD 11." *Current Opinion in Psychiatry*, 30(4), 227–237. https://doi:10.1097/YCO.0000000000000332

Saunders, K. J. (1923). "Buddhism in China: A Historical Sketch." *Journal of Religion*, 3(3), 256–275. http://www.jstor.org/stable/1195251

Saunders, K. J. (1924). *Epochs in Buddhist History: The Haskell Lectures, 1921*. Chicago: University of Chicago Press.

Scaratti, C., Leonardi, M., Silvaggi, F., Ávila, C. C., Muñoz-Murillo, A., Stavroussi, P., . . . Ferraina, S. (2018). "Mapping European Welfare Models: State of the Art of Strategies for Professional Integration and Reintegration of Persons with Chronic Diseases." *International Journal of Environmental Research and Public Health*, 15(4), Article: 781. https://doi:10.3390/ijerph15040781

Schaffner, K. F. (Ed.) (1985). *Logic of Discovery and Diagnosis in Medicine*. Berkeley: University of California Press.

Schaffner, K. F. (1993). *Discovery and Explanation in Biology and Medicine*. Chicago: University of Chicago Press.

Schaffner, K. F. (2016). *Behaving: What's Genetic, What's Not, and Why Should We Care?* New York: Oxford University Press.

Schaler, J. A. (Ed.) (2004). *Szasz under Fire: A Psychiatric Abolitionist Faces His Critics*. Chicago/La Salle, IL: Open Court Publishing.

Scheerenberger, R. C. (1987). *A History of Mental Retardation: A Quarter Century of Promise*. Baltimore: Paul H. Brookes Publishing Co.

Schiavone, S. K., & Jeglic, E. L. (2009). "Public Perception of Sex Offender Social Policies and the Impact on Sex Offenders." *International Journal of Offender Therapy and Comparative Criminology*, 53(6), 679–695. https://doi:10.1177/0306624x08323454

Schiltz, K., Witzel, J., Northoff, G., Zierhut, K., Gubka, U., Fellmann, H., . . . Bogerts, B. (2007). "Brain Pathology in Pedophilic Offenders: Evidence of Volume Reduction in the Right Amygdala and Related Diencephalic Structures." *Archives of General Psychiatry*, 64(6), 737–746. https://doi:10.1001/archpsyc.64.6.737

Schmitter, A. M. (2021). "17th and 18th Century Theories of Emotions." In E. N. Zalta (Ed.), *The Stanford Encyclopedia of Philosophy* (Summer 2021 ed.). Stanford, CA: Metaphysics Research Lab, Stanford University. https://plato.stanford.edu/archives/sum2021/entries emotions-17th18th/

Schouten, B., Vlug-Mahabali, M., Hermanns, S., Spijker, E., & van Weert, J. (2014). "To Be Involved or Not to Be Involved? Using Entertainment-Education in an HIV-Prevention Program for Youngsters." *Health Communication*, 29(8), 762–772. https://doi:10.1080/10410236.2013.781938

Schuster, E. (1989). "In Pursuit of Cultural Literacy." *The Phi Delta Kappan*, 70(7), 539–542. http: www.jstor.org/stable/20403954

Schwartz, M. A., & Wiggins, O. P. (1986). "Logical Empiricism and Psychiatric Classification." *Comprehensive Psychiatry*, 27(2), 101–114. https://doi:10.1016/0010-440X(86)90019-2

Schwartz, M. A., & Wiggins, O. P. (1987a). "Diagnosis and Ideal Types: A Contribution to Psychiatric Classification." *Comprehensive Psychiatry*, 28(4), 277–291. https://doi:10.1016/0010-440X(87)90064-2

Schwartz, M. A., & Wiggins, O. P. (1987b). "Typifications: The First Step for Clinical Diagnosis in Psychiatry." *Journal of Nervous and Mental Disease*, 175(2), 65–77. https://journals.lww.com/jonmd/Fulltext/1987/02000/Typifications__The_First_Step_for_Clinical.1.aspx

Schwartz, M. A., & Wiggins, O. P. (1988a). "Scientific and Humanistic Medicine: A Theory of Clinical Methods." In K. L. White (Ed.), *The Task of Medicine: Dialogue at Wickenburg* (pp. 137–177). Menlo Park, CA: Henry J. Kaiser Family Foundation.

Schwartz, M. A., & Wiggins, O. P. (1988b). "Perspectivism and the Methods of Psychiatry." *Comprehensive Psychiatry*, 29(3), 237–251. https://doi:10.1016/0010-440X(88)90047-8

Schwartz, M. A., & Wiggins, O. P. (2002). "The Hegemony of the DSMs." In J. Z. Sadler (Ed.), *Descriptions and Prescriptions: Values, Mental Disorders, and the DSMs* (pp. 199–209). Baltimore: Johns Hopkins University Press.

Scull, A. T. (1977). *Decarceration: Community Treatment and the Deviant–A Radical View*. Englewood Cliffs, NJ: Prentice-Hall.

Scull, A. T. (1979). *Museums of Madness: The Social Organization of Insanity in Nineteenth-Century England*. London: Allen Lane.

Scull, A. T. (Ed.) (1981). *Madhouses, Mad-Doctors, and Madmen: The Social History of Psychiatry in the Victorian Era*. Philadelphia: University of Pennsylvania Press.

Scull, A. T. (1989). *Social Order/Mental Disorder: Anglo-American Psychiatry in Historical Perspective*. Berkeley: University of California Press. http://ark.cdlib.org/ark:/13030/ft9r29p2x5

Scull, A. T. (1991a). "Psychiatry and Social Control in the Nineteenth and Twentieth Centuries." *History of Psychiatry, 2*(6, Pt 2), 149–169. https://doi:10.1177/0957154X9100200603

Scull, A. T. (1991b). "Psychiatry and Its Historians." *History of Psychiatry, 2*(7, Pt 3), 239–250. https://doi:10.1177/0957154X9100200701

Scull, A. T. (1999). "Rethinking the History of Asylumdom." In J. Melling & B. Forsythe (Eds.), *Insanity, Institutions and Society, 1800-1914: A Social History of Madness in Comparative Perspective* (pp. 295–315). London: Routledge.

Scull, A. T. (2000). "The Madhouse of Dr. Monro: How the Inmates of Bedlam Were Treated." *The Times Literary Supplement, 5091*, 14–15.

Scull, A. T. (2004). "The Insanity of Place." *History of Psychiatry, 15*(4), 417–436. https://doi:10.1177/0957154X04044084

Scull, A. T. (2005). *Madhouse: A Tragic Tale of Megalomania and Modern Medicine*. New Haven, CT: Yale University Press.

Scull, A. T. (2010). "The Art of Medicine: A Psychiatric Revolution." *The Lancet, 375*(9722), 1246–1247. https://doi:10.1016/S0140-6736(10)60532-6

Scull, A. T. (2018). "Creating a New Psychiatry: On the Origins of Non-Institutional Psychiatry in the USA, 1900–50." *History of Psychiatry, 29*(4), 389–408. https://doi:10.1177/0957154x18793596

Scull, A. T. (2021). "American Psychiatry in the New Millennium: A Critical Appraisal." *Psychological Medicine, 51*(16), 2752–2770. https://doi:10.1017/S0033291721001975

Scull, A. T., MacKenzie, C., & Hervey, N. (1996). *Masters of Bedlam: The Transformation of the Mad-Doctoring Trade*. Princeton, NJ: Princeton University Press.

Scurlock, J. A., & Andersen, B. R. (2005). *Diagnoses in Assyrian and Babylonian Medicine: Ancient Sources, Translations, and Modern Medical Analyses*. Urbana/Chicago: University of Illinois Press. https://muse.jhu.edu/book/21624

Searle, J. R. (1992). *The Rediscovery of the Mind*. Cambridge, MA: MIT Press.

Seeskin, K. (2021). "Maimonides." In E. N. Zalta (Ed.), *The Stanford Encyclopedia of Philosophy* (Spring 2021 ed.). Stanford, CA: Metaphysics Research Lab, Stanford University. https://plato.stanford.edu/archives/spr2021/entries/maimonides/

Segal, G. M. A. (2013). "Alcoholism, Disease, and Insanity." *Philosophy, Psychiatry, & Psychology, 20*(4), 297–315. https://doi:10.1353/ppp.2013.0059

Seidentop, L. (2014). *Inventing the Individual: The Origins of Western Liberalism*. Cambridge, MA: Belknap/Harvard University Press.

Seidman, S., Fischer, N., & Meeks, C. (Eds.) (2006). *Handbook of the New Sexuality Studies*. London/New York: Routledge.

Seldin, D. W. (1977). "The Medical Model: Biomedical Science as the Basis of Medicine." In *Beyond Tomorrow: Trends and Prospects in Medical Science* (pp. 31–40). New York: Rockefeller University Press.

Seto, M. C. (2012). "Is Pedophilia a Sexual Orientation?" *Archives of Sexual Behavior, 41*(1), 231–236. https://doi:10.1007/s10508-011-9882-6

Seto, M. C. (2022). "Clinical and Conceptual Problems with Pedophilic Disorder in the DSM-5-TR." *Archives of Sexual Behavior, 51*(4), 1833–1837. https://doi:10.1007/s10508-022-02336-1

Seto, M. C., Cantor, J. M., & Blanchard, R. (2006). "Child Pornography Offenses Are a Valid Diagnostic Indicator of Pedophilia." *Journal of Abnormal Psychology, 115*(3), 610–615. https://doi:10.1037/0021-843X.115.3.610

Shakespeare, W. (2005). *The Yale Shakespeare: The Complete Works.* Edited by W. L. Cross & T. Brooke. New York: Barnes and Noble.

Shanafelt, T. D. (2009). "Enhancing Meaning in Work: A Prescription for Preventing Physician Burnout and Promoting Patient-Centered Care." *JAMA, 302*(12), 1338–1340. https://doi:10.1001/jama.2009.1385

Sharples, R. W. (1995). "Stoicism." In T. Honderich (Ed.), *The Oxford Companion to Philosophy* (pp. 852–853). Oxford: Oxford University Press.

Shaw, E., Pereboom, D., & Caruso, G. D. (Eds.) (2019). *Free Will Skepticism in Law and Society: Challenging Retributive Justice.* Cambridge: Cambridge University Press.

Shaw, I., & Middleton, H. (2016). *Understanding Treatment without Consent: An Analysis of the Work of the Mental Health Act Commission.* London: Routledge.

Shear, M. K., Simon, N., Wall, M., Zisook, S., Neimeyer, R., Duan, N., . . . Keshaviah, A. (2011). "Complicated Grief and Related Bereavement Issues for DSM-5." *Depression and Anxiety, 28*(2), 103–117. https://doi:10.1002/da.20780

Shelp, E. E. (Ed.) (1983). *The Clinical Encounter: The Moral Fabric of the Patient-Physician Relationship* (Philosophy and Medicine series). Dordrecht/Boston/Lancaster: D. Reidel Publishing Company.

Shorter, E. (1997). *A History of Psychiatry: From the Era of the Asylum to the Age of Prozac.* New York: John Wiley & Sons.

Shorter, E., & Fink, M. (2010). *Endocrine Psychiatry: Solving the Riddle of Melancholia.* New York/Oxford: Oxford University Press.

Shrage, L. (2017). "Race, Health Disparities, Incarceration, and Structural Inequality." In N. Zack (Ed.), *The Oxford Handbook of Philosophy and Race* (pp. 449–462). Oxford: Oxford University Press.

Shuman, D. W. (1989). "The Diagnostic and Statistical Manual of Mental Disorders in the Courts." *The Bulletin of the American Academy of Psychiatry & the Law, 17*(1), 25–32. http://jaapl.org/content/17/1/25

Shuman, D. W. (2001). "Expertise in Law, Medicine, and Health Care." *Journal of Health Politics, Policy and Law, 26*(2), 267–290. https://doi:10.1215/03616878-26-2-267

Shuman, D. W. (2002). "Retrospective Assessment of Mental States and the Law." In R. I. Simon & D. W. Shuman (Eds.), *Retrospective Assessment of Mental States in Litigation: Predicting the Past* (pp. 21–46). Washington, DC: American Psychiatric Association Publishing.

Sidgwick, H. (1888). *Outlines of the History of Ethics for English Readers.* London: MacMillan & Co.

Sieff, E. (2003). "Media Frames of Mental Illnesses: The Potential Impact of Negative Frames." *Journal of Mental Health, 12*(3), 259–269. https://doi:10.1080/0963823031000118249

Siegel, L. J. (2006). *Criminology: Theories, Patterns, and Typologies.* Belmont, CA: Wadsworth, Cengage Learning.

Sigerist, H. E. (1951). *A History of Medicine* (Vol. 1, Primitive and Archaic Medicine). New York: Oxford University Press.

Sigerist, H. E. (1961). *A History of Medicine* (Vol. 2, Early Greek, Hindu, and Persian Medicine). Oxford: Oxford University Press.

Sighart, J. (1876). *Albert the Great, of the Order of Friar-Preachers: His Life and Scholastic Labours.* Translated by T. A. Dixon. London: R. Washbourne.

Silva, J. A., Ferrari, M. M., & Leong, G. B. (2002). "The Case of Jeffrey Dahmer: Sexual Serial Homicide from a Neuropsychiatric Developmental Perspective." *Journal of Forensic Sciences, 47*(6), 1347–1359.

Silver, E., Cirincione, C., & Steadman, H. J. (1994). "Demythologizing Inaccurate Perceptions of the Insanity Defense." *Law and Human Behavior, 18*(1), 63–70. https://doi:10.1007/BF01499144

Silver, E., Felson, R. B., & VanEseltine, M. (2008). "The Relationship between Mental Health Problems and Violence among Criminal Offenders." *Criminal Justice and Behavior, 35*(4), 405–426. https://doi:10.1177/0093854807312851

Simon, B. (1980). *Mind and Madness in Ancient Greece: The Classical Roots of Modern Psychiatry.* Ithaca, NY/London: Cornell University Press.

Simon, B. (2008). "Mind and Madness in Classical Antiquity." In E. R. Wallace & J. Gach (Eds.), *History of Psychiatry and Medical Psychology: With an Epilogue on Psychiatry and the Mind-Body Relation* (pp. 175–197). Boston: Springer.

Simon, L., Beckmann, D., Stone, M., Williams, R., Cohen, M., & Tobey, M. (2020). "Clinician Experiences of Care Provision in the Correctional Setting: A Scoping Review." *Journal of Correctional Health Care, 26*(4), 301–314. https://doi:10.1177/1078345820953154

Simon, R. I., & Shuman, D. W. (Eds.) (2002). *Retrospective Assessment of Mental States in Litigation: Predicting the Past*. Washington, DC: American Psychiatric Association Publishing.

Singy, P. (2009). *A History of Violence: Sadism and the Emergence of Sexuality*. Unpublished Paper Presented at Columbia University, 12 November 2009.

Sircar, M. (1933a). "Social and Moral Ideas in the Upanishads." *International Journal of Ethics, 44*(1), 94–105. https://doi:10.1086/intejethi.44.1.2377993

Sircar, M. (1933b). "Reality in Indian Thought." *Philosophical Review, 42*(3), 249–271. https://doi:10.2307/2180322

Sklar, M., Groessl, E. J., O'Connell, M., Davidson, L., & Aarons, G. A. (2013). "Instruments for Measuring Mental Health Recovery: A Systematic Review." *Clinical Psychology Review, 33*(8), 1082–1095. https://doi:10.1016/j.cpr.2013.08.002

Skodol, A. E., & Bender, D. S. (2009). "The Future of Personality Disorders in DSM-V?" *American Journal of Psychiatry, 166*(4), 388–391. https://doi:10.1176/appi.ajp.2009.09010090

Skodol, A. E., Morey, L. C., Bender, D. S., & Oldham, J. M. (2015). "The Alternative DSM-5 Model for Personality Disorders: A Clinical Application." *American Journal of Psychiatry, 172*(7), 606–613. https://doi:10.1176/appi.ajp.2015.14101220

Slate, R. N., & Johnson, W. W. (2008). *The Criminalization of Mental Illness: Crisis and Opportunity for the Justice System*. Durham, NC: Carolina Academic Press.

Slater, D., & Hans, V. P. (1984). "Public Opinion of Forensic Psychiatry Following the Hinckley Verdict." *American Journal of Psychiatry, 141*(5), 675–679. https://doi:10.1176/ajp.141.5.675

Slater, E., & Beard, A. W. (1963). "The Schizophrenia-Like Psychoses of Epilepsy." *British Journal of Psychiatry, 109*(458), 95–112. https://doi:10.1192/bjp.109.458.95

Slobogin, C. (1998). "Psychiatric Evidence in Criminal Trials: To Junk or Not to Junk." *William & Mary Law Review, 40*(1), Article 2. https://scholarship.law.wm.edu/wmlr/vol40/iss1/2

Slobogin, C. (2003). "The Structure of Expertise in Criminal Cases." *Seton Hall Law Review, 34*, 105–126.

Slopen, N. B., Watson, A. C., Gracia, G., & Corrigan, P. W. (2007). "Age Analysis of Newspaper Coverage of Mental Illness." *Journal of Health Communication, 12*(1), 3–15. https://doi:10.1080/10810730601091292

Slovenko, R. (2002). *Psychiatry in Law / Law in Psychiatry*. New York: Brunner-Routledge.

Smith, J. (1988). "Cultural Literacy and the Academic 'Left.'" *Profession, 1988*, 25–28. http://www.jstor.org/stable/25595415

Smith, P., Cullen, F. T., & Latessa, E. J. (2009). "Can 14,737 Women Be Wrong? A Meta-Analysis of the LSI-R and Recidivism for Female Offenders." *Criminology & Public Policy, 8*(1), 183–208. https://doi:10.1111/j.1745-9133.2009.00551.x

Smith, P., Gendreau, P., & Swartz, K. (2009). "Validating the Principles of Effective Intervention: A Systematic Review of the Contributions of Meta-Analysis in the Field of Corrections." *Victims & Offenders, 4*(2), 148–169. https://doi:10.1080/15564880802612581

Sophocles. (2009). *Antigone, Oedipus the King and Electra*. Translated by H. D. F. Kitto. Edited by E. Hall. Oxford: Oxford University Press.

Spence, D. P. (1984). *Narrative Truth and Historical Truth: Meaning and Interpretation in Psychoanalysis*. New York/London: W.W. Norton & Company.

Spierenburg, P. (1995). "The Body and the State: Early Modern Europe." In N. Morris & D. J. Rothman (Eds.), *The Oxford History of the Prison: The Practice of Punishment in Western Society* (pp. 44–70). Oxford: Oxford University Press.

Spinoza, B. (1883). *The Ethics (Ethica Ordine Geometrico Demonstrata)*. Translated by R. H. M. Elwes. The Project Gutenberg. https://www.gutenberg.org/files/3800/3800-h/3800-h.htm

Spitzer, R. L., & Wakefield, J. C. (1999). "DSM-IV Diagnostic Criterion for Clinical Significance: Does It Help Solve the False Positives Problem?" *American Journal of Psychiatry, 156*(12), 1856–1864. https://doi:10.1176/ajp.156.12.1856

Spitzer, R. L., Williams, J. B., & Skodol, A. E. (1980). DSM-III: The Major Achievements and an Overview." *The American Journal of Psychiatry, 137*(2), 151–164. https://doi:10.1176/ajp.137.2.151

Stacy, T. (1991). "The Search for the Truth in Constitutional Criminal Procedure." *Columbia Law Review, 91*(6), 1369–1451. https://doi:10.2307/1123065

Stanghellini, G. (2004). *Disembodied Spirits and Deanimated Bodies: The Psychopathology of Common Sense.* Oxford: Oxford University Press.

Stanghellini, G. (2016). *Lost in dialogue: anthropology, psychopathology, and care.* Oxford: Oxford University Press.

Stanghellini, G., Broome, M., Raballo, A., Fernandez, A. V., Fusar-Poli, P., & Rosfort, R. (Eds.) (2019). *The Oxford Handbook of Phenomenological Psychopathology.* Oxford: Oxford University Press.

Stanghellini, G., & Fuchs, T. (Eds.) (2013). *One Century of Karl Jaspers' General Psychopathology.* Oxford: Oxford University Press.

Stansfield, R., O'Connor, T., Duncan, J., & Hall, S. (2020). "Comparing Recidivism of Sexual and Nonsexual Offenders: The Role of Humanist, Spiritual, and Religious Involvement." *Sexual Abuse, 32*(6), 634–656. https://doi:10.1177/1079063219843903

Steadman, H. J. (1981). "Critically Reassessing the Accuracy of Public Perceptions of the Dangerousness of the Mentally Ill." *Journal of Health and Social Behavior, 22*(3), 310–316. https://doi:10.2307/2136524

Steadman, H. J., & Braff, J. (1983). "Defendants Not Guilty by Reason of Insanity." In J. Monahan & H. J. Steadman (Eds.), *Mentally Disordered Offenders: Perspectives from Law and Social Science* (pp. 109–129). New York: Springer.

Steadman, H. J., & Cocozza, J. J. (1977). "Selective Reporting and the Public's Misconceptions of the Criminally Insane." *Public Opinion Quarterly, 41*(4), 523–533. https://doi:10.1086/268412

Steadman, H. J., & Cocozza, J. J. (1978). "Psychiatry, Dangerousness and the Repetitively Violent Offender." *Journal of Criminal Law and Criminology (1973-), 69*(2), 226–231. https://doi:10.2307/1142396

Steadman, H. J., & Felson, R. B. (1984). "Self Reports of Violence: Ex-Mental Patients, Ex-Offenders, and the General Population." *Criminology, 22*(3), 321–342. https://doi:10.1111/j.1745-9125.1984.tb00303.x

Steadman, H. J., Mulvey, E. P., Monahan, J., Robbins, P. C., Appelbaum, P. S., Grisso, T., . . . Silver, E. (1998). "Violence by People Discharged from Acute Psychiatric Inpatient Facilities and by Others in the Same Neighborhoods." *Archives of General Psychiatry, 55*(5), 393–401. https://doi:10.1001/archpsyc.55.5.393

Steadman, H. J., Robbins, P. C., Silver, E., Mulvey, E. P., Roth, L. H., Monahan, J., . . . Grisso, T. (1999). "Violence in the Mentally Ill: Questions Remain—Reply." *Archives of General Psychiatry, 56*(2), 193–194. https: jamanetwork.com/journals/jamapsychiatry/article-abstract/204677

Stein, D. J., Black, D. W., & Pienaar, W. (2000). "Sexual Disorders Not Otherwise Specified: Compulsive, Addictive, or Impulsive?" *CNS Spectrums, 5*(1), 60–66. https://doi:10.1017/S1092852900012670

Stein, D. J., Hugo, F., Oosthuizen, P., Hawkridge, S. M., & van Heerden, B. (2000). "Neuropsychiatry of Hypersexuality." *CNS Spectrums, 5*(1), 36–46. https://doi:10.1017/S1092852900012657

Stein, D. J., Phillips, K. A., Bolton, D., Fulford, K. W. M., Sadler, J. Z., & Kendler, K. S. (2010). "What Is a Mental/Psychiatric Disorder? From DSN-IV to DSM-V." *Psychological Medicine, 40*(11), 1759–1765. https://doi:10.1017/S0033291709992261

Stekel, W. (1911). "The Sexual Root of Kleptomania." *Journal of the American Institute of Criminal Law and Criminology, 2*(2), 239–246. http://www.jstor.org/stable/1132956

Steury, E. H. (1993). "Criminal Defendants with Psychiatric Impairment: Prevalence, Probabilities and Rates." *Journal of Criminal Law and Criminology, 84*(2), 352–376. https://doi:10.2307/1143818

Stevens, A. J. (2004). "The Enactment of Bayh–Dole." *Journal of Technology Transfer, 29*(1), 93–99. https://doi:10.1023/B:JOTT.0000011183.40867.52

Stevens, R. A. (2008). "History and Health Policy in the United States: The Making of a Health Care Industry, 1948-2008." *Social History of Medicine, 21*(3), 461–483. https://doi:10.1093/shm/hkn063

Stinson, J. D., & Becker, J. V. (2016). "Pedophilic Disorder." In A. Phenix & H. M. Hoberman (Eds.), *Sexual Offending: Predisposing Antecedents, Assessments and Management* (pp. 15–27). New York: Springer.

Stoller, R. J. (1986). *Perversion: The Erotic Form of Hatred*. London: Routledge.

Stone, A. A. (1984). "The Ethical Boundaries of Forensic Psychiatry: A View from the Ivory Tower." *Bulletin of the American Academy of Psychiatry & the Law, 12*(3), 209–219.

Stone, A. A. (2008). "The Ethical Boundaries of Forensic Psychiatry: A View from the Ivory Tower." *Journal of the American Academy of Psychiatry and the Law Online, 36*(2), 167–174. http://jaapl.org/content jaapl/36/2/167.full.pdf

Stout, P. A., Villegas, J., & Jennings, N. A. (2004). "Images of Mental Illness in the Media: Identifying Gaps in the Research." *Schizophrenia Bulletin, 30*(3), 543–561. https://doi:10.1093/oxfordjournals.schbul.a007099

Straus, S. E., Glasziou, P., Richardson, W. S., & Haynes, R. B. (2018). *Evidence-Based Medicine: How to Practice and Teach EBM, 5th ed.* New York: Elsevier.

Stringaris, A., Baroni, A., Haimm, C., Brotman, M., Lowe, C. H., Myers, F., . . . Leibenluft, E. (2010). "Pediatric Bipolar Disorder versus Severe Mood Dysregulation: Risk for Manic Episodes on Follow-Up." *Journal of the American Academy of Child & Adolescent Psychiatry, 49*(4), 397–405. https://doi:10.1016/j.jaac.2010.01.013

Stroud, S., & Svirsky, L. (2021). "Weakness of Will." In E. N. Zalta (Ed.), *The Stanford Encyclopedia of Philosophy* (Winter 2021 ed.). Stanford, CA: Metaphysics Research Lab, Stanford University.https://plato.stanford.edu/archives/win2021/entries/weakness-will/

Stroud, S., and Tappolet, C. (Eds.), (2003). *Weakness of Will and Practical Irrationality*. Oxford: Clarendon Press.

Stuart, H. (2003). "Violence and Mental Illness: An Overview." *World Psychiatry: Official Journal of the World Psychiatric Association (WPA), 2*(2), 121–124. http://www.ncbi.nlm.nih.gov/pmc/articles/PMC1525086/

Stuart, H. (2006). "Media Portrayal of Mental Illness and Its Treatments: What Effect Does It Have on People with Mental Illness?" *CNS Drugs, 20*(2), 99–106. https://doi:10.2165/00023210-200620020-00002

Stucky, E. R., Dresselhaus, T. R., Dollarhide, A., Shively, M., Maynard, G., Jain, S., . . . Rutledge, T. (2009). "Intern to Attending: Assessing Stress among Physicians." *Academic Medicine, 84*(2), 251–257. https://doi:10.1097/ACM.0b013e3181938aad

Stuntz, W. J. (1997). "The Uneasy Relationship between Criminal Procedure and Criminal Justice." *Yale Law Journal, 107*(1), 1–76. https://doi:10.2307/797276

Stuntz, W. J. (2006). "The Political Constitution of Criminal Justice." *Harvard Law Review, 119*(3), 780–851. http://www.jstor.org/stable/4093592

Sturmberg, J., & Topolski, S. (2014). "For Every Complex Problem, There Is an Answer That Is Clear, Simple and Wrong." *Journal of Evaluation in Clinical Practice, 20*(6), 1017–1025. https://doi:10.1111/jep.12156

Summers, M. (2010). " Suitable Care of the African When Afflicted With Insanity": *Race, Madness, and Social Order in Comparative Perspective*. Bulletin of the History of Medicine 84 (1): 58–91.

Sundararaman, R. (2009). *The U.S. Mental Health Delivery System Infrastructure: A Primer* (CRS Report for Congress, R40536). Washington, DC: Congressional Research Service. https://fas.org/sgp/crs/misc/R40536.pdf

Sunstein, C. R. (2017). *#Republic: Divided Democracy in the Age of Social Media*. Princeton, NJ: Princeton University Press.

Surden, H. (2020). "The Ethics of Artificial Intelligence in Law: Basic Questions." In *Forthcoming Chapter in Oxford Handbook of Ethics in AI. University of Colorado Law Legal Studies Research Paper No. 19-29.* https://papers.ssrn.com/sol3/papers.cfm?abstract_id=3441303

Svenaeus, F. (2000). "Hermeneutics of Clinical Practice: The Question of Textuality." *Theoretical Medicine and Bioethics, 21*(2), 171–189. https://doi:10.1023/A:1009942926545

Sverdlik, S. (1988). "Punishment." *Law and Philosophy, 7*(2), 179–201. https://doi:10.1007/BF00144155

Sverdlik, S. (2014). "Punishment and Reform." *Criminal Law and Philosophy, 8*(3), 619–633. https://doi:10.1007/s11572-013-9226-9

Swaminath, G. (2008). "Internet Addiction Disorder: Fact or Fad? Nosing into Nosology." *Indian Journal of Psychiatry, 50*(3), 158–160. https://doi:10.4103/0019-5545.43622

Swanson, J. W., Swartz, M. S., Essock, S. M., Osher, F. C., Wagner, H. R., Goodman, L. A., . . . Meador, K. G. (2002). "The Social–Environmental Context of Violent Behavior in Persons Treated for Severe Mental Illness." *American Journal of Public Health, 92*(9), 1523–1531. https://doi:10.2105/ajph.92.9.1523

Swanson, J. W., Swartz, M. S., Van Dorn, R. A., Elbogen, E. B., Wagner, H. R., Rosenheck, R. A., . . . Lieberman, J. A. (2006). "A National Study of Violent Behavior in Persons with Schizophrenia." *Archives of General Psychiatry, 63*(5), 490–499. https://doi:10.1001/archpsyc.63.5.490

Sward, E. E. (1989). "Values, Ideology, and the Evolution of the Adversary System." *Indiana Law Journal, 64*(2). https://ssrn.com/abstract=2238681

Szasz, T. (1961). *The Myth of Mental Illness: Foundations of a Theory of Personal Conduct.* New York: Hoeber-Harper.

Szasz, T. (1974). *The Myth of Mental Illness: Foundations of a Theory of Personal Conduct.* New York: Harper & Row.

Szasz, T. S. (1960). "The Myth of Mental Illness." *American Psychologist, 15*(2), 113–118. https://doi:10.1037/h0046535

Szasz, T. S. (1963). *Law, Liberty, and Psychiatry: An Inquiry into the Social Uses of Mental Health Practices.* New York: Macmillan.

Szasz, T. S. (1977). *Schizophrenia: The Sacred Symbol of Psychiatry.* New York: Basic Books.

Szasz, T. S. (1991). *Ideology and Insanity: Essays on the Psychiatric Dehumanization of Man.* Syracuse, NY: Syracuse University Press.

Tadros, V. (2011). *The Ends of Harm: The Moral Foundations of Criminal Law.* New York: Oxford University Press.

Takahashi, S. (2013). "Heterogeneity of Schizophrenia: Genetic and Symptomatic Factors." *American Journal of Medical Genetics Part B: Neuropsychiatric Genetics, 162*(7), 648–652. https://doi:10.1002/ajmg.b.32161

Talbott, J. A. (2004). "Deinstitutionalization: Avoiding the Disasters of the Past." *Psychiatric Services, 55*(10), 1112–1115. https://doi:10.1176/appi.ps.55.10.1112

Tanenhaus, D. S. (2002). "The Evolution of Juvenile Courts in the Early Twentieth Century: Beyond the Myth of Immaculate Construction." In M. K. Rosenheim, F. E. Zimring, D. S. Tanenhaus, & B. Dohrn (Eds.), *A Century of Juvenile Justice* (pp. 42–73). Chicago: University of Chicago Press.

Tanguay-Renaud, F. (2013). "Victor's Justice: The Next Best Moral Theory of Criminal Punishment?" *Law and Philosophy, 32*(1), 129–157. https://doi:10.1007/s10982-012-9159-9

Tate, D. F., & Zabinski, M. F. (2004). "Computer and Internet Applications for Psychological Treatment: Update for Clinicians." *Journal of Clinical Psychology, 60*(2), 209–220. https://doi:10.1002/jclp.10247

Taylor, C. C. W. (2005). "Democritus." In C. Rowe & M. Schofield (Eds.), *The Cambridge History of Greek and Roman Political Thought* (pp. 122–129). Cambridge, MA: Cambridge University Press.

Taylor, J. L. (2002). "A Review of the Assessment and Treatment of Anger and Aggression in Offenders with Intellectual Disability." *Journal of Intellectual Disability Research, 46*(Suppl 1), 57–73. https://doi:10.1046/j.1365-2788.2002.00005.x

Teeple, J. B. (2006). *Timelines of World History.* New York: Dorling Kindersley Publishing.

Tekin, Ş. (2014). "A Perfect Storm: Health, Disorder, Culture, and the Self." *Philosophy, Psychiatry, & Psychology, 21*(2), 165–168. https://doi:10.1353/ppp.2014.0024

Tekin, Ş., & Mosko, M. (2015). Hyponarrativity and Context-Specific Limitations of the DSM-5. *Public Affairs Quarterly, 29*(1), 109–134. https://www.jstor.org/stable/43574516

Tengström, A., Hodgins, S., Grann, M., Långström, N., & Kullgren, G. (2004). "Schizophrenia and Criminal Offending: The Role of Psychopathy and Substance Use Disorders." *Criminal Justice and Behavior, 31*(4), 367–391. https://doi:10.1177/0093854804265173

Teplin, L. A. (1984). "Criminalizing Mental Disorder. The Comparative Arrest Rate of the Mentally Ill." *American Psychologist, 39*(7), 794–803. https://doi:10.1037/0003-066x.39.7.794

Testa, M., & West, S. G. (2010). "Civil Commitment in the United States." *Psychiatry (Edgmont), 7*(10), 30–40. https://pubmed.ncbi.nlm.nih.gov/22778709

Tewksbury, R. (2005). "Collateral Consequences of Sex Offender Registration." *Journal of Contemporary Criminal Justice, 21*(1), 67–81. https://doi:10.1177/1043986204271704

Tewksbury, R., & Lees, M. (2006). "Perceptions of Sex Offender Registration: Collateral Consequences and Community Experiences." *Sociological Spectrum*, 26(3), 309–334. https://doi:10.1080/027321 70500524246

Thomasma, D. C. (1994). "Clinical Ethics as Medical Hermeneutics." *Theoretical Medicine*, 15(2), 93–111. https://doi:10.1007/bf00994019

Thompson, A., Issakidis, C., & Hunt, C. (2008). "Delay to Seek Treatment for Anxiety and Mood Disorders in an Australian Clinical Sample." *Behaviour Change*, 25(2), 71–84. https://doi:10.1375/bech.25.2.71

Thompson, T. L. ([1974]2002). *The Historicity of the Patriarchal Narratives: The Quest for the Historical Abraham*. (1974 version published by De Gruyter, Berlin). Valley Forge, PA: Trinity Press International. https://doi.org/10.1515/9783110841442

Thomson, O. (1993). *A History of Sin*. Edinburgh: Canongate Press.

Thornicroft, A., Goulden, R., Shefer, G., Rhydderch, D., Rose, D., Williams, P., . . . Henderson, C. (2013). "Newspaper Coverage of Mental Illness in England 2008-2011." *British Journal of Psychiatry*, 202(s55), s64–s69. https://doi:10.1192/bjp.bp.112.112920

Thornton, D. (2010). "Evidence Regarding the Need for a Diagnostic Category for a Coercive Paraphilia." *Archives of Sexual Behavior*, 39(2), 411–418. https://doi:10.1007/s10508-009-9583-6

Thornton, T. (2017). "Cross-Cultural Psychiatry and Validity in DSM-5." In R. G. White, S. Jain, D. M. R. Orr, & U. M. Read (Eds.), *The Palgrave Handbook of Sociocultural Perspectives on Global Mental Health* (pp. 51–69). London: Palgrave Macmillan.

Thurman, R. A. F. (2006). *Anger* (Vol. 3 of The Seven Deadly Sins series). New York: Oxford University Press.

Tighe, J. A. (1983). "Francis Wharton and the Nineteenth-Century Insanity Defense: The Origins of a Reform Tradition." *American Journal of Legal History*, 27(3), 223–253. https://doi:10.2307/845155

Tillman, R. (1987). "The Size of the 'Criminal Population': The Prevalence and Incidence of Adult Arrest." *Criminology*, 25(3), 561–580. https://doi:10.1111/j.1745-9125.1987.tb00811.x

Timasheff, N. S. (1937). "The Retributive Structure of Punishment." *Journal of Criminal Law and Criminology (1931-1951)*, 28(3), 396–405. https://doi:10.2307/1136721

Timonen, M., Miettunen, J., Hakko, H., Zitting, P., Veijola, J., von Wendt, L., & Räsänen, P. (2002). "The Association of Preceding Traumatic Brain Injury with Mental Disorders, Alcoholism and Criminality: The Northern Finland 1966 Birth Cohort Study." *Psychiatry Research*, 113(3), 217–226. https://doi:10.1016/S0165-1781(02)00269-X

Tondora, J., Miller, R., Slade, M., & Davidson, L. (2014). *Partnering for Recovery in Mental Health: A Practical Guide to Person-Centered Planning*. Hoboken, NJ: John Wiley & Sons.

Tonry, M. (2004). "Moral Panics and 'Windows of Opportunity'." In M. Tonry (Ed.), *Thinking about Crime: Sense and Sensibility in American Penal Culture* (pp. 85–96). Oxford/New York: Oxford University Press.

Tonry, M. (2006). *Thinking about Crime: Sense and Sensibility in American Penal Culture*. New York: Oxford University Press.

Tonry, M. (2011a). "Crime and Criminal Justice." In M. Tonry (Ed.), *The Oxford Handbook of Crime and Criminal Justice* (pp. 3–25). Oxford: Oxford University Press.

Tonry, M. (2011b). "Punishment." In M. Tonry (Ed.), *The Oxford Handbook of Crime and Criminal Justice* (pp. 95–125). Oxford: Oxford University Press.

Tonry, M. & Nagin, D. S. (Eds.) (2017). *Reinventing American Criminal Justice* (Vol. 46 of Crime and Justice: A Review of Research series). Chicago: University of Chicago Press.

Towbin, K., Axelson, D., Leibenluft, E., & Birmaher, B. (2013). "Differentiating Bipolar Disorder–Not Otherwise Specified and Severe Mood Dysregulation." *Journal of the American Academy of Child and Adolescent Psychiatry*, 52(5), 466–481. https://doi:10.1016/j.jaac.2013.02.006

Trent Jr., J. W. (1994). *Inventing the Feeble Mind: A History of Mental Retardation in the United States*. Berkeley/Los Angeles: University of California Press.

Trimbur, M., Amad, A., Horn, M., Thomas, P., & Fovet, T. (2021). "Are Radicalization and Terrorism Associated with Psychiatric Disorders? A Systematic Review." *Journal of Psychiatric Research*, 141, 214–222. https://doi:10.1016/j.jpsychires.2021.07.002

Trinkaus, C. (1949). "The Problem of Free Will in the Renaissance and the Reformation." *Journal of the History of Ideas*, 10(1), 51–62. https://doi:10.2307/2707199

Trotter, G. (2020). "The Authority of the Common Morality." *Journal of Medicine and Philosophy: A Forum for Bioethics and Philosophy of Medicine, 45*(4–5), 427–440. https://doi:10.1093/jmp/jhaa015

Truskinovsky, A. M. (2002). "Literary Psychiatric Observation and Diagnosis through the Ages: King Lear Revisited." *Southern Medical Journal, 95*(3), 343–352. https://doi:10.1097/00007611-200203 000-00012

Tsai, D. F. C. (2005). "The Bioethical Principles and Confucius' Moral Philosophy." *Journal of Medical Ethics, 31*(3), 159–163. https://doi:10.1136/jme.2002.002113

Tucker, G. J. (1998). "Putting DSM-IV in Perspective." *American Journal of Psychiatry, 155*(2), 159–161. https://doi: 10.1176/ajp.155.2.159

Tuckness, A. (2020). "Locke's Political Philosophy." In E. N. Zalta (Ed.), *The Stanford Encyclopedia of Philosophy* (Winter 2020 ed.). Stanford, CA: Metaphysics Research Lab, Stanford University. https:// plato.stanford.edu/archives/win2020/entries/locke-political/

Turner, L. (2003). "Zones of Consensus and Zones of Conflict: Questioning the 'Common Morality' Presumption in Bioethics." *Kennedy Institute of Ethics Journal, 13*(3), 193–218. https://doi:10.1353/ ken.2003.0023

Tyrer, P. (2005). "The Problem of Severity in the Classification of Personality Disorder." *Journal of Personality Disorders, 19*(3), 309–314. https://doi:10.1521/pedi.2005.19.3.309

US Bureau of Justice Statistics (2006). *Mental Health Problems of Prison and Jail Inmates.* NCJ213600. https: bjs.ojp.gov/library/publications/mental-health-problems-prison-and-jail-inmates

US Bureau of Justice Statistics (2017). *Indicators of Mental Health Problems Reported by Prisoners and Jail Inmates, 2011-2012.* NCJ 250612. https://bjs.ojp.gov/content/pub/pdf/imhprpji1112_sum.pdf

Unger, R. H., & Scherer, P. E. (2010). "Gluttony, Sloth and the Metabolic Syndrome: A Roadmap to Lipotoxicity." *Trends in Endocrinology & Metabolism, 21*(6), 345–352. https://doi:10.1016/ j.tem.2010.01.009

United Network for Organ Sharing (UNOS) (undated). "History of Transplantation." https://unos.org/ transplant/history/

Vaillant, G. E. (1984). "The Disadvantages of DSM-III Outweigh Its Advantages." *American Journal of Psychiatry, 141*(4), 542–545. https://doi:10.1176/ajp.141.4.542

van Dijk, N., Hooft, L., & Wieringa-de Waard, M. (2010). "What Are the Barriers to Residents' Practicing Evidence-Based Medicine? A Systematic Review." *Academic Medicine, 85*(7), 1163–1170. https://doi:10.1097/ACM.0b013e3181d4152f

Van Dorn, R., Volavka, J., & Johnson, N. (2012). "Mental Disorder and Violence: Is There a Relationship Beyond Substance Use?" *Social Psychiatry and Psychiatric Epidemiology, 47*(3), 487–503. https:// doi:10.1007/s00127-011-0356-x

Varga, S. (2014). "Self, Narrative, and the Culture of Therapy." *Philosophy, Psychiatry, & Psychology, 21*(2), 161–163. https://doi:10.1353/ppp.2014.0022

Veatch, R. M. (2003). "Is There a Common Morality?" *Kennedy Institute of Ethics Journal, 13*(3), 189–192. https://doi:10.1353/ken.2003.0024

Verdun-Jones, S. N. (2000). "Forensic Psychiatry, Ethics and Protective Sentencing: What Are the Limits of Psychiatric Participation in the Criminal Justice Process?" *Acta Psychiatrica Scandinavica, 101*(399), 77–82. https://doi:10.1111/j.0902-4441.2000.007s020[dash]18.x

Vidal, S., Skeem, J., & Camp, J. (2010). "Emotional Intelligence: Painting Different Paths for Low-Anxious and High-Anxious Psychopathic Variants." *Law and Human Behavior, 34*(2), 150–163. https://doi:10.1007/s10979-009-9175-y

Viki, G. T., Fullerton, I., Raggett, H., Tait, F., & Wiltshire, S. (2012). "The Role of Dehumanization in Attitudes toward the Social Exclusion and Rehabilitation of Sex Offenders." *Journal of Applied Social Psychology, 42*(10), 2349–2367. https://doi:10.1111/j.1559-1816.2012.00944.x

Visootsak, J., & Sherman, S. (2007). "Neuropsychiatric and Behavioral Aspects of Trisomy 21." *Current Psychiatry Reports, 9*(2), 135–140. https://doi:10.1007/s11920-007-0083-x

Vita, A., & Barlati, S. (2019). "The Implementation of Evidence-Based Psychiatric Rehabilitation: Challenges and Opportunities for Mental Health Services." *Frontiers in Psychiatry, 10*(147). https:// doi:10.3389/fpsyt.2019.00147

Vogel, J., & Theorell, T. (2006). "Social Welfare Models, Labor Markets, and Health Outcomes." In J. Heyman, C. Hertzman, M. L. Barer, & R. G. Evans (Eds.), *Healthier Societies. From Analysis to Action* (pp. 267–295). Oxford: Oxford University Press.

von Bertalanffy, L. (1969). *General System Theory: Foundations, Development, Applications.* New York: George Braziller.

von Staden, H. (1989). *Herophilus: The Art of Medicine in Early Alexandria: ed., Translation and Essays.* Cambridge: Cambridge University Press.

Vose, B., Cullen, F. T., & Smith, P. (2008). "The Empirical Status of the Level of Service Inventory." *Federal Probation, 72*(3), 22–29.

Wahl, O. F. (1992). "Mass Media Images of Mental Illness: A Review of the Literature." *Journal of Community Psychology, 20*(4), 343–352. https://doi:10.1002/1520-6629(199210)20:4<343::Aid-Jco p2290200408>3.0.Co;2-2

Wakefield, J. C. (2011). "DSM-5 Proposed Diagnostic Criteria for Sexual Paraphilias: Tensions between Diagnostic Validity and Forensic Utility." *International Journal of Law and Psychiatry, 34*(3), 195–209. https://doi:10.1016/j.ijlp.2011.04.012

Wakefield, J. C., Schmitz, M. F., & Baer, J. C. (2010). "Does the DSM-IV Clinical Significance Criterion for Major Depression Reduce False Positives? Evidence from the National Comorbidity Survey Replication." *American Journal of Psychiatry, 167*(3), 298–304. https://doi:10.1176/appi. ajp.2009.09040553

Wallace, E. R. (1994). "Psychiatry and Its Nosology: A Historico-Philosophical Overview." In J. Z. Sadler, O. P. Wiggins, & M. A. Schwartz (Eds.), *Philosophical Perspectives on Psychiatric Diagnostic Classification* (pp. 16–86). Baltimore: Johns Hopkins University Press.

Wallace, E. R. (2008a). "Freud on 'Mind-Body' I: The Psychoneurobiological and 'Instinctualist' Stance; with Implications for Chapter 24, and Two Postscripts." In E. R. Wallace & J. Gach (Eds.), *History of Psychiatry and Medical Psychology* (pp. 725–756). New York: Springer.

Wallace, E. R. (2008b). "Two 'Mind'-'Body' Models for a Holistic Psychiatry." In E. R. Wallace & J. Gach (Eds.), *History of Psychiatry and Medical Psychology* (pp. 695–723). New York: Springer.

Waller, B. N. (2011). *Against Moral Responsibility.* Cambridge, MA: MIT Press.

Waller, B. N. (2015). *The Stubborn System of Moral Responsibility.* Cambridge, MA: MIT Press.

Waller, B. N. (2017). *The Injustice of Punishment.* London: Routledge.

Waller, B. N. (2020). "Beyond Moral Responsibility to a System That Works." *Neuroethics, 13*(1), 5–12. https://doi:10.1007/s12152-017-9351-6

Waller, D. A. (1983). "Obstacles to the Treatment of Munchausen by Proxy Syndrome." *Journal of the American Academy of Child Psychiatry, 22*(1), 80–85. https://doi:10.1097/00004583-198301 000-00013

Walter, M., Witzel, J., Wiebking, C., Gubka, U., Rotte, M., Schiltz, K., . . . Northoff, G. (2007). "Pedophilia Is Linked to Reduced Activation in Hypothalamus and Lateral Prefrontal Cortex During Visual Erotic Stimulation." *Biological Psychiatry, 62*(6), 698–701. https://doi:10.1016/j.biops ych.2006.10.018

Wang, P. S., Angermeyer, M., Borges, G., Bruffaerts, R., Chiu, W. T., De Girolamo, G., . . . on behalf of The WHO World Mental Health Survey Consortium (2007). "Delay and Failure in Treatment Seeking after First Onset of Mental Disorders in the World Health Organization's World Mental Health Survey Initiative." *World Psychiatry, 6*(3), 177–185. https://www.ncbi.nlm.nih.gov/pmc/artic les/PMC2174579/

Ward, T. (2010). "The Good Lives Model of Offender Rehabilitation: Basic Assumptions, Aetiological Commitments, and Practice Implications." In F. McNeill, P. Raynor, & C. Trotter (Eds.), *Offender Supervision* (pp. 41–64). New York: Routledge.

Ward, T., & Brown, M. (2004). "The Good Lives Model and Conceptual Issues in Offender Rehabilitation." *Psychology, Crime & Law, 10*(3), 243–257. https://doi:10.1080/1068316041000 1662744

Ward, T., Collie, R. M., & Bourke, P. (2009). "Models of Offender Rehabilitation: The Good Lives Model and the Risk-Need-Responsivity Model." In A. R. Beech, E. Craig, & K. D. Browne (Eds.), *Assessment and Treatment of Sex Offenders: A Handbook* (pp. 293–310). Hoboken, NJ: Wiley-Blackwell.

Ward, T., Mann, R. E., & Gannon, T. A. (2007). "The Good Lives Model of Offender Rehabilitation: Clinical Implications." *Aggression and Violent Behavior, 12*(1), 87–107. https://doi:10.1016/ j.avb.2006.03.004

Washington Post (2007). http://media.washingtonpost.com/wp-srv/metro/pdf/cho_mentalhealth.pdf

Watson, A. S. (1992). "The Evolution of Legal Methods for Dealing with Mind-State in Crimes." *Bulletin of the American Academy of Psychiatry and the Law, 20*(2), 211–220.

Watson, J. D. (1990). "The Human Genome Project: Past, Present, and Future." *Science, 248*(4951), 44–49. https://doi:10.1126/science.2181665

Wattles, J. (1996). *The Golden Rule.* New York/Oxford: Oxford University Press.

Weckowicz, T. E., & Liebel-Weckowicz, H. P. (1990). *A History of Great Ideas in Abnormal Psychology* (Vol. 66 of Advances in Psychology). New York: Elsevier.

Weiner, D. (2007). "Phillipe Pinel." In W. F. Bynum & H. Bynum (Eds.), *Dictionary of Medical Biography* (pp. 1008–1013). Westport, CT: Greenwood Press.

Weiner, D. B. (2008a). "The Madman in the Light of Reason: Enlightenment Psychiatry." In E. R. Wallace & J. Gach (Eds.), *History of Psychiatry and Medical Psychology* (pp. 255–277). New York: Springer.

Weiner, D. B. (2008b). "Phillipe Pinel in the Twenty-First Century." In E. R. Wallace & J. Gach (Eds.), *History of Psychiatry and Medical Psychology* (pp. 305–312). New York: Springer.

Weisburd, D., Farrington, D. P., & Gill, C. (Eds.) (2016). *What Works in Crime Prevention and Rehabilitation: Lessons from Systematic Reviews.* New York: Springer.

Weisburd, D., Farrington, D. P., & Gill, C. (2017). "What Works in Crime Prevention and Rehabilitation." *Criminology & Public Policy, 16*(2), 415–449. https://doi:10.1111/1745-9133.12298

Weiss, R. L. (1991). *Maimonides' Ethics: The Encounter of Philosophic and Religious Morality.* Chicago: University of Chicago Press.

Wender, P. H. (1971). *Minimal Brain Dysfunction in Children* (First ed.). New York: Wiley-Interscience.

West, C. P., Dyrbye, L. N., & Shanafelt, T. D. (2009). "Burnout in Medical School Deans." *Academic Medicine, 84*(1), 6. https://doi:10.1097/ACM.0b013e318190147a

West, C. P., Dyrbye, L. N., Sinsky, C., Trockel, M., Tutty, M., Nedelec, L., . . . Shanafelt, T. D. (2020). "Resilience and Burnout among Physicians and the General U.S. Working Population." *JAMA Network Open, 3*(7), e209385–e209385. https://doi:10.1001/jamanetworkopen.2020.9385

Westerhof, G., & Keyes, C. L. M. (2010). "Mental Illness and Mental Health: The Two Continua Model across the Lifespan." *Journal of Adult Development, 17*(2), 110–119. https://doi:10.1007/s10804-009-9082-y

Whelton, W. J. (2004). "Emotional Processes in Psychotherapy: Evidence across Therapeutic Modalities." *Clinical Psychology & Psychotherapy, 11*(1), 58–71. https://doi:10.1002/cpp.392

White, G. D. (2004). "Political Apathy Disorder: Proposal for a New DSM Diagnostic Category." *Journal of Humanistic Psychology, 44*(1), 47–57. https://doi:10.1177/0022167803259255

White, S. M. (2002). "Preventive Detention Must Be Resisted by the Medical Profession." *Journal of Medical Ethics, 28*(2), 95–98.

Whitehead, A. N. (1925). *Science and the Modern World.* Cambridge: Cambridge University Press.

Whiting, D., Lichtenstein, P., & Fazel, S. (2020). "Violence and Mental Disorders: A Structured Review of Associations by Individual Diagnoses, Risk Factors, and Risk Assessment." *The Lancet Psychiatry, 8*(2), 150–161. https://doi:10.1016/S2215-0366(20)30262-5

Widiger, T. A. (2006). "Psychopathy and DSM-IV Psychopathology." In C. J. Patrick (Ed.), *Handbook of Psychopathy, Second ed.* (pp. 156–171). New York: Guilford Press.

Widiger, T. A., & Frances, A. (1987). "Interviews and Inventories for the Measurement of Personality Disorders." *Clinical Psychology Review, 7*(1), 49–75. https://doi:10.1016/0272-7358(87)90004-3

Widiger, T. A., & Frances, A. J. (2002). "Toward a Dimensional Model for the Personality Disorders." In P. T. Costa & T. A. Widiger (Eds.), *Personality Disorders and the Five-Factor Model of Personality, Second ed.* (pp. 23–44). Washington, DC: American Psychological Association.

Widiger, T. A., Frances, A. J., Pincus, H. A., Davis, W. W., & First, M. B. (1991). "Toward an Empirical Classification for the DSM-IV." *Journal of Abnormal Psychology, 100*(3), 280–288. https://doi:10.1037/0021-843X.100.3.280

Wiggins, O. P., & Schwartz, M. A. (1997). "Edmund Husserl's Influence on Karl Jaspers's Phenomenology." *Philosophy, Psychiatry, & Psychology, 4*(1), 15–36. https://doi:10.1353/ppp.1997.0011

Wikipedia Contributors. (2021). "Three Treasures (Taoism)." Page Version ID: 1025960510. Wikipedia, The Free Encyclopedia. https://en.wikipedia.org/w/index.php?title=Three_Treasures_(Taoism)&oldid=1025960510

Wikipedia Contributors (2022). "Little Children (Film)." Page Version ID: 1090883538. Wikipedia, The Free Encyclopedia. https://en.wikipedia.org/w/index.php?title=Little_Children_(film)&oldid=1090883538

Wikipedia Contributors (2021). "Seung-Hui Cho." Page Version ID: 1035354981. Wikipedia, The Free Encyclopedia. https://en.wikipedia.org/w/index.php?title=Seung-Hui_Cho&oldid=1035354981

Wikler, D. (2002). "Personal and Social Responsibility for Health." *Ethics & International Affairs, 16*(2), 47–55. https://doi:10.1111/j.1747-7093.2002.tb00396.x

Wilkinson, S. (2000). "Is 'Normal Grief' a Mental Disorder?" *The Philosophical Quarterly, 50*(200), 289–304. https://doi:10.1111/j.0031-8094.2000.00186.x

Williams, A. (2014). *Forensic Criminology* (First ed.). (pp. 454). London: Routledge. https://doi:10.4324/9780202101148

Willner, P. (1997). "Animal Models of Addiction." *Human Psychopharmacology, 12*(S2), S59–S68. https://doi:10.1002/(SICI)1099-1077(199706)12:2+<S59::AID-HUP903>3.0.CO;2-0

Wilson, M. (1994). "American Psychiatry's Transformation Following the Publication of DSM-III (Dr. Wilson Replies)." *American Journal of Psychiatry, 151*(3), 460.

Wilson, R. J., & Yates, P. M. (2009). "Effective Interventions and the Good Lives Model: Maximizing Treatment Gains for Sexual Offenders." *Aggression and Violent Behavior, 14*(3), 157–161. https://doi:10.1016/j.avb.2009.01.007

Winance, M., & Bertrand, L. (2022). "The Personalisation of Social Care: How Can a Healthcare System Be Adapted to the Specific Characteristics of People with Multiple Impairments? The Case of the Care of People with 'Rare Disabilities' in France." *Journal of Social Policy, First View, 49*(1), 1–18. https://doi:10.1017/S0047279422000411

Winick, B. J., & LaFond, J. Q. (Eds.) (2003). *Protecting Society from Sexually Dangerous Offenders: Law, Justice, and Therapy.* Washington, DC: American Psychological Association.

Winkler, P., Barrett, B., McCrone, P., Csémy, L., Janousková, M., & Höschl, C. (2016). "Deinstitutionalised Patients, Homelessness and Imprisonment: Systematic Review." *British Journal of Psychiatry, 208*(5), 421–428. https://doi:10.1192/bjp.bp.114.161943

Winter, A. (2004). "Screening Selves: Sciences of Memory and Identity on Film, 1930–1960." *History of Psychology, 7*(4), 367–401. https://doi:10.1037/1093-4510.7.4.367

Wittgenstein, L. (Ed.) (1953). *Philosophical Investigations* (First ed.). New York: Macmillan Publishing Company.

Wollert, R., & Cramer, E. (2011). "Sampling Extreme Groups Invalidates Research on the Paraphilias: Implications for DSM-5 and Sex Offender Risk Assessments." *Behavioral Sciences & the Law, 29*(4), 554–565. https://doi:10.1002/bsl.992

Woolhouse, R. (2005). "John Locke." In T. Honderich (Ed.), *The Oxford Companion to Philosophy, New ed.* (pp. 525–529). Oxford: Oxford University Press.

Worchester (MA) Lunatic Hospital (1893). *Sixtieth Annual Report of the Trustees of the Worcester Lunatic Hospital, and Fifteenth Annual Report of the Trustees of the Worcester Insane Asylum at Worcester, for the Year Ending Sept. 30, 1892.* Public Document (Massachusetts) 23. Boston: Wright & Potter Printing Co. http://archives.lib.state.ma.us/handle/2452/781503

Worden, J. W. (2009). *Grief Counseling and Grief Therapy: A Handbook for the Mental Health Practitioner* (Fourth ed.). New York: Springer.

World Health Organization (1992). *The ICD-10 Classification of Mental and Behavioural Disorders: Clinical Descriptions and Diagnostic Guidelines.* Geneva, Switzerland: World Health Organization. https://apps.who.int/iris/handle/10665/37958

World Health Organization (2014). "Mental Health." https://www.who.int/news-room/facts-in-pictures/detail/mental-health

World Prison Brief (2019). "World Prison Brief Data." https://www.prisonstudies.org/country/united-states-america

Wright, P., Nobrega, J., Langevin, R., & Wortzman, G. (1990). "Brain Density and Symmetry in Pedophilic and Sexually Aggressive Offenders." *Annals of Sex Research, 3*(3), 319–328. https://doi:10.1007/BF00849186

Wright, R. (2014). *Sex Offender Laws: Failed Policies, New Directions.* New York: Springer.

Yang, Y., Raine, A., Narr, K. L., Colletti, P., & Toga, A. W. (2009). "Localization of Deformations within the Amygdala in Individuals with Psychopathy." *Archives of General Psychiatry, 66*(9), 986–994. https://doi:10.1001/archgenpsychiatry.2009.110

Yarvis, R. M. (1995). "Diagnostic Patterns among Three Violent Offender Types." *Journal of the American Academy of Psychiatry and the Law, 23*(3), 411–419. http://jaapl.org/content/23/3/411

Youpa, A. (2016). "Leibniz's Ethics." In E. N. Zalta (Ed.), *The Stanford Encyclopedia of Philosophy* (Winter 2016 ed.). Stanford, CA: Metaphysics Research Lab, Stanford University.https://plato.stanford.edu/archives/win2016/entries/leibniz-ethics/

Yuste, P., Garrido, Á., & Finkel, I. L. (2010). "Adad-Apla-Iddina, Esagil-Kīn-Apli, and the Series SA.GIG." In E. Leichty, M. Ellis, & P. Gerardi (Eds.), *A Scientific Humanist: Studies in Memory of Abraham Sachs* (pp. 143–159). Philadelphia: Occasional Publication of the Samuel Noah Kramer Fund 9.

Zachar, P. (2000). "Psychiatric Disorders Are Not Natural Kinds." *Philosophy, Psychiatry, & Psychology, 7*(3), 167–182.

Zachar, P. (2000). *Psychological Concepts and Biological Psychiatry: A Philosophical Analysis* (Vol. 28). Amsterdam/Philadelphia: John Benjamins Publishing.

Zachar, P. (2014). *A Metaphysics of Psychopathology*. Cambridge, MA: MIT Press.

Zachar, P., & Kendler, K. S. (2007). "Psychiatric Disorders: A Conceptual Taxonomy." *American Journal of Psychiatry, 164*(4), 557–565. https://doi:10.1176/ajp.2007.164.4.557

Zachar, P., Krueger, R. F., & Kendler, K. S. (2016). "Personality Disorder in DSM-5: An Oral History." *Psychological Medicine, 46*(1), 1–10. https://doi:10.1017/S0033291715001543

Zachar, P., & Potter, N. N. (2010). "Personality Disorders: Moral or Medical Kinds—or Both?" *Philosophy, Psychiatry, & Psychology, 17*(2), 101–117. https://doi:10.1353/ppp.0.0290

Zachar, P., Regier, D. A., & Kendler, K. S. (2019). "The Aspirations for a Paradigm Shift in DSM-5: An Oral History." *Journal of Nervous and Mental Disease, 207*(9), 778–784. https://doi:10.1097/nmd.0000000000001063

Zaibert, L. (2013). "The Instruments of Abolition, or Why Retributivism Is the Only Real Justification of Punishment." *Law and Philosophy, 32*(1), 33–58. https://doi:10.1007/s10982-012-9156-z

Zaner, R. M. (1990). "Medicine and Dialogue." *Journal of Medicine and Philosophy: A Forum for Bioethics and Philosophy of Medicine, 15*(3), 303–325. https://doi:10.1093/jmp/15.3.303

Zeccola, J., Kelty, S. F., & Boer, D. (2021). "Does the Good Lives Model Work? A Systematic Review of the Recidivism Evidence." *The Journal of Forensic Psychiatry, 23*(3), 285–300. https://doi:10.1108/JFP-03-2021-0010

Zilboorg, G., in collaboration with G. W. Henry. (1941). *A History of Medical Psychology*. New York: W.W. Norton & Company.

Zimmerman, M. (1994). *Interview Guide for Evaluating DSM-IV Psychiatric Disorders and the Mental Status Examination* (First ed.). East Greenwich, RI: Psych Products Press.

Zimring, F. E. (2006). *The Great American Decline*. New York/Oxford: Oxford University Press.

Zinik, G., & Padilla, J. (2016). "Rape and Paraphilic Coercive Disorder." In A. Phenix & H. M. Hoberman (Eds.), *Sexual Offending: Predisposing Antecedents, Assessments and Management* (pp. 45–66). New York: Springer.

Ziv, R. (2017). *The Future of Correctional Rehabilitation: Moving Beyond the RNR Model and Good Lives Model Debate*. New York: Routledge.

Zonana, H. V. & Norko, M. A. (1999). "Sexual Predators." *Psychiatric Clinics of North America, 22*(1), 109–127. https://doi: 10.1016/S0193-953X(05)70063-0

Author index

For the benefit of digital users, indexed terms that span two pages (e.g., 52–53) may, on occasion, appear on only one of those pages.

Subject index

For the benefit of digital users, indexed terms that span two pages (e.g., 52–53) may, on occasion, appear on only one of those pages.